Elsevier's Veterinary Assisting Textbook

Elsevier's Veterinary Assisting Textbook

Second Edition

Margi Sirois, EdD, MS, RVT, LAT

Program Director, Veterinary Technician Program
Ashworth College
Norcross, Georgia

With 672 illustrations

ELSEVIER

ELSEVIER

3251 Riverport Lane
St. Louis, Missouri 63043

ELSEVIER'S VETERINARY ASSISTING TEXTBOOK, SECOND EDITION   ISBN: 978-0-323-35922-1

Notices

Previous edition copyrighted 2013

Library of Congress Cataloging-in-Publication Data

Names: Sirois, Margi, author.
Title: Elsevier's veterinary assisting textbook / Margi Sirois.
Other titles: Veterinary assisting textbook
Description: Second edition. | St. Louis, Missouri : Elsevier, [2017] |
    Includes bibliographical references and index.
Identifiers: LCCN 2015036606 | ISBN 9780323359221 (hardcover)
Subjects: LCSH: Veterinary medicine. | Veterinary nursing. | MESH: Veterinary
    Medicine--methods. | Animal Technicians.
Classification: LCC SF745 .S56 2016 | NLM SF 745 | DDC 636.089--dc23
LC record available at http://lccn.loc.gov/2015036606

Content Strategist: Shelly Stringer
Senior Content Development Specialist: Diane Chatman
Publishing Services Manager: Patricia Tannian
Senior Project Manager: Cindy Thoms
Book Designer: Ashley Miner

Printed in China

Last digit is the print number: 9 8 7 6 5 4

Working together to grow libraries in developing countries

www.elsevier.com • www.bookaid.org

For my family – especially Dan (the wonder husband),
Jen, and Daniel

Contributors to the First Edition

Joanna M. Bassert, VMD
Professor and Director
Program of Veterinary Technology
Manor College
Jenkintown, Pennsylvania

Thomas Colville, DVM, MSc
Red River Zoo
Fargo, North Dakota

Charles M. Hendrix, DVM, PhD
Professor, Department of Pathobiology
College of Veterinary Medicine
Auburn University
Auburn, Alabama

Phillip Lerche, BVSc, PhD, Dipl ACVA
Assistant Professor
Department of Veterinary Clinical Sciences
Ohio State University
Columbus, Ohio

Kathy Lockett Massey, LVMT
Veterinary Technology Department
Columbia State Community College
Columbia, Tennessee

Dennis M. McCurnin, DVM, MS, Dipl ACVS
Professor of Surgery and Management
Director of Continuing Education
Veterinary Clinical Sciences
School of Veterinary Medicine
Louisiana State University
Baton Rouge, Louisiana

Heather Prendergast, BS, AS, RVT, CVPM
Certified Practice Manager
Jornada Veterinary Clinic
Las Cruces, New Mexico

Ed Robinson, CVT
Shakespeare Veterinary Hospital
Veterinary Technology Program Instructor
Penn Foster College
Fairfield, Connecticut

C.C. Sheldon, DVM, MS
Program Director
Veterinary Technician and Laboratory Animal Technician
   Programs
Madison Area Technical College
Madison, Wisconsin

Teresa Sonsthagen, BS, RVT
Instructor, Veterinary Technology Program
North Dakota State University
Fargo, North Dakota

Margi Sirois, EdD, MS, RVT, LAT
Program Director, Veterinary Technician Program
Ashworth College
Norcross, Georgia

Marianne Tear, MS, LVT
Program Director
Veterinary Technology Program
Baker College
Clinton Township, Michigan

John A. Thomas, DVM
Assistant Professor, Veterinary Technology
Cuyahoga Community College
Cleveland, Ohio

James Topel, CVT
Instructor
Veterinary Technician and Laboratory Animal Technician
   Programs
Madison Area Technical College
Madison, Wisconsin

Boyce P. Wanamaker, DVM, MS
Director, Veterinary Technology Program
Columbia State Community College
Columbia, Tennessee

Veterinary assistants play a vital role on the veterinary health care team. An educated assistant working directly with a credentialed veterinary technician can help create a powerful team that greatly improves the ability of the veterinarian to attend to animals in their care. Veterinary assistants are also involved in many of the business aspects of veterinary practice and often work closely with management staff in the practice. This book was designed to aid the veterinary assistant in obtaining the knowledge and skill required to assist the veterinary technician and veterinarian in the care of animals, as well as skills needed to contribute to the smooth functioning of the business side of a companion animal veterinary practice.

Veterinary assistants are most effective when they have a strong understanding of the flow of work in the practice and the roles of each of the members of the veterinary health care team. This information is contained in each chapter. Each chapter begins with learning objectives, a chapter outline, and key words. "Critical Concepts" throughout each chapter highlight important points and provide helpful tips to improve knowledge and skills. Recommended readings provide additional sources of detailed information on the topics. Step-by-step procedures are included for all commonly performed skills expected of veterinary assistants. Ample illustrations are included and tables are used to provide a summary and handy reference for vital information.

The majority of the material for the text is derived from published material in several other textbooks, including *Principles and Practice of Veterinary Technology,* 3rd edition, *Front Office Management for the Veterinary Team, Laboratory Procedures for Veterinary Technicians,* 6th edition, *Animal Restraint for Veterinary Professionals, McCurnin's Clinical Textbook for Veterinary Technicians,* 7th edition, *Diagnostic Parasitology for Veterinary Technicians,* 4th edition, and *Clinical Anatomy and Physiology for Veterinary Technicians,* 2nd edition.

The text is designed to adhere to the model curricula for veterinary assistant training as published by the Association of Veterinary Technician Educators (AVTE) and the National Association of Veterinary Technicians in America (NAVTA). Programs for training of veterinary assistants will find this a valuable resource for providing details on tasks performed by veterinary assistants as well as the roles of all the members of the veterinary health care team.

Workbook

The accompanying workbook includes definitions of key terms, review questions, case presentations, clinical applications, illustration labeling and identification, photo-based quizzes, matching questions, completion questions (fill-in-the-blank type), multiple-choice questions, and other student games and exercises. Each chapter in the workbook corresponds to a chapter in the textbook and reinforces the essential information of the chapter through the use of various exercises and test questions. Students are encouraged to read and review the chapter before attempting to work through the related exercises in the workbook. Chapter objectives provided in the textbook are reiterated in the workbook to help students focus on the material and concepts that they are expected to learn and to understand how this is to be applied in the veterinary clinic setting.

Evolve Assets for Instructors

Instructors can activate the complete teaching experience that comes with this book by registering at http://evolve.elsevier.com/Sirois/vetassisting. New to this edition are TEACH Lesson Plans, a popular and useful resource providing one-stop classroom planning with lectures, activities, and more. Register today and also gain access to the electronic image collection, test bank, PowerPoint lecture outlines, and workbook answer key.

Acknowledgments

This book would not have been possible without the hard work of the many authors and contributors to the previously published textbooks from which much of this volume is derived. I thank them all for their efforts. I am especially grateful to Shelly Stringer and Diane Chatman for their expert assistance.

Margi Sirois

Contents

1 Overview of the Veterinary Profession, 1

2 Office Procedures and Client Relations, 25

3 Medical Terminology, 57

4 Anatomy and Physiology, 69

5 Pharmacology and Pharmacy, 104

6 Animal Behavior and Restraint, 131

7 Animal Husbandry and Nutrition, 171

8 Animal Care and Nursing, 208

9 Anesthesia and Surgical Assisting, 242

10 Laboratory Procedures, 284

11 Diagnostic Imaging, 336

12 Avian and Exotic Animal Care and Nursing, 360

13 Large Animal Nursing and Husbandry, 408

Glossary, 447
Appendices, 471

Overview of the Veterinary Profession[1]

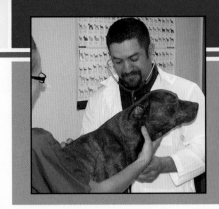

OUTLINE

History of Veterinary Medicine, *2*
Veterinary Health Care Team, *2*
Members of the Veterinary Health Care Team, *3*
Personal Qualifications, *9*
Professional Organizations and Resources, *9*
Types of Veterinary Practices, *9*
Companion Animal Practice, *9*
Mobile Pet Practice, *9*
Referral Practice, *9*
Exotic Animal Practice, *9*
Mixed Practice, *11*
Veterinary Practice Design, *11*
Creating Comfortable Reception Areas, *11*
Creating Comfortable Examination Rooms, *12*
Consultation Rooms, *12*
Retail Area, *12*
Middle Area, *12*
Treatment Area, *12*
Ethics, *14*
Ethics of Working With Animals, *14*
Ethics of the Veterinary Profession, *15*
Laws, *15*

Laws That Ensure the Quality of Veterinary Service, *16*
Common Law Malpractice, *16*
Laws That Provide a Safe Business Environment, *16*
Laws That Maintain a Nonhostile Working
     Environment, *17*
Laws That Govern Labor, *18*
Laws Governing Controlled Substances, *18*
**Occupational Health and Safety in Veterinary
     Practice,** *18*
Safety in the Workplace, *18*
Lifting, *18*
Hazards of Animal Handling, *19*
Hazards of Bathing and Dipping, *20*
Zoonotic Hazards, *20*
Radiation Hazards, *21*
Anesthetic Hazards, *21*
Hazards of Compressed Gases, *22*
Hazards of Sharp Objects, *22*
Chemical Hazards, *22*
Electrical Hazards, *23*
Personal Safety, *24*

LEARNING OBJECTIVES

After reviewing this chapter, the reader will be able to:

1. Describe educational requirements of veterinary team members.
2. Define appropriate nomenclature describing veterinary personnel.
3. Identify the duties of the members of the veterinary health care team.
4. Recognize professional organizations supporting veterinary medicine.
5. Discuss ethical issues and guidelines relevant to the veterinary profession.
6. List and describe general categories of laws relevant to the veterinary profession.
7. Define laws protecting veterinary employees against physical injury, sexual harassment, and discrimination.
8. Explain laws relating to ensuring quality veterinary service.

[1]Elsevier and the author acknowledge and appreciate the original contributions from Sirois M: Principles and practice of veterinary technology, ed 3, St Louis, 2011, Mosby; and Prendergast H: Front office management for the veterinary team, St Louis, 2011, Saunders, whose work forms the heart of this chapter.

KEY TERMS

Academy
American Veterinary Medical Association
American Veterinary Medical Association's Professional Liability Insurance Trust
Board of Veterinary Medical Examiners
Companion Animal Practice
Comprehensive Drug Abuse Prevention and Control Act
Controlled Substance Act
Department of Labor

Dosimetry badge
Drug Enforcement Agency
Employee handbook
Equal Employment Opportunity
Ethics
Ethylene oxide
Fomite
Groomer
Hazardous materials plan
Human-animal bond
Kennel assistant

Malpractice or professional negligence
Material Safety Data Sheet
National Association of Veterinary Technicians in America
Negligence
Nonexempt employees
Occupational Safety and Health Act
Office manager
Personal protective equipment

Practice manager
Receptionist
Right to Know Law
Scavenging system
Veterinarian
Veterinary assistant
Veterinary State Practice Act
Veterinary technician
Veterinary Technician National Examination
Veterinary technologist
Zoonotic diseases

HISTORY OF VETERINARY MEDICINE

Although there are references to animal doctors in ancient literature, modern programs for educating of **veterinarians** did not begin until 1761. The first veterinary college was founded in Lyon, France. Programs to educate veterinarians in the United States were first developed in the 1850s, but the first college program was not established until 1879 at Iowa State University. In the 1800s and early 1900s, most veterinarians were involved with the treatment of livestock. They played an integral role in food safety and developed programs to control diseases that affected humans and the food supply.

As veterinarians became more involved with treatment of pet animals, the need for educated support staff became apparent. The first programs to train veterinary assistants began in 1908 in England at the Canine Nurse's Institute. Programs for educating **veterinary technicians** in the United States began in 1961 with the establishment of the veterinary technician program at the State University of New York (SUNY) Delhi. The U.S. Army also started a program that same year for educating the Veterinary Specialist–Animal Care Specialist personnel at Walter Reed Army Institute of Research in Washington, DC. Today, there are hundreds of programs for education of veterinary technicians and assistants.

VETERINARY HEALTH CARE TEAM

CRITICAL CONCEPT

The goal of every veterinary health care team member is to provide excellent medical care to patients and outstanding customer service to clients.

The veterinary practice can be a highly structured environment that provides an excellent career for all team members. The goal of every practice should be to provide the best medical care to patients and outstanding customer service to clients while providing a workplace that is friendly, efficient, and safe. Each team member contributes to the success of the practice. Veterinarians are responsible for providing the guidelines of medical care, and assistants and technicians are responsible for following these guidelines to provide excellent care.

Clients expect outstanding customer service from veterinary practices. It can take weeks to receive laboratory results in human medicine, and often the physician doesn't call the patient with the results. In veterinary medicine, clients expect veterinarians to call the following day with results and often are upset if the results are not available sooner. Opinion polls conducted in the past have placed veterinarians higher than physicians when respondents were asked to rank professions and the value that they place on each. Some individuals value their veterinarians more than their physicians because the level of care that they receive from their veterinary practice far exceeds the care they receive from their own physicians.

A key ingredient to teamwork is open and honest communication among employees, managers, and owners. The second ingredient for a successful team is developing and embracing respect for one another. When teamwork is evident, clients notice and recommend the friendly, honest, genuine service that a veterinary practice can provide.

The veterinary health care team involves all members of the staff. Each person plays a significant role in a successful practice. Roles and duties vary by practice and typically are defined in an employee manual. Team members working together as a group provide better patient and client care than those who work as individuals. Team members may include, but are not limited to, students, **groomers**, **kennel assistants**, **veterinary assistants**, credentialed veterinary technicians, veterinary technician specialists, **veterinary technologists**, **receptionists**, veterinarians, **office managers**, and **practice managers** (Box 1-1). Many clinics also have specializations within each team member position. Having a team leader can significantly improve communication and accountability.

BOX 1-1	Members of the Veterinary Health Care Team

- Veterinarians
- Veterinary technologists
- Credentialed veterinary technicians
- Veterinary technicians specialists
- Veterinary assistants
- Groomers
- Kennel assistants
- Students
- Receptionists
- Office managers
- Practice managers

Larger practices may have a structured hierarchy, with each team member having a specific role in the practice. Some staff members may be limited to care of hospitalized patients, surgical recovery, or laboratory, whereas others may be assigned to outpatient visits only. Smaller practices have assistants and technicians assigned to all areas of the practice at the same time. Each area requires special knowledge and education and must not be overlooked when completing duties in various areas of the practice.

MEMBERS OF THE VETERINARY HEALTH CARE TEAM

STUDENTS

Students may function as observers or hold paid positions within a hospital. Many students must complete externships as part of an educational program. High school students can earn grades while completing a required number of hours at the job site, and veterinary assistant and technician students may fulfill hours required for their coursework. Students may be assigned tasks by the school that must be done before course completion, which aids in the training process. Task lists can be used as a guide for the practice and the student.

Many veterinary schools have in-clinic prerequisites that must be completed before application and/or admission. Veterinary students can also complete an externship in a private practice to obtain more experience before graduating from a professional program.

GROOMERS

Groomers perform technical skills that they have acquired to care for patients and satisfy clients. This takes patience. They must take precautions to prevent injury to animals and themselves. Animals can become scared and aggressive while being groomed. Clippers are loud and tables can scare pets, causing them to become more aggressive than usual.

Several courses are available to learn how to groom; on-the-job training is also available. The National Dog Groomers Association works with groomers throughout the country to promote and encourage professionalism and education to maintain the image of the pet grooming profession. Their goal is to unite groomers through membership, promote

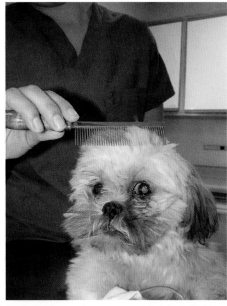

FIGURE 1-1 Groomers play an important role in the veterinary practice. (From Prendergast H: Front office management for the veterinary team, St Louis, 2011, Saunders.)

BOX 1-2	Responsibilities of Groomers

Successful groomers must:
- Have patience.
- Have excellent customer service skills.
- Communicate clearly with clients.
- Be flexible.
- Know when new products are available.
- Know about skin diseases and infections.
- Be aware of communicable and zoonotic diseases.
- Obtain continuing education to serve their patients better.

From Prendergast H: Front office management for the veterinary team, St Louis, 2011, Saunders.

communication with colleagues, set recognized grooming standards, and offer those seeking a higher level of professional recognition the opportunity to have their grooming skills certified. In some states, licensure or certification is required.

At times, groomers are the first to recognize abnormalities that should be further investigated by a veterinarian. Abnormal anal glands, masses, and ear infections are often detected by groomers while they care for pets. Owners appreciate and respect groomers' opinions when these abnormalities are found and often follow up with a visit to a veterinary practice.

Groomers need to communicate clearly and professionally as a part of retaining clients. Some clients require extra time because they expect the best for their pets. Pets may become uncooperative, resulting in a less-than-perfect cut; this can upset clients. Any grooming mistakes reflect negatively on the groomers and the veterinary practice, who must be able to communicate well to handle dissatisfied clients.

Grooming can be an extremely satisfying career for many team members because results of an excellent job can be viewed immediately (Fig. 1-1; Box 1-2).

BOX 1-7 | Veterinary Technician Specialties

- Academy of Veterinary Emergency and Critical Care Technicians (AVECCT)
- Academy of Veterinary Technician Anesthetists (AVTA)
- Academy of Veterinary Dental Technicians (AVDT)
- Academy of Internal Medicine for Veterinary Technicians (AIMVT)
- Academy of Veterinary Zoological Medical Technicians (AVZMT)
- Academy of Veterinary Surgical Technicians (AVST)
- Academy of Veterinary Technicians in Clinical Practice (AVTCP)
- Academy of Veterinary Nutrition Technicians (AVNT)
- Academy of American Association of Equine Veterinary Nursing Technicians (AAEVT)
- Academy of Veterinary Behavior Technicians (AVBT)
- Academy of Veterinary Clinical Pathology Technicians (AVCPT)
- Academy of Dermatology Veterinary Technicians (ADVT)

From Prendergast H: Front office management for the veterinary team, St Louis, 2011, Saunders.

VETERINARY TECHNICIAN SPECIALISTS

Veterinary technicians may decide to focus on a specific area of care. The term society is defined as a group of individuals, veterinary technicians, hospital staff, and veterinarians interested in a specific discipline or area of veterinary medicine. An **academy** is the term selected by the NAVTA to designate a group receiving recognition as a specialty (Box 1-7).

Technicians who choose to specialize must accumulate a specific number of hours within a particular specialty during a set number of years. For example, the Academy of Internal Medicine for Veterinary Technicians requires a minimum of 3 years' experience, with 6000 hours of experience as a credentialed veterinary technician in the field of internal medicine. All experience must be completed within 5 years before application. Candidates are also expected to have a minimum of 40 hours of continuing education on internal medicine before application submission. Candidates also submit case reports and case logs to document their advanced skill level. Once all requirements are met, the technician is permitted to take the examination in the specialty area.

Whether a veterinary assistant, veterinary technician, or technologist, every team member should be educated in basic laboratory work performed in a hospital. Veterinary technicians and technologists must be able to prepare and read blood smears, cytology preparations, urine samples, and fecal smears. Veterinary assistants may become proficient at running chemistry panels and preparing samples for complete blood cell counts on in-house laboratory equipment. All assistants and technicians should become proficient at radiology and learn the safety issues associated with all laboratory and radiology equipment. A veterinarian's productivity increases by delegating tasks associated with patient care to veterinary technicians and assistants. This allows the

---

BOX 1-8 | Responsibilities of Receptionists

Successful receptionists must:
- Have patience.
- Communicate well with team members and clients.
- Provide exceptional service to every client.
- Determine wants and needs of every client and patient.
- Have respect for others.
- Educate clients on the phone.
- Promote products and services provided by the practice.
- Listen to clients.

From Prendergast H: Front office management for the veterinary team, St Louis, 2011, Saunders.

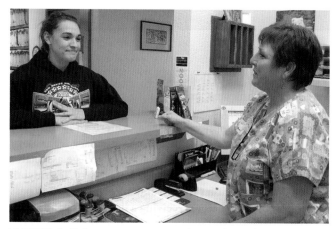

FIGURE 1-4 A receptionist greets a client with a smile, giving a positive first impression of the veterinary practice. (From Prendergast H: Front office management for the veterinary team, St Louis, 2011, Saunders.)

veterinarian to concentrate on diagnosing, prescribing medication, and performing surgeries.

RECEPTIONISTS

Receptionists are often the "face" of the veterinary practice (Box 1-8). They play a significant role in the success of a practice and must appear professional, polite, and caring. They must listen to client stories, show empathy when needed, and be able to collect money from clients under difficult circumstances (Fig. 1-4).

Receptionists greet clients, detail and clarify invoices, and receive money. They answer the phone and can turn an inquiring phone call into an appointment. Receptionists acknowledge clients when they walk in and out of the practice. They make the first impression on a client, whether on the phone or at the front desk.

OFFICE MANAGERS

The office manager is generally responsible for overseeing the front office staff and training receptionists to excel at customer service and public relations (Box 1-9). An office manager may allow a client to charge services and generally oversees accounts receivable. An office manager's realm of authority and decision making may be broad or limited,

BOX 1-9	Responsibilities of Office Managers

Successful office managers must:
- Be a successful receptionist.
- Educate team members.
- Develop coping strategies to handle angry clients.
- Handle accounts receivable with a smile.
- Determine if and when clients may be charged for services rendered.

From Prendergast H: Front office management for the veterinary team, St Louis, 2011, Saunders.

BOX 1-10	Responsibilities of Practice Managers

Successful practice managers must:
- Have patience.
- Lead the team in a positive manner.
- Address conflict immediately.
- Develop training protocols for the entire team.
- Develop client communication strategies.
- Develop sales strategies to increase revenue.
- Hire, fire, and train in a legal manner.
- Determine efficient methods for completion of tasks and procedures.

From Prendergast H: Front office management for the veterinary team, St Louis, 2011, Saunders.

BOX 1-11	Responsibilities of Hospital Administrators

Successful hospital administrators must:
- Have patience.
- Lead the team in a positive manner.
- Oversee each department.
- Develop, implement, and enforce budgets.
- Develop and implement sales strategies to increase revenue.
- Scrutinize medical records for completeness and quality medicine.
- Ensure that practice policies and procedures are being followed by each team member.
- Attend continuing education seminars to improve the quality of the practice.

From Prendergast H: Front office management for the veterinary team, St Louis, 2011, Saunders.

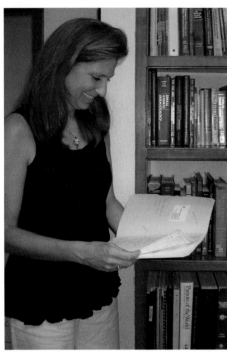

FIGURE 1-5 Office managers ensure that the front office is operating effectively. They must display a friendly attitude and a professional appearance. (From Prendergast H: Front office management for the veterinary team, St Louis, 2011, Saunders.)

depending on the administrative needs and criteria established by the practice. Many office managers are responsible for bank deposit preparation and account management. An office manager is courteous, friendly, and professional (Fig. 1-5). His or her demeanor, whether positive or negative, trickles down through the rest of the team.

PRACTICE MANAGERS

A practice manager helps keep the entire team working together and often reports to a hospital administrator. Practice managers generally handle client and personnel issues, supervise training sessions for team members, and hold team members accountable for their actions. Duties may also include reviewing records for completeness, observing for missed charges, and ensuring that policies are followed correctly. New strategies may be implemented by the practice manager to increase business as well as introduce new products to the clinic. Most practice managers hold a bachelor's degree in science or business administration; others hold an associate's degree in veterinary technology. Practice managers benefit from either type of degree, which allows them to excel at managing a veterinary hospital.

A practice manager may have to wear many hats while on the job, such as copier repair technician, computer technician, plumber, veterinary technician, kennel assistant, and/or counselor. Just as with the office manager, the practice manager must have a positive, friendly attitude with an open door policy for all team members. Great attitudes encourage a professional and successful atmosphere (Box 1-10).

HOSPITAL ADMINISTRATORS

A hospital administrator may be a veterinarian, veterinary technician, or a business manager. She or he generally has complete authority over the operation of the business and practice. This position is responsible for setting budgets, paying bills, creating organizational structure, and planning events (Box 1-11). A typical administrator is responsible for all the duties of the office manager and practice manager. Although a hospital administrator may not be a veterinarian,

BOX 1-12	Responsibilities of Veterinarians

Successful veterinarians must:
- Practice quality and current medicine.
- Communicate well with clients and team members.
- Educate clients and team members.
- Attend continuing education seminars on a regular basis.
- Have patience.
- Have a positive attitude.
- Delegate tasks.
- Diagnose disease, prescribe treatment, and perform surgery.

From Prendergast H: Front office management for the veterinary team, St Louis, 2011, Saunders.

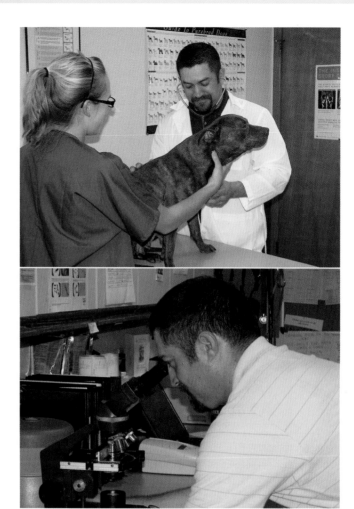

FIGURE 1-6 Veterinarians diagnose disease, prescribe treatment, and perform surgery. (From Prendergast H: Front office management for the veterinary team, St Louis, 2011, Saunders.)

this person should have general knowledge of quality assurance and performance in veterinary medicine and may act in an advisory role in helping establish and supervise protocols of the practice. A hospital administrator may report to the owner or shareholders if the practice is owned by multiple members. Hospital administrators often make the final purchasing decisions.

VETERINARIANS

Veterinarians are the only members of the team allowed to diagnose disease, prescribe treatment, and perform surgery on patients (Box 1-12). They have completed a professional course of study at an accredited college of veterinary medicine. Veterinarians must be licensed in the state where they work and must pass national and state examinations before receiving licensure. In most states, veterinarians are required to complete a minimum number of hours in continuing education each year and must report their hours to the state veterinary board. These requirements ensure veterinarians offer the best medical care available to patients and clients (Fig. 1-6).

TEAM

All roles on a veterinary team are important. All members contribute significantly (Fig. 1-7). As is often said, there is no "I" in "team." Each team member must help others complete tasks in the most efficient manner (Box 1-13). Kennel assistants may need to help a technician restrain a patient for laboratory work, and a technician may need to clean kennels; a veterinarian may need to answer the phone when all receptionists are working actively with clients. This is why cross-training employees in all areas of the practice is crucial. Information and communication can be accessed and shared more easily when team members are knowledgeable in several areas of the practice. When a team environment is created, any role in the veterinary health care team is rewarding. Patients receive better care, clients receive better communication, and employees enjoy coming to work. When employees enjoy their jobs, they work harder and more efficiently and strive to achieve higher goals. Every practice can benefit from a team attitude.

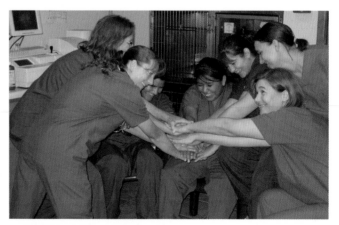

FIGURE 1-7 All team players need to be knowledgeable in several areas of responsibility and work together to keep the practice running smoothly. (From Prendergast H: Front office management for the veterinary team, St Louis, 2011, Saunders.)

BOX 1-13	Characteristics of Successful Team Environments

- Team members understand one another's priorities and difficulties and offer help when the opportunity arises.
- Open communication exists among all employees, managers, and owners.
- Problem solving occurs as a team.
- The team is recognized for outstanding results, as are individuals for their personal contributions.
- Team members are encouraged to make suggestions and test their abilities to improve the quality and quantity of work.

From Prendergast H: Front office management for the veterinary team, St Louis, 2011, Saunders.

PERSONAL QUALIFICATIONS

A genuine desire to care for animals is a common characteristic of those in the veterinary profession. However, the veterinary practice provides both care of animals and service to clients. Veterinary health care team members must also enjoy working with people. A pleasant and cheerful demeanor and the ability to remain calm during unexpected crises are important as well. The veterinary clinic can be a stressful environment, and the team must be ready to handle the emotional stress of working with animals that cannot be cured. The work can also be physically demanding. Walking and standing for long periods of time, reaching, bending, climbing, and the ability to lift and carry 50 pounds without assistance are common requirements. Vision, speech, and hearing must be sufficient to communicate effectively as well as perform observations and other essential skills with animals. Arm and hand steadiness and finger dexterity must be sufficient to operate equipment and perform other essential tasks.

Veterinary support staff members are expected to present themselves in neat, clean, and appropriate attire. Most veterinary hospital staff members wear surgical scrub suits or laboratory jackets. This dress is appropriate for animal medical duties and reflects your position in the medical field and the high value of your services. Large earrings can be a hazard. Facial piercings and tattoos are generally not suitable.

CRITICAL CONCEPT

All veterinary health care team members must present a professional appearance and enjoy working with people.

PROFESSIONAL ORGANIZATIONS AND RESOURCES

Your career will reach new heights when you actively participate in professional organizations. Professionalism, effective communication, networking, and outstanding technical skills in your career choice will make you stand out above the rest. There are a number of groups to choose from that will elevate your status, and the choices are growing at a rapid rate. When you join, you increase the membership base and open many doors for networking and other positive outcomes. Each association has its own mission, vision, and values. State and National organizations also have defined purposes and goals. Research the many organizations that align with your values and support your career. Box 1-14 lists a few of the national groups, organizations, and sites that support veterinary medical professionals and a brief synopsis of the benefits to members.

TYPES OF VETERINARY PRACTICES

A veterinarian may work exclusively with companion animals, work with just one species, or be involved in one specific area of medicine. Each practice type may be structured differently and have differences in the numbers and titles of the support staff team.

COMPANION ANIMAL PRACTICE

Most veterinarians are involved in treating family pets, especially dogs and cats. Some **companion animal practices** will also treat small mammals, such as guinea pigs and rabbits. The term small animal practice may also be used to describe this type of facility.

Companion animal practices generally employ a large support staff team. They are likely to employ two to three veterinary technicians and two to three veterinary assistants for each veterinarian in the practice. Additional personnel include the kennel workers, receptionists, and office manager. In small practices, a veterinary technician or assistant may also perform some of the duties of the receptionist.

MOBILE PET PRACTICE

Many of the same services offered to clients at a companion animal clinic can be offered in a mobile pet practice. The veterinarian will usually have an agreement with a local companion animal practice to provide services that require specialized equipment that cannot be incorporated into the mobile clinic. The mobile clinic is usually a converted recreational vehicle that travels directly to the client's home. A veterinarian in a mobile pet practice may employ a veterinary technician or veterinary assistant to accompany them to the client's home.

REFERRAL PRACTICE

Veterinarians who have special expertise in one aspect of medicine may offer services in a referral practice. The referral practice, also called a specialty practice, may consist of groups of veterinarians with different specializations. Companion animal veterinarians often refer patients that need more advanced care to a specialist.

EXOTIC ANIMAL PRACTICE

Some veterinarians work exclusively with pet birds, reptiles, and small mammals. These species are commonly referred to as exotic pets. The unique anatomy and physiology of these

BOX 1-14 | Groups, Organizations, and Websites That Support the Veterinary Health Care Team

AAHA: Created in 1933, the American Animal Hospital Association accredits almost 14% of veterinary hospitals serving approximately 6000 practice teams. The standards of excellence expected in veterinary medicine and practice management are high. Students and veterinary technicians can also become members of AAHA, even if the veterinary hospital where they work is not a member. Continuing education, career center, and bookstore discounts are a few of the benefits of membership (http://www.aahanet.org).

AAVSB: The American Association of Veterinary State Boards recently became the owner of the Veterinary Technician National Examination (VTNE). The examination is offered during three examination periods each year. This organization helps transfer scores, offers mock examinations, lists state technician associations, and has a list of preparation reading resources for the examination (http://www.aavsb.org).

AVMA: Created in 1863, the American Veterinary Medical Association currently has 68,000 members. They have a committee that accredits veterinary technician programs around the United States and Canada (CVTEA). The AVMA acts as the collective voice for the veterinary profession. It lists state VMAs and may help you find your state VTA (http://www.avma.org).

AVTE: The Association of Veterinary Technician Educators offers a biennial symposium, continuing education, career links, recommended review materials for the VTNE, and newsletters (http://www.avte.net).

BLS.GOV: The Bureau of Labor Statistics provides information about average technician salaries, projections, and more (http://www.bls.gov).

CAAHTT: The Canadian Association of Animal Health Technologists and Technicians has resources that include a career center, VTNE study guide, list of technician programs, and continuing education (http://www.caahtt-acttsa.ca).

CVMA: The Canadian Veterinary Medical Association has resources that include accredited programs and a career center (http://canadianveterinarians.net).

DVM360: This website offers access to a number of journals, such as Firstline, Veterinary Economics, DVM Newsmagazine, and Veterinary Medicine (http://www.vm360.com).

FINANCIAL SIMULATOR PROGRAM: Originally created for veterinary students, this website provides access to an exceptionally valuable personal budget program at the website. It was created by the hospital director at the University of Minnesota College of Veterinary Medicine. The various elements of this budget program can be used by technicians and students and include help to establish personal budgets, make plans to repay education and/or other loans, purchase or lease vehicles, buy homes, and plan for retirement (http://www.finsim.umn.edu).

IVNTA: The International Veterinary Nurses and Technicians Association consists of member countries that seek to foster and promote links with veterinary nursing and veterinary technician staff worldwide by communication and cooperation (http://www.ivnta.org).

MYVETERINARYCAREER: Created in 2007, this website provides personal career management and recruitment. Through their personalized approach, individual preference review, and your identified values, their team will help match you to a veterinary hospital that aligns with your personal mission, goals, and values (http://www.myveterinarycareer.com).

NAVTA: The National Association of Veterinary Technicians in America was created in 1981 to be the national voice of the veterinary technician. Currently, there are 4800 members. It is their goal to influence the future of NAVTA members' professional goals, foster high standards of veterinary care, and promote the veterinary health care team. The website has resources that include a career center, continuing education, state representative contacts, specialty section, quarterly journal (TNJ), and information on student chapters (SCNAVTA) and National Veterinary Technician Week (NVTW) (http//:www.navta.net).

NCVEI: Founded in 2000 by the American Veterinary Medical Association, the American Animal Hospital Association, and the American Association of Veterinary Medical Colleges, and supported by corporate sponsorships, the National Commission on Veterinary Economic Issues offers benchmarking tools and other resources for veterinary practices. Recent articles include "Weathering the Economy" and "The Veterinarian's Guide to Pet Health Insurance." Technicians are greater assets to their veterinary practice if they have a basic understanding of business, profit and loss, and budgeting (http://www.ncvei.org).

NETVET: This is a veterinary resource site for veterinary professionals and animal owners (http://netvet.wustl.edu).

SAFETYVET: Created by a veterinary technician in 1998, this site has resources that include information on OSHA requirements, safety procedures, your rights as an employee, team training, controlled substance logging, radiation exposure, and pregnancy precautions (http://www.safetyvet.com).

SALARYEXPERT: This website allows for geographic research of veterinary professional salaries (http://www.salaryexpert.com).

VETLEARN: This website offers access to numerous journals such as Veterinary Technician, Compendium, Product Forum, and Market News (http://www.vetlearn.com).

VETMEDTEAM: Created as the first website offering continuing education to the entire health care team, VetMedTeam offers VTNE reviews, membership polls, advanced course studies, and practice management and assistant classes (http://www.vetmedteam.com).

VETPARTNERS: VetPartners is a resource for veterinary consultants that include veterinarians, veterinary technicians, practice managers, industry leaders, lawyers, and business associates. Review their site if you wish to become a consultant, want to network with consultants, or need to hire a consultant (http://www.vetpartners.org).

VHMA: Created in 1981, the membership of Veterinary Hospital Managers Association, currently 1500, includes a number of veterinary technicians; 25% of certified veterinary practice managers (CVPM) are veterinary technicians. This organization offers continuing education courses, maintains certification for practice managers, conducts surveys, generates a monthly newsletter, and is growing rapidly (http://www.vhma.org).

VSPN: The Veterinary Support Personnel Network was founded in 1996 and is supported by the Veterinary Information Network (VIN). Membership is free. It offers resources that include online continuing education (since 2001), live chats, surveys, and a bookstore (http://www.vspn.org).

WHERETECHSCONNECT: The largest career center for veterinary technicians and staff, this website was created in 2001. You can post your resume, review career tips, view hospitals seeking

technicians, and participate in their discussion board, all free services for veterinary technicians. Resources for continuing education are also posted (http://www.wheretechsconnect.com).

Adapted from Sirois M: Principles and practice of veterinary technology, ed 3, St Louis, 2011, Mosby.

animals requires specialized expertise in order to handle and treat them in a safe manner that avoids injury to both the animal and the handler. Equipment used for handling, restraint, and treatment of these animals is also unique.

MIXED PRACTICE

Some veterinary facilities treat companion animals and large animals. These facilities may have modifications to allow for treatment of some large animals on site or may incorporate a mobile practice and travel to farms.

CRITICAL CONCEPT

The specific duties of each member of the veterinary health care team will vary depending on the size and type of practice.

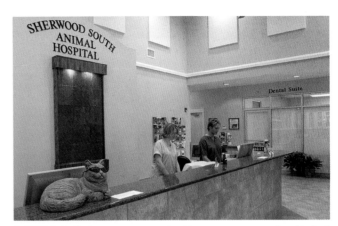

FIGURE 1-8 A reception area should give a warm, comfortable feeling to clients and staff. (From Bassert JM, McCurnin DM: McCurnin's clinical textbook for veterinary technicians, ed 7, St Louis, 2010, Saunders Elsevier.)

VETERINARY PRACTICE DESIGN

Veterinary clinics have a number of specialized areas for examination and treatment of patients. Some areas are designated for patients that must be hospitalized (inpatients) whereas others are for those that do not require hospitalization (outpatients). Additional areas are present that support the office management–related functions and personnel needs.

The size, type of practice, and services offered are three main factors that affect the design and efficiency of a hospital. The primary goal is to develop a solution that optimizes the efficiency of the team while providing clients and patients with a high standard of care.

Most practices are divided into three parts: the front, middle, and back. The front generally consists of the reception area and examination room. The middle refers to the laboratory, pharmacy, and treatment areas, and the back refers to kennel wards and storage area.

CREATING COMFORTABLE RECEPTION AREAS

The reception area is the gateway to the practice and provides the clients with the first impression of the hospital (Fig. 1-8). Overcrowding and congestion always occur in the reception area, especially as clients arrive for appointments and to pick up patients or medications. Congestion doubles as clients check out with their pets. This congestion can lead to undesirable pet interaction and client dissatisfaction.

It is advisable to develop separate waiting areas for dog and cat patients, thereby reducing the stress on the owners and pets. A practice may also have separate check-in and check-out areas, reducing the congestion associated with both procedures. If a practice boards or grooms patients, a separate entrance may benefit clients and team members.

A warm atmosphere can be created with comfortable chairs, nice artwork on the walls, and plants. Chairs should be made of a material that is easy to clean, does not stain, and is durable. Seats should have some space between them. Clients do not like to sit right next to each other, especially those with large dogs. Plants should be hung from the ceiling or on the wall to prevent dogs from urinating on them. A restroom should be provided off the reception area for the convenience of clients.

Photo albums can be created of team members and their pets. Photos may include professional portraits and spontaneous pictures, showing activities in which team members participate with their pets outside the office. Photo albums can also be created of clients and their pets. Clients should be asked for permission to place photos in the album. A practice photo album can also be created, showing different rooms of the practice, activities that occur in those rooms, and team members performing activities. Many clients wonder what it looks like behind the scenes and what happens once their pet leaves the examination room; this is a wonderful way to satisfy them. Picture collages also warm up rooms, giving clients something to look at while they wait.

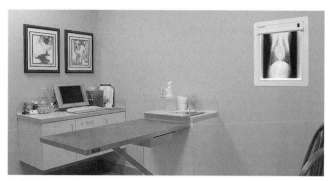

FIGURE 1-9 Examination rooms should be warmly decorated, clean, and in excellent condition. (From Bassert JM, McCurnin DM: McCurnin's clinical textbook for veterinary technicians, ed 7, St Louis, 2010, Saunders Elsevier.)

CREATING COMFORTABLE EXAMINATION ROOMS

Cleanliness of examination rooms is imperative to owners and should be to the entire team. Rooms should be swept and mopped after each patient to decrease the chance of transmitting disease. Cleanliness also prevents the transmission of odors. Warm neutral tones calm clients. A practice may add nicely framed pictures or client education posters. Thumb tacks or push pins should not be used to hang posters; holes in the wall and torn posters devalue the practice. Wall borders also add a nice touch to rooms, along with comfortable chairs that allow clients to sit near patients on the examination table. Rooms should not be cluttered with models, treats, or diagnostic equipment (Fig. 1-9). Countertops and sinks should be clean at all times.

CONSULTATION ROOMS

Consultation rooms are nice for clients who arrive at the practice and need to discuss patient care with veterinarians and technicians. They can also be used for euthanasia. Rooms should be quiet, away from high-traffic areas, and provide a sense of comfort. Nicely framed pictures may line the room, and a comfortable couch or chair should be present. A radiograph viewer may be added for consultation purposes, as well as models for client education. Examination room tables may be left out, because this room is strictly for consultations, not examinations. If euthanasia is performed, the patient may lie on a comfortable blanket on the floor or be held in the arms of the client.

When developing, designing, or remodeling a practice, the Americans with Disabilities Act must be considered. This act is a federal law that protects those with disabilities, including team members and clients. Features must be put in place that allow clients full access to the facility, including parking lot ramps, bathroom access (including wide doors and handrails), and wide doors for wheelchair access to all rooms.

Team members with disabilities cannot be discriminated against if they can complete the job requirements as listed in the job description section of the employee manual. By law, employers may be required to provide reasonable accommodations to enable the employee to perform the listed job

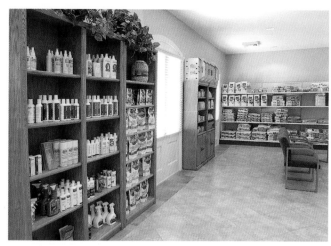

FIGURE 1-10 Professional display in reception area. (From Bassert JM, McCurnin DM: McCurnin's clinical textbook for veterinary technicians, ed 7, St Louis, 2010, Saunders Elsevier.)

duties. Reasonable accommodations may include making existing facilities used by employees readily accessible and usable by individuals with disabilities.

RETAIL AREA

Retail areas are useful for drawing attention to products that the practice promotes; however, extra attention needs to be given to this area to prevent theft (Fig. 1-10). Retail areas that can be placed behind the reception area may hold more valuable items such as collars or leashes; less expensive toys and smaller items can be placed in the reception area. Therapeutic (prescription) diets should be placed behind the counter, allowing maintenance diets to remain in the reception area. Many practices have limited space to carry excess products, so care must be taken when choosing which products will be carried. It should be determined what and how the practice will benefit if it chooses to carry a product. However, clients look to the veterinary practice for recommendations of products to purchase, food, and toys that should be allowed for their pet. An appropriate balance must be determined in each practice.

MIDDLE AREA

The middle area of a veterinary practice generally includes the pharmacy and laboratory areas, which must also function in an efficient manner (Figs. 1-11 and 1-12). If the pharmacy and laboratory share the same space, there must be enough room for computers, laboratory equipment, prescription filling, and a location to write on records. Equipment should be placed in ergonomically efficient locations, reducing the workload of team members as they complete tasks associated with the laboratory area. Laboratory equipment must be placed far enough apart to allow fans to cool the equipment efficiently. Electrical outlets should not be overloaded, which could cause a fire hazard.

TREATMENT AREA

The treatment area is generally referred to as the back of the practice and encompasses radiology (Fig. 1-13), surgery and

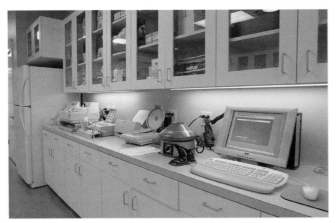

FIGURE 1-11 The laboratory is located just beyond the examination rooms. (From Bassert JM, McCurnin DM: McCurnin's clinical textbook for veterinary technicians, ed 7, St Louis, 2010, Saunders Elsevier.)

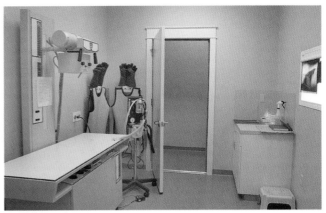

FIGURE 1-13 Radiology room with x-ray machine and protective equipment hanging on the wall. The automatic film processor is not visible through the open door. (From Bassert JM, McCurnin DM: McCurnin's clinical textbook for veterinary technicians, ed 7, St Louis, 2010, Saunders Elsevier.)

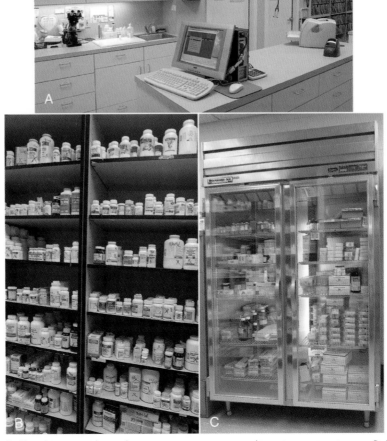

FIGURE 1-12 A, The pharmacy is located near examination rooms and inpatient treatment areas. B, Drug shelf storage in pharmacy. C, Glass door refrigerator for storage of vaccines and biologics. (From Bassert JM, McCurnin DM: McCurnin's clinical textbook for veterinary technicians, ed 7, St Louis, 2010, Saunders Elsevier.)

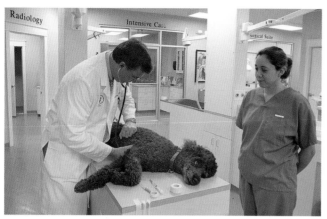

FIGURE 1-14 Centralized treatment area accommodates outpatient and inpatient treatment. (From Bassert JM, McCurnin DM: McCurnin's clinical textbook for veterinary technicians, ed 7, St Louis, 2010, Saunders Elsevier.)

treatment space (Fig. 1-14), the kennel, and isolation wards. Floors should have an antislip surface, reducing accidental slipping on wet floors. The treatment area should be set up to allow traffic to flow freely and uncongested. Treatment tables should be positioned to allow team members to work from any angle. Placement of tables in the center of a room works well. Electrical outlets can be placed in the ceiling, if needed, reducing the number of cords on which a team member might trip (Fig. 1-15). The treatment area must remain clutter-free, allowing the team to work efficiently, especially when space is limited.

ETHICS

Our lives are governed by rules and laws. As children, we are taught the difference between acceptable and unacceptable behavior. We soon learn the standards by which to judge the actions of others and ourselves and easily recognize negative behavior when we encounter it. As adults, we intuitively know what is right, what is fair, and what is honest.

Our society sets specific standards for proper living. An ethical person lives by these standards. Laws set the maximum limits from which we can deviate from the acceptable norm, established by the people and for the people, and made law through legislation. When someone does something unethical, is it something illegal? Not necessarily. **Ethics** are usually based on higher principles than the minimal requirements of the law and, as a member of a profession, we are expected to adhere to ethical standards above those acceptable for the populace. Ethics can be defined as the system of moral principles that determines appropriate behavior and actions within a specific group. Members of the medical profession are expected to adhere to the highest ethical standards. The public accepts, without question, the decisions and judgments made by medical professionals because of their education and expertise.

This text was written for those who work in the veterinary profession. We serve the public and the animal kingdom. A veterinary professional should have a profound commitment

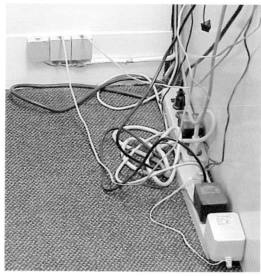

FIGURE 1-15 Overloaded surge suppressors or extension cords can start a fire. (From Bassert JM, McCurnin DM: McCurnin's clinical textbook for veterinary technicians, ed 7, St Louis, 2010, Saunders Elsevier.)

to honesty, compassion, proficiency, and hard work. Individuals with high ethical standards fit perfectly into the veterinary community.

> **CRITICAL CONCEPT**
>
> Ethics is a system of moral principles that guide appropriate behavior and actions.

ETHICS OF WORKING WITH ANIMALS

The use and abuse of animals has been well documented throughout history. Practices such as rat baiting, dog fights and cockfights, and the pointless slaughter of animals for sport have passed from commonplace to criminal acts. The American Society for the Prevention of Cruelty to Animals (ASPCA) was created in 1866, and anticruelty laws were passed the same year.

Our culture demands that we treat animals with kindness, respect, and compassion. Animals once thought to exist only for our use and pleasure are now known to feel pain and experience stress. Nowhere is this concept more important than in the veterinary profession. The **human-animal bond**, a real and maturing concept, defines the special, healthy relationship between people and their pets.

Some people ask whether the rights of an animal should be the same as for humans; they believe that animals should not be used for any purpose. People, they maintain, are merely the highest form of animal life, and all life is important and equal. If you would not do something to a person, they argue, it should not be done to an animal. Animal rights activists question the use of animals for food, clothing, entertainment, and biomedical research. Some even question keeping animals as pets. They question whether owning a pet is the same as slavery in people. However, most people believe in regulated forms of animal use as long as it is compassionate, humane, and not of trivial importance.

Although the public accepts the concept of animal use, it demands nothing less than exemplary care for animals. This is shown in many ways. The public has no tolerance for a dog owner who criminally starves a pet, a commercial puppy mill that houses puppies in unsanitary conditions, or a biomedical facility that violates federal laws that govern the care and use of animals in research. Society considers it a privilege to own an animal. This privilege can be taken away if the owner does not adhere to acceptable standards of animal care.

As your career evolves, you may observe unsatisfactory care and abuse of an animal. Know and understand the state and local laws regarding your obligation as a veterinary professional to report animal abuse to the authorities. There is well-documented evidence that links animal abuse and family violence. The presence of animal cruelty in a household often indicates abuse of other family members. If a veterinary team member is suspicious that an animal has been abused, speak promptly with your veterinarian and local authorities. To learn more, contact your local law enforcement agencies, humane society, or veterinary medical association for proper training.

ETHICS OF THE VETERINARY PROFESSION

Questions of ethics in the veterinary community tend to fall into several major categories. We will look at some of these more closely to understand the ethical challenges that can occur within the veterinary profession.

PROFESSIONAL ETHICS

Medicine will always be an art as well as a science. Professional judgment is the freedom given to all veterinarians to treat a case in a manner that they think best. Sometimes, the choices made by the professional are not those that others in the profession would commonly choose. There may be a fine line between freedom and standard of care. Who decides the difference?

Each state government has created laws for the veterinary profession that are written into the **Veterinary State Practice Act**. The **Board of Veterinary Medical Examiners**, made up of a combination of veterinary professionals and nonveterinarians, is responsible for interpreting the law and standards of care offered to veterinary patients. The board's mission is to protect the consumer and review cases brought against a licensed professional. It is the board's job to determine whether there was medical **negligence** or malpractice. The Board of Examiners, created through government funding, may impose penalties on a veterinarian or technician when they have determined **malpractice or professional negligence**. The veterinary medical board may impose penalties and fines, require further education in record keeping, send letters of guidance or admonition, and/or mandate retraining to avoid future complaints. Suspension of a license to practice is the final tool that a state board uses to ensure that all individuals are practicing to a high standard.

As an employee, you have an ethical obligation to discuss any matter concerning animal care that troubles you with the veterinarian. Keep an open mind. Often, what may appear as inappropriate action by the veterinarian may be satisfactorily explained with a frank dialogue. In most cases, honest discussion will resolve the problem. In extreme cases, staff members may have to discuss their concerns with another veterinarian or the Board of Veterinary Medical Examiners. Cases brought to the board are critiqued objectively and fairly. Accurate records and documentation of conversations, dates, times, and witnesses are needed to create a solid complaint.

ETHICS OF SERVICE TO THE PUBLIC

People who work in the veterinary profession are obligated to serve the public and in so doing, to provide medical care and treatment at a level consistent with the standards of the profession. Members of the profession are morally compelled to report abuses inflicted on animals and legally responsible for reporting public health problems.

It is well understood that the public pays veterinarians and their staff for their services. In essence, the veterinary hospital enters into a contract with the pet owner, wherein specific services are rendered for a certain amount of money. The owner is legally responsible for paying the bill. What are the obligations of the veterinary hospital? Aside from legal obligations of the hospital to render the service competently, the hospital is also morally responsible for treating the animal with care and compassion.

Should the presence or absence of a fee determine whether a sick animal is treated? Ethically, the veterinarian and the supporting staff are obligated to provide at least basic lifesaving treatment and pain relief whenever possible to any animal in its care. This may include performing euthanasia on a badly injured stray in obvious pain.

Veterinary professionals also act as teachers. There is an obligation to communicate with the public in clear, easy to understand language. The subjects may be as diverse as the care of an animal with diabetes, the correct use of dispensed medication, or nutritional tips. We are obligated to communicate and inform. Consent forms can be used as an educational tool and help define the veterinarian-client-patient relationship. Because of concerns regarding this special relationship, the AVMA has defined the relationship regarding the use of dispensing prescribed medications and establishing treatment plans.

LAWS

In the daily practice of veterinary medicine, the veterinary practice team is confronted with a wide variety of legal issues that affect their professional or business decisions. Bodies of law governing daily practices occurring within a veterinary clinic often overlap and fall into one of four categories—federal law, state law, local or municipal law, or common law. Federal, state, and local or municipal laws constitute legislative or written laws. Relevant governmental authorities and agencies enforce these laws, and violations may be punishable by fines and/or jail sentences. In contrast, common law is a body of unwritten law (legal interpretation) that has evolved from use and custom and by judicial decisions establishing precedential case law. Government authorities or agencies do not enforce common law in the same way as legislative laws. Common law is enforced by the judicial system when citizens who may have been injured by a violation of the law file civil lawsuits against the violators.

The laws affecting a veterinary practice can be divided into two groups: (1) laws that ensure the quality of veterinary service to patients; and (2) laws that provide a nonhostile and safe environment for employees, clients, and the public.

CRITICAL CONCEPT

Veterinary practice acts contain the laws that define the practice of veterinary medicine in a particular state.

LAWS THAT ENSURE THE QUALITY OF VETERINARY SERVICE

PRACTICE ACTS

The veterinary practice act of each state and province defines which persons may practice veterinary medicine and surgery in the state and under which conditions. Although practice acts vary in different states and provinces, they generally define the practice of veterinary medicine—making it illegal to practice without a license, stating the qualifications for receiving a license, stating the conditions under which a license can be revoked, and establishing penalties for violating the act.

The practice acts generally define the practice of veterinary medicine and surgery as diagnosing, treating, prescribing, operating on, testing for the presence of animal disease, and making the public aware of your services as a licensed practitioner. Embryo transfer, dentistry, and alternative forms of therapy, such as acupuncture, massage, chiropractic, and holistic medicine, are generally regarded within this definition of veterinary medicine and surgery, although this may vary in different locations.

Allowing only licensed veterinarians to practice veterinary medicine legally may raise questions about the duties performed by veterinary technicians and veterinary assistants. After all, many of the procedures performed routinely by technicians and assistants fall literally within the scope of the practice of veterinary medicine and surgery, such as inserting an intravenous catheter, inducing general anesthesia, and extracting teeth (outlined in some practice acts). However, as long as the staff member is under the direction and responsible supervision of a licensed veterinarian and the staff member does not make decisions requiring a veterinary license, the licensed veterinarian, and not the staff member, is practicing veterinary medicine in such instances. Read your governing body's practice act. Inquiry is your best option; ask that your governing board inform you about your duties and responsibilities by providing updated literature.

Whether a staff member is under the direction and responsible supervision of a licensed veterinarian is a subjective determination that takes into account the degree of experience and competence of the staff member, the task being performed, and the risks to the patient. Regardless of how experienced the staff member may be, in some states the veterinarian must be on the premises or reachable by telephone or two-way radio communication during and for a reasonable time after any veterinary procedure. Although the remainder of this section describes specific laws relevant to the United States, Canada and most other countries have similar laws and regulations.

COMMON LAW MALPRACTICE

When a veterinarian agrees to treat a client's animal, common law automatically imposes on that veterinarian a legal duty to provide medical or surgical care to that client's animal in accordance with that of a reasonably prudent veterinary practitioner of comparable training under the same or similar circumstances.

A veterinarian's failure to live up to this particular duty constitutes negligence, which may also be referred to as malpractice or professional negligence.

For malpractice to be subject to litigation, the plaintiff must prove three elements: (1) the veterinarian agreed to treat the patient; (2) the veterinarian failed to exercise the necessary legal obligation of skill and diligence in treating the patient (negligence); and (3) the negligence caused injury to the patient.

Veterinarians can be found negligent and guilty of malpractice for the injurious actions of a technician or assistant under the common law doctrine of respondeat superior. For example, if a technician mistakenly gave twice the recommended dosage of anesthesia to a patient and this doubled dose caused the death of the animal, the veterinarian may be found negligent and guilty of malpractice, the same as if the veterinarian had given the wrong dosage. If the technician is licensed in the state, the license may also be revoked.

LAWS THAT PROVIDE A SAFE BUSINESS ENVIRONMENT

Federal, state, and common laws exist to help ensure safe and nonhostile working conditions for employees of a veterinary practice, as well as safe conditions for the public.

OCCUPATIONAL SAFETY AND HEALTH ACT

Every employer with one or more employees must operate in compliance with the **Occupational Safety and Health Act (OSHA)** of 1970. OSHA regulations are designed to provide a safe workplace for all persons working in any business affecting commerce. The broad judicial interpretation of commerce includes the business of practicing veterinary medicine and surgery. OSHA requires that all employers "shall furnish to each of his employees employment and a place of employment which are free from recognized hazards that are causing or are likely to cause death or serious physical harm to his employees."

To view the official OSHA site, go to http://www.osha.gov. A complete manual is easily downloaded. **Material Safety Data Sheets**, training, state rules and regulations, fines, and reporting information is located on the site. For example, information regarding personal protective equipment for occupational exposure to Ebola virus can be easily downloaded.

COMMON LAW ORDINARY NEGLIGENCE

Common law establishes for every business owner a legal duty to provide a reasonably safe work environment for employees, as well as a reasonably safe place for clients. Failure to provide this safe environment may constitute ordinary negligence on the part of the veterinarian or business owner. This ordinary negligence is distinguished from malpractice, which is negligence associated with the rendering of professional veterinary medical services. As with malpractice, however, ordinary negligence is not subject to legal action unless it causes injury to a client or employee. For example, if a practice owner provides poor ventilation in a surgical suite and an employee becomes drowsy from anesthetic gases, the employee could not sue and recover damages from the veterinarian unless he or she experiences injury as a consequence (e.g., faints and hits his or her head on the countertop).

In meeting the obligation to provide a safe environment for employees and clients, a veterinarian has a common law duty to supervise proper restraint of any animal under the veterinarian's control. When a client's animal is being examined and the client restrains the animal, it is the veterinarian and not the client who is primarily responsible for proper restraint of that animal. A veterinarian may be found guilty of ordinary negligence if she or he fails to use reasonable care to avoid foreseeable harm to the restrainer or to other people in the vicinity. The definition of reasonable care or foreseeable harm varies, depending on the experience or training of the veterinarian and the animal handler and the procedure done on the animal. Veterinarians have been sued by clients because the client restrained his or her own animal during a procedure and the animal bit the client. To avoid a possible lawsuit, do not allow owners to restrain their own animal within a veterinary hospital.

MEDICAL WASTE MANAGEMENT LAWS

Veterinarians who own or operate a veterinary practice may be subject to the requirements of state law governing management and disposal of medical wastes (Fig. 1-16). Local laws may impose additional restrictions on what types of waste transporters and disposal facilities may be acceptable. Typical waste included under these acts are discarded needles and syringes, vials containing attenuated or live vaccines, culture plates, and animal carcasses exposed to or infected with pathogens infectious to humans or euthanized with a barbiturate. State and local law may extend these categories of regulated veterinary medical waste to include all carcasses, animal blood, bedding, and pathology waste.

Review your state and local regulations to determine which requirements govern your veterinary hospital. Companies specializing in the disposal of medical waste can also provide accurate information. Added cost of proper disposal must be addressed because overhead generally increases as

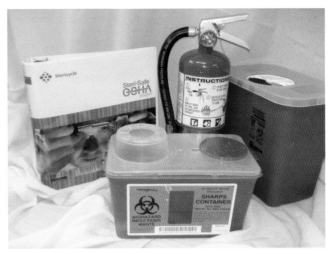

FIGURE 1-16 Syringes and needles must be discarded in a sharps container. (From Sirois M: Principles and practice of veterinary technology, ed 3, St Louis, 2011, Mosby.)

a result of the direct cost of the regulation. Hospital policy manuals may outline how to identify hazardous waste and how to dispose of it properly.

LAWS THAT MAINTAIN A NONHOSTILE WORKING ENVIRONMENT

There is a body of federal, state, and common law that restricts a veterinarian, as the owner of a business, from engaging in hiring or firing practices that wrongfully discriminate against individuals. Firing an individual for discriminatory reasons constitutes a violation of the federal or state **Equal Employment Opportunity (EEO)** laws and may provide a basis for the terminated employee to sue the employer under common law for wrongful termination of employment.

According to federal EEO laws, an employer of 15 or more employees may not discriminate against employees in hiring or firing practices (or in any practice, for that matter) on the basis of race, color, religion, gender, or national origin. Sexual harassment and discrimination on the basis of pregnancy or childbirth are forms of sex discrimination made illegal under federal law. Employers also cannot discriminate against individuals in hiring and firing of employees on the basis of age between 40 and 70 years or on the basis of disabilities, including AIDS and rehabilitated drug abuse. At time of hire a manager and new employee may review the **employee handbook** together, discussing the hospital's philosophies and policies. An acknowledgment of receipt may be signed and placed in the new employee's file.

Common law also protects employees because it prohibits an employer from terminating that employee for discriminatory reasons or other reasons violating public policy. Under the common law tort of wrongful termination, an employee can sue an employer directly for firing the employee on the basis of gender, race, or religious discrimination, or on the basis that the employee is a whistleblower (i.e., has complained of sexual harassment or other violations of the law).

LAWS THAT GOVERN LABOR

The Fair Labor Standard Act (FLSA) establishes minimum wage, overtime, record-keeping, and youth employment standards for employees working in the private sector and in government. As a veterinary practice team member, you generally fall under the nonexempt category (unless you are promoted to an administrative position). At the time of your hire the manager will discuss time cards, overtime, vacation time, benefits, and employment category. **Nonexempt employees** are entitled to paid overtime when working more than 40 hours in a work week, even those on salary. Visit the **Department of Labor** website at http://www.dol.gov to find information related to careers in the veterinary industry.

LAWS GOVERNING CONTROLLED SUBSTANCES

Controlled substances are drugs that may be subject to abuse by team members, clients, and those who rob or burglarize a veterinary hospital. Federal and state laws have been adopted to govern their manufacture, sale, and distribution. In 1970, Congress passed the **Comprehensive Drug Abuse Prevention and Control Act,** regulating the manufacturing, distribution, dispensing, and delivery of certain drugs that have the potential for abuse. Title 2, known as the **Controlled Substance Act (CSA),** is the section most applicable to the veterinary community. The **Drug Enforcement Agency (DEA)** is the primary federal law enforcement agency responsible for combating the abuse of controlled drugs. State and provincial laws differ regarding the regulations of controlled substances. Identify the laws governing veterinary hospitals and controlled drugs in the state or province in which you work.

Classifications of controlled substances are outlined in Chapter 5. Carefully follow all record-keeping, storage, and ordering guidelines related to controlled substances (Fig. 1-17). Report possible abuse or tampering with controlled drugs to your supervisor, hospital manager, or veterinarian.

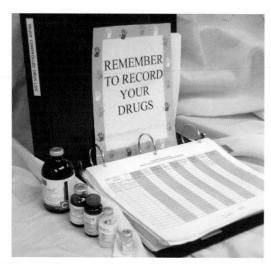

FIGURE 1-17 The Controlled Substances Act describes record-keeping requirements for certain medications. (From Sirois M: Principles and practice of veterinary technology, ed 3, St Louis, 2011, Mosby.)

OCCUPATIONAL HEALTH AND SAFETY IN VETERINARY PRACTICE

As a veterinary health care team member, you may be exposed to many hazards in your daily routine and in the performance of nonroutine functions. Hazards can include exposure to pathogenic microorganisms, chemicals, or radiation in addition to the obvious physical dangers. When properly identified, however, these hazards can be controlled and your risk of injury minimized. Your veterinary hospital will offer training specific to the exposure in your workplace. When you are hired, be sure you discuss personnel protective equipment, evacuation routes and gathering place, safety meetings, and emergency contacts, as outlined in the employee handbook. The **American Veterinary Medical Association's Professional Liability Insurance Trust (AVMAPLIT;** http://www.avmaplit.com) has published a safety manual for veterinary hospitals. In every state, an employee can be legally disciplined, including being terminated, for failure to follow safety rules for the workplace.

SAFETY IN THE WORKPLACE
MACHINERY AND MOVING PARTS

Equipment such as fans, chutes, and dryers have moving parts that can cause severe injury. Never operate machinery or equipment without all the proper guards in place. Long hair should be tied back to prevent it from getting caught in fans or other moving objects. Avoid wearing excessive jewelry, very loose-fitting clothing, or open-toed shoes. If you become aware of an unsafe condition, report it to your supervisor immediately.

SLIPS AND FALLS

You can reduce the chance of personal injury from slips and falls by wearing slip-proof shoes and using nonslip mats or strips in wet areas. Be especially cautious when walking on uneven or wet floors. Never run inside the hospital or on uneven flooring.

LIFTING

When lifting patients, supplies, or equipment, remember to keep your back straight and lift with your legs. Never bend over to lift an object; squat and use your knees when lifting objects. If a motorized lift table is not available, recruit help when lifting patients weighing more than 40 pounds. Remember to follow sound ergonomic principles when positioning or restraining, especially when working with horses or food animals.

STORING SUPPLIES

Store heavy supplies or equipment on the lower shelves to prevent unnecessary strains. Never use stairways as storage areas. Do not overload shelves or cabinets. Store liquids in containers with tight-fitting lids. When possible, store chemicals on shelves at or below eye level. Never climb on cabinets, shelves, chairs, buckets, or comparable items to reach high locations; use an appropriate ladder or stepstool.

TOXIC SUBSTANCES

Eat or drink only in areas free of toxic and biologically harmful substances as outlined in the employee handbook. Keep the staff coffeepot and utensils well away from sources of possible contamination, such as the laboratory, the treatment area, or bathing tub. Ensure that the cabinets above a coffee or food area contain no hazardous chemicals or supplies that could spill on the area. Store food, drinks, condiments, and snacks in a refrigerator free from biologic or chemical hazards; vaccines, drugs, and laboratory samples are all potential contamination sources. It is best to have a minimum of two refrigerators, one for biologic substances and one for employees' food.

HEATING DEVICES

When using equipment such as an autoclave, microwave oven, cautery iron, or other heating device, take time to learn the rules for safe operation. Burns, especially from steam, are painful and serious and can almost always be prevented. Autoclaves also present a danger from the pressure that is used for proper sterilization. When opening an autoclave, first release the pressure with the vent device and let the steam rise completely before opening the door fully. Always assume that cautery devices and branding irons are hot, and use the insulated handle whenever you handle them. Never place heated irons on any surface where they could overheat and start a fire or where someone could touch them accidentally. Microwaves installed overhead may lead to serious injuries.

EYE SAFETY

Familiarize yourself with the locations and use of eye wash stations. Always use safety glasses and other personal protective equipment when required. An employer is required by law to provide this equipment when appropriate.

Be sure you know where the eye wash device is before you need to use it. If you splash a chemical in your eyes, do not rub your eyes with your hands. Immediately call for help. With a coworker's assistance, go to the eye wash station and flush both eyes, even if only one eye is affected. Avoid using the spray attachments for tubs and sinks because the water pressure is unregulated and the streams of water from these devices can be fine enough to lacerate the cornea. Contact lenses should not be worn when working with chemicals because the contact lens will impair the ability of the eye wash to remove any splashed chemicals.

HAZARDS OF ANIMAL HANDLING

Here is the most important rule to follow:
• Do not allow clients to restrain their own animals.

The second rule to follow when working around animals is to stay alert. Sudden noises, movements, or even light can cause an animal to react. If you are the primary restraint person, focus your attention on the animal's reactions and not on the procedure being performed. Learn the correct restraint positions for each species that you handle regularly.

PROTECTIVE GEAR

Your employer is obligated to provide you with **personal protective equipment (PPE**; Fig. 1-18). Some hazards that you may be exposed to when working in a veterinary hospital and the required PPE are listed in Table 1-1.

Make use of any available capture or restraint equipment, such as cages, snares, cat bags, and poles. Wear examination gloves and a surgical mask when handling a stray, wild, or unvaccinated animal. Maintain an appropriate distance from the work area or animal; for example, do not place your face close to the mouth of the animal (see section below,

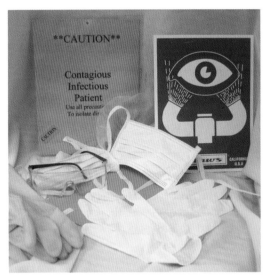

FIGURE 1-18 Personal protective equipment includes gloves, masks, and goggles. (From Sirois M: Principles and practice of veterinary technology, ed 3, St Louis, 2011, Mosby.)

TABLE 1-1	Hazards and Personal Protective Equipment	
POTENTIAL HAZARDS	**PROTECTIVE EQUIPMENT**	
Radiation exposure while taking x-rays	Lead aprons, gloves, thyroid collars	
Bites and scratches	Leashes, muzzles, bags, towels	
Bacterial exposure	Safety glasses, eye shields	
Exposure to hazardous chemical fumes	Masks	
Exposure to hazardous, caustic solutions	Examination gloves, rubber gloves	
Loud noises	Ear plugs	
Burns	Oven mitts and hot pads	

From Sirois M: Principles and practice of veterinary technology, ed 3, St Louis, 2011, Mosby.

"Zoonotic Hazards"). Wear protective leather gloves when handling a fractious animal.

Barking dogs can be a threat to hearing, especially in indoor kennels. Noise levels in canine wards can reach 110 decibels (dB). Exposure to these noise levels for a short time, such as going into the kennel to retrieve a patient, poses no serious damage to your hearing, but excessive or long-term exposure can contribute to hearing loss. When working in noisy areas for extended periods (e.g., when cleaning cages), always wear personal hearing protectors rated to filter the noise by at least 20 dB. (The package label indicates the rating.)

HAZARDS OF BATHING AND DIPPING

VENTILATION

Always use the ventilation fan when bathing or dipping patients. This will keep fumes from shampoos and dips at a safe level. Be sure to wear appropriate protective gear that includes safety glasses, gloves, and apron.

CHEMICAL STORAGE

Chemicals used for bathing and dipping animals can be harmful and must be stored properly. Bottles of dips, shampoos, and parasiticides should be stored in a cabinet at or below eye level. The bottle should be properly labeled, including contents and any appropriate hazard warning (see section below, "Chemical Hazards").

ZOONOTIC HAZARDS

When handling specimens such as fecal samples, laboratory samples, or wound exudates, wear protective gloves and always wash your hands immediately after completing the procedure. Contamination with these types of materials can usually be cleaned up with paper towels soaked in an appropriate disinfecting solution. Latex gloves should be worn and then discarded with the cleaned-up materials.

When treating patients with diseases that are infectious to people or other animals (**zoonotic diseases**), wear a protective apron, examination gloves, face mask, and eye protection. Thoroughly wash your hands with a disinfecting agent, such as chlorhexidine or povidone-iodine scrub, at the completion of treatment. Any clothing that has been contaminated should be changed immediately.

RABIES

Rabies is a serious, usually fatal, viral disease that can affect any warm-blooded animal, including humans. Rabies virus is spread by contact with an infected animal's saliva. Usually, an uninfected animal becomes infected through the bite of a rabid (infected) animal. The disease can also be transmitted by saliva that contaminates an open wound or contacts the mucous membranes, even the residue left on a dog's bowl after eating.

The primary barrier to the spread of rabies from the wild animal population to humans is vaccination of pets and other domestic animals. When you must handle an unvaccinated, wild, or stray animal, always wear protective examination gloves and perhaps even a protective gown and goggles.

A safe and effective human vaccine is available for those who work with animals. Ask your administrator about the hospital's policy on rabies vaccination and employee exposure.

BACTERIAL INFECTIONS

Bacterial infections are certainly possible in the veterinary environment. Aside from the common bacteria that all animals harbor naturally, injury and disease in veterinary patients can expose you to serious pathogens such as *Pasteurella, Salmonella, Escherichia coli,* and *Pseudomonas.* These bacterial agents are capable of causing serious infections in humans. Bacteria are most commonly transferred by direct contact with the animal or its excretions, especially if you have a cut or open sore. Some bacteria are easily aerosolized or released into the air, where they can be inhaled or absorbed through your mucous membranes. The best protection from exposure to bacteria is good personal hygiene and washing your hands after exposure. Always cover any wounds to prevent transmission of bacteria into the wound.

FUNGAL INFECTIONS

Ringworm is a superficial skin infection caused by a fungus, such as *Microsporum canis.* Ringworm is easily transmitted from animals to humans. The most effective protection from ringworm is to wear examination gloves when handling or treating animals with ringworm and to practice good personal hygiene by washing your hands after exposure.

PARASITISM

When the eggs of common internal parasites, such as roundworms and hookworms, infect humans, they usually do not mature to adult parasites but can cause other problems. Some species of roundworm larvae can migrate to almost any organ in the body and cause a condition known as visceral larva migrans. If this condition develops in a vital organ, such as the eye or brain, severe problems can result. The Companion Animal Parasite Council (http://www.capcvet.org) offers literature for veterinary professionals, including articles on internal and external parasites.

Hookworms can cause a condition known as cutaneous larval migrans. This particularly affects children who play in areas in which pets defecate frequently, such as a sandbox. Unlike the visceral cysts caused by roundworm larvae, the lesions of cutaneous larval migrans are relatively easy to visualize. These usually appear as red serpentine lines on the skin of the feet or lower legs.

Borreliosis, or Lyme disease, a bacterial infection transmitted by deer ticks, has become a serious concern for pets and people. When an infected deer tick bites a host (animal or person) during feeding, the bacterium *Borrelia burgdorferi* is transferred to the host. Lyme disease in humans is characterized by joint pain, fever, and other flulike symptoms. The best defense against borreliosis is to check your body for ticks after venturing outdoors and remove them promptly.

Mites causing sarcoptic mange can easily infest people. When treating animals with sarcoptic mange, always wear gloves and a protective gown and wash your hands thoroughly with disinfecting soap immediately after the procedure.

The coccidian parasite *Toxoplasma gondii* can infect cats and humans. Although it is usually not harmful to healthy people, it might cause serious problems to the fetus of pregnant women. Toxoplasmosis is spread from cats to people, usually by ingestion of the infectious oocysts in cat feces, but most humans contract the disease by eating undercooked meat. Pregnant women should avoid cleaning cat litter pans.

BIOLOGICS

Vials containing biologics, such as vaccines and bacterins, usually are not considered hazardous unless the agent can infect humans. For example, vials containing agents such as canine distemper virus or feline calicivirus are not usually considered a danger to humans, but vials containing biologically hazardous agents, such as brucellosis bacterins, must be treated as potentially infectious during and after use. Read the manufacture's insert on proper sterilization and disposal of brucellosis bacterins.

RADIATION HAZARDS

Infrequent exposure to small amounts of radiation, such as routine thoracic or dental x-rays, poses little threat to your overall health. However, long-term exposure to small doses of radiation has been linked to genetic, cutaneous, glandular, and other disorders. Exposure to large doses of radiation can cause skin changes, cell damage, and gastrointestinal and bone marrow disorders that can be fatal.

RADIATION SAFETY

When using radiographic equipment, never place any part of your body in the primary beam, even a hand wearing a lead-lined glove. Always wear the appropriate protective equipment, such as lead-lined aprons, thyroid collar, and lead gloves. Lead-impregnated glasses are also recommended. Always use the collimator to restrict the primary beam to an area smaller than the size of the cassette, creating a clear border around all four sides of the film. Digital radiographs add safety protection in that fewer x-rays are taken because the film can be digitally enhanced or altered. However, proper exposure techniques are still necessary to provide diagnostic-quality images and reduce exposure to radiation.

Portable x-ray machines, such as those used for dental radiography and in mobile practices, can be particularly dangerous because the primary beam of these machines can be aimed in any direction. When using a portable machine, always be sure that there is no human body part in the path of the primary beam, even at a distance. Never hold a cassette during the radiograph procedure, whether wearing lead-lined gloves or not; always use a cassette-holding device. Also, wear a lead-lined apron, thyroid collar, and gloves.

Everyone involved with radiography must wear a **dosimetry badge**. This badge must always be worn during radiographic procedures to measure any scatter radiation that you may receive during the procedure. Your supervisor or hospital administrator will regularly advise you of the readings from your personal dosimetry badge. These reports, required by law, are designed as a warning system to alert you and your supervisor if your exposure to radiation reaches a hazardous level. Because your dosimetry badge number follows you wherever you are employed, it gives an accurate lifetime exposure reading. Follow the manufacturer's directions regarding placement of the dosimeter and transferring your badge number to another hospital.

DEVELOPING CHEMICALS

X-ray developing chemicals, developer and fixer, can be corrosive to materials and human tissue. Take extreme care when mixing, transferring, agitating, or transporting these chemicals, and do this only in a well-ventilated area. Always turn on the exhaust fan when you are in a darkroom. Use protective gloves and goggles when mixing or pouring chemicals. For manual processing tanks, stir chemicals with care and avoid splashing. After handling radiographic developing chemicals, always wash your hands. See Chapter 11 for detailed information on radiation safety.

ANESTHETIC HAZARDS

Long-term exposure to waste anesthetic gases has been linked to congenital abnormalities in children, spontaneous abortions, and liver and kidney damage. OSHA has set the safe exposure limit for halogenated anesthetic agents (e.g., isoflurane) at 2 parts per million (ppm).

According to some sources, as much as 90% of the anesthetic gas levels found in the surgery room during a procedure can be attributed to leaks in anesthesia machines. Thus, always check for leaks in the hoses and anesthetic machine before use. Use hoses and rebreathing bags that are the correct size and consider inflating the endotracheal tube cuff before connecting the patient to the machine. Start the flow of anesthetic gas after connecting the patient to the machine. Before disconnecting the patient, continue oxygen flow until the remaining anesthesia gas has been flushed through the scavenging system. Have anesthetic machines professionally serviced on an annual basis.

A well-designed **scavenging system** captures excess gases directly at the source and transports them to a safe exhaust port, usually outside the building. This is the most effective means of reducing exposure of waste anesthetic gases in the workplace. Scavenger units (canisters) can be purchased and used on machines.

When refilling the anesthetic machine vaporizer, move the machine to a well-ventilated area. Use a pouring funnel and avoid overfilling the vaporizer or spilling the liquid anesthetic. If you accidentally break a bottle of liquid anesthetic, immediately evacuate all people from the area. Open the window and turn on the exhaust fans. Control the liquid with a spill kit absorbent or a generous amount of cat litter. Pick up the contaminated absorbent or cat litter with a dustpan, and place it in a plastic trash bag.

Some procedures, such as mask or tank induction, create additional challenges in collection of waste gases. In these cases, be sure that the room is well ventilated. Exhaust fans for evacuating room air to the outside are recommended. Air-handling systems that recirculate the air can expose others in the hospital to anesthetic gases. Induction chambers can be connected to the scavenging system or an absorption canister to reduce levels of escaping gases.

When changing the soda lime (carbon dioxide absorbent) in anesthetic machines, wear examination gloves. When the soda lime is wet, as it often is from humidity in the patient's breath, it can be caustic to tissues and some metals. Place used soda lime granules in a plastic trash bag and dispose of these in the regular trash. Read the manufacturer's instructions to determine when to change soda lime.

If you are a woman and become pregnant, discuss the anesthetic exposure risk with your physician as soon as possible and notify your supervisor immediately. Follow established policies regarding safety precautions while pregnant in your place of employment.

HAZARDS OF COMPRESSED GASES

Store cylinders of compressed gas (e.g., oxygen) in a dry, cool place, away from potential heat sources such as furnaces, water heaters, and direct sunlight. Always secure the tanks in an upright position by means of a chain or strap, including small tanks. Transportation carts and floor-mounting collars are also acceptable methods of securing compressed gas cylinders. If the cylinder is equipped with a protective cap (usually the large ones are so equipped), it must be firmly screwed in place when the cylinder is not in use. If you must move a large cylinder, do not roll or drag it; always use a hand truck, dolly, or cart and strap the tank to the cart before moving. Always wear impact-resistant protective goggles when connecting or disconnecting tanks, because air escaping from tanks can cause trauma to the cornea of your eyes.

More details on safety issues related to anesthetic procedures are presented in Chapter 9.

HAZARDS OF SHARP OBJECTS

The most serious hazard of sharp objects (termed sharps) in a veterinary environment is from the physical trauma and possible bacterial infection caused by a puncture or laceration. To prevent accidents from punctures or lacerations, always keep needles, scalpel blades, and other sharps capped or sheathed until ready for use. When practical, place the sharp in a red sharps container immediately after use. Do not attempt to recap the needle unless the physical danger from sticks or lacerations cannot be avoided by any other means.

When necessary, needles may be recapped using the one-handed method. Place the cap on a flat surface (table or counter). With one hand, thread the needle into the cap. The cap may then be firmly seated using both hands. The needle should not be removed from the syringe, but the entire unit should be disposed of in the red sharps container. When full, the sharps container must be sealed and disposed of following the hospital's prescribed policy.

Ordinary plastic milk containers are not appropriate sharps collection containers; a 22-gauge needle can easily penetrate them. The containers made for this specific purpose (usually red and labeled with a biohazard symbol) are the most effective and are usually inexpensive (see Fig 1-16). State and local laws may prevent your hospital from using inappropriate sharps containers, and fines may be levied against the hospital if they do not meet established standards.

Cutting off the ends of needles before disposal increases the potential for aerosolization of the liquid involved. Collecting sharps in a smaller container and transferring them to a larger container for disposal places someone at an increased risk of exposure. Neither of these practices is recommended.

Never throw needles or other sharps directly into regular trash containers, regardless of whether or not they are capped. Never open a used sharps container. Never insert your fingers into a sharps container for any reason.

> ### CRITICAL CONCEPT
> View the OSHA website at http://www.osha.gov to print regulations, standards, fact sheets, forms, chemical labeling, and the small business handbook. Also go to http://www.safetyvet.com for more information directly related to veterinary hospitals.

CHEMICAL HAZARDS

Many products you use every day can be hazardous. Every chemical, even common ones such as cleaning supplies, can cause harm. Some chemicals can contribute to health problems, whereas others may be flammable and pose a fire threat. The most common chemicals used in the veterinary workplace are insecticides, medications, and cleaning agents.

Veterinary hospitals must follow the guidelines of OSHA's **Right to Know Law**. This law requires that you be informed about all chemicals to which you may be exposed while doing your job. The Right to Know Law also requires you to wear all safety equipment that is prescribed by the manufacturer when handling a chemical. The safety equipment must be provided by the employer at no cost to you. It is not optional; you must wear what is prescribed.

HAZARDOUS MATERIALS PLAN

A strategic component of the Right to Know Law is the **hazardous materials plan**. This plan describes the details of the practice's **Material Safety Data Sheet (MSDS)** filing system and the secondary container labeling system (Fig. 1-19). The plan also lists the person responsible for ensuring that all employees have received the necessary safety training. You have a right to review any of these materials, so ask your supervisor where your plan is located.

Part of the planning process includes knowing exactly which chemicals are present in the workplace. There must be an up-to-date list of chemicals that are known to be on the hospital premises. It surprises some people to learn that the average veterinary hospital has more than 200 hazardous chemicals present at any time.

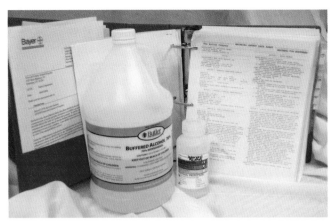

FIGURE 1-19 Material Safety Data Sheets and secondary container labels are important components of the Right to Know Law. (From Sirois M: Principles and practice of veterinary technology, ed 3, St Louis, 2011, Mosby.)

CRITICAL CONCEPT

Use the MSDS website (http://www.MSDSonline.com) to search millions of documents. It's easy to use and can simplify compliance.

MATERIAL SAFETY DATA SHEET SYSTEM

More detailed information about every chemical can be found in the MSDS filing system. When you are hired, your manager will inform you where the MSDS log is kept. When OSHA does its inspection, inspectors will ask where the MSDS log is kept. MSDS documents may look complicated at first glance, but the information that is important to you is easy to find.

CONTAINER LABELS

When you receive a supply of chemicals from the distributor, every bottle is identified with a label containing directions and appropriate warnings. Always read, understand, and follow these directions and warnings printed on the label. When possible, keep this label intact and readable. Sometimes it is necessary to dilute a chemical or pour it into smaller bottles for use. These smaller bottles are known as secondary containers. All secondary containers must have a label that indicates the contents and appropriate safety warnings.

CONTAINER CAPS

Always remember to replace the cap on a chemical bottle after use. Bottles of chemicals should always have tight-fitting, screw-on lids. Always store chemical bottles at or below eye level in a closed cabinet. Never store or use chemicals near food or beverages.

MIXING CHEMICALS

Be cautious when mixing or diluting chemicals. Always wear gloves and protective goggles. Never mix any chemicals unless you know it is safe to do so according to the label or MSDS. Mixing often creates a new, sometimes very dangerous chemi-cal. When making dilute solutions from a concentrate, always start with the correct quantity of water and then add the concentrate. Never add the water to the concentrate, because the chemical may splash or may not react as you expect.

CHEMICAL SPILLS

Minor spills of most chemicals can be cleaned up with paper towels or other absorbent material, such as kitty litter, and disposed of in the trash or sanitary sewer. However, some very dangerous chemicals, such as formaldehyde or ethylene oxide, require special procedures. Before you use a chemical with which you are unfamiliar, review the MSDS and learn the procedures you must follow for cleaning up a spill. When cleaning up any spill, always wear gloves and any other protective equipment specified on the MSDS. Unless prohibited by the instructions on the MSDS, wash the spill site and any contaminated equipment with a detergent soap and water.

HANDLING ETHYLENE OXIDE

Many hospitals use **ethylene oxide** gas to sterilize items that would be damaged by other sterilization procedures. Ethylene oxide is a potent human carcinogen. Take the following precautions when handling or using ethylene oxide:
- Carefully read the MSDS for ethylene oxide.
- Store the ethylene oxide in a safe place.
- Use only approved devices to perform ethylene oxide sterilization.
- Read, understand, and follow all written procedures and safety precautions.
- Know the emergency procedures.
- Be aware of monitoring levels.
- Keep ethylene oxide away from flames and sparks because it is highly flammable.

HANDLING FORMALIN

Liquid or gaseous formaldehyde and formalin are serious health hazards in veterinary hospitals. Because formaldehyde is a known human carcinogen, OSHA monitors its use:
- Carefully read the MSDS for formaldehyde and formalin.
- Store formalin containers safely, including specimen jars.
- Use formalin only with good ventilation; avoid breathing vapors.
- Wear goggles and gloves; avoid skin and eye contact.

Exposure to formalin can be minimized by use of premixed, premeasured vials of formalin for specimens. Veterinary hospitals that still use bulk formalin for diagnostic laboratory tests (e.g., Knott's test) should consider switching to a newer, less hazardous method of testing.

ELECTRICAL HAZARDS

Do not remove light switch or electrical outlet covers. Always keep circuit breaker boxes closed. Only persons trained to perform maintenance duties should repair electrical outlets, switches, fixtures, or breakers. If you must use a portable dryer or other electrical equipment in a wet area, it must be properly grounded and should only be plugged into a ground fault circuit interrupter (GFCI) type of outlet.

Extension cords should be used only for temporary supply applications and should always be of the three-conductor, grounded type. Never run extension cords through windows or doors that could close and damage the wires. Never run extension cords across aisles or floors, which create a tripping hazard. When an extension cord is necessary, it should be adequate for the electrical load. Generally, extension cords longer than 4 feet should not be used for loads greater than 6 A (amps) at 120 V AC or 3 A at 240 V AC.

Equipment with grounded plugs must never be used with adapters or nongrounded extension cords. Never alter or remove the ground terminals on plugs. Appliances or equipment with defective ground terminals or plugs should not be used until repaired.

FIRE AND EVACUATION

When you are hired, review fire safety and locate fire extinguishers with your manager. Read hospital policy on emergency evacuations in your employee handbook. Safety training may include fire or chemical spill drills. Discuss personal safety, emergency evacuation protocols, and animal safety with the hospital administrator.

Always store flammables properly. Materials such as gasoline, paint thinner, and ether should never be stored inside the hospital, except in an approved storage cabinet designed for flammables. Some components of specialty dental and large animal acrylic repair kits are also flammable. Very small amounts of these components can usually be safely stored in an area with good ventilation, free from flames or sparks.

Be alert for situations that could cause a fire. Flammable items, particularly newspapers, boxes, and cleaning chemicals, must always be stored at least 3 feet away from any ignition source, such as a water heater, furnace, or stove. Always use extra care when using portable heaters. Never leave portable heaters unattended and always be sure that they are placed no closer than 3 feet from any wall, furniture, or other flammable material.

Know the location of all fire extinguishers on the premises and how to use them. Before you decide to use a fire extinguisher, be sure that the fire alarm has been sounded, everyone has left the building (or is in the process of leaving), and the fire department has been called. The National Fire Protection Association (NFPA) recommends that you never attempt to fight a fire if any of the following conditions apply:

- The fire is spreading beyond the immediate area where it started or has already become a large fire.
- The fire could block your escape route.

- You are unsure of the proper operation of the extinguisher.
- You doubt that the extinguisher is designed for the type of fire at hand or is large enough to suppress the fire.

Know where the designated emergency exits are. Make sure that emergency exits are always unlocked and free from obstructions. If you must work in a building during nonoperational hours (when security warrants that the doors be locked), be sure you that have at least two clear exits from the building that can be opened without a key.

PERSONAL SAFETY

Workers in emergency or 24-hour practices should use the barriers that are usually available. Use the buzzer to control access through the front door and one-way locks on the remaining doors. This lets you out in case of an emergency but keeps the door locked from the outside. These personal safety techniques are essential in these environments.

In any practice, the potential for robbery is always present. In any situation in which someone demands money or drugs while threatening your personal safety, do not attempt to withhold whatever they demand. Cooperate with the demands, but do not go with the person, even to the parking lot. Attempt to remember every detail of the person's appearance and demeanor. This greatly increases the likelihood that the police will locate the person. As soon as safely possible, let everyone else know of the situation. Attempt to contact the police if this can be done safely without the intruder's knowledge; otherwise, do it immediately after the intruder has left the premises.

RECOMMENDED READINGS

King LJ: *Veterinary medicine and public health at CDC*, http://www.cdc.gov/mmwr/preview/mmwrhtml/su5502a4.htm, 2006.

Prendergast H: *Front office management for the veterinary team*, ed 2, St Louis, 2014, Saunders.

Rose R, Smith C: *Career choices for veterinary technicians: Opportunities for animal lovers*, Lakewood, CO, 2009, AAHA Press.

Seibert Jr PJ: *The complete veterinary practice regulatory manual*, ed 2, Calhoun, TN, 2003, SafetyVet.

Sirois M, editor: *Principles and practice of veterinary technology*, ed 3, St Louis, 2011, Elsevier.

Wilson JF: *Law and ethics of the veterinary profession*, Yardley, PA, 1993, Priority Press.

Wilson JF, Lacroix C: *Legal consent forms for veterinary practices*, Lakewood, CO, 2001, AAHA Press.

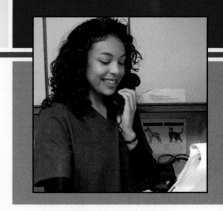

2

Office Procedures and Client Relations[1]

OUTLINE

Front Office Procedures, 26
Telephone Etiquette, 26
Scheduling Appointments, 27
Reminders and Recall Systems, 28
Greeting Clients, 30
Cleanliness, 30
Commonly Used Forms, 30
Invoicing Clients, 35
Managing and Processing Mail, 37
The Office Visit, 38
Admitting Patients, 38
Discharging Patients, 38
Pet Health Insurance, 40
Medical Records, 41
Record Format, 42

Standard Operating Procedures, 46
Inventory Management, 46
Reorder Point, 46
Product Pricing, 47
Labeling Prescription Items, 47
Computer and Software Management, 48
Client Relations, 48
Body Language, 49
The Human-Animal Bond, 50
Grief Counseling, 51
Effects of Patient Loss on Staff, 54
Compounded Loss, 55

LEARNING OBJECTIVES

After reviewing this chapter, the reader will be able to:

1. Describe the importance of informed consent.
2. Clarify admitting and discharge instructions.
3. Identify effective and professional discharge sheets.
4. Define and educate clients regarding pet health insurance.
5. Identify a completed medical record.
6. Identify and use problem-oriented medical record (POMR) and subjective, objective, assessment, and plan (SOAP) record formats.
7. Identify methods used to maintain inventory accurately and efficiently.
8. Develop effective phone techniques.
9. Identify techniques for handling multiple phone lines.
10. Describe methods to greet clients effectively.
11. Differentiate forms used in the veterinary practice.

KEY TERMS

Anesthetic consent form
Client and patient
  information sheet
Co-pay
Deductible
Dispensing fee
Etiquette

Euthanasia release form
Fair Debt Collections
  Practices Act
Indemnity insurance
Informed consent
Interstate health certificate
Markup

Master problem list
Medical records
Minimum prescription fee
Premium
Problem-oriented medical
  record (POMR)
Rabies certificates

Reorder point
Shrinkage
Standard operating procedure
  (SOP)
Subjective, objective, assess-
  ment, and plan (SOAP)

[1]Elsevier and the author acknowledge and appreciate the original contributions from Sirois M: Principles and practice of veterinary technology, ed 3, St Louis, 2011, Mosby; and Prendergast H: Front office management for the veterinary team, St Louis, 2011, Saunders, whose work forms the heart of this chapter.

FRONT OFFICE PROCEDURES

Many practices and policies come into play with the receptionist, assistants, and technicians in the front office. Clients must receive a warm welcome and be able to approach team members comfortably (Fig. 2-1).

Clients should feel that they can ask questions, regardless of the topic. The reception team makes the first impression on every client, which often begins with the phone call. If clients think that they are rushed on the phone, they may think that the practice does not have time for them. Team members should be able to turn each phone call into an appointment while being able to schedule the appointment correctly and efficiently.

A client's experience starts with the first impression and ends when the practice has followed up with the visit. A client may call a practice for the first time to make an appointment, establishing the first impression. The client may choose to make an appointment or call another practice based on the information received. For clients who have made an appointment, the second impression begins when they enter the practice. They should be greeted by a warm, sincere individual who has a genuine concern for them and their pet. A negative impression may be developed if they are ignored or have to wait an excessive amount of time, or if the practice exhibits a dirty appearance. The next impression will be set by the veterinary team. If laboratory samples were submitted, a follow-up call would be expected from the veterinarian. If the client has to call the practice to receive results, another negative impression may be made. A team member has the ability to make all these situations a positive experience for the client and should strive to do so for all clients.

> ### CRITICAL CONCEPT
> Clients must be greeted and acknowledged when they enter the practice.

Teamwork helps facilitate positive experiences for clients and employees. Clients perceive a positive atmosphere in a practice when a team works together. Teams can be developed to work harmoniously and efficiently. These teams satisfy client needs and wants with relative ease.

TELEPHONE ETIQUETTE

Every telephone call must be handled as if it were the client's first call, using proper telephone **etiquette**. The receptionist should answer the phone within three rings; if the receptionist team is busy, another member of the team should receive the phone call. The receptionist should speak slowly and clearly, with correct enunciation. Excellent verbal skills will facilitate client retention, education, and compliance.

The human voice has four components—volume, tone, rate, and quality. The volume of the receptionist's voice should make listeners comfortable, adding to the quality of the conversation. If a person's voice is too loud, listeners (in this case, clients) may pull the phone away from their ear, preventing them from hearing all of a conversation. If a receptionist's volume is too low, clients may be too embarrassed to ask for clarification of something that they did not hear well. Correct volume is essential to a successful phone experience.

The tone of a voice is also referred to as pitch. Some speakers have a low, comforting tone, which increases the quality of the conversation. Others may have a high, squeaky pitch. Some clients may be unable to understand a squeaky voice and become irritated. The tone of voice that a receptionist uses to answer the phone can give a client a lasting impression. Team members should have a pleasant, confident, and understandable voice. Tones can indicate "I am too busy to take your call right now" or "I am at your service today. How may I help you?" Team members should smile as they answer the phone; the tone of that smile will come across the phone line (Fig. 2-2).

The rate of speaking can greatly affect a conversation. The receptionist must be efficient and knowledgeable and speak

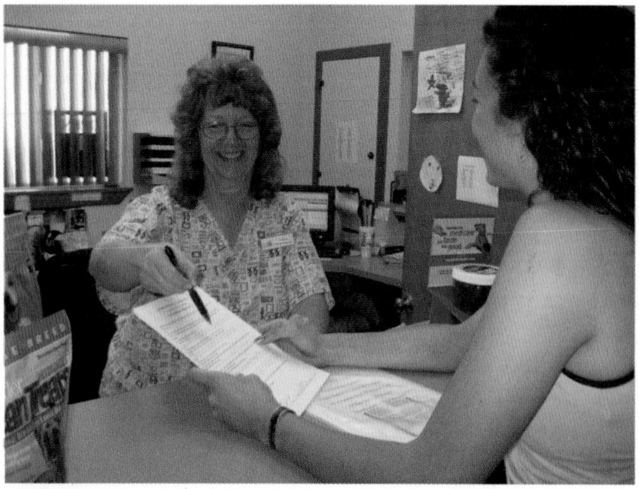

FIGURE 2-1 Greeting a client at the front counter. (From Sirois M: Principles and practice of veterinary technology, ed 3, St Louis, 2011, Mosby.)

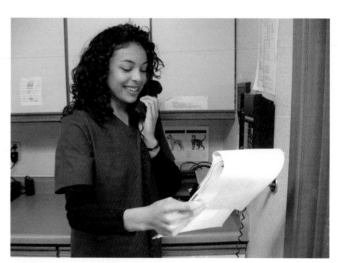

FIGURE 2-2 Answering the phone with a smile projects a friendly attitude that can be detected by the listener. (From Prendergast H: Front office management for the veterinary team, St Louis, 2011, Saunders.)

slowly and clearly. Speaking too quickly can leave the listener confused and unable to follow instructions. People who naturally speak quickly should often remind themselves to slow their speaking rate. Older clients may not hear well and may not be able to understand a team member who is speaking rapidly. This can also imply that the practice is busy and that the receptionist does not have time for the client.

The quality of voice is a combination of clarity, volume, rate, and tone. All four factors are interrelated and have compounding effects on each other. Tape-recording telephone conversations can help team members realize what they sound like on a phone and help improve skills and telephone etiquette.

Team members should answer the phone by introducing themselves; this makes the client aware of with whom they are speaking and quickly develops a relationship. "Good morning, ABC Animal Clinic, this is Teresa. How may I help you?" is a good example.

If a client asks a question that the receptionist cannot answer, the receptionist should ask the client if the call can be placed on hold, allowing the correct answer to be determined. If the answer will take time to receive, the client can be called back. Clients should never be told, "I don't know" or given an incorrect answer. The practice may lose a client if the information is not provided and can be held liable for incorrect information given over the phone.

It is important not to leave callers on hold for longer than 1 minute. Most current phone systems sound an alert after 1 minute; at this time, clients should be told that the team member helping them will return momentarily. If the client will be on hold more than 1 or 2 minutes, the client should be asked if a team member can return the call as soon as the requested information is available. One minute on hold can seem like 5 minutes to a client.

Often, clients call for advice over the phone and do not want to bring a pet in; unfortunately, in today's society, any information can be misinterpreted. A pet's condition cannot be diagnosed over the phone, and team members cannot recommend treatments to clients without illegally diagnosing a disease or condition. If a client is concerned enough to place a call to the practice, he or she should be advised to bring the pet in to be examined by the veterinarian. If the wrong treatment is advised to the client, the practice can be held liable. If the veterinarian allows a recommendation to be given to the client over the phone, it must be documented in the medical record.

> **CRITICAL CONCEPT**
>
> Smiling while answering the phone relays a positive tone of voice to the client.

When clients call to ask questions regarding health care, the receptionist should always end the call by scheduling an appointment. Many clients may be comparison shopping for services. With correct client education, an appointment can be made.

SCHEDULING APPOINTMENTS

Many factors contribute to appointment scheduling. Veterinary practice management software systems usually have a template that has already been created to accommodate the schedule that the practice has deemed appropriate (Fig. 2-3).

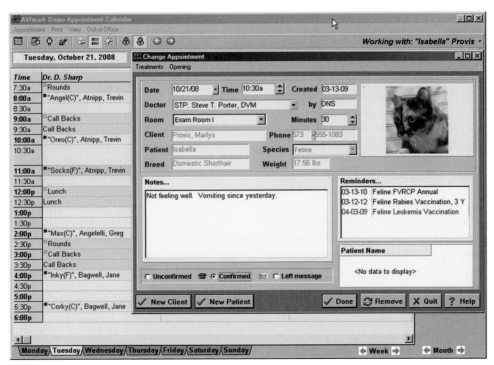

FIGURE 2-3 Computer screen shot: AVImark appointment scheduler. (From Sirois M: Principles and practice of veterinary technology, ed 3, St Louis, 2011, Mosby.)

If paper schedules are used, appropriate lunch break and surgery schedules must be entered.

Appointment schedules should be developed to maximize production while minimizing client wait time. A wait time of 5 minutes can seem to be 15 minutes to the client. The client's time is just as valuable as the practice time and should be understood as such. If the appointment schedule is running behind, clients should be notified immediately. If enough time permits, clients can be called to be notified of the delay; clients who have already arrived at the practice should be updated frequently.

The length of time for an appointment should depend on the reason for the appointment. An orthopedic appointment (e.g., limping dog) will likely take longer for the examination and radiographs than a yearly examination with vaccinations. A senior patient's wellness examination may take longer than a standard regular examination because recommendations for laboratory diagnostics may be made. The practice should develop acceptable time frames for the most common conditions seen in the examination room.

> **CRITICAL CONCEPT**
> Veterinary technician appointments can be made for nail trims, anal gland expressions, laboratory diagnostics, and client education.

Appointments for client education, nail trims, and anal gland expressions can be made with veterinary technicians, allowing the veterinarian(s) to see cases that need to be diagnosed. The experience and education that credentialed technicians possess is an asset to every practice, and maximum use of skills enhances practice efficiency.

Many items are needed when an appointment is made for a client. If a paper schedule is used, more information will need to be requested. Computer-based appointment schedulers will automatically populate the information for current clients. The client's first and last names, pet's name, and reason for the appointment will be required for both systems. The computer will populate the species, age, and client phone number. Client phone numbers should be verified, allowing the practice to call in case of emergency or a change in the schedule.

All those scheduled for appointments and surgeries should be called and reminded of their appointment 1 day prior. This allows the team members to remind clients of special instructions, such as no food or water before surgery. Many practices recommend that clients bring a fresh fecal or urine sample, and team members can kindly remind clients of this service.

If a recheck, follow-up appointment, or booster vaccination is required, the appointment should be made for the client before she or he leaves the practice. Clients will return for appointments that have been made, but less frequently return calls to make appointments. If a practice has a high number of clients who wish to call back to make an appointment, teams may want to keep a running list and call those clients who have not done so or who have not returned for their follow-up examination.

> **CRITICAL CONCEPT**
> Follow-up appointments should be scheduled for clients before they leave the practice.

Often, appointment slots fill up and clients are unable to obtain the appointment that they desire. To fulfill clients' expectations, they may be asked to drop off their pets. This allows the patient to be worked in between existing appointments. If additional diagnostics are required, the client can be called, given an estimate, and asked to approve additional testing. When the pet is ready, the owner can be called and the case can be discussed on the phone or once he or she arrives. Dropping off patients allows clients to have their pet seen, preventing the frustration of waiting an excess amount of time or delaying the appointment schedule. The veterinary technicians must ensure that an accurate history is obtained before the client leaves and that any treatments or anesthesia that may be required are authorized.

REMINDERS AND RECALL SYSTEMS

A reminder and recall system can also be used with computer software systems that will print reports of noncompliant clients. Many software programs can automatically generate reminders and recalls for the veterinary team. Smaller practices may hand-write reminders on a monthly basis. Reminders are simply that: they remind owners that pets are due for a procedure. Practices may elect to send out reminders for a variety of services, including yearly examinations and/or vaccines (based on the current vaccination protocol), heartworm testing, and/or a fecal analysis. Practices may also send out reminders for annual laboratory work, including testing for hypothyroidism, phenobarbital levels, or bile acids for patients that are on long-term medications that may have potential side effects if not monitored closely. Communications can also be sent to remind clients to refill their pets' medication, including heartworm prevention and medications that treat hypothyroidism or hyperthyroidism, seizures, and/or allergies.

Reminders must be clear, concise, and to the point. If a client must make an appointment for an examination, the reminder must clearly indicate that necessity; otherwise, a client may walk into the practice without an appointment for an examination. Grammar and spelling must be correct, and the message must be inviting. A simple reminder can help maintain the relationship that the practice has worked hard to establish with a client (Fig. 2-4).

Reminder cards can be ordered from a variety of software companies or supply houses. Some systems may require a specific type of card to fit system or printer requirements; however, a variety of choices are available. Dogs, cats, puppies, and horses posing in different outfits and performing different tricks should grab a client's attention. Some product

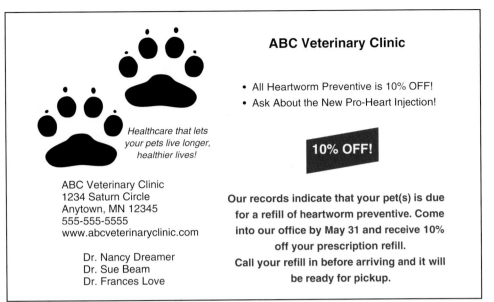

ABC Veterinary Clinic

- All Heartworm Preventive is 10% OFF!
- Ask About the New Pro-Heart Injection!

10% OFF!

Our records indicate that your pet(s) is due for a refill of heartworm preventive. Come into our office by May 31 and receive 10% off your prescription refill.
Call your refill in before arriving and it will be ready for pickup.

Healthcare that lets your pets live longer, healthier lives!

ABC Veterinary Clinic
1234 Saturn Circle
Anytown, MN 12345
555-555-5555
www.abcveterinaryclinic.com

Dr. Nancy Dreamer
Dr. Sue Beam
Dr. Frances Love

FIGURE 2-4 Reminder cards are a good way to maintain client relationships. (From Prendergast H: Front office management for the veterinary team, St Louis, 2011, Saunders.)

Recall List					ABC Animal Clinic
Printed for dates 3/3/09-3/3/09					
Account #	Client	Patient	Phone	Procedure	Doctor
428	Sharon Bean	Miss Kitty	123-458-0901	Fe OVH	ND
17266	Steve Doolittle	Lucky	345-234-1234	K9 OVH	ND
17266	Steve Doolittle	Cookie	345-234-1234	K9 OVH	ND
3427	Desiree Cloud	Scamp	456-123-1234	Dental	SM
6785	Nancy Shade	Wheeler	123-567-8901	K9 OVH	ND

FIGURE 2-5 Recall lists remind staff members to call and check on patients. (From Prendergast H: Front office management for the veterinary team, St Louis, 2011, Saunders.)

manufacturers and vendors also supply reminders for their particular product or service.

Reminders can also come in the form of phone calls. Clients should be called the day before their appointments to remind them of surgical procedures or appointments that have been scheduled. Clients can be reminded of the surgical protocol to follow at that time as well. Those whose pets are due for yearly examinations, laboratory work, and vaccinations should also be called as a friendly reminder. If a client needs to reschedule his or her appointment, it can be done at that time, allowing the team to fill the appointment spot with another patient.

Reminder systems, whether manual or automatic, must be programmed to remove patients once they have died. It is emotionally distressing for a client to receive a reminder for a pet that has died, especially if the loss occurred at the veterinary hospital. It is not uncommon for a pet to suddenly die at home and for the owner not to inform the hospital of the death until receiving an appointment reminder. Team members should be empathetic, apologize,

and guarantee that the owner will not receive another reminder.

In today's high-tech world, veterinary practices can send reminders by email, text messages, and cell phones. This is a relatively inexpensive way to connect with clients and remind them of services that are due for their pets. Computer software systems can be programmed to send printed cards or email reminders, allowing many reminders to be sent at once. Follow-up reminders can then be generated for those who did not respond to the initial notice.

Recalls are lists that are generated by veterinary software systems to remind staff to call certain clients to check on patients (Fig. 2-5). Recalls can be created for surgical patients, pets that have received vaccines, or any patient that has been in the hospital for a period of time. Software systems allow team members to set a specific number of days for the recall to be generated. Certain charged services can also be linked to a recall generator, thereby creating a recall each time one of those services is entered. Each day, reception teams can print lists and call clients to see how patients are progressing.

This is a good time to ensure that the client was satisfied with the services and answer any remaining questions. If the client has any concerns or the pet has not progressed as expected, an appointment can be made with a specific veterinarian to recheck the patient. Always document the telephone conversation and how the pet is recovering in the record. This allows team members to follow the case if the client needs to return for a recheck.

Manual recall lists can also be generated by practices that do not use specialized software. A list can be kept in a small notebook with the client information and a brief reminder of the procedure. This is a well-organized way to help follow up with clients. Again, appointments can be made at this time, if needed, and these conversations must be documented in the record.

GREETING CLIENTS

Clients must always be acknowledged when they arrive to the practice. A client greeter is an excellent resource and one who can help clients with their pets. Not all practices can have the luxury of a client greeter; therefore, the receptionist team must greet clients as they enter. If a receptionist is on the phone, a wave and a smile let clients know that they have been recognized and that a team member will help them shortly. This also applies to team members who are assisting other clients; a quick greeting notifies clients that they have been recognized, without interrupting the initial client.

CLEANLINESS

The receptionist team is responsible for maintaining the reception area. The team should notify another team member about a soiled reception area or clean the area immediately. Bowel movements, urination, and anal gland odors quickly spread, which can damage a client's first impression of the facility. Hair and dirt should also be swept up immediately. Sweeping and mopping of the reception floor should occur more than once a day because odors will penetrate the walls and disseminate rapidly throughout the practice.

Products, shelves, and pictures must be dusted regularly, along with ceiling fan blades, blinds, and window sills. Walls should be washed on a regular basis and chairs cleaned each night. Team members should take a few minutes out of each day to sit in the reception and examination room chairs and look around the room; dirty objects, walls, and items that need to be cleaned can thus be easily identified.

COMMONLY USED FORMS

Clients will be asked to fill out forms when they arrive at the practice for the first visit. A client form requesting the name, contact information, and driver's license number should be filled out and signed by the client. Most forms include a statement indicating that the client is financially responsible for the patient and understands that all services must be paid for once they are rendered (Fig. 2-6). The receptionist must

make sure that this form is completed; the phone number is important, allowing client communication, as is the driver's license number in case the client must be turned over to a collection agency for nonpayment of services.

> **CRITICAL CONCEPT**
>
> Contact information and driver's license numbers are essential pieces of information on client-patient forms.

Patient history forms are critical for new patients. Each new patient form should include the name of the client and patient's name, age, breed, gender, whether the pet has been spayed or neutered, and a medical history, including current medications that the pet is receiving. Clients may become frustrated when completing forms; however, a complete history is imperative for quality medicine (Fig. 2-7).

Practices that are not paperless will use paper records, which are generally kept in an 8½- × 11-inch file folder, with patient separators. Each client has a file folder and patients are separated with index cards or colored paper (see section below, "Medical Records"). Each patient's medical record must include the client's name, contact information, and patient information, including the pet's name, species, breed, gender, and age (Figs. 2-8 and 2-9). Each entry should be dated and initialed by the individual making the entry.

Clients must sign release forms for any treatment or procedure that is authorized. **Anesthesia consent forms**, treatment forms, and euthanasia forms are a few examples of forms that clients must sign. A signed **informed consent** form (Fig. 2-10) is defined as a form signed by the client after all information regarding the procedure has been provided and the client has had the opportunity to ask questions. Information that must be documented for clients includes any risks of the procedure (including death, if that is a risk), the potential outcomes of the procedure, and any alternative procedures that are available, along with an estimate of the costs associated with those procedures. Once the client has been informed about all of these, the client can sign the form. Blanket consent (Fig. 2-11) forms are defined as a consent form that authorizes any procedure but does not include the risks, benefits, outcomes, or estimates. Blanket consent forms are not recommended in practice but are often the sole source of consent forms used. All consent forms must state the client's name, patient's name, name of the procedure, and date.

> **CRITICAL CONCEPT**
>
> Blanket consent forms should be replaced with informed consent forms.

Just as with other consent forms, **euthanasia release forms** must be signed by the owner of the patient. The consent form must state that the pet's death will result. If a necropsy is requested by the pet's owner, the consent form may

ABC Animal Clinic
555 Uptown Circle
Anytown, MN 89000
314-134-4431

Please print clearly

Date _____

Name _____

Mailing Address_____ Zip Code_____

Street Address_____ Zip Code_____

Home Phone _____ Work Phone _____

Drivers License # _____ State _____

Animals:

Name	Date of Birth	Species	Breed	Color	Gender	Spayed or Neutered?
_____	_____	_____	_____	_____	_____	_____
_____	_____	_____	_____	_____	_____	_____
_____	_____	_____	_____	_____	_____	_____

I understand that payment is required in full on the same date that services are rendered.

_____
Signature

FIGURE 2-6 Client and patient information sheet. (From Sirois M: Principles and practice of veterinary technology, ed 3, St Louis, 2011, Mosby.)

Arroyo Vista Animal Clinic
2303 Inspiration Lane

Owners Name _____ Spouse _____

Address _____

Home Telephone _____ Work Telephone _____

Employer's Name and Address _____

Spouse's Employer and Address _____

Best time to call regarding your pet _____ Phone Number _____

In case of emergency, please call _____

WRITTEN ESTIMATES ARE AVAILABLE UPON REQUEST. Please ask the receptionist if an estimate is needed. **ALL FEES ARE DUE AT THE TIME SERVICES ARE RENDERED.** If you plan to pay with check or credit card, please complete the following:

MC   Visa   Exp Date _____

Drivers License Number _____ State _____ Expires _____

How did you hear of Arroyo Vista Animal Clinic?

Yellow Pages _____ Referral (Name)_____ Other _____

Number and type of pets in your household? _____

Pet's Origin: Humane Society   Pet Shop   Kennel   Breeder   Friend   Stray   Other

Please see back of sheet for more information.

FIGURE 2-7 Patient history form. (From Sirois M: Principles and practice of veterinary technology, ed 3, St Louis, 2011, Mosby.)

Continued

	Pet #1	Pet #2	Pet #3
Name			
Species (Dog, Cat)			
Breed			
Color			
Age			
Date of Birth			
Sex			
Length of Time Owned			
Spayed or Neutered			
Vitamins? (Type)			
Diet (Kind of Food)			
Type of Grooming Products			
Inside or Outside?			
Last Rabies Vaccine?			
Last DHLP Vaccine? (Dog)			
Last Parvo Vaccine? (Dog)			
Last FVRCP Vaccine? (Cat)			
Last FeLV Vaccine? (Cat)			
Last Leukemia Test? (Cat)			
Last Heartworm Test? (Dog)			
Heartworm Prevention?			
Last Fecal Exam?			
Last Dental?			
Prior Illness?			
Prior Surgery?			

FIGURE 2-7, Cont'd.

Patient Medical Record

Client Name _____ Telephone Number _____

Address _____ Client Number _____

Pet Name _____ Breed _____ Color _____

Sex _____ Altered _____ DOB _____ Age _____ Species _____

Date		Charges

FIGURE 2-8 Medical record. (From Sirois M: Principles and practice of veterinary technology, ed 3, St Louis, 2011, Mosby.)

Arroyo Vista Animal Clinic
2303 Inspiration Lane

Owner's Name _____ Patient's Name _____

Breed _____ Color _____ Sex _____ Species _____

Date	SOAP	

FIGURE 2-9 SOAP format medical record. (From Sirois M: Principles and practice of veterinary technology, ed 3, St Louis, 2011, Mosby.)

ABC Veterinary Clinic
Surgery, Anesthesia, and Treatment Consent Form

Client Name _____ Patient Name _____

Date _____ Procedure _____ Male / Female

Your pet has been scheduled for a procedure requiring sedation or anesthesia. By signing this form, you authorize ABC Veterinary Clinic and its agents to administer tranquilizers, anesthetics, and analgesia medication that are deemed appropriate. Please be aware that all drugs have a potential for adverse side effects in any particular animal. The chances of such occurrence are extremely small; however, death can result in any anesthetized patient.

Owner Initials _____ Tech Initials _____

In an effort to insure your pet's safety and to anticipate any problems before they occur, we advise pre-anesthetic blood work and electrocardiogram prior to anesthesia. Blood work will determine the kidney and liver functions, which participate in the metabolism of anesthesia. An electrocardiogram can detect abnormal arrhythmias, heart rate, and conductivity.

I Accept/Decline blood work   I Accept/Decline an electrocardiogram

Owner Initials _____ Tech Initials _____

IV fluids are advised for all patients undergoing anesthesia. IV fluids help maintain blood pressure of the patient, while offering support for the kidney's to metabolize the medications. Pets may take longer to recover without IV fluids.

I Accept/Decline IV Fluids

Owner Initials _____ Tech Initials _____

Heartworm tests are recommended for our canine companions older than 6 months of age. Heartworm disease can cause anesthetic complications. We advise FeLV/FIV test for our feline companions. FeLV or FIV infection can delay healing of any surgical site.

I Accept/Decline Heartworm Test   I Accept/Decline FeLV/FIV Test

Owner Initials _____ Tech Initials _____

Vaccinations are important for disease prevention in your pet. We advise that pets be current on vaccines. Rabies is required by law; every pet must have a rabies vaccine.

Vaccines due: DHPP FVRCP FeLV Rabies

Owner Initials _____ Tech Initials _____

Booster?

FIGURE 2-10 Informed consent form. (From Sirois M: Principles and practice of veterinary technology, ed 3, St Louis, 2011, Mosby.)

Continued

Did pet eat this morning?	Yes	No
Has pet had any allergies or vaccine reactions in the past?	Yes	No
Are we declawing the pet?	Yes	No
Are we removing dewclaws?	Yes	No
Does the pet have 2 testicles?	Yes	No
If the pet is pregnant can we continue with surgery?	Yes	No
Does the pet have an umbilical hernia?	Yes	No
May we repair?	Yes	No
Does the pet have retained teeth?	Yes	No
May we remove?	Yes	No
Does the pet need an e-collar?	Yes	No

Dentals: OK to extract teeth?	Yes	No
OK to take dental radiographs if indicated?	Yes	No
OK to apply Doxirobe if indicated?	Yes	No
Is pet currently on antibiotics?	Yes	No

When was last dose?_____

How many pills are left?_____

Growth Removal: Histopath?	Yes	No

Location of growths:

You may contact me TODAY at: _____

Alternative contact phone number: _____

I understand that anesthesia is a risk and authorize the above procedures. I understand that I will be contacted first if any changes in our discussed protocol occur.

Client Signature_____

FIGURE 2-10, cont'd.

ABC Veterinary Clinic
Surgery/Anesthesia Consent Form

Client Name_____ Date _____

Pet's Name_____

Your pet has been scheduled for a procedure requiring sedation or anesthesia. By signing this form, you authorize ABC Veterinary Clinic and its agents to administer tranquilizers, anesthetics, and/or analgesics that are deemed appropriate for your pet. Please be aware that all drugs have the potential for adverse side affects in any particular animal. The chances of such occurrence are extremely small.

I am aware that staff is not on premises after hours, and I agree to indemnify ABC Veterinary Clinic and its agents harmless from and against any and all liability arising from the care that is provided.

In an effort to insure your pet's safety, and to anticipate any problems before they may occur, we have available pre-anesthetic electrocardiogram and blood testing capabilities to detect hidden heart, liver, kidney or other problems which may increase the risk to your pet. The testing is available for an additional charge. If abnormalities are detected, we will attempt to notify you, and the anesthetic procedure may be delayed or modified. Please verify the procedures being performed and indicate your wishes concerning the option of pre-anesthetic testing. If you have any questions, please ask BEFORE signing this form.

Procedures scheduled _____

Routine surgical procedures are painful. We recommend postoperative pain medication for each procedure. Pain medication is automatically dispensed for each patient. If YOU DECLINE POSTOPERATIVE PAIN MEDICATION, PLEASE SIGN HERE

_____

How may we contact you TODAY?

Home phone_____ Work phone_____

Cell phone/pager_____ Client signature _____

FIGURE 2-11 Blanket consent form. (From Sirois M: Principles and practice of veterinary technology, ed 3, St Louis, 2011, Mosby.)

include the appropriate information, as well as the request for disposal of the body (Fig. 2-12).

Rabies certificates are most often computer generated (Fig. 2-13); however, a practice without a computer system must complete the certificates manually (Fig. 2-14). Rabies certificates include the client's name, contact information, patient's name, species, breed, gender, and age. Vaccination information, including the manufacturer of the vaccine, vaccine expiration date, lot number, and tag number are also included. The veterinarian administering the vaccination must sign the certificate. Often, a stamp is used in place of the original signature.

Health certificates are issued by the state and the U.S. Department of Agriculture (USDA). Small animals flying within the United States may require an **interstate health certificate**, whereas those traveling outside the United States will be required to have an international health certificate. Different countries have different requirements for animal importation, and each country should be researched for its rules and regulations. Most current regulations can be found on the website of the USDA.

INVOICING CLIENTS

Invoicing can become a difficult situation for clients who cannot afford the medical care that is recommended. Estimates should always be given to clients, whether on the phone or in the hospital, for every procedure. This prevents clients from being surprised at the time of collection and helps prevent them from arguing about the total cost while informing them that the entire amount will be due at the time the service is rendered.

> **CRITICAL CONCEPT**
>
> Every client should receive an estimate for procedures and sign a copy for the medical record.

Invoices should be detailed for clients. A client will not perceive the value of the service if a total amount is presented without explanation. For example, many clients perceive that a DHLPP injection has only one component because it is only one injection. The invoice should list all five vaccine components of the injection—distemper, hepatitis, leptospirosis, parainfluenza, parvovirus—allowing the client to understand the value of this injection. Once the receptionist can detail the entire invoice for the client, the client will understand the total value of the visit.

Because of the number of outstanding accounts in veterinary medicine, extending credit to clients should not be allowed. Accounts receivable totals should never exceed 2% to 3% of the total gross revenue amount for the practice. Many veterinarians want to be able to extend the offer of credit to clients. Unfortunately, most clients do not extend the courtesy of repayment to the veterinarian.

Payments made on an account can be processed with a variety of methods. Most practices accept cash, checks, debit cards, and credit cards. Credit cards may include Visa, MasterCard, Discover, and American Express. The credit cards that the practice agrees to accept are up to the practice. Businesses must pay a percentage of the total month's charges of each credit card accepted to the credit card agency. This is considered a hidden overhead expense that the practice must recover.

> **CRITICAL CONCEPT**
>
> All credit card and check transactions should be verified with a driver's license or picture ID.

Team members must verify client identification when they accept credit cards or checks. Fraud is increasing across the United States, and it is up to the practice to prevent it. Often, driver's license numbers must be written on checks to be accepted. This allows the district attorney's office to prosecute fraudulent check writers if needed. If a check verification process is used, a driver's license number must match the checking account information or the check may be declined.

Euthanasia Release

I, the undersigned, do hereby certify that I am the owner of the animal, and hereby give ABC Veterinary Clinic full and complete authority to euthanize the animal in whatever manner the doctor shall deem fit. I hereby release the doctors and staff from any and all liabilities for euthanizing said animal. I understand that euthanasia results in death.

I do also certify that the said animal has not bitten any person or animal during the last 15 days and to the best of my knowledge has not been exposed to Rabies.

Date_____ Signature of owner _____

FIGURE 2-12 Euthanasia form. (From Prendergast H: Front Office Management for the Veterinary Team, St Louis, 2011, Saunders.)

RABIES VACCINATION CERTIFICATE *NASPHV FORM 51 (Revised 2007)* Owner's Name & Address		Print Clearly			RABIES TAG NUMBER 2590 MICROCHIP NUMBER 4944047932
LAST Montoya		FIRST Teresa		M.I.	TELEPHONE (575)526-7170
NO STREET 4364 Lost Lane			CITY Las Cruces	STATE NM	ZIP 88007
SPECIES Dog ☒ Cat ☐ Other ☐ (Specify)	SEX Male ☒ Female ☐ Neuter ☒	AGE Months ☐ 6 Years ☒	SIZE Under 20 lbs ☐ 20 - 50 lbs ☐ Over 50 lbs ☒	PREDOMINANT BREED Labrador Ret Mix NAME Blue	PREDOMINANT COLORS/MARKINGS Yellow
	Animal Control License ☐ 1 Yr ☐ 3 Yr ☐ Other___				
DATE VACCINATED 10/24/2008 NEXT VACCINATION DUE BY: 10/24/2011	PRODUCT NAME MANUFACTURER (First 3 Letters) P F I ☐ 1 yr USDA Licensed Vaccine ☒ 3 yr USDA Licensed Vaccine ☐ 4 yr USDA Licensed Vaccine ☐ Initial dose ☐ Booster dose Vacc. Serial (Lot) No.			Veterinarian: Frances S. Bowling License No: Veterinarian's Signature Address Jomada Veterinary Clinic 2399 Saturn Circle Las Cruces, NM 88012	

FIGURE 2-13 Rabies certificate, computer-generated. (From Sirois M: Principles and practice of veterinary technology, ed 3, St Louis, 2011, Mosby.)

OWNER'S COPY **RABIES VACCINATION CERTIFICATE** *NASPHV Form #51* Owner's Name and Address **Print - use ball point pen or type**					Rabies Tag Number
PRINT - Last		First		M.I.	Telephone
No. Street			City	State	Zip
Species: Dog ☐ Cat ☐ Other: ☐ (Specify)	Sex: Male ☐ Female ☐ Neutered ☐	Age: 3 mo to 12 mo ☐ 12 mo or older ☐ Actual Age___	Size: Under 20 lbs. ☐ 20 - 50 lbs. ☐ Over 50 lbs. ☐ Actual___lbs.	Predominant Breed: ___ Name:	Colors:
DATE VACCINATED: Month Day Year VACCINATION EXPIRED: Month Day Year	Producer: ☐☐☐ (First 3 letters) ☐ 1 yr. Lic./Vacc. ☐ 3 yr. Lic./Vacc. ___ Other Vacc. Serial (lot) no.			Veterinarian's: # ___ (License No.) (Signature) Address:	

FIGURE 2-14 Rabies certificate, handwritten. (From Sirois M: Principles and practice of veterinary technology, ed 3, St Louis, 2011, Mosby.)

Credit card machines and check verification systems are an excellent asset to veterinary medicine. They are easy to use and help prevent fraud and bad checks. Both systems use the electronic funds transfer (EFT), in which the total amount is deducted from the client's account at the time of the service. The amount is then deposited into the practice's account.

CareCredit is a type of third-party payment system used exclusively for medical expenses. Clients must fill out an application in the practice, and team members must verify identification before application acceptance. Once the application is complete, a team member can call in the application or enter the information online. Credit decisions are generally received via fax or email within 15 minutes of submission.

MONTHLY STATEMENTS

For the few clients who are allowed to charge, monthly statements must be sent. These statements should include a statement charge, which covers the time required for the team

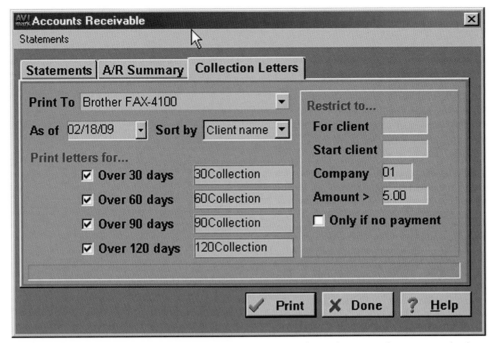

FIGURE 2-15 AVImark collections, screen shot. (From Sirois M: Principles and practice of veterinary technology, ed 3, St Louis, 2011, Mosby.)

to print and send statements. A minimum of 5 dollars should be charged for this (Fig. 2-15). Many practices may also institute a finance charge, which charges the client a percentage of the total amount due. Regulations vary regarding finance fees; therefore, regulations must be confirmed before the institution of such fees. Notice of such fees must also be clearly posted for clients to see and they should be documented in the statement.

OUTSTANDING DEBT COLLECTION

Accounts that are allowed to age to 30, 60, or 90 days postservice can become difficult to collect. The longer the invoice ages, the less likely the invoice will be collected. Team members must be diligent when trying to collect accounts and must be most active in the early age process (less than 45 days). Those responsible for collecting accounts should become familiar with the **Fair Debt Collections Practices Act**, which prevents someone from using unruly tactics when trying to collect on an overdue account. Phone calls cannot be made before 8 AM or after 9 PM, and the account balance cannot be discussed with anyone other than the person who owes on the account (Box 2-1).

Accounts that cannot be collected by team members must be turned over to a collection agency. These agents are occasionally able to collect accounts with which team members have not had success because clients do not want their credit scores negatively affected. A report to a collection agency can remain on a client's credit report for 7 years; therefore, he or she may be more willing to pay the debt. The sooner the overdue amount is turned in to collection agents, the easier they can collect the account. Often, client addresses and phone numbers change; however, if a collection agency has the driver's license number of the client, an infraction can be reported

BOX 2-1	Fair Debt Rules

- Debtors cannot be subjected to harassment, oppressive tactics, or abusive treatment.
- The law prohibits the collector from making any false statements to the client, such as claiming to be a lawyer or government agency.
- Clients may not be called at work if the employer or client objects, or be called at inconvenient times or places, such as before 8 AM and after 9 PM.
- Delinquent payments can only be discussed with the client themselves.

From Sirois M: Principles and practice of veterinary technology, ed 3, St Louis, 2011, Mosby.

to the credit bureau. This is why it is critical to have a driver's license number on the client-patient information form.

MANAGING AND PROCESSING MAIL

Veterinary practices receive many pieces of literature on a daily basis. Some is junk mail, but the majority consists of statements, laboratory reports, information on upcoming continuing education opportunities, or ads for the release of new products and books. All mail must be given to the person to whom it is addressed. Some veterinarians and technicians may want their mail to be opened, allowing greater efficiency in sorting, but others may prefer to keep their privacy. Statements and invoices should be given to the manager in charge of paying bills; all statements must be reviewed for correct charges. All laboratory reports should be placed on the veterinarian's desk for review and then placed in the client's record. Magazines and journals must be given to the subscriber. Continuing education brochures should be posted, allowing the entire team to note the opportunities available to further their knowledge.

THE OFFICE VISIT

The office visit for a client begins when he or she enters the practice. After clients have been greeted by the receptionist team, they are generally placed in an examination room. Usually, an assistant or technician will take a medical history of the patient. A medical history includes each patient's weight and vital signs, which should include the temperature, pulse, and heart and respiratory rates. If any laboratory samples will be needed, the veterinary health care team may confirm the proper sampling technique, equipment, or products needed and ask the veterinarian for authorization to obtain the samples. More information on examination procedures is given in Chapter 8.

The office visit is the perfect time for technicians to educate clients. Puppy and kitten owners should be informed about vaccination schedules, heartworm and intestinal worm prevention, flea and tick disease and prevention, dental disease, and nutrition (Fig. 2-16). Because vaccine boosters must be given, information can be spread over several visits. The goal of each visit is not to overwhelm the client with too much information but to provide enough that they understand the value of the services provided.

Clients with adult patients arriving for yearly examinations must be reminded of heartworm, flea and tick disease and prevention, provided with nutrition guidance, and given information on dental disease prevention. Clients look to the veterinary team for guidance and education, and the team must take the time to educate clients during each visit. Box 2-2 provides client education topics that can be covered during office visits.

ADMITTING PATIENTS

If patients will need to be admitted to the hospital for treatment, team members should follow a protocol that helps develop consistency for clients and patients. As noted, a treatment consent form must be given to the owner to sign. The client must be informed of risks, prognosis, and alternative treatments that are available. An estimate should also be provided for the client, highlighting all possible treatments, procedures, medications, or services that are recommended for the owner. Once the client has been informed, she or he can sign the consent form and estimate, indicating the services that the client authorizes.

If a patient is being admitted for boarding, a separate form should be available for clients to complete (Fig. 2-17). These forms should include emergency and alternative contact information, as well as any pertinent information regarding the pet. This information should include current diet, amount fed per feeding, when the pet is fed, what medications the pet receives, and at what time those mediations are administered. If a blanket, toy, collars, or leash is left, a clear description should be indicated on the admitting sheet.

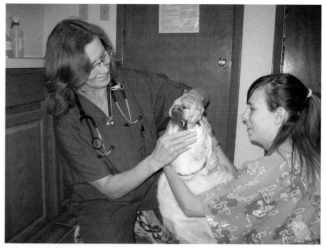

FIGURE 2-16 Veterinarian examining a patient. (From Sirois M: Principles and practice of veterinary technology, ed 3, St Louis, 2011, Mosby.)

BOX 2-2	Education Topics for Puppies, Kittens, Adults, and Seniors

- Vaccine schedule
- Vaccination reactions
- Intestinal parasites
- Nutrition
- Dental disease prevention
- Heartworm prevention
- Flea and tick disease and prevention
- Spay or neuter procedure
- Obesity prevention or management
- Dental disease
- Aging process and laboratory diagnostics

From Sirois M: Principles and practice of veterinary technology, ed 3, St Louis, 2011, Mosby.

Clients may also be asked if they would prefer any additional services or treatments to be performed on their pet while in the boarding facility. Often, dental prophylaxis, bathing, dipping, or grooming are services clients choose for their pets.

DISCHARGING PATIENTS

Patients discharged from the hospital must be released with written instructions (Fig. 2-18). Verbal instructions are not acceptable. Often, clients are given too much information when they arrive to pick up their pets, and they forget most of this information. Distractions, such as other pets, clients, and team members, can prevent clients from paying attention to the release information; therefore, discharge instructions may not be followed.

Invoices and discharge instructions should be detailed with clients before the pet is brought to the owner. (See earlier section, "Invoicing Clients," regarding collection and payment.) Once a pet has been brought to the owner, the owner is more interested in the pet than the release instructions.

Arroyo Vista Animal Clinic

2303 Inspiration Lane, Anywhere, USA

Dr. Larsen, Dr. Cooke, and Dr. Thompson

Boarding Admission Form

Owner _____ Date _____

Address _____ Phone _____

City _____ In case of emergency, please call _____

Pet's Name _____ Breed _____ Sex ____ Age ____ Color ____

Date of last vaccine: _____ Please circle which vaccine: DHPP FVRCP FeLV

Date of last Rabies _____ Date of last Bordetella _____

Medications while boarding _____

Belongings _____

Pet's Name _____ Breed _____ Sex ____ Age ____ Color ____

Date of last vaccine: _____ Please circle which vaccine: DHPP FVRCP FeLV

Date of last Rabies _____ Date of last Bordetella _____

Medications while boarding _____

Belongings _____

Pet's Name _____ Breed _____ Sex ____ Age ____ Color ____

Date of last vaccine: _____ Please circle which vaccine: DHPP FVRCP FeLV

Date of last Rabies _____ Date of last Bordetella _____

Medications while boarding _____

Belongings _____

While boarding, please perform the following procedures:

Physical Exam _____ Vaccinations _____

Heartworm Test _____ Bath _____ Dip _____ Nail Trim _____

Other: 1: _____

2: _____

3: _____

4: _____

All animals entering the hospital must be up to date on vaccination and free of external parasites (fleas, ticks) or they will be treated upon admission at the owner's expense.

I authorize Arroyo Vista Animal Clinic to treat my pet(s) in case an emergency situation should arise.

Pets are released only during the regular office hours. It is my responsibility to inform the hospital if I will be delayed in picking up my pets; I will assume all costs associated with an extended stay.

Owner's signature _____ Date _____

FIGURE 2-17 Boarding form. (From Sirois M: Principles and practice of veterinary technology, ed 3, St Louis, 2011, Mosby.)

FIGURE 2-18 Discharge instructions. (From Sirois M: Principles and practice of veterinary technology, ed 3, St Louis, 2011, Mosby.)

CRITICAL CONCEPT

Written discharge instructions should be sent home with every patient.

Discharge instructions must include any recommended restrictions for food, activity, or therapy and should indicate when to start medication. Doses and instructions for medications should also be included. If a pet has been diagnosed with a particular disease or condition, the client should also be given written materials regarding the diagnosis. The more information that is given to clients, the more satisfied they will be when following the recommendations of the team.

Many computer programs include client education handouts. When selected, they will print the owner's, patient's, and veterinarian's names on each handout. If a computer handout is not available, a practice manager may create a client handout covering the most common diseases and conditions. Literature must appear professional, be error-free, and be written in a client-oriented manner. Clients must be able to understand the information presented to them; copies of information from veterinary texts are often too advanced and can overwhelm the client.

PET HEALTH INSURANCE

Pet health insurance has been available for longer than 20 years but has not been a popular choice among owners until recently. Insurance is a method whereby pet owners can manage the risks of expensive health care. Accidents and diseases are an unexpected cost for owners, and insurance allows them to provide the best treatment available. Many pet owners are forced to make treatment decisions based on cost alone. Pet insurance allows owners the financial resources that they may need to provide lifesaving treatment that they would otherwise not consider.

The National Commission on Veterinary Economic Issues (NCVEI) released a landmark study in 1999 indicating that the increased use of veterinary pet health insurance could increase the demand for service, therefore decreasing the euthanasia rate in the United States. Studies have indicated that pet owners look to their veterinarians for education regarding pet health and insurance for their pets. It is imperative that the entire staff understand the concept of pet insurance and offer it to all clients.

Clients should be made aware of the various companies that offer pet health insurance. Plans and companies vary in different regions; therefore, each policy should be reviewed carefully. Terms that should be considered include whether hereditary conditions are covered and whether benefit schedules or exclusions are listed in the policy. Some benefit schedules only cover a small percentage of what would be considered a reasonable expense for a condition. Some companies may not use a benefit schedule and set payout limits instead, regardless of illness or condition. Most pet insurance companies set high dollar amounts for reasonable expenses; they do not want to set prices for veterinary practices, nor do they want to dissuade owners from purchasing an insurance package.

Indemnity insurance offers compensation for the treatment of injured and sick pets. Owners purchase a policy directly from a pet health insurance company and are eligible for compensation based on the care provided and policy terms. Policies are available for comprehensive illness, standard care, and accident coverage and may cover pet species ranging from dogs and cats to small mammals and birds.

A **premium** is defined as the amount an owner pays monthly or annually to maintain an insurance policy for a pet. Premium amounts are affected by a number of factors, including the **deductible**, **co-pay**, and per-incident, annual, or lifetime limit payout. The age, species, and breed of the animal also affect the cost of the premium, as well as if the pet is spayed or neutered and geographic location of the owner in the United States.

> **CRITICAL CONCEPT**
> Pet health insurance can increase client compliance and retention.

A deductible is the amount an owner must pay before the insurance company will offer compensation. Insurance companies vary and offer either a per-incident deductible or annual deductible. Per-incident deductibles refer to the owner paying the chosen deductible amount each time an incident occurs with the pet. An annual deductible refers to an owner paying the chosen deductible once annually. Once the annual deductible amount has been met, the owner does not have to pay a deductible until the following year. A co-pay is the percentage that the owner is responsible for after the deductible has been met. Lower co-pays increase the amount of the premium and generally range from 10% to 20%.

Some insurance companies offer clients a choice of an annual policy or per-incident limit; others offer one or the other. Annual limits refer to the maximum amount that the insurance company will pay for a condition or illness during the policy term. Per-incident limits refer to the maximum amount an insurance company will pay each time a new problem or disease occurs. Lifetime limits refer to the maximum amount an insurance company will pay during the pet's lifetime.

A preexisting health condition is defined as any accident or illness contracted, manifested, or incurred before the policy effective date. The pet may be enrolled; however, any preexisting condition may be excluded from coverage. It is highly recommended to enroll puppies and kittens before any conditions arise.

Purebred pets known to have congenital and hereditary conditions may also have coverage excluded for those conditions depending on insurance company policy. A congenital condition is generally referred to as an abnormality present at birth, whether apparent or not, that can cause illness or disease. A hereditary condition is an abnormality that is transmitted by genes from the parent to the offspring, whether apparent or not, that can cause disease or illness. Some companies may also argue that some congenital defects are hereditary, therefore excluding coverage of the condition. A portosystemic shunt may be an example of such a condition. Policies must be reviewed carefully for such exemptions.

Many companies have a list of exclusions; diseases, conditions, or treatments that are excluded from policies. Behavior counseling and medications are usually not covered, along with compounded medications, nutraceuticals, or diets. Exclusions should be carefully reviewed before choosing a policy.

MEDICAL RECORDS

Medical records are a major component of the veterinary practice. A medical record is a legal document that must be complete, legible, and made available to clients at their request. Inactive client records must be maintained for 3 years. As a practical matter, most practices maintain medical records for a much longer period, often for years after a client relationship is terminated or after the patient dies.

> **CRITICAL CONCEPT**
> Medical records must be complete and legible.

Completed records must include client contact information, patient name and information, and the date that the service(s) were rendered. The person who made entries in the medical record must initial each entry. Written medical records must be legible; anyone must be able to decipher abbreviations and/or words. Illegible records may lead to incorrect treatments, incorrect client diagnosis, and/or incorrect client education. If a record must be presented in a court of law and a judge cannot read the record, the practice may be at fault and held liable for the presenting claim. If cases are referred to a veterinary specialist and the record is not legible, the specialist may not be able to interpret the record, resulting in communication and diagnostic errors.

Medical records are the legal property of the practice; however, clients may request to have copies for themselves, for a referral, or for a new veterinarian. It is illegal to prevent clients from receiving their records. The practice is permitted to charge a fee to cover the cost of creating duplicate records.

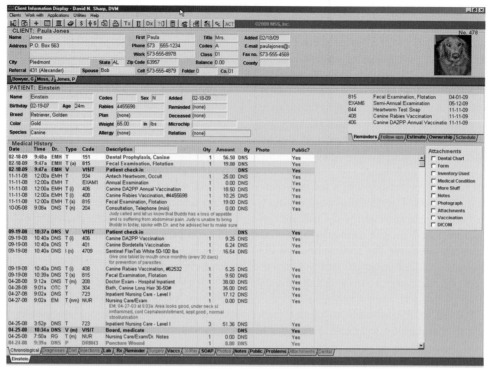

FIGURE 2-19   AVImark medical records screen shot. (From Sirois M: Principles and practice of veterinary technology, ed 3, St Louis, 2011, Mosby.)

Medical records and client-patient information is also confidential; cases should never be discussed by name, and client information should never be released to anyone other than the pet owner.

If medical records need to be copied for a referral veterinarian, the veterinary staff must copy laboratory results that are pertinent to the case and a copy of the records. If radiographs are requested and a digital radiograph machine is used, a CD or DVD of the radiographs can be given to the owner or referring veterinarian. If a standard radiograph machine is used, the radiographs must be checked out to the owner or referral veterinarian. A log should clearly indicate the date, who checked out the radiographs (the owner, or if they were mailed to the referral veterinarian), and the technician assisting the case. Once the radiographs are returned, they can be crossed off the log with a single line strike. This allows radiographs to be tracked if they cannot be located in the practice. Owners or referral veterinarians may fail to return radiographs, and this allows protection of the general practice.

Medical records may be written or a practice may be paperless. Paperless medical records must also be complete and initialed by the author (Fig. 2-19). Many programs will automatically time-stamp entries when they are made, along with the team members' initials. Software programs must ensure record safety, preventing record alteration. Some programs can be programmed with a lockout period, preventing record alteration after a 12- or 24-hour period. If any changes need to be made, a second entry can be made, indicating the change.

All entries in written medical records must be in permanent ink and cannot be altered; instead, the mistake

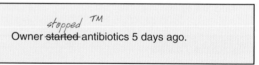

FIGURE 2-20   Example of strike. (From Sirois M: Principles and practice of veterinary technology, ed 3, St Louis, 2011, Mosby.)

should be crossed out with a one-line strike. Liquid correction fluid must never be used in a medical record. Mistakes should be initialed and dated, with the change to follow (Fig. 2-20). This allows an observer to note the nature of the error and to be assured that important evidence has not been destroyed.

Master lists are often used to summarize patient histories. An individual patient record should include a master sheet listing species, gender, breed, age, diet, allergies, unique behaviors, and annual vaccination and parasite control documentation. The master sheet should include a major problem and drug list for which refills are indicated. The master sheet chronologically lists visits, treatments, and client communications (Fig. 2-21).

RECORD FORMAT

Written medical records are generally held in a clasp-type 8½- × 11-inch file folder. Each client has one folder, and all patients owned by that client are clipped within the folder. Patients are separated with color-coded tabs. Clinics often find a smaller paper size to be inadequate and may have incomplete records. Other hospitals maintain entirely computerized medical and financial records for each client. Regardless of the format, the record must be accurate, complete, and secure.

Master Problem List

Client Name _____ Telephone Number _____

Address _____ Client Number _____

Pet Name _____ Breed _____ Color _____

Sex _____ Altered _____ DOB _____ Age _____

	Date Received	Date Received	Date Received	Date Recieved
DHLPP				
FVRCP				
FeLV				
Rabies				
HWT				
FeLV/FIV				

Chronic Diseases/Date of Onset: _____

_____

_____

_____

Current Medications and Directions: _____

_____

_____

_____

FIGURE 2-21 Master sheet. (From Sirois M: Principles and practice of veterinary technology, ed 3, St Louis, 2011, Mosby.)

Storage and retrieval must be convenient and well organized. Various design formats are commercially available to minimize misfiling by incorporating color-coded tabs. If computerized records are used, meticulous accuracy is necessary for all data entries; incorrectly entered computer records may never be retrieved.

POMR AND SOAP

Completed medical records must follow a format, especially those with American Animal Hospital Association (AAHA) accreditation. A **problem-oriented medical record (POMR)** is the most commonly used format in veterinary practice. Each entry follows a distinct format; defined database, **master problem list** (also referred to as master list),

plan, and progress sections. Within the progress section, a standard SOAP format is followed.

SOAP is an acronym that stands for **subjective, objective, assessment, and plan**. Subjective is the most important element and is obtained from the client by the reception staff, veterinary technicians, and assistants. Subjective information includes reason for the office visit, patient history, and observations made by the client. Most subjective information is the opinion(s) and perception(s) of the client (Fig. 2-22).

Objective information is gathered directly from the patient; the physical examination, diagnostic workup, and interpretation are included in this section of the medical record. Objective information is factual information. Veterinary technicians and assistants compile most of the objective information.

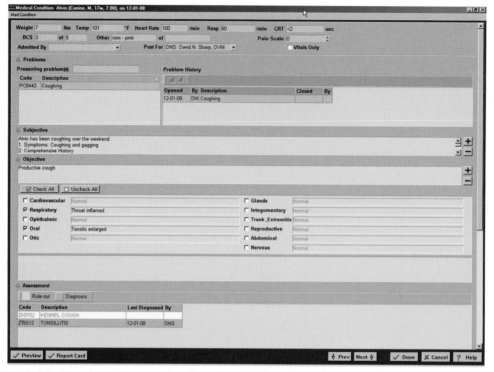

FIGURE 2-22 AVImark SOAP screen shot. (From Sirois M: Principles and practice of veterinary technology, ed 3, St Louis, 2011, Mosby.)

The assessment section includes any conclusions reached by the veterinarian from the subjective and objective section; it also includes a definitive diagnosis. If there are multiple diagnoses or a tentative diagnosis, this can all be documented here, along with a list of rule-ins or rule-outs (R/I or R/O, respectively). Rule-ins can be classified as any disease that the patient could possibly have. Diagnostic work must be done to rule out those particular diseases.

A plan is developed by the veterinarian based on the assessment and includes any treatment, surgery, medication, intended diagnostics, or intended communications with the owner. This can also be a list of options that will be presented to the client.

Commonly overlooked errors and incomplete medical records can be caught before the record has been filed by diligent team members. Some of the most common incomplete errors include laboratory work interpretation, progress notes while the patient is hospitalized, preoperative physical examinations, anesthetic drugs, and initials of the author(s) writing in the record. Laboratory results must be documented, along with any comments on abnormalities. If previous laboratory work is also being compared, this is also an excellent place to write the comparison. Veterinarians must interpret the results, not just document the results. Interpretation is defined as analyzing the results and explaining why those abnormalities may be present. The list of R/I and R/O can be completed with the analysis of pending laboratory work. Animals should have a daily physical examination while they are hospitalized. Results of the physical examination, any medications administered,

and any urination, bowel movements, or vomiting must be documented in the progress notes. Hospitalization sheets should be used to help keep track of patients' status while hospitalized (Fig. 2-23).

Surgical patients must be examined within 12 hours prior to administration of anesthesia, and the examination must be documented in the medical record. Anesthetic drugs, details of the procedure, and the patient's response to and/or complications from the procedure must also be documented. The most common error made is not documenting the communication with the owner regarding the prognosis of the patient. The medical record must clearly state whether the prognosis is poor, guarded, fair, or excellent.

Medication names, strength, and route given must be accurately written in the medical records. For example, 0.2 mL cefazolin IV would be incorrect. This description does not indicate how many milligrams (mg) were given. The entry should read "0.2 mL cefazolin (100 mg/mL) given IV," or it may read "20 mg cefazolin, given IV." Many drugs are available in different strengths, and it is important to identify and document the correct strength of medication. The same drug can also be administered by different routes. Some drugs will have a different dose, depending on the route administered. It is therefore important to document the route by which the medication was administered.

If the legibility and completeness of the medical record is a problem in practice, labels may be used. Labels can be used for examinations, dental prophylaxis, or surgeries, and be developed by the practice manager or ordered from standard office supply and label catalogues (Fig. 2-24).

Client's last name:						Working diagnosis:								
Pet name:						Primary doctor:								

Date:	8am	9	10	11	12	1	2	3	4	5	6	7	8
Feed													
Water													
Walk/litter													
Temperature													
Weight													
Appetite?													
Attitude?													
Urine?													
BM or diarrhea													
Vomit?													

FIGURE 2-23 Hospitalization sheet. (From Sirois M: Principles and practice of veterinary technology, ed 3, St Louis, 2011, Mosby.)

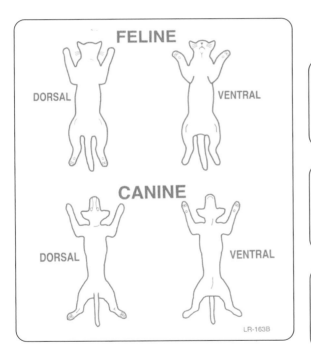

Feline Castration:

Using autoligation technique. No skin closure.
Surgery and recovery uneventful.

Canine and Feline OVH:
Ventral midline incision; _____Polysorb Double ligatures ovarian pedicles; _____Polysorb Double ligature encircling uterine body; _____ Polysorb Simple continuous body wall; _____Polysorb Simple cont. double layer; SubQ / subcut. closure. Surgery and recovery uneventful.

Canine Neuter:
Open/closed technique. Pre-scrotal incision, double ligate testicular artery, vein, and vas deferns with_____Polysorb. Subcutaneous and subcuticular layers closed simple continuous with _____Polysorb. Surgery/recovery uneventful.

Feline Declaw:

Using Roscoe blades, P3 was amputated and sealed with tissue adhesive.

Urinalysis
Source_____   Crystals_____
S.G._____   Glu_____   Casts_____
pH_____   Ket_____   WBC_____
Leuk_____   Uro_____   RBC_____
Nit_____   Bili_____   Epith_____
Protein_____   Blood_____   Bact_____

FIGURE 2-24 Examples of labels (From Prendergast H: Front office management for the veterinary team, ed. 2 St Louis, 2015, Saunders.)

STANDARD OPERATING PROCEDURES

Standard operating procedure (SOP) descriptions may be written for all standardized procedures used in the practice, and a loose-leaf binder may be used to store SOP sheets in a central location. SOP descriptions may also be used for front office staff, including which type of questions may be answered by staff, check-in and release procedures, and front office record-keeping procedures. Annual reviews and updates of SOP descriptions are important. Once the SOP binder is in place, one may reference all standardized procedures by "procedure name, SOP" as the patient medical records are completed.

INVENTORY MANAGEMENT

Inventory is one of the largest expenses of the practice. The ultimate goal should be to maintain inventory costs between 12% and 15% of the overall income of the practice. It is imperative that an inventory manager be well organized, motivated, and willing to make changes and improvements on a routine basis. A large amount of money can be lost in inventoried products through shrinkage, product expiration, or missed charges. **Shrinkage** is defined as the loss of a product without explanation. Shrinkage may result from employee theft. Products that expire are a large loss. If a bottle has not been opened, some manufacturers may exchange the product; others will not and the practice must take the loss. Missed charges account for a large portion of lost revenue and can be tracked easily with the correct training and monitoring.

> **CRITICAL CONCEPT**
> Inventory costs should not exceed 15% of the overall practice income.

The inventory manager should determine a day that is appropriate to place an order. An order should be developed that encompasses the practice's needs for the following 1- or 2-week period. The order must be called in to the distributor before the cutoff period, allowing the shipping department to pack the order appropriately and ship via the least expensive route (Fig. 2-25).

Ordering products should be based on the economic order quantity, reorder point, and number of inventory turns that the product takes within a year. The combination of all three factors will help control inventory, which is commonly a place of missed charges and shrinkage. One must manage inventory well to prevent such losses. Economic order quantity represents the costs related to ordering the item, sales of the item, and purchase price. Inventory turns per year refers to the number of times inventory turns over in a practice, in a specified time. This helps determine correct reorder quantities and points. Each practice should set a goal of 8 to 12 turns per year.

REORDER POINT

A **reorder point** is defined as the point that a stock level reaches before reordering. The average shelf life of an item should not exceed 3 months. Anything longer than 3 months decreases the profits of the veterinary hospital and increases the risk of the product expiring, as well as of theft or damage

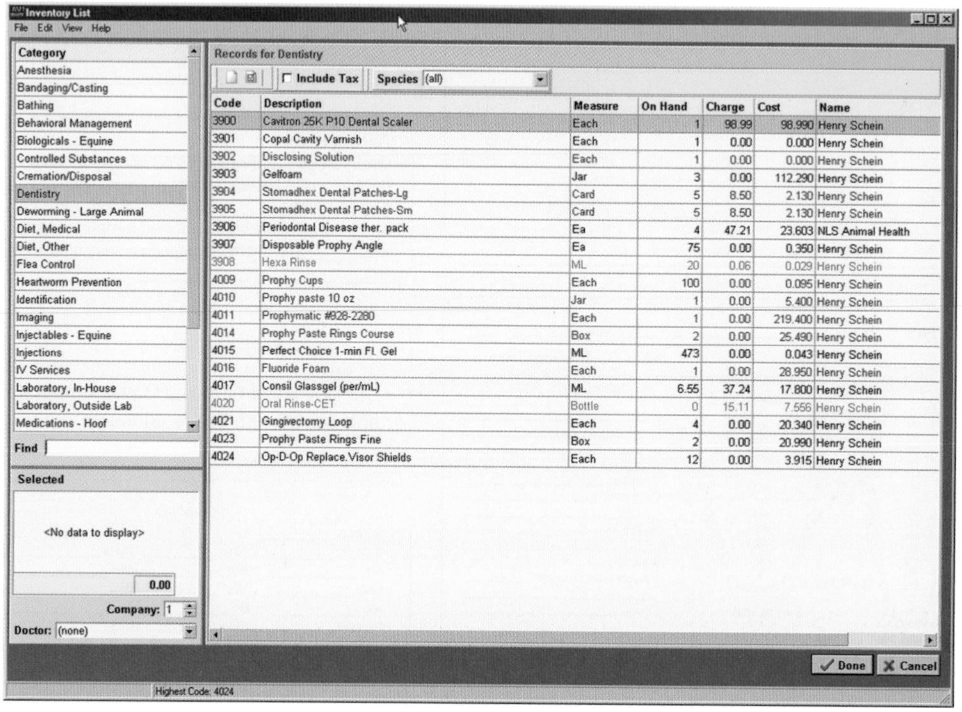

FIGURE 2-25 AVImark inventory screen shot. (From Sirois M: Principles and practice of veterinary technology, ed 3, St Louis, 2011, Mosby.)

to the product. Practices may wish to keep as little inventory on hand as possible. This can be an advantage because it can lower holding costs (costs associated with holding product on the shelf, such as taxes and insurance) and prevent shrinkage (unexplained loss of inventory). However, it can contribute to product shortage, which causes the practice to lose clients and money because the product is unavailable for resale.

If a product is used infrequently and expires before the entire amount can be dispensed, the practice may want to consider writing a prescription for the medication. It is less costly to prescribe certain products than for the practice to continue losing profits to satisfy a few clients or passing the extra costs on to the client. Clients will appreciate the lower cost of purchasing the product elsewhere.

Computer systems are extremely efficient at aiding in inventory management, production of reports, and decreasing loss. However, physical inventory must be taken at the beginning or end of each year, and spot checks should be performed throughout the year. It is also advised to make spot checks when placing orders to verify quantities on the shelf in case of error in the inventory system.

Items should be checked when they are received. Expiration dates, correct product, strength, and count should all be verified against the order book and invoice. Items that are received with a short expiration date should be returned unless they will be used immediately. Short-dated bottles should not be opened. Most inventory products must be returned unopened and free of tampering to be eligible for replacement or credit.

PRODUCT PRICING

The **markup** of a product is defined as the cost of the product multiplied by a percentage to recover hidden costs associated with inventory management. Many practices will mark products up by 100% to 200%. A product markup must be at least 40% to break even.

Practices may add a product **dispensing fee** as well as a minimum prescription charge. The average dispensing fee ranges from $6.00 to $14.00 to cover the cost of the label, pill vial, and time used to count the medication. If a bottle of shampoo or full bottle of medication is dispensed, the average dispensing fee ranges from $3.00 to $5.00. Many practices initiate a **minimum prescription fee** of $11.00 to $13.00 to help recover hidden pharmacy costs (Box 2-3).

BOX 2-3	Example of Prescription Product Markup

28 cephalexin capsules cost $0.40 each; product markup is 200%; dispensing fee is $11.95.

$$\$0.40 \times 200\% = \$0.80$$
$$(\$0.80 \times 28) + \$11.95 = \$22.40 + \$11.95 = \$34.35$$

From Sirois M: Principles and practice of veterinary technology, ed 3, St Louis, 2011, Mosby.

Hidden pharmacy costs include costs associated with expired medications, ordering and shipping costs, and insurance and taxes on products and supplies. These costs can increase rapidly and must be recovered.

Pricing for items (e.g., injections, single-dose items) used in the hospital or administered to patients while in the examination room must also be considered. Common methods include charging a flat fee for injections (e.g., $12.00 per injection) or adding a surcharge for very expensive drugs, such as some postoperative analgesics. In-hospital tablet administration frequently is priced to include drug, labor, and record-keeping costs, such as $3.00 per administration.

Over-the-counter (OTC) products do not require a prescription and can be sold to clients without a client-patient relationship. A prescription product can only be sold on the order of a veterinarian, wherein a current client-patient relationship exists. State practice acts may define the term current and dictate how long a client-patient-veterinary relationship exists after the last examination. A client-patient relationship is defined as the relationship shared by the veterinarian, client, and patient. The veterinarian must be familiar with the case, patient, and client. It is illegal to sell a prescription product when a current relationship does not exist. Veterinarians can receive heavy fines and license revocation for failure to comply.

CRITICAL CONCEPT

A valid client-patient relationship must exist for a veterinarian to dispense prescription products.

Manufacturers may dictate that some products are not prescription products but can only be sold through a veterinarian, wherein a client-patient relationship exists. Examples of such products include some heartworm preventive medications and therapeutic diets such as Purina NF, Waltham S/O, and Hills K/D.

LABELING PRESCRIPTION ITEMS

Every item that is a prescription product must have a label before it leaves the practice. Labels must include the practice name, address, and phone number, veterinarian's name, date of the prescription, client's last name and patient's name, name and strength of the drug (in milligrams [mg] or grams [g]), number of items dispensed (tablets, capsules, or volume in milliliters [mL]), and expiration date of the product. Finally, and most important, the directions of the product must be clear. "Give one capsule by mouth every 8 hours for 7 days" clearly states that one capsule should be given in the mouth, every 8 hours for 7 days. A label that reads "Give one capsule every 8 hours" can be interpreted, for example, as one capsule can be placed on the open wound, over food, or in the water. Clients may also think that, because the presenting symptoms have visually cleared, they do not need to continue giving the antibiotic until it is gone. Directions must be detailed and specific.

COMPUTER AND SOFTWARE MANAGEMENT

Computers are an excellent asset to every veterinary practice. Most practices use computers to a certain extent but may not be using them to their fullest potential. Computers can greatly increase the efficiency of every team member, lower the amount of missed charges, provide professional-appearing client educational materials, maintain inventory and accounts receivable, and provide paperless medical records.

Computers and software can be a great expense, but the rewards far exceed the cost of the equipment. Team members should brainstorm and determine the best location for computer terminals in the practice. Many practices use computers in examination rooms, laboratory areas, pharmacy counters, veterinarian's office, and reception area. This allows data to be entered in multiple locations of the practice. Pharmacy labels can be generated at any terminal and printed in the pharmacy area. Invoices can also be generated at any location and printed at the reception desk.

Team members should also determine which software applications would meet the expectations of team members. In addition to the features listed, veterinary software can aid in invoice development, client education, practice management, and/or digital radiology. Veterinary software manufacturers and distributors should provide the team with demonstrations and/or practice modules, allowing the team to determine which software will meet their needs.

Team members should remember to choose a reputable company that has been in the industry for many years, offering continuous updates and new programs. Software companies strive to provide the most useful features and answer requests from practices, including those regarding safety and security of information.

Advanced software technology must use advanced computers. One cannot expect to run new software on old computers. Software has been developed to run fast and efficiently, and new computers with large amounts of RAM, memory, and storage must be purchased. Many software companies will not guarantee their products without installation on new computers.

As with every situation, a backup plan must exist with the use of computers. Fire, theft, or natural disasters can destroy a practice in a matter of minutes, as can computer viruses or a hacked computer system. It is imperative that security measures be taken to prevent a virus from entering the system. Internet access should be limited to a few individuals, and policies should be instituted regarding Internet sites. Regular scanning of the system to detect evidence of computer viruses or malware is vital to ensuring safety and security of records.

Computer systems should be backed up nightly, on and off premises. On-premise system backup may include a rewritable disk or zip drive. Off-premise system backup can be done through the veterinary software website or another location, such as with cloud computing. Backing up documents offsite prevents thieves from stealing the most current copy of data from the practice if they are removing all the computer equipment. If a fire or natural disaster occurs, the data are also protected.

Computers will not survive a lifetime. Many computers function optimally for only 5 or 6 years and then need to be replaced. Computers often give signals as they are slowly fading. At this point, management must locate a backup computer so that when the computer fails, an alternative computer is ready to take its place. This prevents team members from panicking when the system is temporarily unavailable. If the main computer that needs to be replaced, the backup data from the previous evening can be uploaded, bringing the system back up and allowing the team to move forward.

CLIENT RELATIONS

Clients draw preliminary conclusions about a practice within the first 2 to 5 minutes of entering the building. This conclusion, especially if it is negative, can continue through the rest of the visit. Team members should always greet clients as they enter the facility, regardless of what other tasks they may be doing. If a receptionist is on the phone, acknowledging clients with a smile and a wave is acceptable. If helping another client, a receptionist can greet the entering client with a smile and say, "Hello, I will be with you in a moment." If the receptionist is working with another team member, that task should be put aside and the client should receive the full attention of both team members. Greeting clients by their names and addressing their pets create a positive first impression (Fig. 2-26).

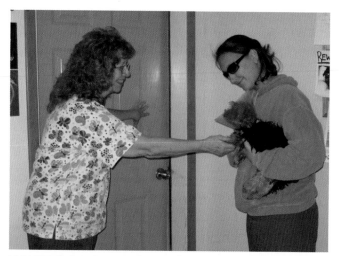

FIGURE 2-26 Greeting clients at the door and addressing them by name makes them feel they are getting personalized attention. (From Prendergast H: Front office management for the veterinary team, St Louis, 2011, Saunders.)

Communication is one of the most important aspects of working with veterinary clients. It is extremely important that clients fully understand procedures that are being performed on their pets. They must also be educated on the proper care of their animals throughout the various life stages. All of this must be relayed in a professional manner.

Client communication comes in a variety of forms. It starts in the front office with the reception team. Greeting clients as they enter the practice indicates that the staff acknowledges their presence. Communication should occur in a positive, friendly manner, which enhances the practice image. Communication includes verbal and written forms in the examination room. The veterinary health care team must educate the client with words that can be understood but must take care to not offend. Many clients want to learn the information but do not understand medical terminology. The amount of information given can be based on the client's knowledge. (Fig. 2-27).

Written communication includes all client educational materials. Clients should take home information with every visit. After puppy and kitten examinations, clients should be sent home with material informing them about internal parasites and vaccination schedules. Clients bringing pets in for follow-up booster examinations may be sent home with information on nutrition and the benefits of spaying and neutering as well as information on the prevention of obesity and dental disease. Yearly examination patients may need to be educated on weight loss programs and nutritional and behavioral issues. Senior patients should be educated about the importance of monitoring blood work and frequent regular examinations. Each client should receive a report card explaining the normal and abnormal findings for his or her pet and which follow-up procedures or treatments are recommended.

Surgical patients must receive postoperative discharge instructions. These instructions may vary by procedure, but all clients must be informed about when to start food, medications, and activity. Boarding clients will appreciate receiving report cards on their pets, which may include information on the pet's appetite, activity level, and attitude. Clients of

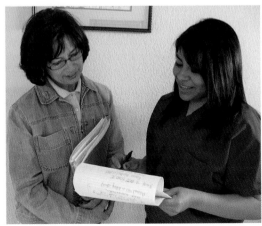

FIGURE 2-27 Technician educating a client. (From Prendergast H: Front office management for the veterinary team, St Louis, 2011, Saunders.)

pets diagnosed with a disease or condition should be given information to take home and review regarding the disease and any treatments available. If the clients have any questions, they can call the practice and verify information before scheduling an appointment for the treatment.

Clients can be pleasant or difficult, depending on the type of person they are, type of day they have had, or type of situation presented to them once they arrive at the practice. If a client has had a bad day, the team may take the brunt of the person's frustration. Team members should remember not to take the comments of these clients personally and instead try to make it a better day for the client.

Receptionists must effectively handle hostile clients on the phone. Although clients may call and be angry with the practice for some reason, the receptionist handling the conversation can turn the call into a positive experience. First, the receptionist should listen to the client. Once the client has finished her or his portion of the conversation, the receptionist should review the facts, ensuring that a miscommunication does not occur. If a manager is available to take the telephone call, the manager and client can discuss the case. If a supervisor is not available, the receptionist can politely state that the manager who can handle the situation is not available at the moment but that he or she will return the call as soon as possible. A delay in the conversation may allow the client to calm down before a manager returns the call, allowing an easier resolution to the issue.

Angry clients at the practice should be taken into an examination room and allowed to vent in private. A team member who simply listens to the client often defuses the situation. The team member can try to offer a solution that is satisfactory to the client to resolve the problem. If the fault lies with the practice, the mistake must be admitted and an apology given. Often, this repairs the situation immediately.

BODY LANGUAGE

The ability to understand a client's body language may help increase client compliance. Body language is a nonverbal form of communication that plays a key role in client education. It accounts for almost 60% of communication. Following are a few key characteristics of body language.

FOLDED ARMS

When a person has folded arms, it generally indicates that he or she is defensive and unwilling to accept recommendations or advice. If a team member is approached by a client and the team member has folded arms, the client may feel uncomfortable about asking questions; role playing will help teach team members remember to unfold arms while in the practice. A client with folded arms may be unwilling to accept recommendations and may have some underlying issues with the service provided. A team member can correct this situation easily by handing the client something to hold. A brochure, a model of a joint (e.g., hip, knee, elbow), or anything else will force the person to unfold the

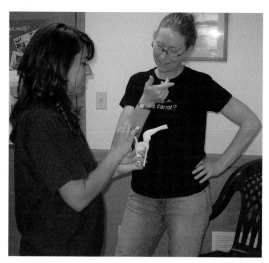

FIGURE 2-28 Technician educating a client by handing her a model. (From Prendergast H: Front office management for the veterinary team, St Louis, 2011, Saunders.)

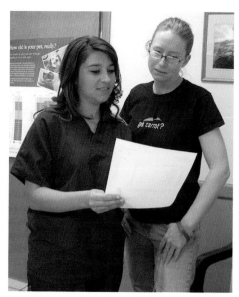

FIGURE 2-29 A professional team member standing up straight with shoulders held back. (From Prendergast H: Front office management for the veterinary team, St Louis, 2011, Saunders.)

arms; this will gradually open the lines for communication (Fig. 2-28). Once this has occurred, the team member can continue educating the client and ask if there is any other information that the client needs. Team members should also make sure at this point that all of the client's concerns have been addressed.

BODY POSTURE

A team member's body posture sends a message to the client. If a team member enters an examination room slumped over, with head down and shoulders folded in, the client is going to think that the team member lacks confidence and skill and does not enjoy his or her job. The client may not accept the recommendations that are given simply because of the team member's poor body posture. Team members who are slumped over are likely to have quiet voices, lack energy, and appear unmotivated. Instead, team members should enter examination rooms with their heads up, a straight body posture, and shoulders back. This attitude will indicate confidence, excitement, and skill. Clients will be more likely to accept the recommendations that are made and develop a strong relationship with the team (Fig. 2-29).

EYE CONTACT

While educating clients, maintain eye contact with them at all times. Lack of eye contact is perceived as diminished skill, knowledge, and confidence. When team members maintain eye contact, the client will feel more comfortable about accepting recommendations.

THE HUMAN-ANIMAL BOND

Over the last century, veterinary medicine has evolved from a focus predominantly on food animals to a companion animal orientation. Pets have moved from the backyard to the house to the bedroom and are perceived as members of the

family. Client expectations are changing as medicine changes and more is learned about the human-animal bond.

> **CRITICAL CONCEPT**
> Many clients consider their pets to be members of the family.

Clients who are not well informed about the human-animal bond may not take into account the impact on household members when making decisions about veterinary care. If there is little bond with the animal, decisions may be influenced more by financial considerations. This is particularly troubling when the decision maker is not as bonded to the pet as other household members. It has been reported that children who are left out of life and death pet care decisions or who are not told the truth by their parents hold lifelong resentment. It is therefore critical for the veterinary team to help the decision maker understand the impact of the human-animal bond and how it may affect household members. It is equally important to involve household members in decisions about pet care. Hospitals should continuously document the relationships and bonds in the household in client records so that all members of the veterinary team can use this information to assist clients and animals.

During a patient's health care crisis, it is a delicate matter to help clients who face difficult decisions. Clients are best served if they consider the human-animal bond in their decisions, but they must not be made to feel guilty or inadequate if financial realities keep them from doing everything that can be offered. The veterinary team's responsibility is to help the animal and prevent suffering, as well as serve the client. Educating clients about the human-animal bond long before there is a crisis and encouraging them to have pet health insurance can help ease the difficult passages.

The opposite extreme from clients who have little appreciation for the human-animal bond is clients who are extremely bonded. These clients are well aware of this bond. They may seek or demand services that have never been requested and that the hospital is not prepared to deliver. Clients such as these actually lead those in the profession to offer new levels of service and veterinary care. The services that your veterinary team performs only for this special client today will be the norm in a few years. Examples are home care by assistants or technicians, respite care, hospice care, and high-technology services such as computed tomography (CT) scanning and magnetic resonance imaging (MRI).

Clients consider companion animals to be members of the family or household, in a role comparable to that of children. They are perceived as helpless innocents who depend on the adults in the house for nurturing and protection. Your goal is to be a partner with the client in helping maintain the bond between them. Part of nurturing the bond is to help clients have realistic expectations of behavior in relation to the species and breed of pet. Also, you must help clients understand animal behavior and learn to communicate with the animal. The greatest number of pets left in animal shelters are there because of behavior problems. These problems are mostly preventable or treatable with client education and animal training. Behavior that goes uncorrected for too long prevents the human-animal bond from forming or breaks the bond and results in the pet being surrendered. An important service you can provide to clients and pets is to be a knowledgeable resource on behavior and training. Recognizing and correcting problem behaviors early in a relationship can be lifesaving for the pet.

It is important to recognize and honor the bond between the client and pet by treating the pet as an individual, not as an example of a particular species or breed. You should try to build on the bond that the pet has already established with the client and form your own bond with the animal. This can be challenging because animals are often stressed just by coming to the hospital and can be more interested in avoiding you than bonding with you. Animals are not all equally lovable and friendly, but as a professional you have an obligation to try to give them all your best care. Remember that the way the animal interacts with the client at home may be completely different from how it interacts with you in the hospital. The careful use of gentle but firm physical restraint, and chemical restraint when needed, will protect you and the animal. It will also reassure the client that the pet is precious to you as well.

Assistance animals such as guide dogs and hearing ear dogs require special care on the part of the veterinary team in recognition of the dependency of the client on the animal and the deep bond between them. You must ask the human companion to direct you and be forthright about any questions or concerns. You must be prepared to alter some of your routine policies and procedures to serve assistance animals best. Avoid separating the person and the animal, if at all possible. You must also discuss in great detail any procedure that may temporarily incapacitate the assistance animal and prevent it from working. Sedation or tranquilization of any type will make it unsafe for the animal to return to work until it has fully recovered.

Hospitalization, which is a routine to people who work in animal hospitals, is stressful to clients who are highly bonded to their pets. They not only miss their pet's companionship but also worry about them, just as parents worry and are distressed by having a child in the hospital. The veterinary team can relieve this strain on the patient and client by making patient visits possible and convenient. Frequent calls to give progress reports also help ease the client's mind.

GRIEF COUNSELING

As pets approach the end of life, clients may begin to recognize how strongly they are bonded and anticipate the loss that they will experience when the pet dies. This realization makes the pet's remaining days more precious than ever. The mission of the veterinary team is to prevent suffering and support the highest quality of life possible during this time before the pet dies or is euthanized. Human hospice offers a model of how to achieve these goals. Hospice endeavors to keep patients in their homes, surrounded by family and friends, pain-free, with their symptoms controlled, so that their last days can be good ones. The patient and family are supported with skilled nursing, respite care for caregivers, and spiritual, psychosocial, and bereavement support. Veterinary hospitals can offer these services by having staff provide home care under the direction of the veterinarian and by finding credentialed psychosocial and spiritual counselors to offer services as needed.

CRITICAL CONCEPT

Assist clients in the bereavement process by suggesting ways to memorialize their pet.

Clients can be assisted in the bereavement process by suggesting ways to memorialize and honor the special relationship they had with their pet. Funeral and burial ceremonies, donations, clay paw prints, pictures, and plantings are all ways of recognizing a special and meaningful relationship. Clients who are most bonded with their animals are at risk of suffering the most grief over their loss. These clients will not get new animals until their grief is resolved, and these are exactly the clients who will provide the best homes for animals and the best veterinary care. It is in the best interest of the client, animal, and veterinarian to help clients through their bereavement.

Clients anticipating or experiencing the loss of a companion animal are emotionally vulnerable. The hospital is also vulnerable. What you do or say to a client while she or he is experiencing the loss of a companion animal can encourage or discourage her or his future relationship with the practice. At such a time, you have the opportunity to provide the best service your hospital has to offer.

The bonds people form with their pets may be deeper than those formed with friends or family members. Pets make us feel better when we are ill, comfort us when we are lonely, accept us when we have made a mistake, and love us unconditionally. This human-animal bond can be broken in many ways. The pet may die of natural causes, run away, or be stolen, killed accidentally, or euthanized. Clients with a deep emotional attachment to their pets can expect to grieve when they lose them.

It is important to respect the feelings of clients experiencing such loss. To do this, you must first understand the stages of grief and determine the significance of the loss to the client. Dr. Elizabeth Kübler-Ross was the first to outline predictable stages of the process of grieving in her book, *On Death and Dying*. Although she wrote about human loss, the stages can be applied to the loss of pets as well.

Loss of a pet elicits a wide range of emotions in clients, which can be associated with certain stages of the grieving process. You can assist the client's smooth transition from one stage to another. The grieving process is not a steady linear ascent from depression to joy; rather, it can be likened to a roller coaster ride, with ups and downs at every turn. At the end of the ride is a state of resolution and acceptance, in which the client is at peace with what went before.

By familiarizing yourself with the characteristics of each stage, you will recognize where your client is in this process and be able to shape your responses appropriately. These responses can facilitate the smooth transition from one stage to the next in the process of grieving.

STAGES OF GRIEF

The stages of grief include denial, bargaining, anger, guilt, sorrow, and resolution. These stages frequently occur in this order, but can occur in other sequences. Some stages may be repeated.

DENIAL. Denial, the first stage of grief, may be played out during the first 24 hours if the animal's death is sudden, or for several days if a terminal illness has been diagnosed. Denial is a coping mechanism that cushions the mind against the shock it has received.

BARGAINING. Clients may bargain with God or another higher entity for the life of a pet, or bargain with the pet itself, trying to make it live. They may offer the pet vitamins, tempt it with its favorite foods, and promise never to scold or neglect it again. Bargaining is a way of keeping hope alive and buying time to fully accept the outcome of the situation. When bargaining does not yield the desired results, anger is a natural response.

ANGER. When faced with the loss of a treasured pet, clients may become angry with the veterinarian, practice staff, family, friends, and themselves. The veterinarian who has failed to "save" the pet, or who has made the diagnosis, may be the initial recipient of the wrath. More often, it is the reception staff members who bear the brunt of the anger, directly or indirectly. Clients may be fearful of alienating

the practitioner on whom they have come to rely. If clients are angry with themselves for overlooking clinical signs or waiting too long to seek care, this self-directed anger, once dissipated, gives way to guilt.

GUILT. Guilt is an unproductive, debilitating emotion that often inhibits progress toward resolution of the loss. It is the enemy of healing and closure and, if excessive, may require the attention of a mental health professional. When guilt subsides, it opens the door for sorrow.

SORROW. Sorrow, or deep sadness, is the core of the grieving process. Although it can be kept at bay during the early stages through the intensity of denial, anger, and guilt, sorrow eventually settles in and permeates all aspects of life.

Sorrow is, in fact, a healing emotion. This is when tears flow freely. Clients feel relief and release from the pent-up emotions of previous days or weeks. Tears may come at work, in the supermarket, or while driving. Clients may report sleep and appetite disturbances at this time. The practitioner may want to remind them, soon after a terminal illness is diagnosed, that adequate rest and nutrition are important. With time, sorrow dissipates, and everyday tasks begin to dominate awareness. Tears no longer break through into daily activities but can surface at more convenient times, such as in the evening after work. Clients then feel more in control and are able to see an end to the intense pain that is true sorrow.

RESOLUTION. In the resolution phase of grieving, clients realize that the pet is gone, that no amount of wishing will make it different, and that they will survive the loss that previously seemed engulfing. Now they can look at photographs of the pet and smile rather than cry, they can remember walks in the park in the summer, instead of anxious trips to the veterinarian, and happy times can be recalled with tenderness rather than despair. During this stage of grief, clients may consider sharing life with another pet for the sheer pleasure of having something warm and furry to hug again.

LONELINESS. Regardless of how a loss occurs and how well prepared a client is, all clients feel their lives touched by loneliness. This can occur in the presence of family and friends, as well as in the company of remaining pets at home. The client shared a relationship with the departed pet that was special and separate from other relationships. Although other pets, family members, and friends can provide company and comfort, they cannot fill the space left by the departed pet. Loneliness arises from this space, and the space fills slowly as the grief process unfolds. Clients may express anger at losing this particular pet while others to whom they are less attached are healthy and well.

An appropriate response from the staff or veterinarian may be, "Even though you have other pets at home, you may still be lonely for Taffy. While you are healing from this loss, your other pets will still be there to love you."

REPLACEMENT. The decision to replace a deceased pet with a new one should be left solely to the individual experiencing the loss. The veterinary staff should not influence the decision in any way. Some pet owners choose to bond with new pets before their older pets die. Others decide that the presence of a new pet in their home would be stressful for the older pet and decide to wait. Some clients may never again adopt new pets. Everyone involved must consider the client's needs, as well as the needs of the current pet. It is important not to try to "fix" the client's loss by suggesting replacement.

If a client is trying to avoid the experience of loss by finding a replacement for the pet, bonding with the new pet usually does not occur. The new pet is not accepted as a unique being if the owner wants it to be just like the deceased pet. Often, these new pets are given away or neglected. Owners may comment that the new Max is nothing like the old Max. Occasionally, a client who had taken good care of a previous pet brings in a pet that has been neglected. This client probably has not bonded successfully with the new pet and may need support in deciding whether to keep it or find it a new home. The client may not have resolved the loss of the previous pet and may need to see a counselor or support group that deals with pet loss issues.

ASSISTING BEREAVED PET OWNERS

Clients grieve in a variety of ways. Some demonstrate their emotions openly, whereas others may show little if any feeling in your presence. Do not assume that a stoic display means that the client is not grieving.

Assess your client's feelings to determine how much support you should provide. When clients show reluctance to accept concerned overtures from you, take a minute to let them know that you care about their well-being. By acknowledging their sadness, you open the door for them to experience their emotions, sending the simple message that it is acceptable to grieve.

Veterinary staff members are in a position to encourage healthy coping skills in their clients. Clients look to the veterinary staff for support, assurance, understanding, and validation when facing a loss. If you can assist your clients in this way, you are building the foundation for natural resolution of the loss. In doing so, you continue to maintain their respect and solidify your working relationship. Recognizing the different stages of grief assists you in providing your clients with the type of support they need.

ACKNOWLEDGING THE LOSS

What a client needs and values most from the staff is their time and presence. In being present with clients during a loss, you help legitimize the grief reaction and give them permission to verbalize their feelings. Many pet owners go to great lengths to appear stoic in the presence of others. In our society, death is often dealt with through denial, so it is vital that you validate the client's loss. The most beneficial thing that a veterinary staff member can do for the client is to let him or her know that grieving for the loss of a pet is perfectly normal.

Sending a card, personal note, or flowers to the client are all ways of expressing condolences. What clients will remember the most is how they were cared for during their loss. Being cared for and acknowledged is something a client will remember long after the flowers have wilted and the note or card has been discarded.

Veterinary staff members may feel uncomfortable in attending a grieving client. Some pet owners attribute unrealistic powers of control over life and death to their veterinarians. This is especially true for veterinarians who are specialists in their fields. A client whose pet has cancer and has been referred to an internist for treatment may have a strong need to believe that this veterinarian with specialized skills can help the pet. This can place the veterinarian in the difficult position of conveying the limitations of treatment to the client.

Being with a client who is very tearful or angry can be an uncomfortable experience. You may worry that you will do or say the wrong thing. You may find it easier to hide behind your professional role and keep the client emotionally at a distance. This often leaves the client feeling neglected and abandoned. A client is less likely to return to an emotionally nonsupportive veterinary facility, even if the very best treatment was provided for the terminally ill pet.

Your responsibility is not to work in the capacity of a therapist or counselor. However, learning and using a variety of counseling and communication skills can enhance your relationships with your clients. By communicating effectively with your clients, you help them accept and resolve their losses sooner than pet owners whose losses have not been properly acknowledged.

Skills and techniques that can be used to assist your clients include attending, effective listening, reflection, and validation. Some clients are easier to help than others, and you must make an extra effort to support the more difficult ones. Demonstrate that you are attempting to understand what the clients are expressing by responding at appropriate intervals to their comments. Avoid using clichés or telling them that you know exactly how they feel; you don't.

Try saying, "What I hear you saying is …." Let the client tell you what the loss means to her or him. Ask the client, "How can I help you? What things have you done in the past that have supported you through a difficult time?"

REFLECTION

Summarizing what the client is expressing is called reflection. When you reflect their underlying concerns, clients believe that you understand what they are saying. In addition, you can reframe the experience of loss and hopelessness into one of hope and possibility.

By establishing open communication, you will be in a position to offer the type of help that clients need. Some clients may only need to hear that they did the right thing and want to be informed of disposing of the remains. Others need emotional support and may be referred to a group or private therapist.

VALIDATING THE LOSS

When your clients tell you what the loss means to them, it is important to let them know that you understand the relationship that they have shared with the pet. In validating the loss, you will discover that a pet can fulfill many needs of pet owners. Be alert for key comments, such as, "We never had any children. Kelsey was like our child," "Buttons was my whole life," or "How will I ever feel safe alone at night without Cole?" A pet may have served as a child to some clients, a best friend to others, or even as a bridge to the past. It may have accompanied the owner from college to career, to marriage, and on through other important life stages. It may have been a source of comfort during a stressful time, such as a divorce, loss of a loved one, a move, or a change in jobs.

ATTENDING

Without realizing it, you can make it difficult for clients to express their feelings and concerns. The way you sit, stand, look at, or speak with them can inhibit or enhance communication. An open posture with uncrossed arms and legs demonstrates to your clients that you are available and ready to listen. Facing them directly while maintaining comfortable eye contact sends the message that you are interested in what they have to say. Avoid standing behind the counter, desk, or examination table when clients are expressing their feelings about their pet to you.

EFFECTIVE LISTENING

Listening effectively is much more than hearing what a client is saying. Listening effectively means giving your complete attention and allowing time for the client to ramble, cry, and show anger. You should learn to tolerate periods of silence from the client. You may feel a strong desire to fill in the silence with words; refrain from doing so. The client needs you to be there silently.

By recognizing the different components of grief, you can accept a client's expressions of anger and denial and be empathetic about the guilt and deep sadness. Whether the client's initial reaction is overt despair or quiet shock, your interactions set the stage for the grieving process that follows.

The current loss can trigger remembrance of past losses, particularly for the older client. This compound effect may threaten to overwhelm the client. Clients can be reminded that this is a common reaction to loss of a pet.

Use your own words to convey messages of understanding and empathy toward your clients. The idea is to listen and then respond to clients by expressing the core significance of the loss. Validating the loss helps the client feel special and cared for by the veterinarian and hospital staff.

ACHIEVING CLOSURE

The perfect way to end a conversation with a grieving client is to give a directive. For example, "I would like you to go home, get some rest, and then think about the options we discussed." Or, you can inform the client about a support group in your area for bereaved pet owners. For example, "There is a place you can go and meet with other pet owners who are sharing similar feelings to yours." You can give the client a brochure or offer to make an appointment for him or her to talk with the support group leader.

Make clients take comfort in thinking about how to honor their pets. For example, clients can donate to a charity in honor of a pet, plant a rosebush near the burial site, or create a scrapbook of memories shared with the pet.

The following suggestions may be helpful in assisting your clients:

- Provide facial tissues.
- Schedule appointment times to allow additional time to be spent with a bereaved pet owner or one whose pet is seriously ill.
- Create a brochure that includes all available support information (e.g., pet loss support groups, private therapists, hotlines, burial information, literature on pet loss). Make the brochure available to clients anticipating a loss as well as to those experiencing one.
- Send a sympathy card or flowers immediately after the loss. Late arrivals can be painful reminders for clients.
- Collect any fees owed before a euthanasia procedure is performed. A client will find it awkward to have to regain composure and pay a bill after the emotional experience of saying goodbye to a beloved pet.
- Let clients know that you and the rest of the staff are available to assist them, before and after the loss of a pet. Most pet owners have questions regarding their pet's illness and need reassurance that they did the right thing.
- If possible, maintain a private area in which clients can say goodbye to the pet, grieve, or regain composure. If such an area is not available, consider allowing extra time in the examination room before or after the loss.
- When attending to the patient, make certain that the owner can tell that the pet is comfortable and cared for. A simple gesture, such as placing a towel on a cold examination table, can demonstrate your compassion for the patient. If you send a final bill to the client, make sure it does not arrive on the same day as the sympathy card or flowers.

EFFECTS OF PATIENT LOSS ON STAFF

As difficult as the loss of a pet may be for a client, the loss of a patient may be difficult for the veterinary health care team as well. Because euthanasia is an acceptable and legal means of terminating an animal's life, veterinary practitioners and their staff face a stress that is unknown to most other medical practitioners.

Each member of the staff has a personal set of beliefs and feelings regarding the issue of loss. Some may feel awkward attending a grieving client. Others may have unresolved feelings about pets that they have lost themselves. Most people in the veterinary field have a love for animals and want to help them. Few consider the effect of the loss of a patient on themselves.

When assisting bereaved pet owners, staff members may feel emotions comparable to those that the client experiences. Learn how to empathize and assist in a caring manner while still maintaining emotional distance.

The following steps will help you in this process:

- Take a team approach to cases in which euthanasia is an option. This can alleviate some of the feelings of failure and grief regarding the loss of a patient.
- Create and participate in a support group for veterinary staff. This is a forum for airing private feelings and receiving feedback from peers.
- Encourage open communication among staff members, confrontation of personal feelings and beliefs surrounding death, and self-examination regarding the emotional reaction to loss of a patient.

When a client is facing the crisis of losing a treasured pet, you can play a positive role in guiding the client through an emotionally difficult time, thereby solidifying your working relationship with the pet owner. Clients who respect the veterinarian and staff will speak highly of them to others, refer other pet owners to the practice, and return with new pets. Pet loss is an opportunity for everyone concerned to grow emotionally and to solidify working relationships.

COMPOUNDED LOSS

When faced with loss of a pet, the owner is often reminded of losses from the past, both human and animal. A compound loss can feel so overpowering that a client may respond in a way that seems out of proportion to the current facts. When this occurs, you might say, "I can see that you are troubled and concerned about Woody. Have you had other experience with loss?"

Sometimes, an invitation to talk about a previous pet loss elicits information regarding past loss of family and friends, the demise of a relationship, or loss of a job. If the information is forthcoming, you can tell the client, "I know that when faced with the loss of a pet that you love, you can be reminded of other previous losses, and this can hurt more than if you were dealing with a single loss. Don't be surprised if you are suddenly recalling sad times from the past. Just know that it is very natural, at a time like this, to remember family and friends who are no longer with you. Try talking things over with a close friend or, if you'd like, I can give you some referrals for counseling that might help you get through this difficult time."

RECOGNIZING AND RESPONDING TO SIGNALS

A client may convey feelings of deep despair verbally or though body language. Such statements as, "Muffin is the only friend I have in the world. I don't know how I can face another day without her by my side," or "Nothing matters now that Jake is dying. It will kill me to bring him in for euthanasia. I might as well be dead, too," should alert you to the need for outside professional evaluation and treatment.

You must determine whether these clients have a reliable, concerned friend or relative who can stay with them, particularly if you have doubts about their safety if left alone. Make appropriate referrals and offer to call for an appointment before they leave the office. Do this openly to encourage trust and open communication. Knowing that an appointment has been arranged can have a calming and reassuring effect. Make every effort to secure the first appointment available and, if possible, telephone the client the next day for a welfare check and reminder of the appointment date and time. Extract a promise from the client that he or she will contact the crisis intervention hotline if he or she experiences overwhelming loneliness and sadness. Make certain that you know the telephone number and that the client has it before leaving your office.

If the client refuses any referrals or assistance and you sense that the client is a danger to himself or herself, you may need to resort to police escort of this client to a local psychiatric clinic for evaluation and treatment. This may be an extreme measure, but it could save a life. Let the veterinarian know about any concerns you may have regarding a client. Develop a protocol for clients experiencing emotional problems surrounding the death or illness of a pet. You might say to the client, "I know that you do not want to accept a referral for help, but I am so concerned about you that I will notify the police for assistance in getting you the help you need. I really do care about you and don't want anything bad to happen to you." Remember that extreme actions displayed by a client sometimes call for extreme reactions by the staff.

> **CRITICAL CONCEPT**
>
> Contact your local mental health department for assistance in compiling a list of mental health professionals and support groups.

REFERRING TO MENTAL HEALTH PROFESSIONALS

Clients experiencing intense anger, despair, and guilt often benefit from professional intervention outside of your office. Maintain a list of counselors and support groups for referral of clients experiencing grief associated with pet loss. A pet loss support group can provide a client with a safe place to express his or her feelings. It offers clients the opportunity to meet with like-minded pet owners with whom to share their fears, tears, memories and, finally, smiles.

When making referrals for group or individual counseling services, you might say something like, "I know you are very sad about Mitzi's ailing health. Here is some information about a support group for people who are struggling with the loss of a pet. This may help you sort out some of your feelings."

Your local mental health department can assist you in compiling a list of mental health professionals and support groups. The Delta Society in Bellevue, Washington (http://www.deltasociety.org) maintains a list of pet loss support counselors and groups throughout the country. It also can provide you with additional books and videotapes on grief counseling. Assembling a community referral file for your clients takes time and effort, but this special service conveys the hospital staff's concern for their safety and well-being.

RECOMMENDED READINGS

AVMA Guidelines on Veterinary Hospice Care. https://www.avma.org/KB/Policies/Pages/Guidelines-for-Veterinary-Hospice-Care.aspx

Bacal R: *Complete idiot's guide to dealing with difficult employees*, Madison, WI, 2000, CWL Publishing.

Fuller G: *The workplace survival guide*, Englewood Cliffs, NJ, 1996, Prentice Hall.

Griffin J, editor: *How to say it at work*, ed 2, New York, 2008, Prentice Hall.

Kübler-Ross E: *On death and dying*, New York, 1969, Collier Books.

Prendergast H, editor: *Front office management for the veterinary team*, ed 2, St Louis, 2014, Saunders.

Sirois M, editor: *Principles and practice of veterinary technology*, ed 3, St Louis, 2011, Elsevier.

3 Medical Terminology[1]

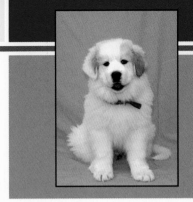

OUTLINE

Introduction to Word Parts, *58*
Prefix, *58*
Root Word, *58*
Combining Form, *58*
Combining Vowel, *58*
Combining Vowel Added to a Suffix, *58*
Compound Word, *58*
Using Word Parts to Form Words, *58*
Use of the Prefix, *58*
Suffix, *58*
Compound Word, *59*
Prefix and Suffix, *59*

Prefix, Root Word, and Suffix, *59*
Defining Medical Terms Using Word Analysis, *59*
Combining Forms for Body Parts and Anatomy, *59*
Suffixes and Prefixes, *61*
Suffixes for Surgical Procedures, *61*
Suffixes for Diseases or Conditions, *61*
Prefixes for Diseases or Conditions, *62*
Plural Endings, *62*
Suffixes for Instruments, Procedures, and Machines, *63*
Terms for Direction, Position, and Movement, *63*
Body Regions, *64*
Dental Terminology, *64*

LEARNING OBJECTIVES

After reviewing this chapter, the reader will be able to:

1. Construct medical terms from word parts.
2. Describe how to construct medical terms.
3. Define the meanings of common prefixes and suffixes used in medical terms.
4. Define terms used for common surgical procedures, diseases, instruments, procedures, and dentistry.
5. Describe anatomic terms for direction.

KEY TERMS

Buccal
Caudal
Combining form
Combining vowel
Compound word
Cranial
Distal

Dorsal
Lateral
Medial
Mesial
Oblique
Occlusal
Palmar

Peripheral
Plantar
Prefix
Proximal
Recumbent
Root word
Rostral

Sagittal
Suffix
Superficial
Supination
Transverse
Ventral

[1]Elsevier and the author acknowledge and appreciate the original contributions from Sirois M: Principles and practice of veterinary technology, ed 3, St Louis, 2011, Mosby, whose work forms the heart of this chapter.

Veterinary medical terminology is the "language" of the veterinary profession. This language is used in everyday speech, recorded in medical records, and used in journal articles and published textbooks for veterinary technicians and veterinarians. The most important goal of this chapter is to learn correct pronunciation and proper spelling of medical terms. Next, you will learn to memorize word parts and their meanings, and then you will be able to recognize and use medical words correctly. To assist with correct pronunciation, accented syllables are printed in UPPER CASE LETTERS. Syllables that are not accented are in lower case letters. In multisyllabic words with primary and secondary accents, the syllable with the primary accent is in **BOLDFACE UPPER CASE LETTERS**, and the syllable with the secondary accent is in UPPER CASE LETTERS. Unaccented syllables are in lower case letters. Words of one syllable are in lower case letters. Multisyllabic words, in which all syllables receive equal stress, are in lower case letters.

INTRODUCTION TO WORD PARTS

PREFIX

A **prefix** is a syllable, group of syllables, or word joined to the beginning of another word to alter its meaning or create a new word. The prefix may indicate position, time, amount, color, or direction to a root word. A prefix is not often used as a word alone unless a hyphen is inserted between it and the following word.

Example: *Pre-* is a prefix meaning "before, in space or in time." When joined to the root word *natal*, meaning "birth," the result becomes the medical word: *PREnatal*. Prenatal means "before birth." The prefix *pre* used alone means nothing to the reader.

ROOT WORD

A **root word** is the subject part of the word consisting of a syllable, group of syllables, or word that is the basis (or word base) for the meaning of the medical word.

Example: *CARdi-* is a root word meaning "heart." The root word used alone means nothing to the reader, as shown in the following example.

Example: The patient was diagnosed with *CARdi*. Now add the suffix *itis* (meaning "inflammation") to the end of the root word. The sentence begins to make sense with this addition. The patient was diagnosed with carDItis, or inflammation of the heart.

COMBINING FORM

A **combining form** is a word or root word that may or may not use the connecting vowel *o* when it is used as an element in a medical word formation. The combining form is the combination of the root word and the combining vowel. It is generally written in the following manner.

Example: CARdi/*o*: The combining form for the heart (root word plus combining vowel)

See combining vowel.

COMBINING VOWEL

A **combining vowel** is a vowel, usually an *o*, used to connect a word or root word to the appropriate suffix or to another root word.

COMBINING VOWEL ADDED TO A SUFFIX

A **suffix** is a syllable, a group of syllables, or a word added at the end of a root word to change its meaning, give it grammatical function, or form a new word. Suffixes normally do not stand alone as words. When they are used alone, a hyphen is used preceding and attached to the suffix.

Example: *-gram* is a suffix meaning "a recording by an instrument." A cardiogram is a recording of heart movement made by an instrument.

COMPOUND WORD

A **compound word** is two or more words or root words combined to make a new word.

Example: *Horse* and *fly* combine to form the word HORSE*fly*.

CRITICAL CONCEPT

Prefixes, root words, and suffixes can be combined to form medical terms.

USING WORD PARTS TO FORM WORDS

USE OF THE PREFIX

A prefix is attached to the beginning of a root word to form a new word.

Example: Prefix + root word = new word

Prefix	Root Word	Combined	Definition
de-	horn	DEhorn	To remove the horns
Semi-	PERmeable	semiPERmeable	Allowing only certain elements or liquids to pass through a membrane

SUFFIX

A suffix is attached to the end of a root word to form a new word.

Example: Root word + suffix = new word

Root Word	Suffix	Combined	Definition
TONsil	-itis	TONsillitis	Inflammation of the tonsils
THYroid	-ectomy	THYroidECtomy	Removal of the thyroid gland

COMPOUND WORD

Two words are joined together to form a new word.

Example: Root word 1 + root word 2 = new word

Word 1	Word 2	Combined	Definition
lock	jaw	LOCKjaw	Common name for the disease tetanus
blood	worms	BLOODworms	Worms (nematodes) that inhabit a main artery of the intestines in horses

There are certain rules peculiar to the use of combining forms and the combining vowel *o*. These rules are as follows.

- If a suffix begins with a consonant, use the combining vowel *o* with the root word (the combining form), to which the suffix will be added.

Example: *CARdi/o* (combining form for heart) plus the suffix *-megaly* (meaning "enlargement of") forms *CARdioMEGaly*, meaning "enlargement of the heart." Note that the combining vowel *o* is retained.

- Do not use the combining vowel *o* when a suffix begins with a vowel.

Example: *HEPat/o* (combining form for liver) plus the suffix *-osis* (meaning "a condition, disease, or morbid process") combine to form *HEPaTOsis*, meaning "a disease occurring in the liver." Note the combining vowel *o* is not used.

- If the suffix begins with the same vowel with which the combining form ends (minus the combining vowel *o*), do not repeat the vowel when forming the new word.

Example: *CARdi/o* minus *o* is *CARdi-*. *CARdi-* plus the suffix *-itis* (meaning "inflammation of") combines to form *carDItis*, meaning "inflammation of the heart." Note, as the rule states, that this word may have only a single *i* because the medical root word joins the suffix.

Combining Forms	Suffix	Combined	Definitions
cardi/o	-logy	CARdiOLogy	Study of heart diseases
mast/o	-itis	masTItis	Inflammation of the mammary glands

PREFIX AND SUFFIX

In this situation, no root word is used. The prefix is added directly to the suffix.

Prefix	Suffix	Combined	Definition
dys-	-uria	dysUria	Trouble urinating
POLy-	-phagia	POLyPHAgia	Eating to excess

PREFIX, ROOT WORD, AND SUFFIX

Words are formed by adding both the prefix and suffix to the root word.

Prefix	Root Word	Suffix	Combined	Definition
un-	sound	-ness	unSOUNDness	A form of physical dysfunction
PERi-	cardi-	-al	PERiCARdial	In the area surrounding the heart

DEFINING MEDICAL TERMS USING WORD ANALYSIS

Analyzing words teaches you to think logically and makes words easier to remember. The process of word analysis is the reverse of word construction. When analyzing a word, start at the end of the word (the suffix) and work toward the beginning (prefix). Analyze the components in sequence.

> **CRITICAL CONCEPT**
>
> Analyze medical terms by defining each word component in sequence starting at the suffix.

Example:
oVARioHYSterECtomy=
ovari/o/hyster/ectomy
4   3   2   1

1. The suffix *-ectomy* means to surgically remove.
2. The root word *hyster* refers to the uterus.
3. The *o* is the combining vowel for the previous root word.
4. The root word *ovari* refers to the ovaries.

Thus, *ovariohysterectomy* means "excision (surgical removal) of the uterus and ovaries." Note that steps 3 and 4 may be combined into one step, using the combining form *ovari/o*, which refers to the ovaries.

COMBINING FORMS FOR BODY PARTS AND ANATOMY

Following is a list of body parts and their respective combining forms. This is not a complete list of combining forms but represents some that are used often in veterinary terminology. To learn these words and their meaning requires memorization. Use handheld flash cards with the combining form on one side and the meaning or body part on the other.

Combining Form	Body Part
abdomin/o	abdomen
aden/o	gland
adren/o	adrenal gland
angi/o	vessel
arteri/o	artery
arthr/o	joint
atri/o	atrium
blephar/o	eyelid, eyelash
bronch/o	bronchus
cardi/o	heart
cephel/o	head
cerebell/o	cerebellum
cervic/o	cervix or neck of an organ
cheil/o	lip
chol/o, chole-	bile
cholecyst/o	gallbladder
chondr/o	cartilage
cili/o	eyelid, eyelash
col/o	colon
colp/o	vagina
cost/o	rib
crani/o	cranium, skull
cyst/o	bladder
cyt/o	cell
dactyl/o	digit, toe
dent/o	tooth, teeth
derm/o, dermat/o	skin
duoden/o	duodenum
encephal/o	brain
enter/o	intestines
epididym/o	epididymis
epis/o, episi/o	vulva
esophag/o	esophagus
faci/o	face
fibr/o	fibers
gastr/o	stomach
gingiv/o	gums
gloss/o	tongue
gnath/o	jaw
hem/o, hemat/o	blood
hepa-, hepat/o	liver
hist/o	tissue
hyster/o	uterus
ile/o	ileum (of intestine)
ili/o	ilium (of pelvis)

Combining Form	Body Part
jejun/o	jejunum
kerat/o	cornea or horny tissue
labi/o	lip
lapar/o	flank, abdomen
laryng/o	larynx
lip/o	fat
lymph/o	lymph
mast/o, mamm/o	mammary glands
mening/o	meninges
metr/o	uterus (special reference to inner lining)
muscul/o, my/o, myos-	muscle
myel/o	bone marrow or spinal cord
nephr/o	kidney, nephron
neur/o	nerve
occipit/o	back of head
ocul/o	eye
odont/o	tooth, teeth
onych/o	claw, hoof
ophthalm/o	eye
orchi/o, orchid/o	testes
or/o	mouth
oste/o, oss/eo, oss/i	bone
ot/o	ear
ovari/o	ovary
palat/o	palate
peritone/o	peritoneum
pharyng/o	pharynx
phleb/o	vein
pil/o	hair
pneum/o	lung, air, breath
pod/o	foot
proct/o	rectum
pulmo-, pulmon/o	lung
pyel/o	pelvis of kidney
rect/o	rectum
ren/o	renal (kidney)
rhin/o	nose
splen/o	spleen
spondyl/o	vertebra, spinal column
steth/o	chest
stomat/o	mouth
tars/o	ankle
ten/o, tend/o	tendon
thorac/o	thorax
thym/o	thymus gland
thyr/o, thyroid-	thyroid gland
tonsill/o	tonsil

Combining Form	Body Part
trache/o	trachea
trich/o	hair
tympan/o	tympanum (middle ear), tympanic membrane, eardrum
ureter/o	ureter
urethr/o	urethra
ur/o	urine
uter/o	uterus
vagin/o	vagina
vas/o	vessel or duct
ven/o	vein
ventricul/o	ventricle
vertebr/o	vertebra
vulv/o	Vulva

Remember, words for some body parts have more than one combining form. Examples from the previous list are the following:

mouth = or/o, stomat/o
teeth = dent/o, odont/o

There are no general rules for when one or the other is used. This must be learned by listening and reading to be aware of how these combining forms are used. You already know some of them. For example, you know that there is oral medication, not stomatal medication. Often, the different combining forms refer to a specific part of a structure or specific use of the structure. *Or/o* often refers to the mouth as the first part of the digestive system, whereas *stomat/o* refers to the lining of the oral cavity or the opening to the oral cavity (e.g., stomatitis, stomatoplasty).

SUFFIXES AND PREFIXES

SUFFIXES FOR SURGICAL PROCEDURES

Following is a list of suffixes for surgical procedures. Using the rules for word construction, you can form words to describe a variety of surgical procedures on various body parts or define these words using the word analysis technique previously described.

Suffix	Meaning	Example and Definition
-centesis	to puncture, perforate, or tap—permitting withdrawal of substances (e.g., fluid, air)	AbDOMinocenTEsis = surgical puncture of the abdomen to remove fluid from the peritoneal cavity
-ectomy	to excise or surgically remove	CHOLecysTECtomy = surgical removal of the gallbladder
-ize	use, subject to	AnEStheTIZE = subject to anesthesia
-pexy	fixation or suturing (a stabilizing type of repair)	GAStroPEXy = fixation of the stomach to the body wall

Suffix	Meaning	Example and Definition
-plasty	to shape, the surgical formation of, or plastic surgery (meaning "to improve function, to relieve pain, or for cosmetic reasons")	CHEIloPLASty = plastic repair of the lips (to improve looks and function)
-rrhaphy	to surgically repair by joining in a seam or by suturing together	HERniORRhaphy = surgical repair of a hernia
-stomy	to make a new, artificial opening in a hollow organ (to the outside of the body), or to make a new opening between two hollow organs	CoLOStomy = surgical creation of a new opening between the colon and the outside of the body GAStroDUodeNOStomy = to create a new opening between the stomach and the duodenum
-tomy	to incise or cut into (making an incision)	LAPaROTomy = surgical incision into the abdomen

SUFFIXES FOR DISEASES OR CONDITIONS

The same rules and procedures used to form and analyze surgical words can be used with suffixes that refer to diseases or conditions to describe a problem affecting a particular organ or body part. Following is a list of these suffixes:

Suffix	Meaning	Example and Definition
-algia	pain	MyALgia = muscular pain
-emesis	vomit	HemateMEsis = vomiting blood
-emia	blood condition	AnEmia = lack of blood
-esis, -iasis, -asis	infestation or infection with, a condition characterized by	ParEsis = partial paralysis Lithlasis = condition characterized by formation of calculi
-genesis	development, origin	CarCINoGENesis = development of cancer
-ism	a state or condition, a fact of being, result of a process	HyperCORtiSONism = condition resulting from excessive cortisone
-itis	inflammation of	TONsilltis = inflammation of the tonsils
-megaly	enlarged	HePAtoMEGaly = enlarged liver
-oma	tumor	LElomyOMa = tumor of smooth muscles
-osis	abnormal condition or process of degeneration	NePHROsis = degenerative disease of the kidneys
-path, -pathy	disease	pathogenic = disease causing
-penia	deficiency or lack of	LEUkoPENia = deficiency of white blood cells
-phage, -phagy	eating	COproPHAgy = eating feces

Suffix	Meaning	Example and Definition
-phobia	abnormal fear or intolerance of	PHOtoPHObia = intolerance of light
-plasia, -plastic, -plasty	forming, growing, changing	ANaPLAsia = changing structure of cells RHInoPLASty = surgical change to the nose
-pnea	breathing	DYSpnea = difficulty breathing
-rrhea	flow or discharge	DIarRHEa = discharge of feces

PREFIXES FOR DISEASES OR CONDITIONS

Following is a list of prefixes used to create words indicating a specific problem within the body or a body system:

Prefix	Meaning	Example and Definition
a-, an-	without or not having	aNEmia = not having enough red blood cells
anti-	against	AntibiOTic = drug that acts against bacteria
brachy-	short	BRAchycePHALic = short head
brady-	slow	BRAdyCARdia = excessively slow heart rate
cata-	down, under, lower, against	CaTAbolism = breaking down
contra-	against, opposed	CONtraINdiCAted = something that is not indicated
crypt/o	hidden	CryptORCHidism = hidden or undescended testis
de-	remove, take away, loss of	deHYdrated = excessive loss of body water
dis-	apart from, free from	DISinFECtion = to free from infection
dolich/o-	long	DOlichocePHALic = long head
dys-	difficult, painful, abnormal	DysPHAgia = difficulty eating or swallowing
e-, ec-, ex-	out of, from, away from	ecTOPic = out of place
eu-	normal, good, true, healthy	EUthanAsia = inducing death painlessly
glyc/o-, gluc/o-	sugar, sweet	HyperglycEMia = a condition of excessive sugar in the blood
hem/a-, hemat/o-, hem/o-	blood	HEmatURia = blood in the urine
hemi-	half	hemiPLEgia = paralysis of one side of the body
hydr/o-	water, fluid	HYdroCEPHalus = fluid in the brain

Prefix	Meaning	Example and Definition
hyper-	high, excessive	HYperTHERmia = body temperature higher than normal
hypo-	low, insufficient	HYpoTHYroidism = deficiency of thyroid activity
macro-	large	MAcrocyte = large cell
mal-	bad, poor	MALocCLUsion = poor fit of upper and lower teeth when jaws close
meg/a-, meg/alo-	large, oversized	MEgaCOLon = abnormally enlarged colon
micro-	small	MIcrophTHALmos = abnormally small eye
necr/o-	death	NEcropsy = examination of dead animal
neo-	new	NeoPLAStic = new tissue growth
olig/o-	few, little	OLigURia = scant urine production
pan-	all, entire	PanzoOtic = throughout an animal population
poly-	many, much	POLyPHAgia = excessive eating
pseudo-	false	PSEUdocyEsis = false pregnancy
py/o-	pus	PYoMEtra = pus in the uterus
tachy-	fast, rapid	TACHyCARdia = excessively fast heart rate
ur/e-, ur/ea-, ur/eo-, ur/in-, ur/ino, ur/o	urine or urea	GlucosURia = sugar in the urine UrEMia = urea in the blood

PLURAL ENDINGS

It is important to understand the methods for converting singular forms of medical words to their plural forms, and vice versa. Following is a list of common singular endings and their corresponding plural endings:

Singular	Plural	Example
-a	-ae	VERtebra, VERtebrae
-anx	-anges	PHAlanx, phaLANges
-en	-ina	LUmen, LUmina
-ex, -ix	-ices	Apex, Apices CERvix, CERvices
-is	-es	TEStis, TEStes
-inx	-inges	MENinx, meNINges
-ma	-mata or -mas	ENema, ENeMAta or ENemas
-um	-a	Ovum, Ova
-ur	-ora	FEMur, FEMora
-us	-i	Uterus, Uteri

SUFFIXES FOR INSTRUMENTS, PROCEDURES, AND MACHINES

Below is a list of suffixes that when added to a combining form of a body part, form a word pertaining to an instrument, procedure, or a machine that looks into, cuts, or measures a body part.

Suffix	Meaning	Example and Definition
-graph	Instrument or machine that writes or records	ELECtroCARdiograph = machine that records electrical impulses produced by the beating heart
-graphy	procedure of using an instrument or machine to record	ELECtroCARdiOGraphy = procedure of using an electrocardiograph to produce an electrocardiogram
-gram	product, written record, "picture," or graph produced	ELECtroCARdiogram (ECG, EKG) = graphic tracing of the electrical currents flowing through the beating heart
-meter	instrument or machine that measures or counts	TherMOmeter = instrument used to measure body temperature
-metry -imetry	procedure of measuring	doSIMetry = act of determining the amount, rate, and distribution of ionizing radiation
-scope	instrument for examining, viewing, or listening	OtoSCOPE = instrument for looking into the ears
-scopy	act of examining or using the scope	LAPaROScopy = procedure of using a laparoscope to view the abdominal cavity
-tome	instrument for cutting, such as into smaller or thinner sections	MicroTOME = instrument for cutting tissues into microthin slices or sections

TERMS FOR DIRECTION, POSITION, AND MOVEMENT

To describe the positions and relationships of body parts, topographic terms must be used. Common words such as up, down, front, back, top, and bottom are not useful because their meanings depend on the orientation of both the animal and the viewer. To be useful, the meanings of directional terms used to describe anatomy must be clear and independent of the body's position and the angle from which it is viewed.

Many directional terms come in pairs that mean they are opposite of each other. Most terms are relative terms that mean they are used in relation to other parts. Left and right always refer to the animal's left and right.

Anatomic terms of direction are used when describing locations of lesions on an animal's body and for positioning animals for radiography.

Following is a list of words used to describe direction or position of a body part relative to other body parts (Fig. 3-1).

abDUCtion: Movement of a limb or part away from the median line or middle of the body.

adDUCtion: Movement of a limb or part toward the median line or middle of the body.

adJAcent: Next to, adjoining, or close. **Example:** The tongue is adjacent to the teeth.

CAUdal: Pertaining to the tail end of the body, or denoting a position more toward the tail or rear of the body than another reference point (body part). **Example:** The tail is **caudal** to the head.

CENtral: Pertaining to or situated near the more proximal areas of the body or a structure; opposite of peripheral. **Example:** The spinal cord is central to the sciatic nerve.

CRAnial: Pertaining to the cranium or head end of the body, or denoting a position more toward the cranium or head end of the body than another reference point (body part). **Example:** The head is **cranial** to the tail.

deep: Situated away from the surface of the body or a structure; opposite of superficial. **Example:** The muscles are deep to the skin.

DIStal: Farther from the center of the body, relative to another body part or location on a body part relative to another closer location. **Example:** The tibia is **distal** to the femur.

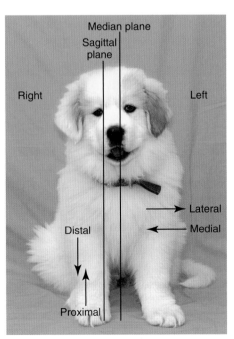

FIGURE 3-1 Anatomic planes and directional terms, dog. (From Colville, Joann, Sharon Oien. Clinical veterinary language, Mosby, 2014.)

DORsal: Pertaining to the back area of a quadruped (animal with four legs), or denoting a position more toward the spine than another reference point (body part). **Example:** The vertebral column is **dorsal** to the abdomen.

exTENsion: The act of straightening, such as a joint; also, the act of pulling two component parts apart to lengthen the whole part.

FLEXion: The act of bending, such as a joint.

LATeral: Denoting a position farther from the median plane of the body or a structure, on the side or toward the side away from the median plane, or pertaining to the side of the body or of a structure. **Example:** The **lateral** surface of the leg is the "outside" surface.

MEdial: Denoting a position closer to the median plane of the body or a structure, toward the middle or median plane, or pertaining to the middle or a position closer to the median plane of the body or a structure. **Example:** The **medial** surface of the leg is the "inside" surface.

obLIQUE: At an angle, or pertaining to an angle. **Example:** The vein crosses **obliquely** from the dorsal left side to the ventral right side.

PALmar: **Palmar** pertains to the caudal surface of the front foot distal to the antebrachiocarpal joint; also pertains to the undersurface of the front foot.

peRIPHeral: Pertaining to or situated near the periphery, the outermost part, or surface of an organ or part. **Example:** The enamel of a tooth is **peripheral** to the dentin and central root canal.

PLANtar: **Plantar** pertains to the caudal surface of the back foot distal to the tarsocrural joint; also pertains to the undersurface of the rear foot.

prone, proNAtion: Lying face down, in ventral recumbency. Pronation is the act of turning the body or a leg so the ventral aspect is down.

PROXimal: Nearer to the center of the body, relative to another body part, or a location on a body part relative to another, more distant, location. **Example:** The humerus is **proximal** to the radius.

reCUMbent: Lying down; a modifying term is needed to describe the surface on which the animal is lying. Example: An animal in dorsal recumbency is lying on its dorsum (back), face up (Fig. 3-2).

ROStral: Pertaining to the nose end of the head or body, or toward the nose. **Example:** The nose is **rostral** to the eyes.

SUperFIcial: Situated near the surface of the body or a structure; opposite of deep. **Example:** The skin is **superficial** to the muscles.

SUpine, SUpinNAtion: Lying face up, in dorsal recumbency. **Supination** is the act of turning the body or a leg so that the ventral aspect is uppermost.

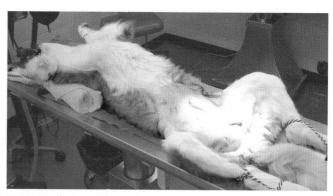

FIGURE 3-2 Dorsal recumbency. (From Colville TP, Bassert JM: Clinical anatomy and physiology laboratory manual for veterinary technicians, St Louis, 2009, Mosby.)

VENtral: Pertaining to the underside of a quadruped, or denoting a position more toward the abdomen than another reference point (body part). **Example:** The intestines are **ventral** to the vertebral column.

BODY REGIONS

Specific locations on an animal's body may sometimes be described using shortcut anatomic terms. For example, the term withers may be used to describe the area dorsal to the scapula. Some of these terms are used universally for all animals. For example, the withers is the withers on all animals. Other terms are used only for specific species. For example, pastern is a term that is used mainly for hoofed animals. This is the area where the leg angles forward, or the area right above the hoof. Table 3-1 lists the commonly used terms that you will have to know to correctly define the regions of an animal's body. Table 3-2 contains terms to describe larger body regions. Table 3-3 contains terms to describe specific animal species and life stages.

DENTAL TERMINOLOGY

The teeth have their own set of positional terms listed below (Fig. 3-3).

ocCLUsal: The chewing or biting surface of teeth; toward the plane between the mandibular and maxillary teeth.

BUccal: Toward the cheek; tooth surface toward the cheek.

LINGual: Pertaining to the tongue; tooth surface toward the tongue.

CONtact: Tooth surface facing an adjacent or opposing tooth.

MEsial: Tooth surface closest to the midline of the dental arcade.

TABLE 3-1	Animal Body Regions		
VETERINARY POSITION OR DIRECTION	**DEFINITION**	**EXAMPLE**	**COMPARABLE HUMAN TERM**
right and left	the animal's right side and left side		right and left
median plane	an imaginary plane that runs down the center of the body lengthwise and divides it into equal left and right halves		median plane
medial	toward the median plane		medial
lateral	away from the median plane		lateral
rostral	toward the tip of the nose when referring to the head		nasal
cranial	toward the head end of the body or in a direction toward the head		superior

Continued

TABLE 3-1	Animal Body Regions—cont'd		
VETERINARY POSITION OR DIRECTION	**DEFINITION**	**EXAMPLE**	**COMPARABLE HUMAN TERM**
	AND on the front of the forelegs above the carpus (the joint corresponding to the human wrist) and on the front of the back legs above the tarsus (the joint corresponding to the human ankle)		anterior
caudal	toward the tail end of the body or in a direction toward the tail		inferior
	AND on the back of the forelegs above the carpus (the joint corresponding to the human wrist) and on the back of the rear legs above the tarsus (the joint corresponding to the human ankle)		posterior
transverse plane	divides the body into cranial (front) and caudal (rear) parts		transverse plane
proximal	a position on a limb that is closer to the point of attachment to the body		proximal
distal	a position on a limb that is farther away from the point of attachment to the body		distal
dorsal	toward the animal's back		posterior

TABLE 3-1	Animal Body Regions—cont'd		
VETERINARY POSITION OR DIRECTION	**DEFINITION**	**EXAMPLE**	**COMPARABLE HUMAN TERM**
	AND the top/front surface of the forelimb distal to the carpus (the joint corresponding to the human wrist) and the top/front surface of the rear legs distal to the tarsus (the joint corresponding to the human ankle)		anterior or the top of the foot
ventral	toward the animal's belly		anterior
dorsal plane	runs lengthwise down the body and divides it into dorsal and ventral portions		frontal plane
palmar	the back of the forefeet distal to the carpus (the joint corresponding to the human wrist)		palmar, or the palm of the hand
plantar	the back of the rear feet distal to the tarsus (the joint corresponding to the human ankle)		plantar, or the bottom of the foot
superficial or external	toward the surface of the body or body part		superficial or external
deep or internal	toward the center of the body or body part		deep or internal
recumbency	lying down		lying down, reclining

Colville, Joann, Sharon Oien: Clinical veterinary language, St Louis, Mosby, 2014.

TABLE 3-2	Larger Body Region Terms
TERM	**MEANING**
Withers	The area dorsal to the shoulder blade (scapula)
Flank	The lateral side of the abdomen between the last rib and the hindlimb
Muzzle	The most rostral portion of the face
Tailhead	Dorsal surface where the tail joins the body
Stifle	Joint of the hindlimb that would be equivalent to the human knee
Hock	Joint of the hindlimb that would be equivalent to the human ankle
Carpus	Joint of the forelimb that would be equivalent to the human wrist
Axilla (axillary region)	Area of the forelimb equivalent to the human armpit
Inguinal region	Groin; site where the upper part of the hindlimb meets the abdomen

TABLE 3-3	Specific Animal Species and Life Stage Terms			
SPECIES	**COMMON NAME**	**FEMALE**	**MALE**	**OFFSPRING**
Canine	Dog	Bitch	Dog/stud	Pup
Feline	Cat	Queen	Tom	Kitten
Equine	Horse	Filly (intact female less than 4 yrs old) Mare (intact female over 4 yrs old)	Colt (intact male less than 4 yrs old) Stallion (intact male over 4 yrs old) Gelding (neutered male horse)	Foal (when gender is unknown) Weanling (young horse less than one year and already weaned)
Bovine	Cattle	Cow (intact female) Heifer (young female before her first calf)	Bull (intact male) Steer (neutered male)	Calf
Ovine	Sheep	Ewe	Ram (intact male) Wether (castrated male)	Lamb

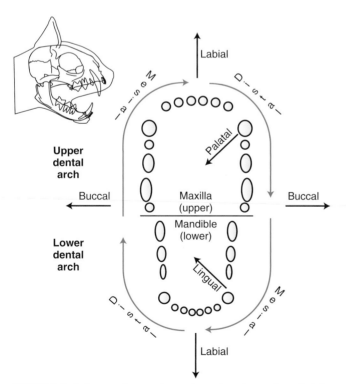

FIGURE 3-3 Positional terminology—the oral road map. (From Colville TP, Bassert JM: *Clinical anatomy and physiology laboratory manual for veterinary technicians*, St Louis, 2009, Mosby.)

RECOMMENDED READINGS

Christenson D: *Veterinary medical terminology*, ed 2, St Louis, 2008, Saunders.

Cohen BJ: *Medical terminology*, ed 5, Philadelphia, 2010, Lippincott.

Colville Joann, Sharon Oien: *Clinical veterinary language*, St Louis, 2014, Mosby.

Leonard PC: *Quick and easy medical terminology*, ed 6, St Louis, 2010, Saunders.

McBride DF: *Learning veterinary terminology*, ed 2, St Louis, 2002, Mosby.

Mosby: *2002 Mosby's medical, nursing & allied health dictionary*, ed 6, St Louis, 2002, Saunders.

Saunders veterinary terminology flash cards, St Louis, 2009, Saunders.

Shiland BJ: *Mastering health care terminology*, ed 3, St Louis, 2010, Mosby.

Sirois M: *Principles and practice of veterinary technology*, ed 3, St Louis, 2011, Elsevier.

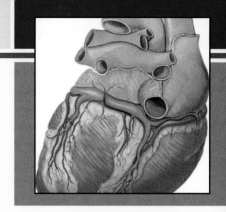

4

Anatomy and Physiology[1]

OUTLINE

Cells, 70
Epithelial Tissue, 70
Connective Tissue, 70
Skeleton, 73
Types of Bones, 73
Common Bone Features, 73
Axial Skeleton, 73
Appendicular Skeleton, 74
Visceral Skeleton, 76
Joints, 76
Integument, 76
Skin, 77
Hair, 78
Claws and Hooves, 79
Circulatory System, 79
Blood Vascular System, 79
Blood Circulation Pathways, 80
Role of White Blood Cells in Immunity, 81
Lymphatic System, 83
Respiratory System, 84
Upper Respiratory Tract, 84
Lower Respiratory Tract, 85
Respiratory Mechanisms, 85
Digestive System, 86
Mouth, 86
Esophagus, 87
Stomach, 87
Intestine, 87
Accessory Digestive Organs, 87

Nervous System, 88
Central Nervous System, 88
Peripheral Nervous System, 89
Autonomic Nervous System, 89
Muscular System, 90
Skeletal Muscle, 90
Cardiac Muscle, 90
Smooth Muscle, 90
Senses, 90
General Senses, 91
Special Senses, 92
Endocrine System, 94
Hypothalamus, 95
Pituitary Gland, 95
Thyroid Gland, 95
Parathyroid Glands, 95
Adrenal Glands, 96
Pancreas, 96
Gonads, 97
Urinary System, 97
Kidneys, 97
Ureters, 98
Urinary Bladder, 98
Urethra, 98
Reproductive System, 98
Male Reproductive System, 98
Female Reproductive System, 99

LEARNING OBJECTIVES

After reviewing this chapter, the reader will be able to:

1. Describe types of cells and tissues of the body.
2. List the names of organs and structures that make up the various body systems.
3. Describe the ways in which organs and body systems function and interact.
4. Describe the general and special senses of the body and their functions.
5. Differentiate between exocrine and endocrine glands.

[1]Elsevier and the author acknowledge and appreciate the original contributions from Sirois M: Principles and practice of veterinary technology, ed 3, St Louis, 2011, Mosby; and Colville T, Bassert JM: Clinical anatomy and physiology for veterinary technicians, ed 2, St Louis, 2008, Mosby, whose work forms the heart of this chapter.

KEY TERMS

Anatomy	Dental formula	Integument	Smooth muscle
Appendicular skeleton	Endocrine glands	Lymphatic system	Special senses
Autonomic nervous system	Endocrine system	Parturition	Tissues
Axial skeleton	Exocrine glands	Physiology	Urinary system
Cardiac cycle	General senses	Reproductive system	
Central nervous system	Gestation	Skeletal muscle	

Studying **anatomy** and **physiology** will help you better understand the wonderful machine that is the animal body. Anatomy is the study of normal structure of various body organs and their location. It tells about the basic similarities or differences within the species. Physiology, on the other hand, describes the mechanism and steps of how the body and its various components function. Although anatomy and physiology are two different sciences, studying them together gives a clearer picture of how the body is organized and how its various components function in a complex, interrelated fashion.

CELLS

Cells are the basic structural and functional units of life. All living things are composed of cells. An animal's body is composed of many different types of cells, each with its own place and function. Each cell relies on the rest of the body to meet its nutritional and waste elimination needs, and the whole body relies on the contribution of all of its cells for its support. This relationship can be summarized by the following formula:

Cell health ↔ tissue health ↔ organ health ↔
system health ↔ body health .

Note that the arrows point in both directions. The health of the cell depends on the health of the **tissues** of which it is part. In turn, the tissues depend on the health of the cells that make them up, and the organs that they are part of, and so on up the line. The degree of health at each level determines whether the body as a whole is healthy.

Unlike single-celled animals, complex (multicelled) organisms have specialized cells that allow the whole body to operate (Fig. 4-1). Groups of specialized cells make up tissues. Four basic types of tissues make up the animal body—epithelial tissue, connective tissue, muscle tissue, and nervous tissue. Functional groupings of tissues make up organs, such as the kidneys, that contain elements of all four basic tissues. Systems are groups of organs that are involved in a common activity. For example, the salivary glands, esophagus, stomach, pancreas, liver, and intestines are all parts of the digestive system.

EPITHELIAL TISSUE

Epithelial tissue covers the interior and exterior surfaces of the body, lines body cavities, and forms glands (Fig. 4-2).

Its function includes protection from physical wear and tear as well as penetration by foreign invaders, selective absorption of substances (e.g., by the intestinal lining), and secretion of various substances. All epithelial tissues share three common features:

- They consist entirely of cells.
- They do not contain blood vessels. Epithelial cells derive nourishment from blood vessels in the connective tissues beneath them.
- At least some epithelial cells are capable of reproducing. Epithelial tissue cells must be capable of compensating for wear and tear, as well as injuries.

> **CRITICAL CONCEPT**
>
> The four basic types of tissues are epithelial tissue, connective tissue, muscle tissue, and nervous tissue.

The covering and lining of epithelial tissue can be simple (one cell layer thick) or stratified (more than one cell layer thick) and can be composed of several different cell types. Simple epithelial tissues are in the kidney tubule and the lining of the blood vessels, intestines, and upper respiratory tract. Skin, ducts of sweat glands, and the lining of the urinary bladder are composed of stratified epithelial tissues.

Glandular epithelium cells are specialized cells that secrete substances directly into the bloodstream or out onto a body surface. The ductless glands that secrete directly into the bloodstream are the **endocrine glands** (e.g., pituitary gland, thyroid, testes, ovaries, adrenal gland). They produce hormones. **Exocrine glands** secrete substances through ducts. They can be simple, with a single duct (e.g., sweat glands), or compound, with a branching duct system (e.g., mammary glands).

CONNECTIVE TISSUE

Connective tissue holds the different tissues together and provides support. It contains fewer cells and more fibers than epithelial tissue. If the body consisted entirely of cells, it would lie like a puddle of gelatin on the ground. Cells are soft in consistency. Firmer connective tissue is necessary to support the cells and allow the body to assume an efficient shape and overall structure.

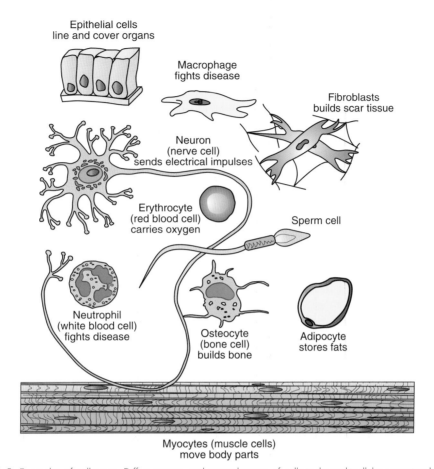

FIGURE 4-1 Examples of cell types. Differentiation and specialization of cells in the multicellular organism have led to a diverse array of cell types. The shape and size of the cell are related to its function. (From Colville TP: Clinical anatomy and physiology for veterinary technicians, ed 2, St Louis, 2008, Mosby.)

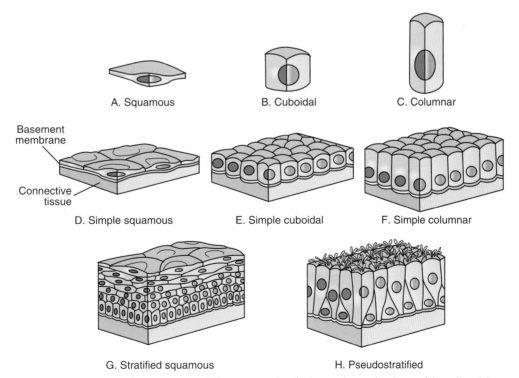

FIGURE 4-2 Classification of epithelia. Epithelial tissues are classified according to the shape of the cell and the way in which cells are arranged. Stratified epithelial tissues are composed of many layers of cells, and each layer of cells may have a different shape. In these cases, tissue is classified according to the shape of the cells on the surface, in the outermost layer. (From Colville TP: Clinical anatomy and physiology for veterinary technicians, ed 2, St Louis, 2008, Mosby.)

The cells of most connective tissues produce nonliving intercellular substances that connect and give support to other cells and tissues. These intercellular substances range from various types of fibers to the firm, mineralized matrix of bone.

Six main types of connective tissues are present in the body—adipose connective tissue, loose connective tissue, dense connective tissue, elastic connective tissue, cartilage, and bone. Blood is also a connective tissue; it will be discussed with the rest of the blood vascular system.

> ### CRITICAL CONCEPT
> Six main types of connective tissues are present in the body—adipose connective tissue, loose connective tissue, dense connective tissue, elastic connective tissue, cartilage, and bone. Blood is also a connective tissue.

Adipose connective tissue consists of collections of lipid-storing cells, what we commonly refer to as fat. It represents the body's storage supply of excess nutrients. When the dietary intake of nutrients exceeds the body's needs, adipose connective tissue proliferates. In leaner times, when the dietary nutrient intake is insufficient, the lipid stored in the adipose connective tissue can be mobilized to meet the body's nutritional needs.

Loose connective tissue is found throughout the body wherever cushioning and flexibility are needed. It is commonly found beneath the skin and around blood vessels, nerves, and muscles. Its main components are fiber-producing cells, fibroblasts, and three types of fibers (collagen fibers, reticular fibers, and elastic fibers). Collagen fibers are predominant and are strong to provide strength to the organs. Reticular fibers form a supportive framework. Elastic fibers are a minor component and provide some degree of elasticity. Both sets of fibers are intertwined in a loose mesh that provides cushioning and flexibility in almost all directions (Fig. 4-3).

Dense connective tissue has the same components as loose connective tissue but is much more densely packed. One variety of dense connective tissue has the fibers arranged in parallel bundles. This type of tissue is regularly arranged. It makes up tendons, which attach muscles to bones, and ligaments, which attach bones to other bones. The other type of tissue is irregularly arranged. It is like a densely compacted version of loose connective tissue. It is found in the capsules that surround and protect many soft internal organs.

Cartilage consists of a few cells, called chondrocytes, and various types and amounts of fibers embedded in a thick, gelatinous, intercellular substance, the matrix. Cartilage is firmer than fibrous tissue, but it is not as hard as bone and contains no blood vessels. Nutrients for chondrocytes must diffuse through the matrix from the periphery of the cartilage. This limits how thick cartilage can become. Hyaline cartilage is smooth and glossy in appearance. It contains more chondrocytes and a few collagen fibers. It is found in the tracheal rings and the articular (joint) surfaces of bones. Fibrous cartilage contains large numbers of densely arranged collagen fibers in its matrix and few chondrocytes, making it very durable. It makes up most of the intervertebral discs,

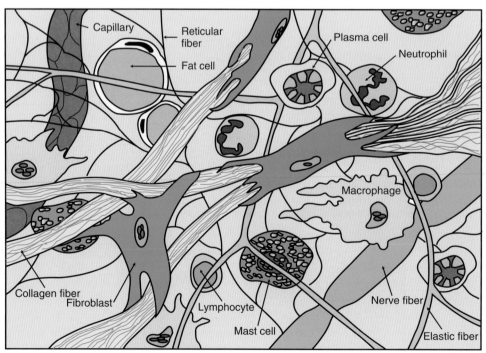

FIGURE 4-3 Loose connective tissue contains all three types of fibers (elastic, collagen, and reticular) and a wide variety of cells (lymphocytes, mast cells, neutrophils, fibroblasts, adipocytes, and plasma cells) suspended in ground substance. These three components—fibers, cells, and ground substance—are found in varying amounts in all connective tissue. (From Colville TP: Clinical anatomy and physiology for veterinary technicians, ed 2, St Louis, 2008, Mosby.)

which cushion the vertebrae. Elastic cartilage contains large numbers of elastic and collagen fibers, giving it more flexibility than the other two cartilage types. It makes up parts of the larynx and most of the ear flap (pinna).

Bone is second only to the enamel of teeth in its hardness. It is composed of a few cells, the osteocytes, embedded in a matrix that has become mineralized through a process called ossification. It is important to note that, despite its hard, dead appearance, bone is living tissue, with an excellent capacity for regeneration and remodeling.

SKELETON

The skeleton is the framework of bones that supports and protects the soft tissues of the body. Some bones, such as the bones of the skull, which enclose and protect the delicate brain, surround sensitive tissues. Most of the bones of the skeleton, however, form the scaffolding around which the rest of the body tissues are arranged. A variety of bone shapes are present in various locations in the body (Fig. 4-4).

TYPES OF BONES
LONG BONES
Long bones have two extremities (epiphyses) and a shaft (diaphysis). A small portion of long bone between the epiphysis and diaphysis at both ends is the metaphysis, which contains a hyaline cartilage or growth plate. It is the part where bone grows in length on both extremities. A long bone contains a medullary cavity filled with a bone marrow. Examples of long bones are the humerus, radius, ulna, metacarpals, femur, tibia, fibula, and metatarsals. Bone marrow contains the stem cells, which produce the blood cells. Bone marrow collection is valuable in the diagnosis of the diseases of blood, especially when blood shows abnormal cells.

FLAT BONES
Flat bones are expanded in two directions to provide maximum area for muscle attachment. Examples of flat bones are the scapula, skull bones, and pelvis.

SMALL BONES
Small bones are cuboidal or approximately equal in all dimensions; they are located at complex joints such as the carpus and hock joint. Examples of small bones are the carpal and tarsal bones.

IRREGULAR BONES
Irregular bones are bones with an irregular shape, such as the vertebrae.

SESAMOID BONES
Sesamoid bones are tiny bones found along the course of the tendons. These bones reduce friction and change the direction of a tendon. Examples of sesamoid bones are the patella and fabella. The patella, or kneecap, is the largest sesamoid bone.

PNEUMATIC BONES
Pneumatic bones contain air spaces to make the skeleton lighter. Most of the bones of a bird's skeleton are pneumatic bones.

COMMON BONE FEATURES
- An articular surface is a surface in which a bone forms a joint with another bone. It is usually smooth and is often covered with a layer of hyaline cartilage.
- A condyle is a large, convex, articular surface usually found on the distal ends of the long bones that make up the limbs.
- A foramen is a hole in a bone through which blood vessels and nerves usually pass.
- A fossa is a depression in a bone usually occupied by a muscle or tendon.
- A facet is a flat and smooth articular area, such as the surface of a tarsal or carpal bone.
- A bone head is a spherical articular projection usually found on the proximal ends of some limb bones.
- The neck of a bone is the often-narrowed area that connects a bone head with the rest of the bone.
- A process, tuber, tubercle, tuberosity, or trochanter is a lump or bump on the surface of a bone. It is usually the site where the tendon of a muscle attaches to a bone. The larger the process, the more powerful the muscle that attaches at the site.

AXIAL SKELETON
The **axial skeleton** is composed of the bones located on the axis or midline of the body. It is composed of the bones of the skull, spinal column, ribs, and sternum (Fig. 4-5).

> *CRITICAL CONCEPT*
> The axial skeleton is composed of the bones of the skull, spinal column, ribs, and sternum.

The skull is composed of many bones, most of which are held together by immovable joints called sutures. The skull bones can be divided into the bones of the cranium and the bones of the face, which extend in a rostral direction from the cranium. The bones of the cranium house and protect the brain, and the bones of the face house mainly digestive and respiratory structures.

The spinal column is composed of a series of individual bones called vertebrae. The vertebrae form a long, flexible tube called the vertebral canal. The vertebral canal houses and protects the spinal cord. The vertebrae are divided into five groups, and each vertebra is numbered within each group from cranial to caudal. The cervical vertebrae (C) are in the neck region. The first cervical vertebra (C1) is the atlas that forms a joint with the skull. The thoracic vertebrae (T) are dorsal to the chest region and form joints with the dorsal ends of the ribs. The lumbar vertebrae (L), which are dorsal to the abdominal region, are fairly large and heavy because they serve as the site of attachment for the large sling muscles that support the abdomen.

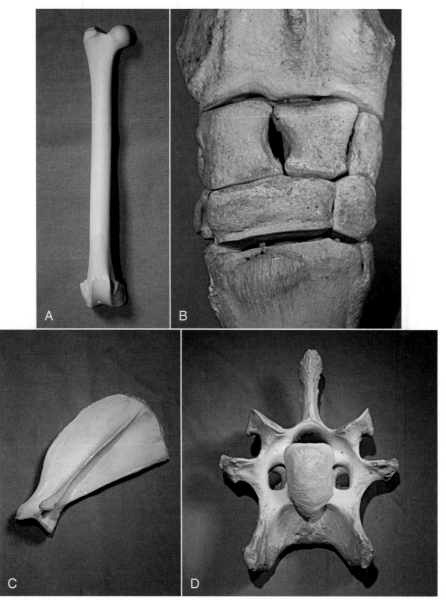

FIGURE 4-4 Bone shapes. **A,** Long bone, feline femur. **B,** Short bones, equine carpus. **C,** Flat bone, canine scapula. **D,** Irregular bone, bovine cervical vertebra. (From Colville TP: Clinical anatomy and physiology for veterinary technicians, ed 2, St Louis, 2008, Mosby.)

The sacral vertebrae (S) in the pelvic region are fused together into a solid structure called the sacrum, which forms a joint with the pelvis. The caudalmost vertebrae, the coccygeal vertebrae (Cy), form the tail. The number of vertebrae in each region varies with species (Table 4-1).

The ribs support and help form the lateral walls of the thorax or chest. Their number varies with the species, but the number of rib pairs is usually the same as the number of thoracic vertebrae. They form joints with the thoracic vertebrae dorsally and are continued ventrally by rods of hyaline cartilage, the costal cartilages. The costal cartilages of ribs at the cranial end of the thorax are connected directly to the sternum at their ventral end. The costal cartilages of the caudal ribs do not reach the sternum; they connect to the costal cartilage cranial to them. The spaces between ribs are referred to as intercostal spaces.

The sternum forms the ventral portion of the thorax. It is composed of a series of rodlike bones called sternebrae. The manubrium sterni is the first (cranialmost) sternebra, and the xiphoid process is the last (caudalmost). These two bones are often used as external landmarks on the animal.

APPENDICULAR SKELETON

The **appendicular skeleton** is composed of the bones of the limbs (Table 4-2). The forelimb is referred to anatomically as the thoracic limb and the hindlimb is called the pelvic limb.

CRITICAL CONCEPT

The forelimb is referred to anatomically as the thoracic limb, and the hindlimb is called the pelvic limb.

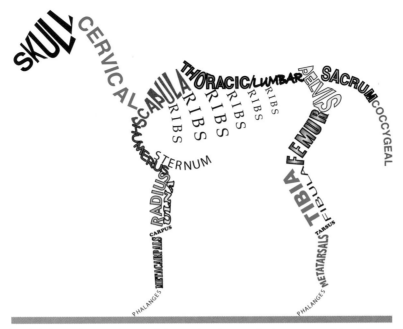

FIGURE 4-5 Word skeleton, the main bones of the axial and appendicular portions of the skeleton. (From Colville TP: Clinical anatomy and physiology for veterinary technicians, ed 2, St Louis, 2008, Mosby.)

TABLE 4-1	Vertebral Formulas for Some Common Species				
SPECIES	**CERVICAL**	**THORACIC**	**LUMBAR**	**SACRAL**	**COCCYGEAL**
Cat	7	13	7	3	5-23
Cattle	7	13	6	5	18-20
Dog	7	13	7	3	20-23
Goat	7	13	7	5	16-18
Horse	7	18	6	5	15-21
Human	7	12	5	5	4-5
Pig	7	14-15	6-7	4	20-23
Sheep	7	13	6-7	4	16-18

From Colville TP: Clinical anatomy and physiology for veterinary technicians, ed 2, St Louis, 2008, Mosby.

TABLE 4-2	Bones of the Limbs (Proximal to Distal)
THORACIC LIMB	**PELVIC LIMB**
Scapula	Pelvis
	Ilium
	Ischium
	Pubis
Humerus	Femur
Radius	Tibia
Ulna	Fibula
Carpal bone (carpus)	Tarsal bones (tarsus)
Metacarpal bones	Metatarsal bones
Phalanges	Phalanges

From Colville TP: Clinical anatomy and physiology for veterinary technicians, ed 2, St Louis, 2008, Mosby.

From proximal to distal, the bones of the thoracic limb are the scapula, humerus, radius and ulna, carpal bones, metacarpal bones, and phalanges. The scapula is the shoulder blade. It is a flat bone with a shelflike spine on its lateral surface. At its distal end, it has a shallow cavity called the glenoid cavity that forms the shoulder joint with the humerus, the long bone of the brachium or upper arm. The proximal end of the humerus is composed of the head, a smooth articular surface that forms the shoulder joint with the scapula, and the greater tubercle, where the powerful shoulder muscles attach. The distal joint surfaces of the humerus, the condyles, form the elbow joint with the radius and ulna, the bones of the antebrachium or forearm.

The radius is the main weight-bearing bone of the antebrachium, and the ulna forms much of the snug-fitting elbow joint with the condyle of the humerus. At the proximal end of the ulna is the olecranon process, the point of the elbow where the powerful triceps brachii muscle attaches.

In animals such as cows and horses, the radius and ulna are fused together.

Located between the radius and ulna and the metacarpal bones is the carpus. It is composed of two rows of short bones and is equivalent to the human wrist. Just distal to the carpus are the metacarpal bones, equivalent to the bones of the human hand between the wrist and fingers. The phalanges are the bones of the digits, equivalent to human fingers. Dogs and cats have five digits (toes) in each forelimb. Each digit is composed of two phalanges (proximal and distal), as in the human thumb, or three phalanges (proximal, middle, and distal), as in human fingers.

The bones of the pelvic limb, from proximal to distal, are the pelvis, femur, patella, tibia and fibula, tarsal bones, metatarsal bones, and phalanges. The pelvis is composed of three pairs of bones that are fused in the adult animal, the ilium, ischium, and pubis. The cranial part of the ilium is the iliac crest, which is one of the sites to aspirate bone marrow. At the junction of the three bones on each side is a deep cavity, the acetabulum, which is the socket portion of the ball and socket hip joint.

The femur is the long bone of the thigh region. The head of the femur forms the ball portion of the hip joint and the greater trochanter is the site of attachment for the powerful gluteal (rump) muscles. At its distal end are the condyles, which form the stifle joint with the tibia, and the trochlear groove, in which the patella rides.

The patella, or kneecap, is the largest sesamoid bone in the body. Sesamoid bones are located in tendons that change direction sharply at joints. The patella helps distribute the force of the quadriceps femoris muscle, the main extensor muscle of the stifle joint.

The tibia is the main weight-bearing bone of the distal leg. The fibula is thin and runs along the entire length of the tibia in dogs and cats. In other species, such as cows and horses, the fibula is a small, sometimes incomplete bone that is primarily a site of muscle attachment.

The tarsus is equivalent to the human ankle and consists of two rows of short bones. The tuberosity of the large calcaneus or fibular tarsal forms the point of the hock joint, equivalent to the human heel bone. The metatarsal bones and phalanges of the pelvic limb are similar to the metacarpal bones and phalanges of the thoracic limb.

VISCERAL SKELETON

The bones of the visceral skeleton, when present, occur in soft tissues of the body. The os penis of the dog is a well-developed bone in the penis.

JOINTS

Bones come together at the joints. Our usual image of joints is that of freely movable joints, such as the elbow or hip. However, joints can be any of three main types; fibrous joints are immovable, cartilaginous joints are slightly movable, and diarthrodial or synovial joints are freely movable.

> ### CRITICAL CONCEPT
> Joints are classified as one of three main types—fibrous joints, cartilaginous joints, and diarthrodial or synovial joints.

Fibrous joints hold bones together but do not allow movement at the joint site. The sutures that hold many of the skull bones together are immovable joints.

Cartilaginous joints allow a slight rocking movement. The cartilaginous intervertebral discs and the symphysis that unites the pubic bones of the pelvis allow a slight amount of movement.

Synovial joints are what people usually think of when they think of joints. They allow free movement between bones in several directions. Synovial joints usually have smooth articular surfaces covered by articular cartilage and a fibrous joint capsule. The inner side of the joint capsule is lined by synovial membrane, which secretes the oily synovial fluid

that covers and protects the articular cartilages from wearing against each other. The normal synovial fluid is clear, sticky, slippery, and viscous. When the joint is inflamed, the fluid becomes thin and less slippery and can no longer protect the cartilage. Many joints also have fibrous ligaments that hold bones together. Most ligaments are extracapsular (located outside the fibrous joint capsule), such as collateral ligaments. Some ligaments are intracapsular (located inside the joint cavity), such as cruciate ligaments, which connect the distal end of the femur to the proximal end of the tibia.

Synovial joints allow some combination of six potential joint movements (Figs. 4-6 and 4-7): flexion, extension, adduction, abduction, rotation, and circumduction. Flexion decreases the angle between two bones; extension increases the angle. Adduction moves the extremity toward the median plane, and abduction moves it away from the median plane. Rotation is a twisting movement of a part on its own axis. The shaking of the head of a wet dog is a rotation movement. Circumduction is a movement in which the distal end of an extremity describes a circle.

INTEGUMENT

The **integument** is the outer covering of the body. It consists primarily of the skin, hair, claws or hooves, and horns. In nonmammalian species it also includes such

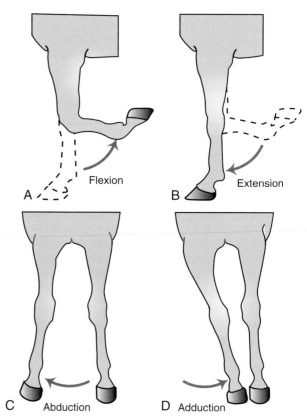

FIGURE 4-6 *Movements of equine front leg.* **A,** *Flexion, lateral view.* **B,** *Extension, lateral view.* **C,** *Abduction, cranial view.* **D,** *Adduction, cranial view.* (From Colville TP: Clinical anatomy and physiology for veterinary technicians, ed 2, St Louis, 2008, Mosby.)

structures as feathers and scales (Fig. 4-8). In addition to its obvious protective role, the integument has several other important functions. Its multitude of sensory receptors makes it one of the most important parts of an animal's sensory system. The integument also helps in regulating body temperature through its ability to adjust blood flow to the skin, adjust the position of hairs, and secrete sweat. The integument also produces vitamin D and secretes and

excretes a number of substances through various types of skin glands.

SKIN

The skin is the largest body organ. It consists of two main layers, the superficial epithelial layer (epidermis) and the deep connective tissue layer (dermis).

The epidermis is composed of keratinized, stratified squamous epithelium (Fig. 4-9). The surface layer of the epidermis dries out and is converted to a tough horny substance called keratin, which also makes up the bulk of hair, claws, hooves, and horns (antlers).

Within the deepest layers of the epidermis of most animals are melanocytes, cells that produce granules of the dark pigment melanin. This pigment gives color to the skin, hair, and other integumentary structures. An albino animal has a total lack of melanin, resulting in pale white skin and hair and unpigmented irises in the eyes.

The dermis layer of skin is composed of collagen, elastic, and reticular fibers. It contains hair follicles, sebaceous glands, sudoriferous glands, and arrector pili muscles. In addition, this layer also contains various sensitive nerve endings and blood vessels. The sebaceous glands are the oil glands of the skin. They secrete oily sebum, which helps waterproof the skin and keep it soft and pliable. Sebum is secreted directly onto the shafts of hairs in the hair follicles. Sudoriferous glands are the sweat glands, which primarily help cool the body. Some animals, such as horses, have sudoriferous glands spread over their entire body. Others, such as dogs and cats, have only a few, clustered in the footpad and nose areas.

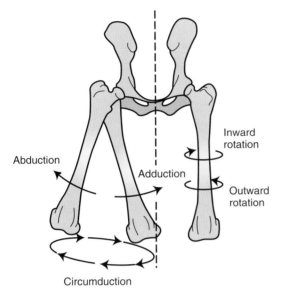

FIGURE 4-7 Movements of canine femurs, cranial view. (From Colville TP: Clinical anatomy and physiology for veterinary technicians, ed 2, St Louis, 2008, Mosby.)

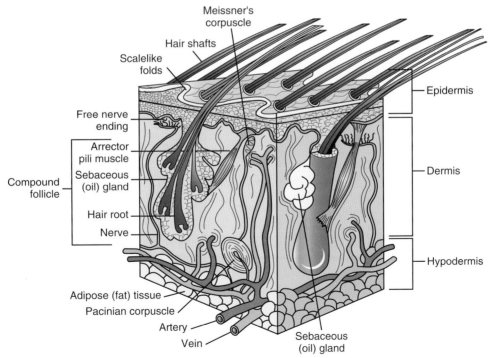

FIGURE 4-8 Cubed section of canine skin and underlying subcutaneous tissue. Note that the epidermis of canine skin includes folds from which compound hairs arise. (From Colville TP: Clinical anatomy and physiology for veterinary technicians, ed 2, St Louis, 2008, Mosby.)

The hypodermis or subcutis is a layer of loose connective tissue just below the dermis, which connects the skin to underlying muscles. It also contains some fat cells. The subcutaneous injection is administered into this layer by lifting a fold of skin.

CRITICAL CONCEPT

The skin consists of two main layers, the superficial epithelial layer (epidermis), and the deep connective tissue layer (dermis).

HAIR

Hair covers most of the body surface of most animals. Hair is composed of densely compacted keratinized cells produced in glandlike structures called hair follicles. Hairs are constantly shed and replaced. The visible part of each hair is referred to as the hair shaft. The portion within the skin is called the hair root. The color of hair results from the granules of melanin that are incorporated into the hairs during the course of their development. At the base of some hair roots, a tiny muscle is attached, the arrector pili muscle. When it

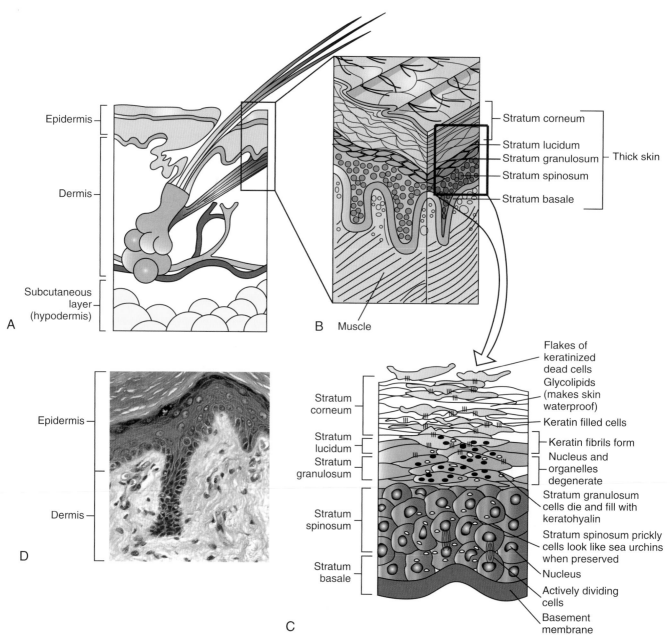

FIGURE 4-9 Layers of epidermis. **A,** Epidermis is the outermost layer of skin. **B,** Thick regions of skin are composed of five layers, whereas thinner regions may contain only three. **C,** Layers of the epidermis. Skin cells actively divide in the stratum basale, where they are supplied with nutrients from blood vessels in the dermis immediately below it. As new cells are produced, older ones are pushed into more superficial layers. By the time they arrive at the skin's surface, they have become little more than thin flakes of keratin. **D,** Light photomicrograph of integument. (From Colville TP: Clinical anatomy and physiology for veterinary technicians, ed 2, St Louis, 2008, Mosby.)

contracts, it pulls the hair into a more upright position. This produces what is called goosebumps or raised hackles. The purpose of erecting the hair generally is to retain heat when an animal is cold by fluffing up the hair coat or to make the animal look larger and more fearsome as a part of the sympathetic nervous system fight-or-flight response.

CLAWS AND HOOVES

Claws and hooves are horny structures that cover the distal ends of the digits. They are composed of parallel bundles of keratinized cells organized into an outer wall and a bottom sole.

CIRCULATORY SYSTEM

The circulatory system is primarily a transport system in the body. It transports a variety of substances throughout the body, such as cells, antibodies, nutrients, oxygen, carbon dioxide, metabolic wastes, and hormones. Its two main divisions are the blood vascular system and lymphatic system.

BLOOD VASCULAR SYSTEM

The blood vascular system consists of a closed system of tubes through which a fluid connective tissue is propelled by a muscular pump. The fluid connective tissue is blood, the tubes are blood vessels, and the pump is the heart (Fig. 4-10).

There are three types of blood vessels—arteries, capillaries, and veins. Arteries carry blood away from the heart to the capillaries. Arteries are large near the heart and gradually branch into smaller and smaller vessels as they course throughout the body. From the arteries blood passes into the extensive networks of tiny capillaries located throughout the body.

Capillaries are porous, composed of a single layer of endothelium, and permit substances to move freely between the extracellular fluid (fluid surrounding cells) and blood. The basic purpose of most of the blood vascular system is to deliver blood to the capillaries, where nutrients, waste products, gases, hormones, and other substances can be exchanged. Substances such as oxygen (O_2) and nutrients move out of the blood and into the cells. Metabolic wastes

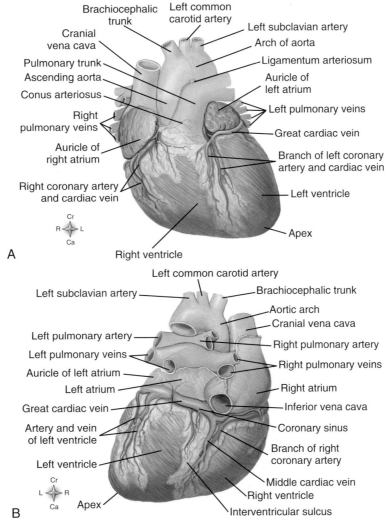

FIGURE 4-10 Heart and great vessels. **A,** Ventral view. **B,** Dorsal view. (From Colville TP: Clinical anatomy and physiology for veterinary technicians, ed 2, St Louis, 2008, Mosby.)

and carbon dioxide (CO_2) move out of the cells and into the blood. From the capillaries the CO_2-laden, waste-filled blood passes first into small venules and then into veins for the return trip to the heart. Many veins contain tiny one-way valves along their length. These one-way valves, assisted by movement of muscles in the area, help propel the blood back toward the heart.

BLOOD CIRCULATION PATHWAYS

SYSTEMIC CIRCULATION

During systemic circulation, blood moves from the heart to the body tissues and back to the heart. The aorta (the largest and main artery) originates from the left ventricle of the heart and carries oxygenated blood to various body tissues. The veins take the blood back to the heart and to the cranial and caudal venae cavae, which open into the right atrium of the heart.

PULMONARY CIRCULATION

During pulmonary circulation, blood moves from the heart to the lungs and back to the heart again. The pulmonary artery carries CO_2-rich blood from the right ventricle of the heart to the lungs for purification (oxygenation). The pulmonary veins bring oxygenated blood from the lungs to the left atrium of heart.

HEART

The heart is a muscular two-way pump that propels blood around the body and receives it back. It consists of dense accumulations of cardiac muscle cells and connective tissue organized into two side by side pumps that together are composed of four chambers (two atria and two ventricles) and four one-way valves.

The heart has four chambers, two atria (right and left atrium) and two ventricles (right and left ventricles):

- Right atrium: The right atrium lies just above the right ventricle and receives CO_2-rich blood from cranial and caudal venae cavae.
- Left atrium: The left atrium lies just above the left ventricle and receives oxygenated blood from the pulmonary veins. It is separated from the right atrium by an interatrial septum.
- Right ventricle: The right ventricle receives blood from the right atrium through the right atrioventricular opening (AV opening), which is guarded by a tricuspid valve. The pulmonary artery originates from the right ventricle, and its opening is guarded by pulmonary semilunar valves.
- Left ventricle: The left ventricle receives blood from the left atrium through the left atrioventricular opening, which is guarded by a bicuspid valve or mitral valve. The aorta originates from the left ventricle, and its opening is guarded by aortic semilunar valves.

CARDIAC CYCLE

The **cardiac cycle** refers to the series of events happening during one heartbeat. It includes the relaxation of the heart

chambers (diastole) to receive the blood and contraction of the heart chambers (systole) to pump the blood into body tissues and lungs (Fig. 4-11).

The receiving chamber of the right side of the heart is the right atrium. Blood flows into it from the venae cavae, the large systemic veins. When the right atrium contracts, it pumps blood through a large one-way valve, the tricuspid valve, into the right ventricle. The tricuspid valve gets its name from its three flaps, or cusps. When the right ventricle contracts, the tricuspid valve closes and blood flows out through the one-way pulmonary valve into the pulmonary artery, which carries blood to the lungs. When the right ventricular contraction is complete, the pulmonary valve closes, preventing blood from flowing back into the right ventricle.

The dynamics are similar on the left side of the heart. Blood flows into the left atrium from the pulmonary veins. When the left atrium contracts, it pumps blood through the mitral valve into the left ventricle. The mitral valve is named for the resemblance (in an ancient anatomist's eye) of its two cusps to the miter worn by bishops. When the left ventricle contracts,

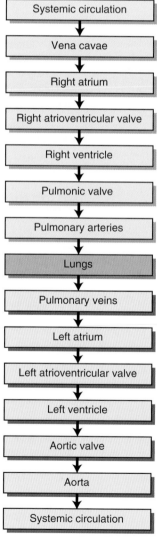

FIGURE 4-11 Adult blood flow summary. (From Christenson DE: Veterinary medical terminology, ed 2, St Louis, 2007, Saunders.)

the mitral valve closes and blood flows out through the aortic valve into the aorta, the beginning of systemic circulation. When left ventricular contraction is complete, the aortic valve closes to prevent the flow of blood back into the ventricle.

Specialized areas and bundles of cardiac muscle cells initiate each heartbeat, but the rate of heartbeat is controlled by the **autonomic nervous system**. By its nature, cardiac muscle contracts without needing external stimuli, but the activity of the many millions of individual cardiac muscle cells must be coordinated for the heart to contract in an organized, efficient manner.

BLOOD

Blood is a specialized connective tissue composed of fluid and cellular portions. The fluid portion is plasma and the cellular portion is composed of red blood cells, white blood cells, and platelets (Fig. 4-12).

Plasma is composed of 91% water, 7% protein molecules, and 2% other substances and electrolytes. It serves to suspend the blood cells and dissolve the many substances that are transported in the blood. If removed from blood vessels, plasma clots. Fibrinogen is one of the proteins in plasma. Fibrinogen is converted through a complex series of steps to strands of fibrin. The fibrin strands form a meshwork that traps the rest of the cellular components and forms what is recognized as a blood clot. This blood-clotting process serves to obstruct leaking blood vessels temporarily and minimize blood loss caused by injury.

Red blood cells (RBCs), also called erythrocytes, are the most numerous of the blood cells, typically numbering in the millions per microliter of blood. In mammalian species RBCs do not normally contain a nucleus and are shaped like biconcave discs resembling tiny pillows. In birds, reptiles, and fish, they are normally nucleated and elliptical. The protein hemoglobin, which gives erythrocytes their red color, also gives them the ability to carry large amounts of O_2 to the body's cells.

White blood cells (WBCs), also called leukocytes, typically number in the tens of thousands per microliter of blood. They are divided into granulocytes (neutrophils, eosinophils, and basophils) and agranulocytes (lymphocytes and monocytes). Granulocytes have stainable granules in their cytoplasm; agranulocytes lack cytoplasmic granules.

ROLE OF WHITE BLOOD CELLS IN IMMUNITY

Each of the white blood cells (leukocytes) has a specific role within the immune system. Most mammals have two types of white blood cells, granulocytes and agranulocytes.

GRANULOCYTES

Granulocytes play a role in the natural defenses and adaptive defenses. Both eosinophils and basophils are involved in the

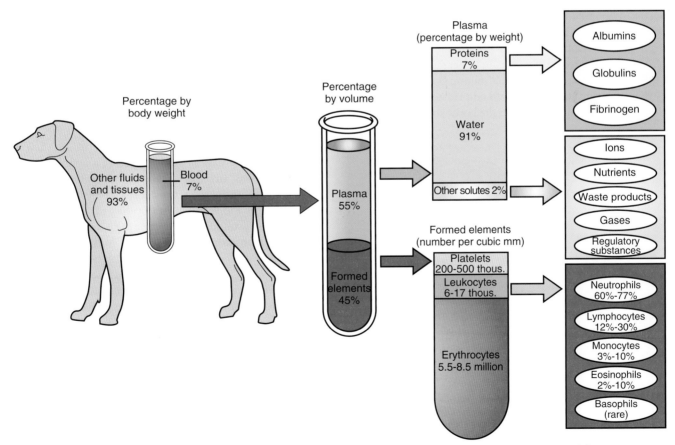

FIGURE 4-12 Composition of blood. Values are approximate for blood components in normal adult dogs. (From Colville TP: Clinical anatomy and physiology for veterinary technicians, ed 2, St Louis, 2008, Mosby.)

inflammatory response generated when an antigen invades the body. Eosinophils and basophils release specific chemicals to help activate other aspects of the immune system. Neutrophils also play a major role in the immune response. The respiratory, digestive, and **urinary systems** contain groups of neutrophils, referred to as resident neutrophils, that act as scavengers and function to phagocytize foreign substances. Phagocytosis literally means "cell-eating." The neutrophils engulf the antigen and then release chemicals that damage the foreign agent (Fig. 4-13). This phagocytic activity is part of the natural defenses. When these defenses are incapable of fully neutralizing the antigen, the neutrophils become active within the adaptive defenses. Specific neutrophils function in the adaptive defenses by processing the antigen and presenting it to a cell that is capable of triggering the cascade of reactions that results in antibody formation. Antigen processing is a complex process that results in exposure of the surface marker protein on the antigen. This allows for recognition of the antigen as a foreign substance. The neutrophil then interacts with another cell that will respond by triggering additional parts of the adaptive defenses.

AGRANULOCYTES

Monocytes and lymphocytes each have unique roles within the immune system. Monocytes act in a manner similar to phagocytic neutrophils. They are often referred to as tissue macrophages and are capable of phagocytosis and antigen processing and presentation. Lymphocytes are the primary cellular components of the antibody-producing systems. Specific subpopulations or subgroups of lymphocytes each play a specific role in this process. These subgroups are referred to as T lymphocytes and B lymphocytes. Although there are no apparent differences in appearance of the cells in different subgroups, they are biochemically and functionally diverse groups that are derived and matured in different ways and in different locations in the body.

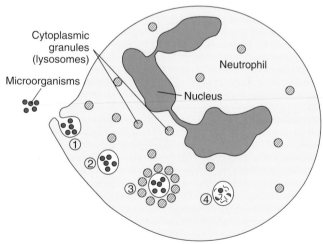

FIGURE 4-13 Phagocytosis and destruction of microorganisms. 1, Neutrophil membrane engulfs microorganisms. 2, Phagocytic vacuole is formed. 3, Cytoplasmic granules (lysosomes) line up around phagocytic vacuole and empty their digestive enzymes into the vacuole. 4, Microorganisms are destroyed. (From Colville TP: Clinical anatomy and physiology for veterinary technicians, ed 2, St Louis, 2008, Mosby.)

T lymphocytes are involved in assisting in full activation of B lymphocytes, although B lymphocytes can be activated without this interaction. B lymphocytes are responsible for the creation and secretion of antibody that is specific for a certain antigen. The process is triggered when an antigen-presenting cell (e.g., macrophage, neutrophil) presents an antigen to a B lymphocyte. That specific B lymphocyte is then sensitized to that particular antigen and begins to synthesize and release antibody. B lymphocytes have an additional capability of memory. As B lymphocytes are maturing, they develop with the capability of producing antibody against a specific antigen that has been presented to them during their maturation. When an antigen that has been previously encountered by a B lymphocyte is encountered again, the B lymphocyte is able to respond more quickly and begin producing antibody almost immediately. The production of a specific antibody is referred to as humoral immunity because the antibody is secreted into the body fluids, or humors. T lymphocytes, in addition to their role in the activation of B lymphocytes, are also capable of direct attack on antigens. This is referred to as cellular immunity.

ANTIBODIES

The production of a specific antibody is a critical part of the immune system response. Antibodies are protein molecules produced by a certain subgroup of B lymphocytes when they are presented with a substance that is recognized as foreign (the antigen).

Antibodies are also referred to as immunoglobulins and are present in several forms in the body. Each type is responsible for a specific activity within the immune system. The five types of antibodies are referred to by the abbreviation Ig, for immunoglobulin, followed by a letter that designates the type of antibody (Fig. 4-14). The five types of antibodies found in most mammalian organisms are IgG, IgM, IgA, IgD, and IgE.

Each antibody is produced at a specific time in the immune system response. Some are also produced when certain types of antigens are involved (e.g., parasites). An immunoassay is any test that uses interactions between antibody and antigen to produce a result. Commercial production of monoclonal antibodies to many different antigens has resulted in a variety of test kits for use in the veterinary laboratory. These specific antibodies to many different antigens can be produced and used in the laboratory for rapid identification of disease-producing organisms. In general, these tests are easy to perform, take minimal time, and are relatively inexpensive.

Antigens are usually present in the blood, so the sample used for immunoassays is often a blood sample. Depending on the test being used, the sample may be whole anticoagulated blood, serum, or plasma. Some immunoassays may use urine, feces, or saliva as the sample. With a few exceptions, in-house immunologic test kits use enzyme-linked immunosorbent assay (ELISA) or immunochromatography (ICT) assay methods. It is vital that veterinary technicians understand the principles of these in-house immunologic tests to avoid false results.(see Chapter 10)

Platelets are not whole cells but are fragments of cytoplasm from large cells (megakaryocytes) in the bone marrow. Their function is to help minimize blood loss from damaged blood vessels by adhering to the injured area and initiating the blood-clotting process.

FETAL CIRCULATION

A fetus developing in the uterus leads a parasitic existence. It derives all its nutrition and O_2 from the mother's blood and sends its metabolic wastes and CO_2 back to the mother's blood for elimination. The placenta is the life support system of the fetus that makes this possible. The fetus is connected to the placenta by the umbilical cord. The placenta surrounds the fetus and attaches to the wall of the uterus so that placental and maternal blood vessels are in close proximity to each other. There is normally no direct mixing of fetal and maternal blood.

The umbilical vein carries nutrient-rich, freshly oxygenated blood from the placenta to the fetus. The fetal heart then pumps the blood throughout the developing fetus, where the blood releases its nutrients and O_2 and picks up wastes and CO_2. The umbilical arteries return this waste-filled blood to the placenta, where it exchanges its wastes for nutrients and O_2.

Because the fetal lungs are essentially nonfunctional until birth, the fetal blood vascular system has two major modifications that divert most of the blood away from the lungs (Fig. 4-15). The foramen ovale is a hole in the interatrial septum of the heart, the wall between the left and right atria. This foramen allows some of the blood returning from the systemic circulation to flow from the right atrium directly into the left atrium, bypassing the lungs. The ductus arteriosus connects the pulmonary artery with the aorta. Most of the blood pumped out of the right ventricle flows through the ductus arteriosus into the aorta and into the system circulation, again bypassing the lungs. The developing lungs need only a small amount of blood flow to meet their metabolic needs. At or soon after birth, the foramen ovale and ductus arteriosus close in response to the sudden pressure changes created by the functioning lungs. Patent ductus arteriosus (PDA) is a common congenital abnormality in dogs when the ductus arteriosus fails to close and persists even after birth. In dogs, another vessel called the ductus venosus connects the portal sinus to the posterior vena cava, diverting the blood away from the liver until birth. Its lumen is obliterated after birth, forming the ligamentum venosum. If this duct persists after birth, it creates a portosystemic shunt.

LYMPHATIC SYSTEM

The lymphatic system is a vascular system that serves to return excess tissue fluid to the blood vascular system. Along the way it filters the tissue fluid, examines it for foreign invaders, and manufactures defensive cells and antibodies to help keep the body healthy.

At the blood capillary level, more fluid flows out of the porous capillaries than returns to them. If not removed somehow, this excess fluid would accumulate in body tissues and cause progressive swelling. Lymph capillaries begin peripherally as blind-ended vessels that pick up this excess fluid, called lymph, and move it toward the thorax. The small lymph vessels merge to form larger vessels. These larger lymph channels contain small one-way valves, similar to the valves in veins. Combined with body movements, these one-way valves help propel the lymph to the thorax, where it is deposited back into the bloodstream.

Along the network of lymph vessels are small lumps of tissue called lymph nodes. These contain large accumulations of one type of white blood cell, lymphocytes, organized into collections called lymph nodules. The lymph nodes filter the lymph, removing debris and foreign invaders, and produce

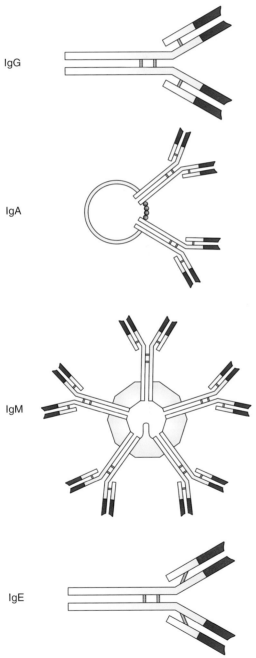

FIGURE 4-14 Schematic representation of IgM (pentamer), IgG and IgE (monomers), and IgA (dimer). (From Sirois M: Principles and practice of veterinary technology, ed 3, St Louis, 2011, Mosby.)

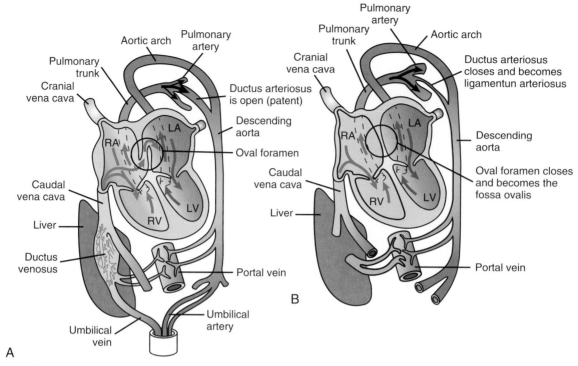

FIGURE 4-15 Circulatory patterns in fetus and in newborn. **A,** Fetal circulation. **B,** Newborn circulation. *LA,* Left atrium; *LV,* left ventricle; *RA,* right atrium; *RV,* right ventricle. (From Colville TP: *Clinical anatomy and physiology for veterinary technicians,* ed 2, St Louis, 2008, Mosby.)

antibody-producing cells that are important components of the body's defense mechanisms.

Lymph nodules are also found in areas of the body other than lymph nodes. The spleen, a large, tongue-shaped organ located near the stomach, is a blood-storage organ, but it also contains large accumulations of lymph nodules. The thymus is a lymphoid organ located in the caudal cervicocranial thoracic region. It is of importance primarily in young animals. It helps jump-start the immune system and then gradually shrinks and disappears around the time of sexual maturity. Accumulations of lymph nodules are also found in the tonsils, scattered in the lining of the intestines.

RESPIRATORY SYSTEM

The primary function of the respiratory system is to exchange O_2 in oxygenated blood for CO_2, which is produced as a waste product by the cells. Secondary functions include vocalization (e.g., barking, mooing), body temperature regulation, and acid-base regulation.

Respiration occurs at two levels in the body. Internal respiration involves gas exchange between the blood and the body's many cells and tissues, and it occurs at the cellular level throughout the body. O_2 carried in the RBCs is exchanged for CO_2 produced by tissue cells. External respiration involves the exchange of gases between blood and the outside air, and it occurs in the lungs. Carbon dioxide in the blood is exchanged for O_2 from the air.

The respiratory system is composed of the upper respiratory tract, which consists of a series of tubes that connect the

lungs with the external environment, and the lower respiratory tract, which consists of structures within the lungs.

UPPER RESPIRATORY TRACT

The upper respiratory tract starts at the tip of the nose (Fig. 4-16). Inhaled air enters the nostrils and passes back through the nasal passages. The lining of the nasal passages contains extensive networks of blood vessels and a ciliated epithelium coated with watery mucus. Blood circulating throughout the

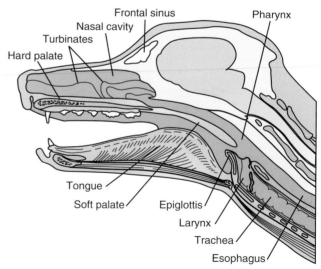

FIGURE 4-16 Longitudinal section of canine upper respiratory tract. (From Colville TP: *Clinical anatomy and physiology for veterinary technicians,* ed 2, St Louis, 2008, Mosby.)

nasal lining warms the incoming air, the watery mucus humidifies it, and the cilia sweep foreign material that has become trapped in the mucus out of the nasal passages. These functions form a conditioning system that supplies the lungs with relatively pure, warm, humidified air.

From the nasal passages, inhaled air passes through the pharynx, or throat. This is a common passageway for the digestive and respiratory systems. Through a series of intricate reflexes, the pharynx and larynx help prevent swallowed material from entering the lower respiratory tract.

The larynx, commonly called the voice box, is a short, irregular tube of cartilage and muscle that connects the pharynx with the trachea. In addition to its voice-producing function, it also acts as a valve to control airflow to and from the lungs. At the junction of the pharynx and larynx is the epiglottis, a flap of cartilage that acts as a trap door to cover the opening of the larynx during swallowing.

Carrying air from the larynx to the lungs is the trachea, or windpipe. The trachea is composed of several C-shaped incomplete rings of hyaline cartilage, which prevent it from collapsing during inhalation. At its caudal end, the trachea divides into the left and right bronchi, which enter the lungs.

LOWER RESPIRATORY TRACT

The bronchi enter the lungs and branch into smaller and smaller air passageways that eventually lead to tiny, grapelike clusters of thin cells called alveoli (Fig. 4-17). The alveolus is the actual site of gas exchange in the lungs. Each alveolus

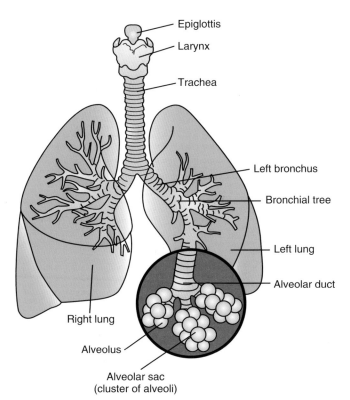

FIGURE 4-17 Lower respiratory tract. (From Colville TP: Clinical anatomy and physiology for veterinary technicians, ed 2, St Louis, 2008, Mosby.)

consists of a tiny, extremely thin-walled sac surrounded by elastic fibers and a network of capillaries.

> ### CRITICAL CONCEPT
> The actual site of gas exchange in the lungs is the alveolus, a tiny, thin-walled sac surrounded by elastic fibers and a network of capillaries.

RESPIRATORY MECHANISMS

The process of external respiration depends on physical mechanisms that allow air to move in and out of the lungs and on control systems that set limits on and adjust the process.

THORAX

The area referred to as the thorax is located between the neck and diaphragm. Normally, there is negative pressure (partial vacuum) in the thorax. Combined with the elasticity and pliable nature of the lungs, this causes the lungs to conform to the size and shape of the thoracic cavity. A small amount of pleural fluid lubricates the lung surfaces and thoracic (pleural) lining. A puncturing wound or gunshot in the thoracic cavity can reduce the negative pressure, leading to collapse of the lungs.

INSPIRATION

Inspiration on inhaling is the process of drawing air into the lungs. It is accomplished by contractions of the diaphragm and other muscles. The diaphragm is a dome-shaped, sheet-like muscle that completely separates the thoracic cavity from the abdominal cavity. The contraction of the diaphragm pushes the abdominal organs down and increases the volume of the thoracic cavity. The lungs expand passively as the thoracic cavity enlarges, and air is drawn into them through the upper respiratory passages.

EXCHANGE OF GASES

Air that is drawn into the alveoli during inspiration contains high levels of O_2 and low levels of CO_2. Blood passing through the capillary networks around the alveoli contains low levels of O_2 and high levels of CO_2. Both gases move from areas of high concentration to areas of low concentration by a process called diffusion. Oxygen diffuses from the alveoli to the blood in the alveolar capillaries. Carbon dioxide diffuses in the other direction, from the blood of the alveolar capillaries to the alveoli.

EXPIRATION

Air rich with carbon dioxide from the alveoli must be eliminated from the lungs so that a fresh breath of O_2-rich air can be inspired. Expiration occurs as muscular contractions compress the thoracic cavity and elastic lung tissue returns to its original shape, expelling air from the lungs.

CONTROL OF BREATHING

Two systems control the process of respiration, a mechanical control system and a chemical control system. The mechanical control system sets normal limits on inspiration and expiration to allow rhythmic, resting respiration. The inspiratory center in the brain initiates impulses at regular intervals. These impulses travel to the diaphragm, allowing it to contract and the lungs to inflate. Stretch receptors in the lungs sense when the preset limit of inflation has been reached. They initiate impulses that travel to the respiratory centers in the brain, stopping inspiration and starting passive expiration. The chemical control system monitors the chemical composition of the blood. If it senses fluctuations in O_2 and CO_2 levels or pH, it initiates adjustments in respiration necessary to restore normal values.

DIGESTIVE SYSTEM

The digestive or alimentary system converts food eaten by an animal into nutrient compounds that body cells can use for metabolic fuel. The digestive system consists of a tube running from the mouth to the anus, with accessory digestive organs attached to it (Fig. 4-18). Food moving through the tube is broken down into smaller, simpler compounds through the process of digestion. These simple compounds then pass through the wall of the digestive tract into the bloodstream through the process of absorption for distribution of nutrients to body cells.

The structure of a species' digestive system is largely dependent on its diet. Nutrients in the plant matter diet of herbivores, such as horses and cattle, are largely incorporated within hard-to-digest cellulose. Herbivores depend on the help of microorganisms, such as protozoa and bacteria, to help break down cellulose through a process called microbial fermentation. At some point in their digestive tract, herbivores have a large fermentation vat, in which cellulose can be broken down into usable nutrients. In cattle this is the rumen; in horses it is the much-enlarged cecum, part of the large intestine. The digestive system of carnivores (meat eaters), such as dogs and cats, is much simpler. Carnivores depend on enzymes to break down easy-to-digest animal source nutrients through the process of enzymatic digestion. Therefore, no large fermentation vat is needed. Omnivores (species eating a mixed diet), such as pigs, are somewhat intermediate. They depend primarily on enzymatic digestion, with a minor amount of microbial fermentation occurring in their large intestine.

MOUTH

The mouth is where food is chewed and mixed with saliva in preparation for swallowing. Four types of teeth, arranged into upper and lower dental arcades, begin the process of digestion by cutting and crushing the food. The most rostral teeth are the incisors (I). Ruminants, such as cattle and sheep, do not have upper incisors. They have a firm, fibrous dental pad instead. The four canines (C), if present, are located at the rostral lateral corners of the mouth, adjacent to the incisors. The premolars (PM) are the rostral cheek teeth, and the molars (M) are the caudal cheek teeth (Fig. 4-19).

Each tooth is composed of three different kinds of firm connective tissue. The exposed portion, the crown, is covered by enamel, the hardest substance in the body. The bulk of the tooth is composed of a dense material called dentin. The root, which helps anchor the tooth in its bony socket, is covered by cementum. The fibers that connect the cementum to the bony socket are called periodontal ligaments. Periodontitis is

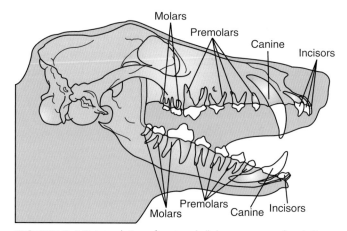

FIGURE 4-19 Lateral view of canine skull showing types of teeth (From Colville TP: Clinical anatomy and physiology for veterinary technicians, ed 2, St Louis, 2008, Mosby.)

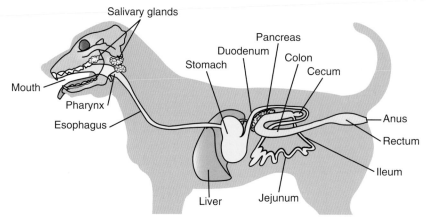

FIGURE 4-18 Schematic representation of the digestive apparatus of the dog. (From Colville TP: Clinical anatomy and physiology for veterinary technicians, ed 2, St Louis, 2008, Mosby.)

the inflammation of these ligaments from the accumulation of plaque and bacterial toxins in gum pockets. It is the most common tooth problem in dogs and cats older than 5 years.

DENTAL FORMULA

A **dental formula** places the teeth in the upper arcade in the numerator position and the teeth in the lower arcade in the denominator position. To get the entire mouth, multiply by 2:

$$\text{Dog}:2\left(I\frac{3}{3},\ C\frac{1}{1},\ PM\frac{4}{4},\ M\frac{2}{3}\right)=42$$

$$\text{Cat}:2\left(I\frac{3}{3},\ C\frac{1}{1},\ PM\frac{3}{2},\ M\frac{1}{1}\right)=30$$

Once the food has been chopped and ground by the teeth and moistened with saliva, it is swallowed. Muscular movements of the tongue and pharynx move the bolus of food back through the pharynx to the opening of the esophagus, where it begins its journey to the stomach and through the remainder of the digestive tract.

ESOPHAGUS

The esophagus is a muscular tube that connects the pharynx with the stomach. Food passes through it quickly on its way to the stomach; no significant digestion or absorption occurs in the esophagus. The size of the opening of the esophagus into the stomach is regulated by the cardiac sphincter. This muscular ring functions as a valve to seal the esophagus off from the stomach. In the normal digestive process, the cardiac sphincter opens only to allow swallowed food to pass into the stomach. It also relaxes to allow food to pass back up the esophagus in species that can vomit or ruminate.

STOMACH

The stomach is an enlarged chamber in which swallowed food is mixed with hydrochloric acid and digestive enzymes. In simple-stomached animals, such as horses and dogs, significant digestion of food begins in the stomach.

The simple stomach of monogastric animals is a single chamber lined with large folds, the rugae, and dense accumulations of gastric glands. The gastric glands secrete hydrochloric acid and various digestive enzymes, which begin the digestion process, and mucus, which coats the stomach lining and keeps it from being digested along with the food. Very little absorption of nutrients occurs in the stomach. The stomach serves mainly to mix the food with the acid and enzymes to begin digestion. By the time the food leaves the stomach through the pyloric sphincter to enter the small intestines, it has been converted into a semiliquid homogeneous material called chyme.

INTESTINE

After leaving the stomach, chyme enters the tubelike intestine. Moved along by muscular contractions, the chyme is further digested by mixing with secretions from the pancreas,

liver, and glands in the intestinal wall. Most absorption of nutrients takes place in the intestines. The large surface area of the intestinal lining aids in nutrient absorption. Countless tiny, fingerlike processes called villi cover the lining. Each villus contains tiny blood and lymph vessels at its center, into which nutrients are absorbed through the simple columnar epithelial covering.

The first portion of the intestine is the small intestine, so named because of its relatively small diameter. It has three segments, the duodenum, jejunum, and ileum. (Note the similarity in name, but difference in spelling, to one of the pelvic bones, the ilium.)

> ### CRITICAL CONCEPT
> The three segments of the small intestine are the duodenum, jejunum, and ileum.

The duodenum is the first, relatively short segment of the small intestine. It receives the chyme through the stomach's pyloric valve. Ducts carrying bile from the liver and digestive enzymes from the pancreas enter the small intestine lumen (interior).

The next segment, the jejunum, is the longest segment of the small intestine. This is where most nutrient absorption takes place. The ileum is the last, relatively short segment of small intestine. It leads to the large intestine.

The large-diameter large intestine receives undigested and unabsorbed food material from the ileum. It absorbs water from the chyme and absorbs any nutrients not previously absorbed by the small intestine. The first segment of the large intestine is the cecum. This blind-ended sac is small in carnivores, such as dogs, and very large in monogastric herbivores, such as horses. Next is the longest segment of the large intestine, the colon. The final intestinal segment is the rectum, which carries its contents, called feces, to the anus for discharge from the body, or defecation.

The anus is the caudal opening of the digestive system to the outside world. It is surrounded by ringlike sphincter muscles that allow the animal to control defecation consciously.

ACCESSORY DIGESTIVE ORGANS

Several sets of salivary glands produce saliva, a watery fluid that is carried from the salivary glands to the mouth by ducts. Although saliva contains small amounts of digestive enzymes, its primary function is to moisten and lubricate food as it is chewed, making it easier to swallow. The drier the diet of the animal, the more saliva is produced.

The pancreas is located near the duodenum and has endocrine and exocrine functions. Its endocrine functions involve the production of two hormones, insulin and glucagon, which help control glucose metabolism in the body. These hormones are discussed later with the **endocrine system**. The exocrine secretion of the pancreas, called pancreatic juice, is involved with digestion. Pancreatic juice is carried to the duodenum through the pancreatic duct(s). The main components of pancreatic juice are sodium bicarbonate, which helps neutralize the very acidic chyme entering the duodenum from the stomach, and a variety of digestive enzymes.

Located just caudal to the diaphragm, the liver is the largest gland in the body. Three important functions of liver are detoxification, storage, and modification of nutrients. It is an important "factory" that assembles simple nutrient molecules into larger compounds, which can be used by the body's cells. The portal vein, which carries nutrient-rich blood from the intestines directly to the liver, supplies the raw materials for the factory. The liver also secretes bile, a greenish fluid that carries waste products of hemoglobin metabolism out of the body and aids in the breakdown and absorption of fats and fat-soluble vitamins from the intestine.

NERVOUS SYSTEM

The nervous system is a complex communication system in the animal body. It detects and processes internal and external information and formulates appropriate responses to changes, threats, and opportunities that the animal continually faces. Almost all conscious and unconscious functions of the body are controlled or influenced by the nervous system.

The basic structural and functional unit of the nervous system is the nerve cell, the neuron. Neurons are specialized cells that respond to stimuli and conduct impulses from one part of a cell to another. Two types of fiberlike processes extend from the cell bodies of neurons, dendrites and axons. Dendrites are often multiple, and they conduct impulses received from other neurons toward the nerve cell body. Axons are usually single, and they conduct impulses away from the cell body to other neurons or the effector organs, such as muscle cells. The junction of an axon with another nerve cell is called a synapse.

CRITICAL CONCEPT

Neurons are specialized cells that respond to stimuli and conduct impulses from one part of a cell to another.

The branched end of an axon is called the telodendron. When a nerve impulse reaches the telodendron, it causes the release of tiny sacs of chemicals called neurotransmitters into the narrow synaptic space. When neurotransmitter molecules diffuse across the synapse to contact the cell membrane of the adjacent nerve cell, they induce a change in the other nerve cell. Enzymes in the synaptic space then quickly inactivate the neurotransmitter molecules.

Neurons have three unique physical characteristics: they do not reproduce, their processes are capable of limited regeneration if damaged, and they have an extremely high oxygen requirement. Their lack of reproductive ability means that any loss of neurons, as from disease or injury, is permanent. Their dendritic and axonic processes sometimes regenerate if the nerve cell body is intact; this may restore function of reattached digits or limbs under some circumstances.

The high oxygen requirement of neurons makes them among the most delicate cells in the body. They begin to suffer permanent damage if deprived of blood for more than a few minutes. This is why cardiopulmonary resuscitation must begin within just a few minutes after cardiac arrest if there is to be any chance of complete recovery.

The main divisions of the nervous system are the **central nervous system**, the peripheral nervous system, and the autonomic nervous system.

CENTRAL NERVOUS SYSTEM

The central nervous system consists of accumulations of nerve cell bodies, nerve fibers (axons), and supporting cells in the brain and spinal cord. The brain, consisting of the cerebrum, cerebellum, and brainstem, is housed in the skull (Fig. 4-20). The spinal cord is housed in the vertebral canal formed by the vertebrae. Together, they form the main control systems for the rest of the body.

Cross sections of the brain and spinal cord reveal two distinctly different-colored areas, the gray matter and white matter. Areas containing accumulations of nerve cell bodies appear grayish and make up the gray matter. Areas containing large accumulations of nerve fibers appear pale and make up the white matter.

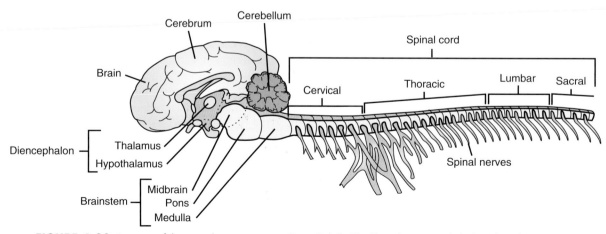

FIGURE 4-20 Anatomy of the central nervous system. (From Colville TP: Clinical anatomy and physiology for veterinary technicians, ed 2, St Louis, 2008, Mosby.)

The cerebrum is the largest, most rostral part of the brain. It consists of two large lateral cerebral hemispheres separated by a deep cleft. Its surface area is increased by systems of folds termed the *gyri* and grooves termed the sulci. The cerebral cortex, or outer layer of the cerebrum, consists of gray matter. The medulla, or inner portion of the cerebrum, consists of white matter. The functions of the cerebrum are complex and poorly understood. It is the center of higher learning and intelligence and it functions in perception, maintenance of consciousness, thinking and reasoning, and initiation of responses to sensory stimuli.

The cerebellum is located just caudal to the cerebrum. Its surface folds are small and packed closely together, giving it a wrinkled appearance. As in the cerebrum, the cerebellar cortex is composed of gray matter and its inner medulla is composed of white matter. The cerebellum does not initiate movements but serves to coordinate, adjust, and generally fine-tune movements directed by the cerebrum.

The brainstem is the most primitive part of the brain. It forms the stem to which the cerebrum, cerebellum, and spinal cord are attached. Color distinctions between gray and white matter are difficult to observe in the brainstem. Functionally, the brainstem maintains the vital functions of the body. Centers in the brainstem control respiration, body temperature, heart rate, gastrointestinal tract function, blood pressure, appetite, thirst, and sleep-wake cycles. Severe damage to vital centers in the brainstem usually results in immediate death.

The spinal cord is the caudal continuation of the brainstem. On cross section, the gray matter forms a butterfly-shaped area in the central area of the spinal cord. The white matter forms the outer cortex. Spinal nerves exit and enter the spinal cord between each set of adjacent vertebrae. They carry information to and from the peripheral portion of the nervous system.

PERIPHERAL NERVOUS SYSTEM

The peripheral nervous system consists of cordlike nerves that run throughout the body. The nerves are actually bundles of axons that carry impulses between the central nervous system and the rest of the body. Nerves that carry only information toward the central nervous system are called sensory nerves. Those that carry only instructions from the central nervous system out to the body are called motor nerves. Most nerves are mixed nerves, a combination of sensory and motor nerves. The peripheral nervous system includes the cranial nerves and spinal nerves.

SPINAL NERVES

Spinal nerves originate as two roots, the dorsal root and ventral root, on either side of the spinal cord. These two roots combine to form the spinal nerve proper. The spinal nerves mainly innervate the striated muscles. Some spinal nerves also carry sympathetic and parasympathetic nerve fibers, which innervate smooth muscle fibers (organs). Spinal nerves from the thoracic and lumber regions of the spinal cord carry sympathetic nerve fibers. Spinal nerves from the sacral region carry parasympathetic nerve fibers.

CRANIAL NERVES

There are 12 pairs of cranial nerves, mainly arising from the ventral surface of the brain. The cranial nerves are designated by their names and numbers (in Roman numerals; Table 4-3). For example, the first cranial nerve (CN) is called the olfactory nerve (CN I), and the second cranial nerve is called the optic nerve (CN II). Cranial nerves usually innervate to the structures in the head and neck area. The exception is the vagus nerve (CN X), which is the longest cranial nerve that innervates many organs of the body.

AUTONOMIC NERVOUS SYSTEM

The autonomic nervous system is the self-governing portion of the nervous system. It operates independently of conscious thought to maintain homeostasis, a constant internal environment in the body. Primarily a motor system, the autonomic nervous system consists of two parts, the sympathetic system and parasympathetic system, which have opposite effects and are in constant balance with each other.

TABLE 4-3	Functions of the 12 Cranial Nerves			
NUMBER	**NAME**	**TYPE**	**KEY FUNCTIONS**
I	Olfactory	Sensory	Smell
II	Optic	Sensory	Vision
III	Oculomotor	Motor	Eye movement, pupil size, focusing lens
IV	Trochlear	Motor	Eye movement
V	Trigeminal	Both sensory and motor	Sensations from the head and teeth, chewing
VI	Abducent	Motor	Eye movement
VII	Facial	Both sensory and motor	Face and scalp movement, salivation, tears, taste
VIII	Vestibulocochlear	Sensory	Balance, hearing
IX	Glossopharyngeal	Both sensory and motor	Tongue movement, swallowing, salivation, taste
X	Vagus (wanderer)	Both sensory and motor	Sensory form gastrointestinal tract and respiratory tree; motor to the larynx, pharynx, parasympathetic; motor to the abdominal and thoracic organs
XI	Accessory	Motor	Head movement, accessory motor with vagus
XII	Hypoglossal	Motor	Tongue movement

From Colville TP: Clinical anatomy and physiology for veterinary technicians, ed 2, St Louis, 2008, Mosby.

The sympathetic system produces the fight-or-flight reaction in response to real or perceived threats. In a time of crisis or physical threat, the heart rate and blood pressure increase, the air passageways in the lungs and the pupils of the eyes dilate, digestive tract activity decreases, and the hairs stand on end, producing what is known as raised hackles. The net effect is to prepare the body for intense physical exertion and to make the animal look larger and more threatening.

The parasympathetic system has the opposite effect. It is the rest and restore system. It predominates during relaxed, routine, business-as-usual states. The heart rate and blood pressure decrease, the air passageways in the lung and the pupils of the eyes constrict, and digestive tract activity increases. The net effect is to allow the body to relax and rejuvenate itself.

MUSCULAR SYSTEM

The general function of muscle is to move the body, internally and externally. The nervous system gives the orders, and the muscular system is among the most important systems that carry them out. There are three distinctly different types of muscle in the body—**skeletal muscle**, cardiac muscle, and **smooth muscle** (Fig. 4-21). All these muscles have the ability to contract and relax, which helps them perform various functions.

CRITICAL CONCEPT

There are three types of muscle in the body—skeletal muscle, cardiac muscle, and smooth muscle.

SKELETAL MUSCLE

Skeletal muscle derives its name from the fact that it moves the skeleton. It is also known as voluntary striated muscle because it is under conscious control and its cells, at the microscopic level, have a striped or striated appearance.

Skeletal muscle cells (myocytes) are shaped like long cylinders or fibers. These large cells usually have multiple nuclei. Most of their mass is composed of smaller myofibrils made up of smaller protein filaments. The net effect is an intricate arrangement of filaments that can slide over each other, shortening the muscle cell when it contracts.

Skeletal muscle fibers respond to impulses delivered by nerves. The connection of a nerve fiber with a skeletal muscle fiber is called the neuromuscular junction. Each nerve fiber supplies more than one muscle fiber. A motor unit is composed of a nerve fiber and all the muscle fibers it supplies. If there is a small number of muscle fibers per nerve fiber, fine delicate movements are possible. The muscles that move the eyeball fall into this category. On the other hand, muscles that must make large, powerful movements, such as the leg muscles, have a large number of muscle fibers supplied by each nerve fiber.

Skeletal muscles are usually attached to bones at both ends by tendons. The more stable of the muscle's attachments is called its origin. The more movable of the attachments is called its insertion.

CARDIAC MUSCLE

Cardiac muscle is found only in the heart. It is also known as involuntary striated muscle because it is not under conscious control and its cells are striped, or striated.

Cardiac muscle cells have no characteristic shape. Rather, they form an intricate branching network in the heart. They are firmly attached to each other, which allows considerable force to be generated as they contract.

Cardiac muscle cells each have an innate contractile rhythm that does not require an external nerve supply. The rhythmic contractions of the heart chambers are coordinated by a system of specialized cardiac muscle cells. The heart does have an autonomic nerve supply. However, it does not initiate contractions of the muscle cells; it modifies them. Sympathetic stimulation increases the rate and force of cardiac muscle contractions. This is part of the fight-or-flight response. Parasympathetic stimulation has the opposite effect—it decreases the rate and force of contraction. Through this autonomic stimulation, the rate and force of cardiac contractions can be adjusted according to the body's needs.

SMOOTH MUSCLE

Smooth muscle is found mainly in internal organs. It is called smooth because its cells do not show any stripes or striations under magnification. It is involuntary muscle because it is not under conscious control.

Cells of smooth muscle are spindle-shaped, wide in the middle and tapered at the ends. Depending on their location, they may be short and thick or long and fiberlike. Two types of smooth muscle are found in the body—visceral smooth muscle, found in hollow abdominal organs, and multiunit smooth muscle, found where fine contractions are needed.

Visceral smooth muscle occurs in large sheets in the walls of the gastrointestinal tract, uterus, and urinary bladder. These muscle cells are linked, so entire areas of cells act as a large unit. Nerve supply is autonomic and serves mainly to modify contractions. Sympathetic stimulation (fight-or-flight) decreases activity, whereas parasympathetic stimulation (rest, rejuvenation) increases it.

Multiunit smooth muscle consists of individual muscle units that each require specific nerve stimulation to contract. Unlike visceral smooth muscle cells, these muscle cells are not linked, so their contractions are localized and discrete. Multiunit smooth muscle is found where fine, although involuntary, movements are needed, such as in the iris and ciliary body of the eye, walls of blood vessels, and walls of tiny air passageways in the lungs.

SENSES

The senses are the means whereby the body monitors its internal and external environment. Sensory receptors are specialized nerve endings that convert mechanical, thermal,

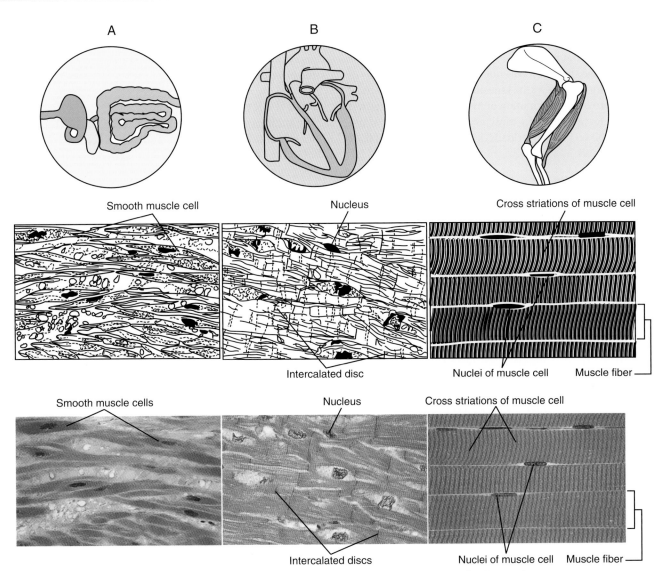

FIGURE 4-21 Types of muscle tissue; photomicrographs and sketches of these cells illustrate the microanatomy. **A,** Smooth muscle. This is nonstriated, involuntary, and composed of small, spindle-shaped cells that lack striations or bands and therefore appear smooth. Each cell has a centrally located nucleus. It is found in the walls of hollow organs such as the esophagus, stomach, intestine, colon, blood vessels, and bladder and in skin attached to hair and in the iris of the eye. It moves food through the digestive tract, regulates the size of an organ, controls light entering the eye, moves fluid through vessels, and causes hair to stand erect. **B,** Cardiac muscle. This is striated and involuntary; cells are cylindrical and branched with a single, centrally located nucleus. Cells form an intricate network and are connected by intercalated discs in a specialized type of gap junction. It is found only in the heart. It pumps blood through the vascular system. Note the intercalated discs unique to the cardiac cell. Each cell contains only one centrally located nucleus. **C,** Skeletal muscle. This is striated and voluntary; cells are striped, long, and cylindrical, each with multiple, eccentrically placed nuclei. It s attached to bone and occasionally to skin, eyeballs, and upper part of the esophagus. It controls voluntary movement of the body, including movement of the eyes and the initial part of swallowing. Note that each cell contains multiple nuclei, which are found along the cell membrane. (From Colville TP: Clinical anatomy and physiology for veterinary technicians, ed 2, St Louis, 2008, Mosby.) (Photomicrograph in **A,** Courtesy Carolina Biological Supply, Burlington, NC, Phototake, New York; photomicrographs in **B** and **C,** courtesy Ed Reschke.)

electromagnetic, and chemical stimuli from the environment into nervous impulses. When sensory impulses reach the central nervous system, they are perceived as sensations such as smell, taste, or sight.

Various sensations are received and interpreted by the central nervous system. The five senses we usually think of (hearing, smell, taste, touch, and sight) are not the only

sensations perceived by the central nervous system. A description of the **general senses** and **special senses** is given in Table 4-4.

GENERAL SENSES

The general senses are so named because they are distributed generally throughout the body or over the entire skin surface.

Their receptors are fairly simple modified nerve endings. The tactile sense, or sense of touch, perceives mechanical contact with the surface of the body. The temperature sense is a thermal sense that perceives hot and cold. The position of the limbs is monitored by the kinesthetic sense, a mechanical sense that provides information on the position of joints and the relative force exerted by muscles and tendons. The sense of pain can be set off by overloads of mechanical, thermal, or chemical stimuli.

SPECIAL SENSES

The special senses are so named because their sensory receptors are concentrated in certain areas, rather than being generally distributed. All receptors for the special senses are located in the head. Also, in several cases, the sensory receptor cells are aided by sophisticated accessory structures.

GUSTATORY SENSE

The gustatory sense, the sense of taste, is a chemical sense. It detects chemical substances in the mouth that are dissolved in saliva. The receptor cells are located in tiny taste buds found mainly on the tongue. Each taste bud has an opening on its surface, the taste pore. Hairlike microvilli from the receptor cells project into the taste pore. When dissolved chemical substances enter the taste pore, their molecules interact with the microvilli, generating impulses that travel to the brain and are interpreted as various tastes.

OLFACTORY SENSE

The olfactory sense, the sense of smell, is also a chemical sense. It detects chemical substances in inhaled air. The receptor cells are located in the epithelium of the nasal passages. Hairlike microvilli from the olfactory cells project up into the mucous

layer that overlies the nasal epithelium. When chemical substances dissolve in the mucus, the microvilli are stimulated and information about odors is transmitted to the brain via the olfactory nerve.

AUDITORY SENSE

The auditory sense is the sense of hearing. Through a complex set of auditory passageways and ear structures, mechanical vibrations of air molecules are converted into impulses that the brain decodes as sounds. Sound waves from the environment are collected by the external ear structures, amplified and transmitted through the middle ear structures, and converted to impulses in the inner ear. Most of the ear structures are located in the temporal bones of the skull (Fig. 4-22).

TABLE 4-4	General and Special Senses	
SENSE	**WHAT IS SENSED**	**TYPE OF STIMULUS**
General Senses		
Visceral sensations	Hunger, thirst, hollow organ fullness	Chemical, mechanical
Touch	Touch and pressure	Mechanical
Temperature	Heat and cold	Thermal
Pain	Intense stimuli of any type	Mechanical, chemical, or thermal
Proprioception	Body position and movement	Mechanical
Special Senses		
Taste	Tastes	Chemical
Smell	Odors	Chemical
Hearing	Sounds	Mechanical
Equilibrium	Balance and head position	Mechanical
Vision	Light	Electromagnetic

From Colville TP: Clinical anatomy and physiology for veterinary technicians, ed 2, St Louis, 2008, Mosby.

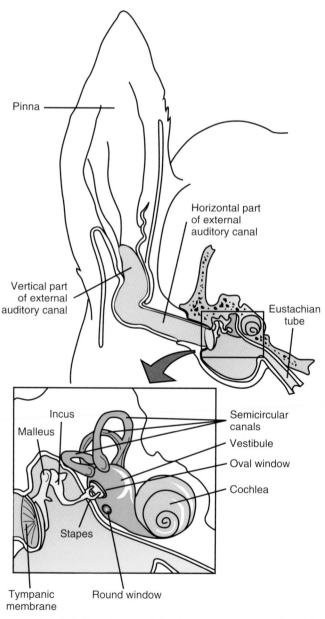

FIGURE 4-22 Cross section of the dog's ear structures, with middle and inner ear regions enlarged. (From Colville TP: Clinical anatomy and physiology for veterinary technicians, ed 2, St Louis, 2008, Mosby.)

The external ear is composed of the pinna (ear flap), external auditory canal, and tympanic membrane (eardrum). The pinna is a cartilaginous funnel that collects sound waves and directs them medially into the external auditory canal, which leads to the tympanic membrane. The tympanic membrane is a thin, connective tissue membrane that is tightly stretched across the opening into the middle ear. Sound waves cause the membrane to vibrate.

Medial to the tympanic membrane is the air-filled middle ear cavity, which transmits vibrations of the tympanic membrane to the inner ear via three tiny bones called ossicles. The first bone, the malleus, is attached to the medial surface of the tympanic membrane. It forms a tiny joint with the second bone, the incus, which forms a joint with the third bone, the stapes, which is in contact with the cochlea of the inner ear. Vibrations of the tympanic membrane are transmitted by the ossicles to the inner ear. Air pressure within the middle ear must equilibrate with the atmospheric pressure of the external air to prevent undue bulging of the tympanic membrane. The eustachian tube, which links the middle ear with the pharynx, accomplishes this pressure equilibration as the animal swallows.

The inner ear contains three structures, the cochlea, vestibule, and semicircular canals. The cochlear is responsible for the sense of hearing, whereas the vestibular part and semicircular canals help in monitoring balance and head position.

The cochlea is a fluid-filled space shaped like a hollow spiral snail shell. Running along its length, like a ribbon, is the organ of Corti, which contains the receptor cells for hearing. When sound wave vibrations are transmitted to the cochlear fluid, the fluid movements distort the microvilli on the receptor cells on the organ of Corti. This generates impulses that are carried to the brain via the cochlear nerve.

VESTIBULAR SENSE

The vestibular sense, also a mechanical sense, monitors balance and head position. Its receptors are contained in two structures of the inner ear, the vestibule and semicircular canals. Together with the cochlea, these structures make up the inner ear. The vestibule consists of two fluid-filled spaces in each inner ear that contain patches of sensory epithelium on their floor. The sensory cells have hairlike microvilli that project into an overlying coat of gelatinous material. This gelatinous layer contains tiny crystals of calcium carbonate, the otoliths. Any tilting or linear motion of the head causes movement of the otoliths, which distorts the microvilli, generating nervous impulses. These vestibular impulses carry information to the brain about changes in the position and linear motion of the head.

The semicircular canals are three fluid-filled canals of semicircular shape on each side of the head. Parts of the semicircular canals are oriented in different planes, at right angles to each other, much like two walls and a ceiling join at a corner. At one end of each canal are the receptors, which contain sensory cells that are similar to those of the vestibule. Hairlike microvilli of the sensory cells project into an overlying layer of gelatinous material. Rotation of the head in any plane moves the fluid in a semicircular canal and stimulates its sensory cells. The resulting impulses carry information to the brain about rotary motion of the head.

VISUAL SENSE

The visual sense (sight) is the only well-developed electromagnetic sense of mammals. Its receptor organ, the eye (Fig. 4-23), has a complex organization of component parts that function together to gather and focus light rays on photoreceptor cells. When stimulated by light, the sensory cells of the inner eye generate impulses to the brain through the optic nerve. The brain interprets these impulses as light.

The outer covering of the eyeball or globe is a dense, fibrous, connective tissue layer that supports it and gives it shape. The clear window on the rostral portion of the eye is the cornea. Light rays enter the eye through the cornea and

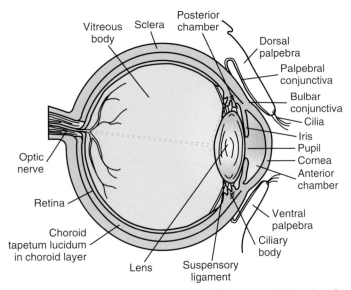

FIGURE 4-23 Sagittal section of the eye. (From Colville TP: Clinical anatomy and physiology for veterinary technicians, ed 2, St Louis, 2008, Mosby.)

are focused on the photoreceptors at the caudal portion of the eye. Although the cornea is composed of fibrous connective tissue, it normally contains just enough water to render it transparent. The sclera makes up the rest of the fibrous outer layer of the globe. Because of its white color, the sclera is commonly referred to as the white of the eye.

Caudal to the cornea is the fluid-filled space called the anterior chamber and the colored iris. The watery fluid that fills the anterior chamber is called the aqueous humor and is produced by cells caudal to the iris. The iris is a muscular diaphragm that controls the size of the aperture at its center, the pupil. In bright light, the parasympathetic system stimulates the iris to contract, reducing the size of the pupil to protect the sensitive photoreceptor cells. In dim light, the sympathetic innervation relaxes the iris muscles, enlarging the pupil to allow more light to enter.

Caudal to the iris is a transparent, biconvex, elastic, crystalline structure called the lens. The lens is responsible for the process of accommodation, focusing the light rays on the photoreceptor cells in the caudal portion of the eye to allow for near and far vision. Around its periphery, the lens is connected to the ciliary body by tiny suspensory ligaments. The ciliary body contains the muscles responsible for changing the shape of the lens as required to focus the light rays. The muscles in the ciliary body are oriented so that when an animal is looking at something very close, they contract and allow the lens to assume its more natural rounded shape, focusing the close-up image on the photoreceptors. For distant objects, the ciliary muscles relax, allowing the globe's natural elasticity to pull the lens into a flattened shape more appropriate for distant vision.

The area caudal to the lens is filled with a transparent gelatinous substance called the vitreous humor. The light rays pass through this substance on their way to the photoreceptor-containing layer, the retina.

The retina is where visual images are formed. It is a complex, multilayered structure that lines most of the interior of the eye caudal to the lens. It is composed of photoreceptor cells termed rods and cones and several layers of nerve cell bodies and synapses that integrate and relay information from the receptor cells to the brain. The rods and cones have different shapes and different functions. The rods are long and narrow and are more sensitive to light than the cones. They do not, however, detect colors or detail well. They are the receptors for dim light vision. The cones are somewhat flask shaped and detect detail and colors well. The area of the retina at which nerve fibers converge to form the optic nerve is called the optic disc. No rods or cones are present there; it is the blind spot of the eye.

The eye is a sensitive organ that is protected by accessory structures. These include the conjunctiva, eyelids, and lacrimal apparatus.

The conjunctiva is a thin membrane that lines the underside of the eyelids and covers the outer aspect of the eyeball. Its transparency allows the sclera of the globe and the blood vessels of the eyelids to show through. Examination of the conjunctiva makes it possible to detect abnormalities such as anemia or jaundice.

The eyelids are dorsal (upper) and ventral (lower) folds of skin lined by conjunctiva that cover and protect the eye when the animal blinks or sleeps. The medial and lateral junctions of the eyelids are the medial canthus and lateral canthus of the eye, respectively. The third eyelid, or nictitating membrane, is a plate of cartilage covered by conjunctiva located medially between the eyelids and eyeball in some species. (Fig. 4-24).

The lacrimal apparatus is concerned with production and drainage of tears from the surface of the eye. The lacrimal glands, which produce tears, are located dorsal to the lateral canthus of the eye. Tears flow down over the surface of the eye, aided by blinking movements of the eyelids. At the medial canthus of the eye are the lacrimal puncta: two small openings, one in the upper lid margin and one in the lower lid margin, that drain tears from the eye. From the lacrimal puncta the tears drain into the lacrimal sac and then into the nasolacrimal duct, which carries the tears into the nasal cavity. The ducts may become blocked because of swelling and mucus accumulation, leading to overflowing of tears.

ENDOCRINE SYSTEM

The endocrine system consists of glands in various parts of the body that secrete minute amounts of chemical substances called hormones directly into the bloodstream, rather than through ducts (Fig. 4-25). These hormones circulate throughout the body and bind to their respective target cells, causing changes in the activity of those cells.

CRITICAL CONCEPT

Glands of the endocrine system secrete hormones directly into the bloodstream.

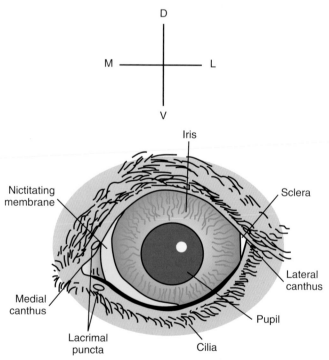

FIGURE 4-24 External view of the dog's left eye. (From Colville TP: *Clinical anatomy and physiology for veterinary technicians*, ed 2, St Louis, 2008, Mosby.)

The endocrine system and nervous system are partners in regulating and controlling functions in an animal's body. The nervous system operates on a short time scale; it can respond rapidly to changes but is not well suited to sustained, long-term activity. The endocrine system does not respond as rapidly as the nervous system but can maintain secretion of hormones for long periods.

Recent studies about the functioning of animal bodies have shown that they are even more complex than earlier thought. Nowhere is this more apparent than in the endocrine system. Hormones of one sort or another are produced throughout the body. Some work locally, whereas others circulate to distant parts of the body. For purposes of clarity and brevity, this chapter deals only with the major endocrine glands (Table 4-5).

HYPOTHALAMUS

The hypothalamus is a part of the brainstem. Together with the pituitary gland, it controls many of the other major endocrine glands. It is extensively connected by nerve fibers to various parts of the brain dorsally and by nerve fibers and blood vessels to the pituitary gland ventrally. It is a vital link between the nervous and endocrine systems.

The hypothalamus influences the pituitary gland by two different mechanisms. It produces hormones called releasing factors and inhibiting factors. These hormones travel down to the anterior part of the pituitary gland through short blood vessels. There, they cause release or inhibition of the anterior pituitary gland's various hormones. The hypothalamus also produces two hormones that are carried down through nerve fibers to the posterior portion of the pituitary gland for storage and release.

PITUITARY GLAND

The pituitary gland is often called the master endocrine gland because many of the hormones it produces direct the activity of other major endocrine glands. The pituitary is a pea-sized

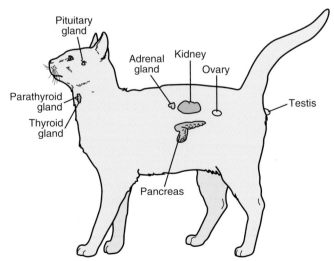

FIGURE 4-25 Relative locations of major endocrine glands in the cat. (From Colville TP: Clinical anatomy and physiology for veterinary technicians, ed 2, St Louis, 2008, Mosby.)

gland connected by a stalk to the hypothalamus. In reality it is two separate glands, the anterior and posterior pituitary glands. These glands are joined physically into one structure.

ANTERIOR PITUITARY GLAND

The anterior pituitary gland produces and releases six hormones—growth hormone (GH), prolactin, thyroid-stimulating hormone (TSH), follicle-stimulating hormone (FSH), luteinizing hormone (LH), and adrenocorticotropic hormone (ACTH).

- Growth hormone, as its name implies, stimulates growth in young animals. It also plays an important role in the general metabolism of body cells in animals of any age.
- Prolactin has a known effect only in females. It helps initiate and maintain milk secretion in the mammary glands.
- Thyroid-stimulating hormone, as its name implies, stimulates the thyroid gland to produce and release hormones.
- Follicle-stimulating hormone derives its name from its effect in females, in which it stimulates production of follicles in the ovary. In males, it stimulates production of spermatozoa in the testes.
- Luteinizing hormone also derives its name from its effect in females, in which it promotes ovulation of a mature ovarian follicle and the follicle's conversion into a corpus luteum. In males, it stimulates the testes to produce testosterone.
- Adrenocorticotropic hormone stimulates the cortex of the adrenal gland to produce and release its hormones.

POSTERIOR PITUITARY GLAND

The posterior pituitary gland does not produce any hormones but stores and releases two hormones produced in the hypothalamus.

Antidiuretic hormone (ADH), also called vasopressin, causes the kidneys to conserve water, producing more concentrated urine. It acts on the distal convoluted tubules and collecting ducts of the kidneys and increases water reabsorption.

The primary effects of oxytocin, the second hormone stored in the posterior pituitary, are to promote uterine contractions at **parturition** and milk let-down from a lactating mammary gland.

THYROID GLAND

The thyroid gland consists of two lobes that may or may not be connected. One lobe is located on either side of the larynx in the neck region. The thyroid gland produces two hormones, thyroxine (T_4) and calcitonin. Thyroxine produces an effect similar to that of growth hormone; it is necessary for normal growth and helps regulate metabolism in the cells of animals of any age. The other thyroid hormone, calcitonin, regulates the blood calcium level and is secreted when blood calcium levels are abnormally high.

PARATHYROID GLANDS

The parathyroid glands are several small nodules located in, on, or near the thyroid gland. The effects of the hormone that

TABLE 4-5	Major Endocrine Glands		
GLAND	**HORMONE**	**TARGET**	**ACTION**
Anterior pituitary	Growth hormone	All body cells	Growth, metabolic regulation
	Prolactin	Female—mammary gland	Lactation
		Male—no known effect	None
	Thyroid-stimulating hormone	Thyroid gland	Thyroid hormone production
	Adrenocorticotropic hormone	Adrenal cortex	Adrenocortical hormone production
	Follicle-stimulating hormone	Female—ovary (follicles)	Oogenesis
		Male—testis (seminiferous tubules)	Spermatogenesis
	Luteinizing hormone	Female—ovary (follicle/ corpus luteum)	Ovulation and corpus luteum production
		Male—testis (interstitial cells)	Testosterone production
	Melanocyte-stimulating hormone	Unknown	Unknown
Posterior pituitary	Antidiuretic hormone	Kidney	Water conservation
	Oxytocin	Female—uterus	Contraction at parturition
		Mammary gland	Milk let-down
		Male—no known effect	No known effect
Thyroid	Thyroid hormone	All body cells	Growth, metabolic regulation
	Calcitonin	Bones	Prevents hypercalcemia
Parathyroid	Parathyroid hormone	Kidneys, intestines, bones	Prevents hypocalcemia
Adrenal cortex	Glucocorticoid hormones	Whole body	Increased blood glucose, blood pressure maintenance
	Mineralocorticoid hormones	Kidneys	Sodium and water retention, potassium elimination
	Sex hormones	Whole body	Minimal effects
Adrenal medulla	Epinephrine and norepinephrine	Whole body	Part of fight-or-flight response
Pancreas (islets)	Insulin	All body cells	Movement of glucose into cells and its use for energy
	Glucagon	Whole body	Increased blood glucose
Testis	Androgens	Whole body	Anabolic effect, development of male secondary sex characteristics
Ovary	Estrogens	Whole body	Preparation for breeding and pregnancy
	Progestins	Uterus	Preparation for and maintenance of pregnancy

they produce, parathormone, oppose those of calcitonin. Parathormone acts to regulate the blood calcium level and is secreted when blood calcium levels become too low.

ADRENAL GLANDS

The adrenal glands are located near the kidneys. They consist of two parts, the cortex and medulla. The adrenal cortex, the outer part of the gland, produces three groups of hormones— glucocorticoids, mineralocorticoids, and sex hormones. The adrenal medulla, the inner part of gland, produces two hormones that are similar to each other, epinephrine and norepinephrine.

ADRENOCORTICAL HORMONES

Glucocorticoid hormones are the basis for cortisone-type drugs. Their primary effects are to increase the blood glucose level through a number of mechanisms, decrease inflammation, and affect the metabolism of fats (mobilization), proteins (catabolism), and carbohydrates (glucose production).

Mineralocorticoid hormones, primarily aldosterone, work mainly in the kidney to promote the retention of water and sodium, which the body needs in large amounts. It does this by promoting elimination of potassium, which the body cannot tolerate in large amounts.

Sex hormones, both estrogens and androgens, are produced in the adrenal cortices of both sexes. The amounts produced are relatively minor.

ADRENAL MEDULLARY HORMONES

The hormones of the adrenal medulla, epinephrine and norepinephrine, are released under control of the sympathetic nervous system as part of the body's fight-or-flight response.

PANCREAS

The pancreas is mainly an accessory digestive organ that serves as an exocrine gland and as an endocrine gland. The exocrine part of the pancreas contains acinar cells that produce enzymes. The enzymes are released in the duodenum through pancreatic ducts. The endocrine part of the pancreas mainly contains small nodules of endocrine cells, the islets of Langerhans. Two hormones are produced in the islets, insulin and glucagon. Insulin is necessary for the body's cells to use glucose for fuel. It prevents abnormally high blood glucose levels and allows glucose to enter the cells for use. A defect in insulin secretion or action leads to diabetes mellitus, characterized by abnormally high blood glucose levels and many metabolic difficulties. The other pancreatic hormone, glucagon, has the opposite effect and tends to increase the blood glucose level.

GONADS

The gonads are the sex cell–producing organs. The male gonads are the testes, and the female gonads are the ovaries. In addition to their sex cell production, the gonads are also endocrine organs.

The main hormone produced in the testes is the male sex hormone, testosterone. Its Leydig cells produce testosterone at a fairly constant level throughout the year. Very small amounts of the female sex hormone, estrogen, are also produced in the testes by Sertoli cells.

Two main hormones produced by the ovaries are estrogen and progesterone. Levels of the hormones produced by the ovaries fluctuate in a cyclical fashion, linked to the development of the follicles and corpora lutea. Under the stimulation of FSH from the pituitary gland, follicles develop in the ovaries. The developing follicles produce the hormone estrogen, which is responsible for the signs of heat, or estrus. After LH from the pituitary gland has caused the follicle to rupture and release its ovum, it stimulates the empty follicle to develop into a solid corpus luteum, which produces progesterone. Progesterone is necessary for the maintenance of pregnancy. If the animal is pregnant, the corpus luteum is retained. If the animal is not pregnant, the corpus luteum lasts for only a short time and then regresses.

URINARY SYSTEM

The many metabolic reactions that take place in the body's cells generate a variety of chemical by-products. Some of these substances are still useful to the body and are recycled, but others would be harmful if allowed to accumulate in the body. These harmful waste products must be eliminated. The urinary system is the primary means whereby waste products are removed from the blood.

The urinary system consists of two kidneys, two ureters, the urinary bladder, and the urethra (Fig. 4-26).

> ### CRITICAL CONCEPT
> The urinary system consists of two kidneys, two ureters, the urinary bladder, and the urethra.

KIDNEYS

The left and right kidneys are located in the dorsal part of the abdominal cavity, just ventral to the most cranial lumbar

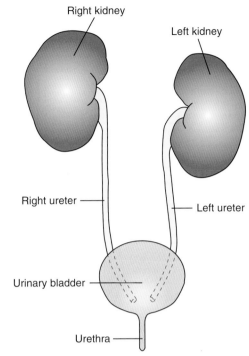

FIGURE 4-26 Parts of the urinary system. The urinary system is made up of two kidneys, two ureters, one urinary bladder, and one urethra. (From Colville TP: Clinical anatomy and physiology for veterinary technicians, ed 2, St Louis, 2008, Mosby.)

vertebrae. Most animals have smooth, bean-shaped kidneys. The right kidney of the horse is heart-shaped. Bovine kidneys have a lobulated appearance. Blood and lymph vessels, nerves, and the ureter enter and leave the kidney through an indented area, the hilus.

A rough-appearing outer cortex is wrapped around a smooth-appearing inner medulla. The area deep to the hilus region is the renal pelvis, the funnel-like beginning of the ureter.

The work of the kidneys is done at the microscopic level in tiny waste disposal units called nephrons. Depending on the animal's size, each kidney may contain from several hundred thousand to several million nephrons. Each nephron is a tube with several bends. This tube has different names because the shape and function of its cells change as it passes through different levels of the kidney matrix. The nephron (tubule) has the following parts: renal corpuscle; proximal convoluted tubule; loop of Henle; distal convoluted tubule; and collecting tubule (Fig. 4-27).

Renal corpuscles are blood filters, located in the renal cortex. Each renal corpuscle is composed of glomeruli surrounded by a Bowman's capsule. Glomeruli are tufts of capillaries interposed between the arterioles entering and leaving the renal corpuscle. A saclike structure called a Bowman's capsule, which is a blind end of each tubule, surrounds the glomerulus. Cells of the glomerulus and Bowman's capsule together make a filtration membrane, which is highly permeable. When blood enters the renal corpuscles, a portion of the plasma, along with its wastes, is filtered out through this filtration membrane into the next portion of the tubule, the proximal convoluted tubule. The balance of

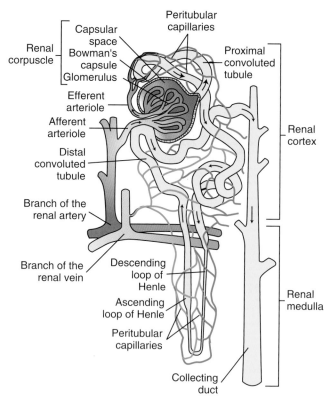

FIGURE 4-27 *Microscopic anatomy of a nephron. Arrows* indicate the direction of fluid flow through the nephron. (From Colville TP: Clinical anatomy and physiology for veterinary technicians, ed 2, St Louis, 2008, Mosby.)

the blood that was not filtered out passes into the capillary network surrounding the rest of the nephron. The filtered fluid passes slowly through the rest of the nephron and is modified as it moves along. From the proximal convoluted tubule, the contents pass to the loop of Henle, which dips deep into the renal medulla. Passing superficially out of the medulla, the loop of Henle continues as the distal convoluted tubule and finally dumps its fluid contents into the collecting tubules, which carry the solution, now called urine, to the renal pelvis.

As the fluid that was filtered out in the renal corpuscle passes through the tubules of the nephron, it is chemically altered. Useful substances, like most of the water, are resorbed back into the blood of the capillary network. Waste products that were resorbed initially are secreted from the capillaries back into the tubules. By the time the fluid in the nephron reaches the collecting tubules, it has become urine. Collecting tubules of all nephrons drain urine into the renal pelvis, the funnel-like opening of the ureter in the kidney.

URETERS

From each renal pelvis, urine is transported to the urinary bladder by the ureters, muscular tubes that conduct the urine by smooth muscle contractions. The ureters enter the bladder at oblique angles, forming valvelike openings that prevent backflow of urine into the ureters as the bladder fills.

URINARY BLADDER

The urinary bladder is a muscular sac that stores urine and releases it periodically to the outside in a process called urination. The kidneys constantly produce urine. As urine accumulates in the urinary bladder, the bladder enlarges and stretch receptors in the bladder wall are activated when the volume reaches a certain point. A spinal reflex then initiates contraction of the smooth muscle in the bladder wall. A voluntarily controlled sphincter muscle around the neck of the urinary bladder enables conscious control of urination.

URETHRA

The urethra is the tube that carries urine from the urinary bladder to the outside of the body. In females, it is relatively short, straight, and wide and has a strictly urinary function. In males, it is relatively long, curved, and narrow, and serves both urinary and reproductive functions.

REPRODUCTIVE SYSTEM

The **reproductive system** is different from other body systems. Whereas most other systems contribute to the survival of the individual animal, the main function of the reproductive system is to help maintain the species. It influences other organ systems, but most parts of the reproductive system are not essential to life. Also, successful functioning of the mammalian reproductive system requires two animals, a male and a female.

MALE REPRODUCTIVE SYSTEM

The male reproductive system is organized to produce male reproductive cells and transmit them to the female. Its main components are the testes, epididymis, vas deferens, accessory sex glands, and penis (Fig. 4-28).

The testes are the male gonads. Their functions include production of the male reproductive cells (spermatozoa) and male sex hormones. Before birth, the testes develop in the abdominal cavity. At or soon after birth they descend through slits in the abdominal muscles called the inguinal rings into a sac of skin called the scrotum. The scrotum houses the testes and helps regulate their temperature. To produce viable spermatozoa, the testes must be maintained at a temperature slightly lower than body temperature. A muscle in the scrotum, the cremaster muscle, acts to raise or lower the testes to adjust their temperature. A network of veins, pampiniform plexuses, surrounding the cranial part of testes also helps lower the temperature of arterial blood coming to testes.

> **CRITICAL CONCEPT**
>
> The main components of the male reproductive system are the testes, epididymis, vas deferens, accessory sex glands, and penis.

Within the testes, spermatogenesis occurs in the seminiferous tubules. Each U-shaped tubule is connected at both ends to efferent ducts. When development of spermatozoa is

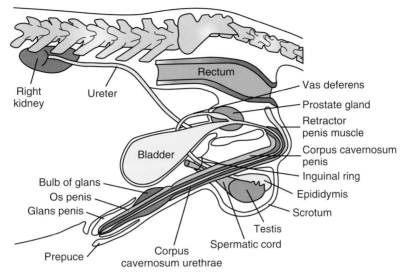

FIGURE 4-28 Male urinary and reproductive organs of the dog, lateral view. (From Colville TP: Clinical anatomy and physiology for veterinary technicians, ed 2, St Louis, 2008, Mosby.)

complete in the seminiferous tubules, the spermatozoa move through the efferent ducts into the epididymis, a long, convoluted tube lying along the surface of the testis. Spermatozoa are stored here until ejaculation. If spermatozoa are not expelled from the epididymis, they die there and are absorbed.

Leading from the epididymis proximally up to the pelvic portion of the urethra is the vas deferens. This muscular tube carries spermatozoa and the fluid in which they are suspended to the urethra for emission as a component of semen.

Also entering the pelvic portion of the urethra are several types of accessory sex glands. The accessory sex gland found in all common mammals is the prostate gland. Other glands, such as the seminal vesicles and bulbourethral glands, are present only in certain species. Each is responsible for adding components of semen to the spermatozoa that are delivered by the vas deferens during ejaculation.

The penis is the male organ of copulation. It consists of roots, which attach it to the brim of the pelvis, a body, which consists primarily of erectile tissue, and the glans, which is the distal free end of the penis that is richly supplied with sensory nerve endings. The erectile tissue is composed of spongy networks of vascular sinuses surrounded by connective tissue.

With appropriate and adequate sensory stimulation, the penis becomes erect and ready for copulation. Through several mechanisms, more blood enters the erectile tissue than leaves it. The result is engorgement and stiffening of the penis, called erection.

Continued stimulation of the penis can produce ejaculation, the reflex expulsion of semen from the urethra. Ejaculation occurs in two rapidly successive stages. First, spermatozoa and seminal fluids are moved into the urethra. Second, semen is expelled from the urethra by rhythmic contractions of the muscles surrounding the urethra.

FEMALE REPRODUCTIVE SYSTEM

The female reproductive system is organized to produce female reproductive cells, accept male reproductive cells

(spermatozoa), allow one sperm cell to unite with each female reproductive cell, and then shelter and nourish the resulting developing fetuses until birth. The organs of the female reproductive system are the ovaries, oviducts, uterus, cervix, vagina, and vulva (Fig. 4-29).

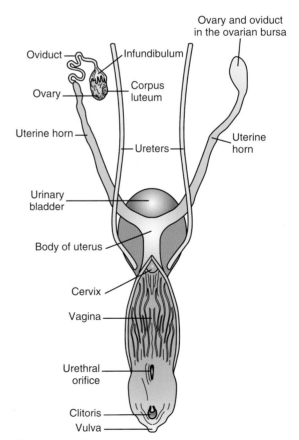

FIGURE 4-29 Reproductive system of bitch, dorsal view. (From Colville TP: Clinical anatomy and physiology for veterinary technicians, ed 2, St Louis, 2008, Mosby.)

The ovaries are the female gonads. Ovaries produce the female reproductive cells (ova) and hormones. Unlike spermatozoa, ova are not continually produced. At or soon after birth, the ovary contains all the ova that it will ever contain. They remain in an immature state until activated by cyclical hormonal cycles.

Under the influence of FSH and LH from the pituitary gland, a few ova at a time develop in the follicles of the ovary. A single layer of flattened follicular cells surrounds the immature ova. When a particular follicle becomes activated, the follicular cells become more cuboidal and multiply to form many layers around the ovum. Spaces gradually form between the follicular cells through secretion of fluid. By the time the follicle is mature, the ovum sits on a tiny hill of follicular cells and is surrounded by the fluid-filled antrum of the follicle. The mature follicle is a large, blisterlike structure that protrudes from the surface of the ovary. As it develops, the follicle secretes increasing amounts of estrogen, which causes the physical and behavioral signs of heat, or estrus.

Release of the ovum, called ovulation, usually occurs as a result of falling FSH levels and peaking LH levels. Ovulation is characterized by the physical rupture of the follicle surface. As the fluid of the antrum rushes out, it carries the ovum with it. After ovulation, the collapsed follicle fills with blood and becomes a corpus hemorrhagicum (CH), which is converted quickly to a corpus luteum (CL), under the influence of LH. The corpus luteum starts producing progesterone, which is necessary for the maintenance of pregnancy. If an animal becomes pregnant, the CL stays on the ovary throughout the pregnancy. If there is no conception and the animal does not become pregnant, the CL regresses and becomes a nonfunctional corpus albicans just before the next heat.

Partially surrounding each ovary, but not physically connected to it, are the oviducts, which are convoluted, tubular extensions of the uterus. At its ovarian end, each oviduct is flared to form the funnel-like infundibulum, which catches ova as they are released from the follicles.

The uterus is a hollow, muscular organ that is continuous with the oviducts cranially and opens, via the cervix, into the vagina caudally. In most common domestic mammals, the uterus consists of two cranial uterine horns that unite in a caudal uterine body.

The cervix is a powerful smooth muscle sphincter that functions to close off the lumen of the uterus from the lumen of the vagina most of the time. The only times the cervix is relaxed and partially dilated are at breeding and parturition.

The vagina is the canal from the cervix to the vulva. It receives the erect penis during copulation and is the birth canal for the newborn at parturition.

The vulva is the external portion of the female genitalia. It consists of the vestibule, the short space between the vagina and labia where the urethra opens, the clitoris, a small, sensitive erectile body homologous to the penis of the male, and the labia, which form the outer boundary of the vulva.

FEMALE REPRODUCTION PHYSIOLOGY: NONPREGNANT ANIMALS

Unlike women and other female primates that have menstrual cycles, with variable levels of sexual receptivity, mammals commonly encountered in veterinary medicine have an estrous cycle, in which the period of sexual receptivity, estrus (heat), is concentrated during a short period, lasting from 1 to several days. During the reminder of the estrous cycle, the female does not accept the male's sexual advances nor allow mating.

The estrous cycle is composed of four or five stages, depending on the species and whether the animal is polyestrous (cycles repeatedly) or monestrous (cycles only once during the breeding season). The stages of estrus are anestrus, proestrus, estrus, metestrus, and diestrus.

ANESTRUS. Anestrus is the period of ovarian inactivity, with no behavioral signs of heat or estrus.

PROESTRUS. Under the influence of gonadotropin-releasing hormone (GnRH) produced in the hypothalamus, FSH is released from the pituitary, acts on the ovary, and causes initial follicle development. These growing follicles produce estrogen, which causes the genital and behavioral changes that attract the male and prepare the female's reproductive tract for mating. Although the proestrus female may show signs of interest in the male, she will not allow mating.

ESTRUS. Estrus is the period of true heat, during which the female allows mating. The estrogen levels peak early in estrus and cause the pituitary to release LH, which further matures the follicles and results in release of the egg(s) at ovulation.

METESTRUS. Metestrus is the short stage during which the female may still attract males but no longer allows mating. During this stage, ovulated follicles metamorphose into corpora lutea, which begin to secrete progesterone. Metestrus is so short in some species that it is not even discussed as a separate stage and is included in diestrus.

DIESTRUS. Diestrus is a stage of ovarian activity without signs of heat. The CL develops fully and produces maximum levels of progesterone to ready the uterus for the conceptus and maintain pregnancy.

If the female does not become pregnant, prostaglandins are released from the uterus, destroying the CL and stopping progesterone production. The female then enters anestrus if it is a monestrous species, such as the dog, or reenters proestrus if it is a polyestrous species, such as the cow. Some polyestrous animals cycle throughout the year (cow), whereas other animals are seasonally polyestrous (e.g., mare, ewe, doe) in response to changing day length.

Seasonally polyestrous animals enter anestrus at the end of the breeding season.

REPRODUCTIVE PHYSIOLOGIC PATTERNS

BITCHES. The bitch (female dog) is a seasonally monestrous animal with a definite anestrous period between cycles. Most bitches come into season approximately once every 6 to 7 months. The heats can occur at any time of the year; however, they seem to be concentrated in the spring and fall. Some female dogs may cycle only once a year, as is the case with the Basenji breed. Other individual dogs may cycle every 4 months and still be considered normal. Bitches reach puberty at 6 to 24 months of age, with an average of 10 to 12 months. Small breeds usually reach puberty earlier than large breeds.

QUEENS. The queen (female cat) is different from other animals discussed earlier in that the others are spontaneous ovulators. That is, they release their eggs at a predetermined time in their cycle, after the appropriate hormonal changes. The queen, on the other hand, is an induced ovulator, meaning coitus (mating) is necessary to stimulate ovulation. The queen is a seasonally polyestrous animal. If not induced to ovulate, she will have several cycles of sexual behavior before being bred and induced to ovulate, or having the follicles regress. Queens have a short anestrous period between October and January, but they then cycle regularly for the rest of the year if they do not conceive. Because the cat is an induced ovulator, the CL is not produced unless coitus has occurred. The cycle lasts approximately 14 days and is composed of 1 to 2 days of proestrus, 3 to 6 days of estrus (heat), and approximately 7 days of metestrus before proestrus occurs again.

FERTILIZATION AND PREGNANCY

At copulation, semen is usually deposited in the proximal vagina. Spermatozoa rapidly move through the cervix, into the uterus, and up the oviducts through a combination of their own swimming actions and contractions of the female reproductive tract. Normally, the spermatozoa arrive at the oviduct before the ovum has entered it. They must spend some time maturing there to improve their capability to fertilize the ovum. This final maturation process is called capacitation.

When the ovum arrives in the oviduct, spermatozoa swarm around it, but only one sperm cell is allowed to penetrate the ovum and fertilize it (Fig. 4-30). Once a single spermatozoon has penetrated the ovum, entry of all others is blocked. Soon after fertilization, the nucleus of the ovum and nucleus of the spermatozoon fuse, or combine. The fertilized ovum now has the full complement of chromosomes and is called a zygote.

The zygote immediately begins the process of cell division, called cleavage, as cells lining the oviduct slowly move it distally toward the uterus. The single cell divides into two cells, the two cells to four, and so on. Cleavage proceeds so rapidly that the cells do not have time to grow larger between divisions. The overall size of the dividing zygote does not increase appreciably during this initial period. When it reaches the uterus, the zygote has formed into a hollow ball of cells, the blastocyst, which is ready to implant itself into the wall of the uterus.

Following implantation, the placenta, the life support system of the developing fetus, develops. The placenta is a multilayered, fluid-filled sac in which the embryo develops. It attaches to the uterine wall so that its blood vessels and the uterine blood vessels are intertwined. Nutrients

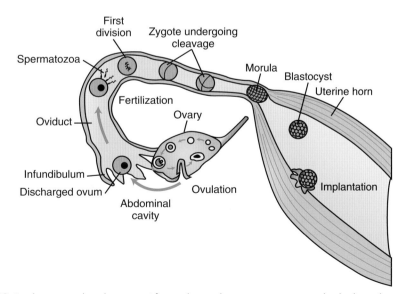

FIGURE 4-30 Fertilization and implantation. After ovulation, the ovum starts moving slowly down the oviduct toward the uterus. A spermatozoon in the oviduct fertilizes the ovum, forming the single-celled zygote. Cleavage of the zygote begins almost immediately as the single cell divides into two cells, two cells divide into four, and so on. After 1 or 2 days, the zygote has formed into a solid mass of cells called the morula. The morula continues to develop into a hollow ball of cells, the blastocyst, which enters the uterus and implants in its wall. (From Colville TP: Clinical anatomy and physiology for veterinary technicians, ed 2, St Louis, 2008, Mosby.)

and gases are exchanged between these maternal and fetal blood vessels. Normally, there is no direct mixing of fetal and maternal blood. The developing fetus is linked with the placenta via the umbilical cord, through which blood in the umbilical arteries and vein flows to and from the fetus.

The time from fertilization of the ovum to delivery of the newborn is referred to as the **gestation** period. It is convenient to divide it into three, often unequal, segments, called trimesters. The first trimester is the period of the embryo, when the newly implanted zygote is getting itself organized and developing its life-supporting placenta. During this period, the developing offspring is often referred to as an embryo. Starting with the second trimester, the developing offspring is generally called a fetus. The second trimester is the fetal development period, when all the various parts of the fetus are taking shape and differentiating from each other. All the body tissues, organs, and systems develop during this period. The third trimester is the period of fetal growth. All parts of the fetus grow dramatically during this last period of development, preparing it to transition from a parasitic to a free-living existence after birth. The lengths of the gestation period in some common species are listed in Table 4-6.

PARTURITION

After the preparatory changes of late pregnancy, which ready the dam and fetus for birth, parturition begins. Parturition has several common names, depending on the species involved. Parturition in the bitch is called whelping. In the cat, it is called kittening or queening.

Parturition is divided into three stages. Stage 1 is preliminary to expulsion of the fetus. During this stage, the uterine muscles undergo rhythmic contractions, which reposition and advance the fetus toward the cervix. In response to these contractions and the pressure of the fetus, the cervix relaxes fully and dilates. The dam in first-stage labor often is anxious and restless and shows evidence of abdominal cramps. Stage 1 ends with delivery of the fetus into the pelvic canal and rupture of the fetal membranes.

Stage 2 is the stage of expulsion of the fetus from the birth canal. Uterine contractions are stronger and accompanied by abdominal straining to help expel the fetus. The importance of abdominal straining versus uterine contractions in the birth process varies among species. With successful delivery of the fetus, the dam completes stage 2 and rests during the first part of stage 3.

Stage 3 of parturition is characterized by expulsion of the placenta. Uterine contractions continue but are not as severe as those in stage 2. The uterus begins to shrink toward its nonpregnant size. In polytocous (litter-bearing) species, the cycle of stages 1 to 3 repeats itself with each fetus. Stages 1 and 2 may occur several times and result in passage of several fetuses before a placenta is passed in stage 3 in these species.

After delivery of the fetus, the dam rests and begins to care for the newborn. She licks it dry, which helps stimulate breathing. She chews off any amniotic membrane remaining on the fetus. The bitch and queen usually chew the umbilical cord to sever the placenta. The cord usually ruptures spontaneously during delivery of the calf or during the mare's or foal's efforts to rise.

It is often difficult to tell when a dam has finished delivering all of the offspring. Prepartum radiographs made 1 week before the due date can determine the exact number of pups or kittens in the dam. The bitch's abdomen may be palpated for more pups, or a finger in a sterile glove may be introduced into the vagina to feel for another pup. X-rays of the abdomen may be necessary. Some bitches and queens eat their neonatal pups, so care must be taken to differentiate fetuses in the stomach from those in the uterus.

MILK PRODUCTION. The mammary glands are specialized skin glands that produce secretions essential for nourishment of the newborn. Mammary glands are found in males and females, but the hormone environment necessary for their full development and milk secretion only occurs near the end of pregnancy in females.

The process of milk production, called lactation, begins toward the end of pregnancy. Several hormones are involved, chiefly prolactin. The initial mammary secretion after parturition is called colostrum and differs from normal milk in composition and appearance. Colostrum has a laxative effect on the newborn and is important in transferring antibodies from the mother to the offspring. The intestine of the newborn can absorb the large antibody molecules in the colostrum for only a few hours after birth, so it is important that a newborn suckle colostrum as soon as possible after birth.

Suckling or milking stimulates continued production of milk. Sensory stimulation of the teat or nipple, either by the offspring's suckling or by milking, causes continued production of the hormones necessary to support lactation.

TABLE 4-6	Gestation Periods of Some Common Species	
SPECIES	**RANGE**	**APPROXIMATE GESTATION PERIOD**
Cats	55-69 days	2 mo
Cattle	271-291 days	9 mo
Dogs	59-68 days	2 mo
Elephants	615-650 days	21 mo
Ferrets	42 days	6 wk
Goats	146-155 days	5 mo
Hamsters	19-20 days	3 wk
Horses	321-346 days	11 mo
Humans	280 days	9 mo
Pigs	110-116 days	3 mo, 3 wk, and 3 days
Rabbits	30-32 days	1 mo
Sheep	143-151 days	5 mo

From Colville TP: Clinical anatomy and physiology for veterinary technicians, ed 2, St Louis, 2008, Mosby.

Stimulation of the teat or nipple causes immediate release of oxytocin from the posterior pituitary gland. Oxytocin has the effect of squeezing milk out of the alveoli and small ducts of the mammary gland into the large ducts and sinuses, where the newborn can extract it by suckling. The immediate effect of suckling or milking is called milk let-down. Cessation of suckling or milking results in the cessation of milk production; the mammary gland dries up.

RECOMMENDED READINGS

Colville T, Bassert JM: *Clinical anatomy and physiology for veterinary technicians*, ed 2, St Louis, 2009, Mosby.

Dyce KM: *Textbook of veterinary anatomy*, ed 4, St Louis, 2010, Saunders.

Feldman EC, Nelson RW: *Canine and feline endocrinology and reproduction*, ed 3, St Louis, 2004, Saunders.

Frandson RD, Fails AD, Wilke WL: *Anatomy and physiology of farm animals*, ed 6, Philadelphia, 2003, Lippincott Williams & Wilkins.

McBride DF: *Learning veterinary terminology*, ed 2, St Louis, 2002, Mosby.

Saunders Veterinary Anatomy Coloring Book, St Louis, 2011, Saunders.

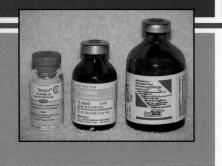

5 Pharmacology and Pharmacy[1]

OUTLINE

Drug Names, 105
Dosage Forms, 106
Solid and Semisolid Dosage Forms, 106
Liquid Dosage Forms, 106
Prescriptions and Dispensing Medication, 108
Writing Prescriptions, 108
Components of a Prescription, 109
Containers for Dispensing Medication, 110
The Metric System, 110
Calculating Drug Doses, 111
Storing and Handling Drugs in the Pharmacy, 112
Storing and Prescribing Controlled Substances, 112
Handling Toxic Drugs, 113
Therapeutic Range, 113
Dosage Regimen, 113
Routes of Administration, 114
Movement of Drug Molecules in the Body, 114
How Drugs Exert Their Effects, 115
Drugs Affecting the Gastrointestinal Tract, 115
Emetics, 115
Antiemetics, 116
Antidiarrheals, 116
Adsorbents and Protectants, 116
Laxatives, Lubricants, and Stool Softeners, 117
Antacids, 117
Antiulcer Drugs, 117
Appetite-Stimulating Drugs, 117
Drugs Affecting the Cardiovascular System, 117
Antiarrhythmic Drugs, 117
Positive Inotropic Agents, 118
Vasodilators, 118
Diuretics, 119
Drugs Affecting the Respiratory System, 119
Antitussives, 119
Mucolytics, Expectorants, and Decongestants, 120
Bronchodilators, 120
Drugs Affecting the Endocrine System, 120
Drugs Used to Treat Hypothyroidism, 120

Drugs Used to Treat Hyperthyroidism, 121
Endocrine Pancreatic Drugs, 121
Drugs Used to Treat Hypoadrenocorticism, 121
Drugs Used to Treat Hyperadrenocorticism, 121
Drugs Affecting Reproduction, 121
Drugs Affecting the Nervous System, 122
Anesthetics, 122
Tranquilizers and Sedatives, 122
Analgesics, 123
Anticonvulsants, 123
Central Nervous System Stimulants, 123
Antimicrobials, 124
Penicillins, 124
Cephalosporins, 124
Bacitracins, 125
Aminoglycosides, 125
Fluoroquinolones, 125
Tetracyclines, 125
Sulfonamides and Potentiated Sulfonamides, 125
Lincosamides, 125
Macrolides, 125
Metronidazole, 125
Nitrofurans, 126
Chloramphenicol and Fluorfenicol, 126
Rifampin, 126
Antifungals, 126
Amphotericin B and Nystatin, 126
Flucytosine, 126
Fluconazole, Ketoconazole, and Itraconazole, 126
Griseofulvin, 126
Antiparasitics, 126
Internal Antiparasitics, 126
External Antiparasitics, 127
Anti-Inflammatories, 128
Glucocorticoids, 128
Nonsteroidal Anti-inflammatory Drugs, 128
Other Anti-Inflammatories, 129

[1]Elsevier and the author acknowledge and appreciate the original contributions from Sirois M: Principles and practice of veterinary technology, ed 3, St Louis, 2011, Mosby and Wanamaker BP, Massey KL: Applied pharmacology for veterinary technicians, ed 4, St Louis, 2009, Saunders, whose work forms the heart of this chapter.

OUTLINE—cont'd

Disinfectants and Antiseptics, *129*
Phenols, *129*
Alcohols, *129*
Quaternary Ammonium Compounds, *129*

Chlorine Compounds, *129*
Iodophors, *130*
Biguanides, *130*

LEARNING OBJECTIVES

After viewing this chapter, the reader will be able to:
1. List the various categories of drugs and their clinical uses.
2. Identify dosage forms in which drugs are available.
3. Calculate drug dosages.
4. List and compare routes by which various types of drugs are administered.
5. Describe ways in which drugs exert their effect and affect body tissue.
6. Explain procedures used to safely store and handle drugs.
7. List the primary drugs affecting various body systems.

KEY TERMS

Analgesics	Continuous rate infusion	Expectorants	Proprietary name
Anthelmintic	Controlled substance	Fungicidal	Residue
Antibiotic	Corticosteroid	Metric system	Sanitizers
Anticonvulsants	Disinfection	Neuroleptanalgesia	Subcutaneous (SC) injection
Anti-inflammatory drugs	Decongestant	NSAIDs	Therapeutic range
Antimicrobial	Diuretic	Osmotic diuretic	Tincture
Antiseptics	Dose	Per os	Vasodilator
Bactericidal	Elixir	Pharmacokinetics	Vermicide
Bacteriostatic	Emetics	Positive inotropic drugs	Virucidal
Bronchodilator	Enteric-coated tablet	Prescription	

DRUG NAMES

Drugs are generally referred to by three different names. The chemical name, such as D-alpha-amino-*p*-hydroxybenzyl-penicillin trihydrate, describes the drug's chemical composition. The nonproprietary name, sometimes called the generic name, is a more concise name given to the specific chemical compound. Examples of nonproprietary names are aspirin, acetaminophen, and amoxicillin. The **proprietary** or trade name is a unique drug name given by a manufacturer to its particular brand of drug. Examples of proprietary or trade names include Excedrin, Tylenol, and Amoxi-Tabs. Because the trade name is a proper noun, it is capitalized, and the superscript ® or ™ is added to signify that the trade name is a registered trademark and cannot be legally used by other manufacturers. Because many drug manufacturers produce similar products, a single generic drug can be sold under a number of trade names. For example, the antibiotic amoxicillin is manufactured by several different companies, each of which has its own trade name for amoxicillin (e.g., Amoxi-Tabs, Robamox-V, Amoxil).

The Center for Veterinary Medicine (CVM) of the U.S. Food and Drug Administration (FDA) requires that drug container labels list specific items, including the generic and trade names of the medication, the drug concentration, the quantity in the drug container, the name and address of the manufacturer, the manufacturer's lot number, and the expiration date of the medication (Fig. 5-1). Instructions for use must also be included, either on the label or in an insert within the package.

> **CRITICAL CONCEPT**
> Most drugs are referred to by the generic name in veterinary clinics.

When a drug company develops and patents a new drug (not just a new trade name for an old drug, but a new chemical) and obtains FDA approval to sell it, the company has the exclusive rights to manufacture this drug for a number of years. During that time, no other drug manufacturer can produce the same drug. This allows the drug company to recover, at the expense of the consumer, the costs of the research, development, and testing that the company has invested to bring the drug to market. After these patent rights expire, other companies can legally produce the drug. These copycat drugs are called generic equivalents, because they have properties equivalent to those of the original compound. Generic equivalents are usually sold at a much lower price than the original manufacturer's product because the generic manufacturer has not had to underwrite the costs for the development of the original drug.

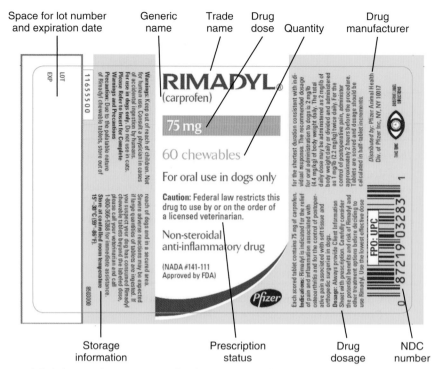

FIGURE 5-1 A label showing the components of a drug as required by the U.S. Food and Drug Administration. (From Wanamaker B, Massey M: Applied pharmacology for veterinary technicians, ed 5, St Louis, 2014, Saunders.)

DOSAGE FORMS

Drugs are also described by their dosage form. The form of a drug is usually solid, semisolid, or liquid (Table 5-1).

SOLID AND SEMISOLID DOSAGE FORMS

Solid dosage forms include tablets, which are powdered drugs compressed into pills or discs, and capsules, which are powdered drugs enclosed within gelatin capsules. **Enteric-coated tablets** have a special covering that protects the drug from the harsh acidic environment of the stomach and prevents the tablet from dissolving until it enters the intestine. Sustained-release forms of oral drugs release small amounts of the drug into the intestinal lumen over an extended period. Suppositories are inserted into the rectum, where they dissolve and release the drug to be absorbed across the membranes of the intestinal wall.

LIQUID DOSAGE FORMS

A solution is a drug dissolved in a liquid vehicle that does not settle out if left standing. In contrast, a suspension contains drug particles that are suspended, but not dissolved, in the liquid vehicle. These drug particles usually settle to the bottom of the container when the container is left standing, so one must shake it back into suspension before administration to ensure consistent dosing. Syrups, such as cough syrups, are solutions of drugs with water and sugar (e.g., 85% sucrose).

Elixirs are solutions of drugs dissolved in sweetened alcohol. Elixirs are used for drugs that do not readily dissolve in water. It is therefore important that you do not dilute an

TABLE 5-1	Dosage Forms	
SOLID FORMS	**SEMISOLID FORMS**	**LIQUID FORMS**
Tablet	Suppositories	Syrup
Capsule	Liniment	Elixir
Enteric-coated tablet	Ointment	Tincture
Sustained release	Cream	Lotion
Implant	Paste	Injectable

From Sirois M: Principles and practice of veterinary technology, ed 3, St Louis, 2011, Mosby.

elixir with water because the water will stratify into a layer separate from the elixir solution.

Tinctures are alcohol solutions meant for topical application (applied onto the skin). Topical products are available as liniments, which contain a drug in an oil base that are rubbed into the skin, or lotions, which are drug suspensions or solutions that are dabbed, brushed, or dripped onto the skin without rubbing (e.g., poison ivy medications).

Ointments, creams, and pastes are semisolid dosage forms that are applied to the skin (ointments, creams) or given orally (pastes). Ointments and creams are designed to liquefy at body temperatures, whereas pastes tend to keep their semisolid form at body temperature.

Repository forms of injectable drugs are formulated to prolong absorption of the drug from the site of administration and thus provide a more sustained effective drug concentration in the body. Implants are solid dosage forms that are injected or inserted under the skin and dissolve or release a drug over an extended period.

INJECTABLE DRUGS: NEEDLES AND SYRINGES

Drugs given by injection are said to be parenterally administered, as opposed to those given enterally via the gastrointestinal tract. Parenteral medications may be supplied in single-dose vials, multidose vials, ampules, or large volume bottles or bags (Fig. 5-2). Injectable drugs are administered via a needle and syringe. Syringes are available in various sizes and styles. The most commonly used sizes are 3, 6, 12, 20, 35, and 60 mL. Syringes may be ordered from the manufacturer with or without an attached needle. The tip of the syringe, where the needle attaches, can be one of four types—Luer-Lok tip (Fig. 5-3, *A*), slip tip (see Fig. 5-3, *B*), eccentric tip (see Fig. 5-3, *C*), or catheter tip (see Fig. 5-3, *D*). A complete syringe consists of a plunger, barrel, hub, needle, and dead space (Fig. 5-4). The area in which fluid remains when the plunger is completely depressed is called the dead space.

SYRINGES

Tuberculin Syringe. A tuberculin syringe (Fig. 5-5) holds up to 1 mL of medication. It usually is available with a 25-gauge or smaller attached needle. This syringe is commonly used for injections of less than 1 mL. Some tuberculin syringes have a dead space. Although the patient receives the proper amount of medicine, some liquid remains in this dead space, thus wasting the drug and costing the practice money. This is also important to remember when a tuberculin syringe is used to draw up controlled substances. The dead space will cause the controlled substance log book to reflect more of the controlled substance than is actually in the vial. Thus, the dead space should be considered when amounts used are documented. Some tuberculin syringes are manufactured with low dead space or no dead space at all. In the case of syringes with no dead space, the needle screws into the tuberculin syringe instead of attaching to the tip.

Insulin Syringe. An insulin syringe (Fig. 5-6) usually is supplied with a 25-gauge needle and, different from other syringes, has no dead space. The syringe is divided into units instead of milliliters and should be used only for insulin injection.

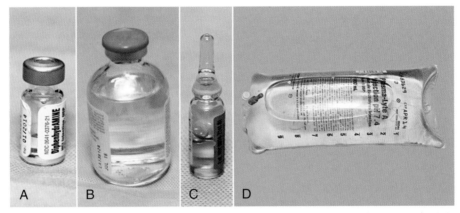

FIGURE 5-2 Parenteral medications are supplied in single-dose vials (**A**), multidose vials (**B**), ampules (**C**), and large-volume bottles or bags used for intravenous administration (**D**). (From Wanamaker B, Massey M: Applied pharmacology for veterinary technicians, ed 5, St Louis, 2014, Saunders.)

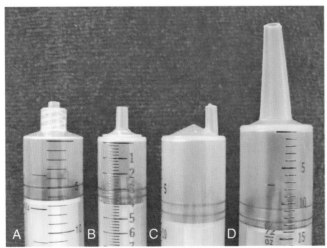

FIGURE 5-3 Syringes are available with different tips, such as a Luer-Lok tip (**A**), slip tip (**B**), eccentric tip (**C**), and catheter tip (**D**).

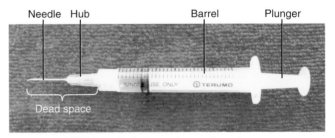

FIGURE 5-4 The parts of a needle and syringe.

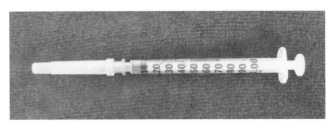

FIGURE 5-5 A tuberculin syringe with needle attached.

Figure 5-7 illustrates the importance of being familiar with the different types of syringes and the units of measurement found on each. This is necessary to ensure that one can draw up an accurate amount of medication.

NEEDLES. Needles are available in various sizes and styles, but all needles have three parts, the hub, shaft, and bevel (Fig. 5-8). Needle sizes vary by gauge and by length. The gauge refers to the inside diameter of the shaft; the larger the gauge number, the smaller the diameter. The length of the needle is measured from the tip of the hub to the end of the shaft. Lengths longer than 1 inch generally are used in large animals and occasionally for biopsy. The bevel is the angle of the opening at the needle tip. It is often helpful when venipuncture is performed to have the beveled side of the needle facing up before the needle is inserted into the patient.

Some drugs may be unstable in solution and may require reconstitution with sterile water or another diluent; these may be used immediately for injection (Procedure 5-1).

PRESCRIPTIONS AND DISPENSING MEDICATION

WRITING PRESCRIPTIONS

A **prescription** is an order from a licensed veterinarian directing a pharmacist to prepare a drug for use in a client's animal. Drugs that do not require a prescription are referred to as over-the-counter (OTC) drugs. When writing prescriptions, veterinarians must adhere to the following guidelines:

* Veterinary prescription drugs must be used only by or on the order of a licensed veterinarian.
* A valid veterinarian-client-patient relationship must exist.
* Veterinary prescription drugs must meet proper requirements for labeling.
* Veterinary prescription drugs should be dispensed only in a quantity necessary for the treatment of the animal(s). Unlimited refills are limited to lifelong treatments to decrease the potential of misuse of the drugs.

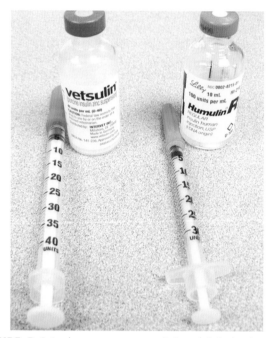

FIGURE 5-6 Insulin syringes come in 0.5- and 0.3-mL volumes and are graded in units. (From Sirois M: Principles and practice of veterinary technology, ed 3, St Louis, 2011, Mosby.)

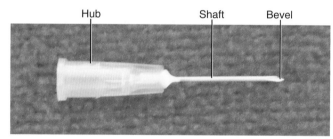

FIGURE 5-8 A needle consists of three parts, the hub, shaft, and bevel.

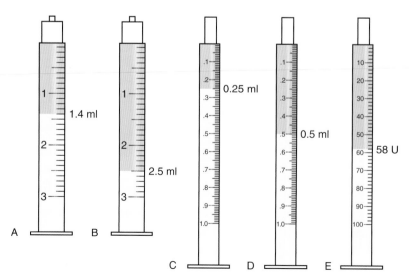

FIGURE 5-7 Examples of how to read amounts of medication contained in a syringe. (From Wanamaker BP, Massey K: Applied pharmacology for veterinary technicians, ed 4, St Louis, 2009, Saunders.)

📋 **PROCEDURE 5-1** RECONSTITUTION OF A MEDICATION

Materials Needed

Syringe of adequate size for the amount of diluent, with a needle attached
70% isopropyl alcohol
Cotton swab

Procedure

1. Clean the rubber diaphragm of the medication vial and the diluent vial with an alcohol swab **(A).**

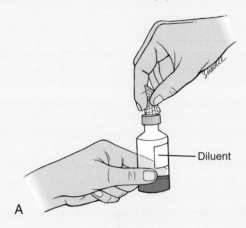

A

2. Remove the needle cap and pull back on the plunger to fill the barrel with air equal to the desired amount of diluent. Inject the air into the vial of diluent to create positive pressure and to ease withdrawal **(B).** Invert the diluent vial and withdraw the desired amount of diluent.

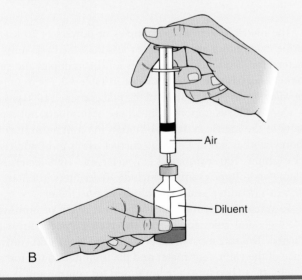

B

3. Inject the diluent into the medication vial and withdraw the syringe and needle. Shake the vial to mix well **(C).**

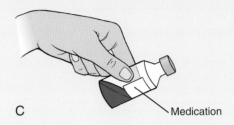

C   — Medication

4. Positive pressure may be created in the freshly mixed medication vial before the desired amount of medication has been withdrawn. Once the medication has been withdrawn **(D),** label the syringe, if needed, or administer the drug to the patient. After withdrawing the patient's medication, dispose of the vial or store it according to the label.

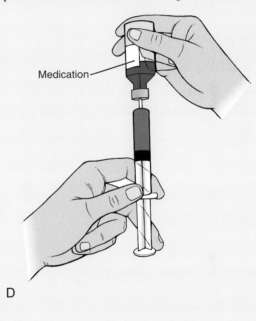

Medication —

D

From Wanamaker, BP, Massey K: Applied pharmacology for veterinary technicians, ed 4, St Louis, 2009, Saunders.

- Appropriate records of all prescriptions issued must be maintained.
- Veterinary prescription drugs must be appropriately handled and stored for safety and security.

CRITICAL CONCEPT

There must be a client-patient-veterinarian relationship for a veterinarian to prescribe medications.

COMPONENTS OF A PRESCRIPTION

A sample prescription is shown in Figure 5-9. Box 5-1 shows common abbreviations used in prescriptions and their meanings. Valid prescriptions must contain the following items:

- Name, address, and telephone number of the person who wrote the prescription
- Date on which the prescription was written
- Owner's name, animal's name, and species of animal

HOMETOWN VETERINARY ASSOCIATES

2000 West Chelsea Ave., Momack, PA

(324) 555-4313

Date: November 22, 2011

Patient: Cricket   **Species:** Canine

Owner: Lee Ann Wozniak   **Phone:** 555-0127

Address: 929 Christopher Robin Lane, Brookside, PA 13235

℞ Amoxicillin tablets 100mg #30 tabs
    Sig: 1 tab q8h POPRN until gone

_____ Andrew Ryan **D.V.M.**

FIGURE 5-9 Typical prescription for a veterinary drug. (From Sirois M: Principles and practice of veterinary technology, ed 3, St Louis, 2011, Mosby.)

BOX 5-1	Abbreviations Commonly Used in Prescriptions

ABBREVIATION	MEANING	ABBREVIATION	MEANING
bid	Twice daily	po	By mouth
cc	Cubic centimeter	prn	As needed
disp	Dispense	q	Every
g	Gram	q8h	Every 8 hours
gm	Gram	qd	Every day
gr	Grain	qid	Four times daily
h	Hour	qod	Every other day
lb	Pound	sid	Once daily
mg	Milligram	stat	Immediately
mL	Milliliter	tid	Three times daily
od	Right eye	tsp	Teaspoon
os	Left eye		

Note: The abbreviation "sid" is rarely used or recognized by pharmacists outside the veterinary profession.
From Sirois M: Principles and practice of veterinary technology, ed 3, St Louis, 2011, Mosby.

- Rx symbol (abbreviation of *recipe*, Latin for "take thou")
- Drug name, concentration, and number of units to be dispensed
- *Sig.* (abbreviation of *signa*, Latin for "write" or "label"), indicating directions for the client in treating the animal
- Signature of the person who wrote the prescription
- U.S. Drug Enforcement Administration (DEA) registration number if the drug is a controlled substance

Many pharmacies will also require the owner's address and phone number.

CRITICAL CONCEPT

Always double-check a prescription label that has been written or printed to make sure that it is accurate.

CONTAINERS FOR DISPENSING MEDICATION

Many veterinary practices dispense tablets and capsules in plastic containers with a childproof lid. If medication is dispensed in a paper envelope and a child becomes poisoned, the veterinarian could be found negligent in dispensing the medication in a manner that placed the child at risk.

Liquids are dispensed in individual syringes or a bottle. The bottle usually has a syringe or dropper to draw up the amount needed at each treatment.

THE METRIC SYSTEM

Although several systems of measurement are used in veterinary medicine, most of the calculations performed in veterinary practice involve units in the **metric system**. The metric system uses powers of 10 as a base for different units in the system. The metric system is a decimal system of notation with only three basic units for weight, volume, and length. Various values can be expressed in the metric system by adding prefixes to the basic units that designate multiples or fractions of the basic units. To work in the metric system, some of the more commonly used prefixes and their abbreviations must be memorized.

The three basic units of measure are summarized below:

Measurement	Unit	Symbol
Length	Meter	m
Mass	Gram	g
Volume	Liter	l or L

The metric system uses multiples or powers of 10 to describe magnitudes greater than or less than the basic units of meter, gram, and liter. The prefixes for the multiples and submultiples of basic units are provided in Table 5-2. For example, the *kilo*gram is 1000 grams and the *milli*gram is 1/1000 gram.

Consistency is important in all use of numbers, but especially in the metric system. Although the unit gram may be abbreviated as gm or Gm, the correct use is g. In addition, for example, 100 *centi*meters is 1 *meter*, and 1000 *meters* is 1 *kilo*meter. Volume examples include 10 *deci*liters in 1 *liter*, 10 *liters* in 1 *deca*liter, and 10 *deca*liters in 1 *hecto*liter.

To minimize errors and misinterpretations of numbers, a few general rules for use of the metric system must be learned. The rule most often encountered is the unit equivalence of the cubic centimeter and the milliliter. In the metric system, these two units are both used for volume and designate the same volume. This is because the metric measure of a liter is defined as a volume of 1000 cubic centimeters (cc) or a volume of 10 cm × 10 cm × 10 cm. Although the terms *milliliter* and *cubic centimeter* are often used interchangeably, milliliter is the correct designation for use in medicine.

As with all decimal units, any decimal number that has no whole number to the left of the decimal point should have a zero inserted as a placeholder. Zeroes should not be added after decimal numbers to avoid confusion in medication orders. Fractions are not written in the metric system. Always use decimal numbers to express numbers that are less than one.

TABLE 5-2	Prefixes for the Multiples and Submultiples of Basic Units	
POWER OF 10	**PREFIX**	**SYMBOL**
10^{12}	tera	T
10^{9}	giga	G
10^{6}	mega	M
10^{3}	kilo	K
10^{2}	hecto	h
10^{1}	deca or deka	da
10^{-1}	deci	d
10^{-2}	centi	c
10^{-3}	milli	m
10^{-6}	micro	mc or μ
10^{-9}	nano	n
10^{-12}	pico	p
10^{-15}	femto	f
10^{-18}	atto	a

From Hendrix CM, Sirois M: Laboratory procedures for veterinary technicians, ed 5, St Louis, 2007, Mosby Elsevier.

CALCULATING DRUG DOSES

Calculating the dose of drug to be administered involves the following steps:

1. Weigh the animal and convert the weight in pounds to kilograms (if necessary).
2. Depending on how the drug is usually dosed (e.g., mg/kg, U/kg), use the animal's weight to calculate the correct dose (e.g., in mg, mL, units, g).
3. Based on the concentration of the drug (e.g., mg of drug/mL of solution or mg of drug/tablet), determine what volume or number of tablets to administer. Simple algebra helps calculate the amount (dose) of drug to be given (e.g., mg or mL) along with the animal's weight and the recommended drug dosage (e.g., mg/kg). You can also calculate the number of units to give (e.g., tablets or mL) if you know the amount of drug in each unit (e.g., mg/mL or mg/tablet) and the duration of treatment (days). Common metric conversion factors used in calculating drug doses are listed in Box 5-2.
   Step 1. Set up an equation so that the units (e.g., kg, lb) are the same on the top (numerator) and bottom (denominator) on both sides of the equation. Then, solve for X (e.g., kg of body weight). This is shown in step 1 of Box 5-3.
   Step 2. Once the animal's weight has been converted to the appropriate units (in this case, kg), determine the amount of drug (dose) to be given. On the left of the equation is the drug dosage (e.g., milligrams of drug/kilogram body weight), and the X you are solving for is the total drug dose (in milligrams). This is shown in step 2 of Box 5-3.
   Step 3. After the total dose is determined (in mg or some other measure), calculate the volume (e.g., mL) or number of solid units (tablets, capsules) to be administered using the concentration of drug in the solution (mg of drug/mL of solution) or in each solid unit

BOX 5-2	Metric Conversion Factors

1 kg = 1000 g = 100,000 milligrams (mg)
1 kg = 2.2 lb
1 gram = 1 gm = 1000 mg = 0.001 kg
1 gram = 1 g = 15.43 grains (gr)
1 grain = 64.8 milligrams (usually rounded to 60 or 65 mg)
1 lb = 0.454 kg = 16 ounces (oz)
1 mg = 0.001 g = 1000 micrograms (μg or mcg)
1 liter (L) = 1000 mL = 10 deciliters (dL)
1 mL = 1 cc = 1000 microliters (μL or mcL)
1 tablespoon (tbsp) = 3 teaspoons (tsp)
1 tsp = 5 mL
1 gallon (gal) = 3.786 L
1 gal = 4 quarts (qt) 8 pints (pt) = 128 fluid ounces (fl oz)
1 pt = 2 cups (C) = 16 fl oz = 473 mL

From Sirois M: Principles and practice of veterinary technology, ed 3, St Louis, 2011, Mosby.

BOX 5-3	Simple Algebraic Calculation Used to Calculate a Drug Dose

What volume of a drug solution should we give to a 44-lb dog if the recommended dosage is 5 mg/kg and the concentration of the solution is 50 mg/mL?

Step 1: Convert pounds to kilograms.

$$X \text{ kg} = \frac{44 \text{ lb}}{2.2\frac{\text{lb}}{\text{kg}}} = 20 \text{ kg}$$

Step 2: Calculate the total drug dose.

$$X \text{ mg} = 5\frac{\text{mg}}{\text{kg}} \times 20 \text{ kg} = 100 \text{ mg}$$

Step 3: Calculate the volume of solution needed.

$$X \text{ mL} = \frac{100 \text{ mg}}{50\frac{\text{mg}}{\text{mL}}} = 2 \text{ mL}$$

From Sirois M: Principles and practice of veterinary technology, ed 3, St Louis, 2011, Mosby.

(mg of drug/tablet), solving for milliliters of liquid or number of tablets. This is shown in step 3 of Box 5-3.

When dispensing solid units (tablets, capsules), round to the nearest unit (or half- or quarter-tablet if the tablet is designed to be broken and greater accuracy is essential). The steps for calculating the total number of solid units required during a course of treatment are detailed in Box 5-4. Always check the rounded dosage with the veterinarian because some drugs have a very narrow margin of safety and may need to be rounded down versus up.

Examples

1. A 50-lb canine is prescribed amoxicillin twice a day for 7 days. Normal dosing is 10 mg/lb and the tablets come in 50, 100, 250, and 500 mg. What is the prescribed dose, and which concentration of tablet should be prescribed?

BOX 5-4 | Calculating the Number of Tablets to Dispense

How many 25-mg tablets should we dispense for a 10-lb cat if the recommended dosage is 5 mg/lb twice daily for 7 days?

Step 1: Calculate the number of tablets needed per dose.

$$10 \text{ lb} \times 5\frac{\text{mg}}{\text{lb}} = 50 \text{ mg per dose}$$

Step 2: Calculate the number of tablets needed daily.

2 tablets per dose × twice daily = 4 tablets daily

Step 3: Calculate the number of tablets needed for 7 days.

4 tablets daily × 7 days = 28 tablets

From Sirois M: Principles and practice of veterinary technology, ed 3, St Louis, 2011, Mosby.

---

a. 10 mg/lb × 50 lb = 500 mg is the dose. Therefore, 500-mg tablets should be prescribed. The prescription would then be one 500-mg tablet orally every 12 hours for 7 days, a total of 14 tablets.

2. A 14-lb feline is prescribed furosemide at 2 mg/kg. This medication comes 12.5- and 50-mg tablets. What is the prescribed dose and which tablet should he get?
   a. 14 lb/(2.2 kg/lb) = 6.36 kg
   b. 2 mg/kg × 6.36 kg = 12.7 mg dosage
   c. The 12.5-mg tablets should be prescribed.

3. A 25-lb canine is prescribed doxycycline at 10 mg/kg. The owners have requested liquid, not pill, form. The doxycycline comes in a 5-mg/mL liquid dosing form.
   a. 25 lb/(2.2 kg/lb) = 11.3 kg
   b. 10 mg/kg × 11.3 kg = 113-mg dose
   c. The liquid is 5 mg/mL so 113 mg/(5 mg/mL) = 22.7 mL of liquid at each dosing.

4. The veterinarian asks you to give a 985-lb equine an injection of Banamine at 1.1 mg/kg. Banamine comes in a 50-mg/mL concentration for injection. How much will you be giving?
   a. 985 lb/(2.2 kg/lb) = 447.7 kg
   b. 1.1 mg/kg × 447.7 kg = 492.5 mg
   c. 492 mg/(50 mg/mL) = 9.85 mL of Banamine

CRITICAL CONCEPT

Become familiar with the medications commonly used in practice so you will have a general idea of the amount that should be given and then catch a mistake in figuring out the dosage if you make one.

STORING AND HANDLING DRUGS IN THE PHARMACY

Drugs that are improperly stored (e.g., exposed to extreme temperature or light) can degenerate or become inactivated, providing little or no benefit to the animal for which they are used. Drugs still on the pharmacy shelf after the listed expiration date on the container may be less effective. In some cases, such as with tetracycline, these expired drugs can become hazardous to the animal. Store drugs at their optimal temperature to prevent damage. Temperatures used for drug storage, according to label specifications, are found in Table 5-3.

Drugs that are sensitive to light are usually kept in a dark amber container. Tablets and powders tend to be sensitive to moisture, and their containers usually contain silica packets to absorb moisture. Some drugs are destroyed by physical stress such as vibrations. Insulin is one such drug that can be inactivated by violent shaking of the vial.

CRITICAL CONCEPT

Make sure drugs are stored properly to ensure their effectiveness.

STORING AND PRESCRIBING CONTROLLED SUBSTANCES

A **controlled substance** is defined by law as a substance with potential for physical addiction, psychological addiction, and/or abuse. Controlled drugs are sometimes called schedule drugs. Controlled substances must be stored securely under lock and key to prevent access by unauthorized personnel. By law, a written record must be kept describing when, for what purpose, and how much of the controlled drug was used. These records must include receipts for the purchase or sale of controlled substances and must be maintained for 2 years.

Drug manufacturers and distributors are required to identify a controlled substance on its label with an upper case C, followed by a Roman numeral (Fig. 5-10), which denotes the drug's theoretical potential for abuse:

- *C-I* denotes extreme potential for abuse, with no approved medicinal purpose in the United States. These include such drugs as heroin, lysergic acid diethylamide (LSD), and marijuana. (There is some controversy about marijuana being in this category, but it has not been changed to a different class at the time of this writing.)
- *C-II* denotes a high potential for abuse. Use may lead to severe physical or psychological dependence. These include such drugs as opium, pentobarbital, and morphine.

TABLE 5-3 | Drug Storage Temperatures

HEAT LEVEL	TEMPERATURE
Cold	Not exceeding 8° C (46° F)
Cool	8°-15° C (46°-59° F)
Room temperature	16°-30° C (60°-86° F)
Warm	31°-40° C (87°-104° F)
Excessive heat	>40° C (104° F)

From Sirois M: Principles and practice of veterinary technology, ed 3, St Louis, 2011, Mosby.

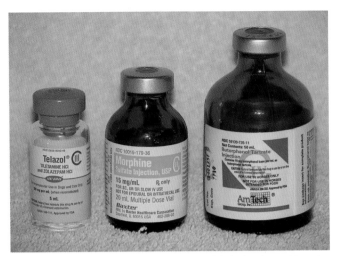

FIGURE 5-10 Controlled substances are labeled with a "C" and a roman numeral. (From Prendergast H: Front office management for the veterinary team, St Louis, 2011, Saunders.)

TABLE 5-4	Commonly Used Controlled Substances in Veterinary Medicine and Their Classifications
CLASSIFICATION OF CONTROLLED SUBSTANCE	**COMMONLY USED DRUGS**
C-I	None used in veterinary medicine
C-II	Pentobarbital, morphine, hydromorphone, fentanyl, oxymorphone
C-III	Ketamine, buprenorphine, tiletamine-zolazepam (Telazol), hydrocodone, testosterone
C-IV	Phenobarbital, diazepam, butorphanol
C-V	Tussigon, codeine products

From Sirois M: Principles and practice of veterinary technology, ed 3, St Louis, 2011, Mosby.

- *C-III* denotes some potential for abuse but less than for C-II drugs. Use may lead to low to moderate physical dependence or high psychological dependence. These include such drugs as ketamine, buprenorphine, and anabolic steroids.
- *C-IV* denotes low potential for abuse. Use may lead to limited physical psychological dependence, including such drugs as phenobarbital and diazepam (Valium).
- *C-V* also denotes low potential for abuse, but these drugs are subject to state and local regulation (e.g., Robitussin AC, which contains small amounts of codeine).

For veterinarians to use, prescribe, or buy a controlled substance legally from an approved manufacturer or distributor, they must have obtained a certification number from the DEA. This DEA certification number must be included on all prescriptions or any order forms for schedule (controlled) drugs. Even with a valid DEA number, veterinarians cannot prescribe Schedule I (C-I) drugs.

Prescriptions for Schedule II (C-II) drugs, which have the most potential for abuse, must be in written form (many states have special forms for C-II drug prescriptions) and cannot be telephoned to a pharmacist. In case of an emergency, when the prescription must be ordered by telephone, the verbal prescription must be followed by a written order within 72 hours. Schedule II drug prescriptions may not be refilled; a new prescription must be written for each treatment period. Table 5-4 lists some commonly used controlled substances in veterinary medicine and their classifications.

HANDLING TOXIC DRUGS

Veterinary professionals may be exposed to toxic drugs in various ways, including the following:
- Absorption through the skin via spillage from a syringe or vial, or other contact
- Inhalation of aerosolized drug as a needle is withdrawn from a vial that is pressurized by injection of air to facilitate removal of the drug

- Ingestion of food contaminated with drug via aerosolization or direct contact
- Inhalation resulting from crushing or breaking of tablets and subsequent aerosolization of drug powder
- Absorption or inhalation during opening of glass ampules containing antineoplastic agents

The best way to avoid exposure is to educate all involved personnel about the safe handling and storage of these drugs. Training may be in-house or formal. Such safety training should be periodically repeated to emphasize the importance of handling precautions and as a refresher for staff members.

THERAPEUTIC RANGE

The concentration of a drug in the body must be such that the detrimental effects are minimized and benefits are maximized. This ideal range of drug concentration is referred to as the **therapeutic range**. If an excessive dose results in accumulation of too much drug in the body, drug concentrations are said to be toxic, and signs of toxicity develop. If a small drug dose does not produce drug concentrations within the therapeutic range, drug concentrations are said to be at subtherapeutic levels, and the drug's beneficial effect is not achieved.

DOSAGE REGIMEN

There are three components of therapeutic administration of drugs—the dose, dosage interval, and route of administration. Altering any of these components can result in drug concentrations that are too high or too low.

A drug's **dose** is the amount of drug administered at one time. For accuracy and clarity in communicating with pharmacists or other veterinary professionals, always state the dose in units of mass (e.g., mg, g, gr). Do not state the dose in number of product units (e.g., tablets or capsules) or volume (mL, L), because manufacturers may produce the same drug in solid dosage forms of various sizes or solutions with various concentrations. For example, writing in an animal's record that the animal received "one tablet of amoxicillin" is of no value because amoxicillin is available in tablet sizes ranging from 50 mg up to 500 mg. The same is true if you state, "Give 3 mL of xylazine," because 3 mL of a xylazine solution with a concentration of 20 mg/mL contains much less xylazine than 3 mL of a solution with a concentration of 100 mg/mL.

The time between the administration of separate drug doses is referred to as the dosage interval. Dosage intervals are often expressed with the Latin abbreviations shown in Box 5-1.

The dose and dosage interval together are often referred to as the dosage regimen. The total amount of drug delivered to the animal in 24 hours is determined by multiplying the dose by the frequency of administration (e.g., 100 mg given four times daily results in a total daily dosage of 400 mg).

CRITICAL CONCEPT

Always record the actual concentration of a drug given because most drugs come in multiple concentrations.

ROUTES OF ADMINISTRATION

The amount of a drug that reaches the target tissues in the body can be significantly altered if the proper route of administration is not used. The route of administration is how the drug enters the body. Drugs given by injection are said to be parenterally administered. Drugs given by mouth, or **per os** (PO), are said to be orally administered. If a drug is applied to the surface of the skin, as with lotions and liniments, it is said to be topically administered.

Parenteral administration of drugs is further broken down into specific routes. Intravenous (IV) administration involves injecting the drug directly into a vein. IV injections can be given as a single volume at one time, called a bolus, or can be slowly injected or dripped into a vein over several seconds, minutes, or even hours as an IV infusion. Drugs that are given over long periods of time ranging from hours to days are referred to as being given by **continuous rate infusion** (CRI). The differences in drug concentrations achieved by these variations of IV administration are shown in Figure 5-11.

Note that IV injection is not the same as intra-arterial injection. Drugs given by intra-arterial injection are injected into an artery (not a vein), quickly producing high concentrations of drug in tissues supplied by that artery. After IV injection, blood containing the drug passes to the heart and is mixed and diluted with the remaining blood in circulation before it is delivered to body tissues. Inadvertent injection of drugs intra-arterially (e.g., injection into the carotid artery instead of the jugular vein) delivers a bolus of a drug directly to tissues. These accidental intra-arterial injections can produce severe effects, such as seizures or respiratory arrest. Injection of a drug outside the blood vessel (not within the vessel lumen) is an extravascular or perivascular injection.

Some drugs cause extreme local inflammation and tissue death if accidentally injected extravascularly. Intramuscular (IM) administration involves injecting the drug into a muscle

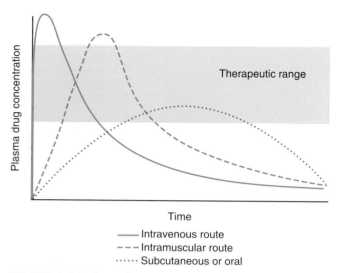

FIGURE 5-11 Plasma drug concentrations attained after intravenous, intramuscular, subcutaneous, and oral administration. (From Sirois M: *Principles and practice of veterinary technology*, ed 3, St Louis, 2011, Mosby.)

mass. **Subcutaneous (SC) injections** are administered deep to (beneath) the skin, into the subcutis. Intradermal (ID) injections are administered within (not beneath) the skin with very small needles. The intradermal route is usually reserved for skin-testing procedures, such as testing for tuberculosis or reaction to allergenic substances. Intraperitoneal (IP) injections are administered into the abdominal body cavity and may be used when IV or IM injections are not practical, as in some laboratory animals, or large volumes of solution must be administered for rapid absorption.

MOVEMENT OF DRUG MOLECULES IN THE BODY

Pharmacokinetics describes how drugs move into, through, and out of the body. Knowledge of a drug's pharmacokinetics facilitates understanding of why the drug must be given by different routes or dosage regimens to achieve therapeutic success under different clinical circumstances. Pharmacokinetics involves absorption, distribution, metabolism, and elimination.

The movement of drug molecules from the site of administration into the systemic circulation is called absorption. After a drug has been ingested, injected, inhaled, or applied to the skin, it must be absorbed into the blood and travel to the body areas where it will have its intended effect (target tissues). IV injections almost instantaneously achieve their peak concentration (highest level) in the blood (see Fig. 5-11). Drugs given by IM administration take some time to diffuse from the injection site in the muscle into the systemic circulation. Drugs given by PO administration and SC injection take longer to be absorbed because they must diffuse farther to reach the systemic circulation (SC injection) or must pass through several barriers to be absorbed (PO administration). Drugs given by the IM, SC, or PO route attain therapeutic concentrations more slowly than drugs given IV.

Distribution describes the movement of a drug from the systemic circulation into tissues. Drugs generally are distributed most rapidly and in greater concentrations to well-perfused (rich blood supply) tissues. Examples of well-perfused tissues include active skeletal muscle, liver, kidney, and brain. In contrast, inactive skeletal muscle and adipose (fat) tissue are relatively poorly perfused, so it takes more time for drugs to be delivered to these tissues. Some drugs bind to proteins in the blood; these protein-bound drug molecules are unable to leave the systemic circulation and so are not distributed to tissues. Thus, a significant portion of a highly protein-bound drug remains in systemic circulation, where these protein-bound drug molecules act as a so-called reservoir of additional drug.

Many drugs are altered by the body before being eliminated. This process is referred to as biotransformation, or drug metabolism. The altered drug molecule is referred to as a metabolite. The liver is the primary organ involved in drug metabolism, or biotransformation. However, other tissues, such as the lung, skin, and intestinal tract, may also biotransform drug molecules. The product of biotransformation (metabolite) is usually readily eliminated by the kidney or liver. Removal of a drug from the body is called drug elimination or excretion. The two major routes of elimination are via the kidney (into the urine) and via the liver (into the bile and subsequently into the feces). Inhalant anesthetics and other volatile agents are mostly eliminated via the lungs, although some inhalant anesthetics (e.g., methoxyflurane, halothane) have some hepatic biotransformation and renal excretion. Drug elimination is greatly affected by dehydration; kidney, liver, or heart disease; age; and other physiologic and pathologic (disease) conditions.

HOW DRUGS EXERT THEIR EFFECTS

For cells to respond to a drug molecule, the drug must usually combine with a specific protein molecule on or in the cell, called a receptor. A given receptor combines only with the molecule of certain drugs, based on their shape or molecular makeup.

This concept is illustrated by a key and lock, in which the drug is the key and the receptor is the lock into which only the correct key will fit (produce an effect). The effect of the correct drug molecule-receptor combination is some cellular change, such as causing the cell to secrete substances, muscle cells to contract, or neuronal cells to depolarize (fire). Cells do not have receptors for all drugs; only certain cells respond to certain drugs.

DRUGS AFFECTING THE GASTROINTESTINAL TRACT

Drugs or functions related to the stomach (gastrointestinal [GI] tract) are called gastric, as in gastric ulcers, gastric blood flow, or gastric emptying. Drugs or functions related to the duodenum, jejunum, or ileum are usually referred to as enteric. Drugs and functions related to the colon are referred to as colonic.

CRITICAL CONCEPT
Gastric, enteric, and colonic all refer to the GI tract.

EMETICS

Emetics are drugs that induce vomiting (Box 5-5). The complex process of emesis is controlled by a group of neurons in the medulla of the brainstem, known as the vomiting center. Emetics are most often used to induce vomiting in animals that have ingested toxic substances. They should not be used in

---

BOX 5-5	Commonly Used Gastrointestinal Drugs

Emetics
Apomorphine
Xylazine
Hydrogen peroxide

Antiemetics
Chlorpromazine
Dimenhydrinate (Dramamine)
Meclizine (e.g., Bonine, Dramamine Less Drowsy)
Maropitant citrate (Cerenia)
Metoclopramide (Reglan)
Cisapride (Propulsid)
Ondansetron (Zofran)

Antidiarrheals
Diphenoxylate (Lomotil)
Loperamide (Imodium)
Bismuth subsalicylate (Pepto-Bismol)

Adsorbents and Protectants
Activated charcoal (Toxiban)
Kaolin pectate (Kaopectate)

Laxatives, Lubricants, and Stool Softeners
Indigestible fiber (bran, Metamucil)
Metamucil
Phosphate salts (Fleet enema)
Psyllium
Mineral oil
Glycerin
Docusate sodium succinate (Colace)
Lactulose

Antacids
OTC products (Tums, Rolaids)
Aluminum products (Amphojel)
Magnesium and aluminum (Maalox)
Ranitidine (Zantac)
Famotidine (Pepcid)

Antiulcer Drugs
Sucralfate (Carafate)
Omeprazole (e.g., Gastrogard, Prilosec OTC)
Misoprostol (Cytotec)

Appetite Stimulants
Cyproheptadine
Diazepam (Valium)

Adapted from Sirois M: Principles and practice of veterinary technology, ed 3, St Louis, 2011, Mosby.

all cases of poisoning, however, because the risk of aspiration (inhalation) of stomach contents into the lungs may outweigh the benefit of induced vomiting. Also, vomiting should not be induced if a corrosive substance or volatile liquid was ingested.

Apomorphine quickly causes emesis in dogs when given by IV or IM injection, or when an apomorphine tablet is placed in the conjunctival sac of the eye. Apomorphine is a less effective emetic in cats. An effective emetic for cats is the sedative xylazine (e.g., Rompun, Anased), which produces emesis within minutes of injection.

Hydromorphone is not commonly used to induce vomiting but does have that side effect, so it has been used. The main side effect of using this medication is significant sedation and possible bradycardia, which are usually not desirable when trying to induce vomiting.

Syrup of ipecac does not produce vomiting until 10 to 30 minutes after administration. This is because the ipecac must pass from the stomach into the intestine to produce the required local irritation (local effect) and also to be absorbed (central effect on the vomiting center). The 10- to 30-minute lag time between ipecac administration and the onset of vomiting can lead uninformed clients or veterinary professionals to believe that the initial dose was ineffective, causing them to administer multiple doses of the drug before vomiting begins. This medication has fallen out of favor because of the lag time and potential for overdosing. Other local emetics include hydrogen peroxide, a warm concentrated solution of salt and water, and a solution of powdered mustard and water. These emetics do not work consistently.

ANTIEMETICS

Antiemetics are drugs that prevent or decrease vomiting (see Box 5-5). Antiemetics should only be used when the vomiting reflex is no longer of benefit to the animal. Phenothiazine tranquilizers, such as acepromazine (PromAce), chlorpromazine (Thorazine), and prochlorperazine (Compazine, Darbazine), are commonly used to combat vomiting caused by motion sickness. The antihistamines meclizine (e.g., Bonine, Dramamine Less Drowsy), dimenhydrinate (Dramamine), and diphenhydramine (Benadryl) are also used occasionally for prevention of motion sickness. Maropitant citrate (Cerenia), a neurokinin receptor antagonist, was approved for use in 2008 to help relieve acute vomiting and vomiting caused by motion sickness. This drug works to block the pharmacologic action of substance P in the central nervous system (CNS).

Atropine, aminopentamide (Centrine), and isopropamide (combined with prochlorperazine in Darbazine) are anticholinergic drugs that prevent vomiting by blocking impulses traveling to the CNS via the vagus nerve and motor impulses traveling via the vagus nerve to the muscles involved with the vomiting reflex. These drugs are used less often because of the availability of other, more locally effective drugs.

Metoclopramide (Reglan) is a centrally acting antiemetic that also has local antiemetic activity. Metoclopramide has been useful for helping animals that vomit because of slowed gut motility. Cisapride (Propulsid) has been used to reduce regurgitation in dogs with megaesophagus (dilated esophagus) and in cats with chronic constipation or cats that frequently vomit hairballs.

Ondansetron (Zofran) is a selective serotonin reuptake inhibitor (also known as a 5-HT3 receptor antagonist). It is unclear as to whether it acts centrally, peripherally, or both because the 5-HT3 receptors for serotonin are located peripherally (the vagus nerve) and centrally (the chemoreceptor trigger zone in the brain). Ondansetron is used when other more widely used antiemetics are not effective because of the expense and limited experience in veterinary medicine.

ANTIDIARRHEALS

Antidiarrheals are drugs used to combat various types of diarrhea (see Box 5-5). Narcotics commonly used to combat diarrhea include diphenoxylate (Lomotil), paregoric (tincture of opium), and loperamide (Imodium). A disadvantage of narcotics when used as antidiarrheals is that their analgesic effect can mask pain that otherwise could be used to monitor progression or resolution of disease. Another disadvantage is that narcotics can cause excitement in cats (so-called morphine mania).

The anticholinergics atropine, propantheline bromide, isopropamide (Darbazine), and aminopentamide (Centrine) are used as antispasmodics because they decrease spastic colonic contractions and combat diarrhea associated with these contractions. These drugs are not particularly effective for most cases of small bowel diarrhea.

Bismuth subsalicylate, the active ingredient in Pepto-Bismol, breaks down in the gut to bismuth carbonate and salicylate. The bismuth tends to coat the intestinal mucosa, perhaps protecting it from enterotoxins, and seems to have some antibacterial activity. The major antisecretory effect, however, is probably from the salicylate (an aspirin-like compound), which decreases inflammation and blocks the formation of prostaglandins that would normally stimulate fluid secretion.

ADSORBENTS AND PROTECTANTS

Locally irritating substances, such as bacterial endotoxins, can produce acute diarrhea. Any drug that prevents these agents from contacting the intestinal mucosa could theoretically reduce the diarrheal response. This is the underlying principle of adsorbents and protectants. An adsorbent causes another substance to adhere to its outer surface, thus reducing contact of that substance with the intestinal tract wall (see Box 5-5).

Activated charcoal adsorbs enterotoxins to its surface, preventing them from contacting the bowel wall. The charcoal and the adsorbed enterotoxin then are excreted in the feces. Activated charcoal comes with or without a sorbitol additive, which is a cathartic. The cathartic helps eliminate the charcoal from the body before it releases the toxin it was bound to. Sorbitol additives should not be used in very dehydrated animals or animals that already have severe diarrhea. Kaolin and pectin (Kaopectate) are often used together for the symptomatic relief of vomiting or diarrhea.

The kaolin-pectin combination is thought to adsorb entero-toxins. It is questionable as to whether kaolin-pectin has any significant effect in controlling diarrhea in veterinary patients.

LAXATIVES, LUBRICANTS, AND STOOL SOFTENERS

Laxatives, cathartics, and purgatives facilitate evacuation of the bowels. Laxatives are considered the most gentle of this class of drugs, whereas cathartics have more of an evacuating effect and purgatives are potent in their actions. Irritant laxatives, including castor oil and phenolphthalein, work by irritating the bowel, resulting in increased peristaltic motility (see Box 5-5).

Bulk laxatives are much gentler than irritant laxatives. These drugs pull water osmotically into the bowel lumen or retain water in the feces. Hydrophilic colloids or indigestible fiber (e.g., bran, methylcellulose, Metamucil) are not digested or adsorbed to any degree and therefore create an osmotic force to produce their laxative effect. Psyllium is a hydrophilic compound that has gained popularity for its supposed health benefits. Hypertonic salts such as magnesium (milk of magnesia, Epsom salts) and phosphate salts (Fleet Enema) are poorly absorbed and create a strong osmotic force that attracts waters into the bowel lumen.

Lubricants (e.g., mineral oil, cod liver oil, white petrolatum, glycerin) are given to make the stool slipperier for easy passage through the bowel. The greatest danger associated with the use of oils is aspiration into the lungs, with subsequent pneumonia. Glycerin is most commonly used as a suppository.

Docusate sodium succinate (Colace) is a stool softener that acts as a wetting agent by reducing the surface tension of feces and allowing water to penetrate the dry stool. Docusate sodium succinate and related calcium and phosphate compounds may also stimulate colonic secretions, resulting in increased fluid content of feces.

Lactulose is another laxative that increases osmotic pressure by drawing water into the colon, which results in fecal material containing more liquid. It can also have an acidifying action that is used in the treatment of hepatic encephalopathy because it traps ammonia in the form of ammonium. It is generally used in small animals with chronic constipation problems. The most common danger with the use of lactulose is excessive fluid loss leading to dehydration. Administering fluids may be warranted with initial use.

ANTACIDS

Antacids reduce the acidity of the stomach or rumen (see Box 5-5). Nonsystemic antacids in liquid or tablet form are composed of calcium, magnesium, or aluminum, and they directly neutralize acid molecules in the stomach or rumen. OTC products such as Tums and Rolaids are nonsystemic antacids made primarily of calcium. Other nonsystemic antacids include magnesium products (Riopan, Carmilax), aluminum products (Amphojel), and combinations of magnesium and aluminum products (Maalox).

Systemic antacids decrease acid production in the stomach. Systemic antacids include cimetidine (Tagamet), ranitidine (Zantac), and famotidine (Pepcid).

ANTIULCER DRUGS

Sucralfate (Carafate) is an antiulcer drug used to treat ulcers of the stomach and upper small intestine. The drug has been referred to as a gastric Band-Aid because it forms a sticky paste and adheres to the ulcer site, protecting it from the acidic environment of the stomach. Omeprazole (e.g., Gastrogard, Prilosec OTC) is a gastric acid pump inhibitor that binds irreversibly to the secretory surface of cells in the stomach. It therefore decreases acid secretion (antacid) and helps support the stomach lining (antiulcer). Misoprostol (Cytotec) is a synthetic prostaglandin that helps decrease acid secretion in the stomach and increases production of the stomach lining (mucosa). Misoprostol is mostly used to combat insults to the stomach caused by nonsteroidal anti-inflammatory drugs (NSAIDs). It only comes in 100- and 200-µg tablets, making it difficult to use in very small animals (see Box 5-5).

APPETITE-STIMULATING DRUGS

Cyproheptadine is a serotonin antagonist antihistamine that is mostly used as an appetite stimulant for cats. Diazepam (Valium), a benzodiazepine, can also be used as an appetite stimulant but, again, only in cats. Neither drug works in other species (see Box 5-5).

DRUGS AFFECTING THE CARDIOVASCULAR SYSTEM

ANTIARRHYTHMIC DRUGS

An arrhythmia is any abnormal pattern of electrical activity in the heart. Arrhythmias are divided into two general groups, arrhythmias that result in an increased heart rate (tachycardia) and those that cause a decreased heart rate (bradycardia). Once the type of arrhythmia has been determined, an effective antiarrhythmic drug (Box 5-6) is used to reestablish a normal conduction sequence (sinus rhythm).

Lidocaine, mexiletine, quinidine, and procainamide reverse arrhythmias primarily by decreasing the rate of movement of sodium into heart cells. Lidocaine, which is also used as a local anesthetic under the name of Xylocaine, is only available in injectable form. Veterinary technicians must realize that lidocaine is packaged in vials with or without epinephrine. Lidocaine with epinephrine is designed for use as a local anesthetic, not as an antiarrhythmic drug. Accidental IV injection of lidocaine containing epinephrine into an animal with an arrhythmia could cause death. Thus, it is important always to check the lidocaine bottle before use in treating arrhythmias to be sure that it does not contain epinephrine.

Procainamide and quinidine are more commonly used for their ventricular antiarrhythmic effects in dogs and cats. Because quinidine and procainamide are available in oral

| BOX 5-6 | Commonly Used Cardiovascular Drugs |

Antiarrhythmic Drugs
Lidocaine
Quinidine
Propanolol
Atenolol
Verapamil
Diltiazem
Amlodipine (hypertension)

Inotropic Agents
Digoxin
Pimobendan

Vasodilators
Hydralazine
Nitroglycerin
Pimobendan (see inotropic drugs)
Enalapril (Enacard)
Benazepril

Diuretics
Furosemide (Lasix)
Spironolactone
Mannitol

Adapted from Sirois M: Principles and practice of veterinary technology, ed 3, St Louis, 2011, Mosby.

forms, they are used for the long-term maintenance of patients with ventricular arrhythmias.

When stimulated by the sympathetic nervous system or by sympathomimetic drugs (drugs that mimic the effects of the sympathetic nervous system), β_1 receptors in the heart cause the heart to beat more rapidly and with greater strength. Such β_1 stimulation can produce arrhythmias. Drugs that block beta receptors are known as beta blockers. Beta blockers cause the heart to contract with less force. Propranolol (Inderal) blocks the stimulation of β_1 receptors by epinephrine, norepinephrine, and other β_1-stimulating drugs. It decreases the heart rate and prevents tachycardia in response to stress, fear, or excitement. Atenolol (Tenormin) and metoprolol (Lopressor) act similarly to propranolol but at high doses the β_1 receptor activity may be lost, causing β_2 blockade. Atenolol and metoprolol are preferred for animals with asthma.

Calcium channel blockers include verapamil and diltiazem. Although calcium channel blockers are not commonly used to treat arrhythmias in veterinary patients, verapamil and diltiazem have been used successfully for the treatment of supraventricular tachycardia, atrial fibrillation, and atrial flutter. A more common use of diltiazem is for cats with hypertrophic cardiomyopathy, in which the heart becomes thickened and enlarged to the point at which it cannot contract efficiently. These drugs combat arrhythmias by blocking calcium channels of cardiac muscle cells, resulting in decreased conduction of depolarization waves and decreased automaticity of parts of the conduction system.

Another calcium channel blocker most commonly used for hypertension in small animals is amlodipine. It dilates the peripheral arteries and thereby reduces afterload. It is eliminated quickly from the system, and hypertension can return rapidly if any doses are missed.

POSITIVE INOTROPIC AGENTS

Drugs that increase the strength of contraction of a weakened heart are referred to as **positive inotropic drugs** (positive inotropes; see Box 5-6). Digoxin is the drug of choice for maintaining long-term positive inotropic effects. Digoxin exerts its positive inotropic effect primarily by making more calcium available for the contractile elements within cardiac muscle cells. Digoxin, available as a tablet and elixir, is often used to control supraventricular tachycardia caused by atrial fibrillation. Digoxin has a small therapeutic index, meaning that therapeutic concentrations are close to toxic concentrations. Early signs of digoxin toxicity include anorexia, vomiting, and diarrhea. Owners of animals receiving digoxin should be instructed to watch for these early signs of toxicity and to contact the veterinarian immediately if they should occur.

Pimobendan is an inodilator because it has both inotropic and **vasodilator** effects. This drug is used in conjunction with other medications in dogs to treat congestive heart failure secondary to dilated cardiomyopathy or chronic mitral valve insufficiency.

Dobutamine is also an inotropic agent that is generally used for the short-term management of heart failure and for shock patients when fluid therapy alone is not working. It is used only as a CRI because of its limited availability and quick metabolization by the system. This drug is most commonly used in the intensive care unit (ICU) setting.

VASODILATORS

Vasoconstriction of peripheral blood vessels is a normal physiologic response to the drop in blood pressure caused by congestive heart failure, hemorrhage, and dehydration. Vasodilators open (dilate) constricted vessels, making it easier for the heart to pump blood through these vessels (see Box 5-6).

Hydralazine is a vasodilator that causes arteriolar smooth muscle to relax, which benefits animals with a poorly functioning left atrioventricular (mitral) valve (mitral insufficiency). Hydralazine allows more blood to flow into the aorta and less to flow back into the left atrium. Although the valve itself remains poorly functional, blood flow through the left heart is improved.

Nitroglycerin relaxes the blood vessels on the venous side of the circulation; it may also help dilate coronary arterioles. The drug is well absorbed through the skin and mucous membranes. In animals nitroglycerin cream and nitroglycerin in patch form are applied to the skin to improve cardiac output and reduce pulmonary edema and ascites (abdominal fluid accumulation). Nitroglycerin cream is applied every 4 to 6 hours to the hairless inner aspect of the pinna, thorax, or groin. A nitroglycerin patch provides drug diffusion for

24 hours and can be cut into small pieces to adjust the dose for smaller patients.

Nitroprusside acts much like nitroglycerin but is usually found only in the ICU setting because of the necessity to monitor blood pressure constantly and the need to give the drug as a CRI.

Other vasodilators are enalapril (Enacard), captopril, and benazepril, which block angiotensin-converting enzyme (ACE) and prevent the formation of angiotensin II (a potent vasoconstrictor) and aldosterone. Therefore, they are sometimes referred to ACE inhibitors. Enalapril, captopril, and benazepril are balanced vasodilators that relax the smooth muscles of arterioles and veins, so they are useful for treating animals with cardiac disease that involves the right and left ventricles (e.g., severe cardiac valvular disease, cardiomyopathy).

DIURETICS

Diuretics are drugs that increase urine formation and promote water loss (diuresis; see Box 5-6). In animals with congestive heart failure, sodium retention from aldosterone secretion and concomitant retention of water in the blood and body tissues lead to pulmonary edema, ascites, and an increased cardiac workload. Removing water from the body with diuretics reduces these harmful conditions. Diuretics should be used cautiously in animals with hypovolemia (low blood volume) or hypotension (low blood pressure) because they further decrease the fluid component of blood and reduce blood pressure.

Loop diuretics such as furosemide (Lasix) produce diuresis by inhibiting sodium resorption from the loop of Henle in nephrons. When sodium resorption is inhibited, osmotic forces are exerted that cause additional water in the urine to be retained. Retention of sodium in the urine that is forming retains water in the urine osmotically and prevents its resorption. In the distal convoluted tubule, potassium is exchanged for sodium so that sodium is still resorbed and conserved by the body to some degree. Because loop diuretics cause potassium to be excreted in the urine, prolonged use of loop diuretics may result in hypokalemia (low blood potassium level).

Thiazide diuretics such as chlorothiazide are not often used in veterinary medicine because of the safety and effectiveness of furosemide. Thiazides are less potent than loop diuretics because of their site of action in the distal convoluted tubule. Thiazide diuretics can cause loss of potassium, with resultant hypokalemia.

Spironolactone is a diuretic that is a competitive antagonist of aldosterone, the hormone that normally causes sodium resorption from the distal renal tubules and collection ducts. When aldosterone is inhibited, more sodium remains in the lumen of the renal tubules, osmotically retaining water and preventing its resorption. Because sodium is excreted and potassium is conserved in the body, drugs such as spironolactone are called potassium-sparing diuretics.

Mannitol is a carbohydrate (sugar) used as an **osmotic diuretic**. Mannitol is poorly resorbed from the renal tubule, thus providing a solute that osmotically retains water in the renal tubular lumen. Mannitol is not used for the treatment of cardiovascular disease but is used to reduce cerebral edema associated with head trauma and as a diuretic for flushing absorbed toxins from the body.

DRUGS AFFECTING THE RESPIRATORY SYSTEM

ANTITUSSIVES

Antitussives are drugs that block the cough reflex, which is coordinated by the cough center in the brainstem (Box 5-7). A productive cough refers to a cough that produces mucus and other inflammatory products that are coughed up into the oral cavity. A nonproductive cough is dry and hacking, and no mucus is coughed up. Antitussives suppress the coughing that normally removes mucus, cellular debris, exudates, and other products that accumulate in the bronchi as a result of infection or inflammation. For this reason, in animals with a productive cough (much mucus is produced), antitussive drugs should be used cautiously and large doses should be avoided. In such cases, suppression of coughing with cough suppressants can result in the accumulation of excessive mucus and debris.

Antitussives should be used for animals with a dry, nonproductive cough producing little or no inspissated mucus. Often, these coughs keep the animal (and owner) awake, preventing the animal from getting the rest it needs to recover. Antitussives are commonly used for treating uncomplicated tracheobronchitis (referred to as kennel cough) in dogs. This retching type of cough is often punctuated by gagging up small amounts of mucus that the owner interprets as vomitus. This type of cough is extremely irritating to the upper

---

BOX 5-7	Commonly Used Respiratory Drugs

Antitussives
Butorphanol (Torbugesic)
Hydrocodone (Hycodan)
Dextromethorphan (Robitussin, other OTC cough medications)

Mucolytic
Acetylcysteine (Mucomyst)

Expectorant
Guaifenesin

Decongestant
Phenylephrine

Bronchodilators
Terbutaline
Albuterol
Clenbuterol
Aminophylline

Adapted from Sirois M: Principles and practice of veterinary technology, ed 3, St Louis, 2011, Mosby.

airway mucosa; such irritation stimulates more coughing, which further irritates the airway. This pattern can continue for weeks if the cough is not treated.

Butorphanol (Torbutrol) is a centrally acting opioid cough suppressant that, unlike most other opioid cough suppressants, is generally not classified as a controlled substance. In antitussive doses, butorphanol causes little sedation as compared with stronger opioid drugs.

Hydrocodone (Hycodan) is a C-III narcotic available only by prescription from a veterinarian with a DEA clearance for writing C-III prescriptions. Sedation is often noted in treated animals, and long-term administration can result in constipation.

Codeine is a relatively weak opioid narcotic that is a component of many cough suppressant preparations. Most products containing codeine are prescription preparations with a C-V controlled substance rating. The sedative effect of codeine is similar to that of hydrocodone, and use of the compound can become habit forming.

Dextromethorphan is a common ingredient in OTC non-prescription cough, flu, and cold preparations. Its actions are similar to those of the more potent narcotic antitussives, but it is not a controlled substance. Dextromethorphan is generally not as effective for controlling coughs in veterinary patients as butorphanol or other prescription antitussives; however, owners often initially use human cold products containing dextromethorphan to curtail coughing in their pets. Although dextromethorphan in OTC products is fairly harmless, the other compounds in cold or flu preparations can cause significant harm to animals (e.g., acetaminophen can be toxic in cats). Therefore, it is unwise to recommend that pet owners use OTC products to control coughing in their animals.

MUCOLYTICS, EXPECTORANTS, AND DECONGESTANTS

Mucolytic agents are designed to break up (lyse) mucus and reduce the viscosity of mucus so that the cilia can move it out of the respiratory tract. Acetylcysteine (Mucomyst) is a mucolytic agent that decreases the viscosity of mucus. Acetylcysteine may be administered by nebulization (inhalation of a fine mist containing the drug) or given PO; however, its taste is awful and it must be masked with flavoring agents or administered by feeding tube). Nebulized saline and other fluids are used to increase the fluid content of respiratory mucus in the lower airways. Acetylcysteine is also used as the treatment for acetaminophen toxicity in cats.

Expectorants are compounds that also increase the fluidity of mucus in the respiratory tract by generating liquid secretions by respiratory tract cells. Guaifenesin (glycerol guaiacolate) and saline expectorants (e.g., ammonium chloride, potassium iodide, sodium citrate) are given PO. The volatile oils, such as terpin hydrate, eucalyptus oil, and pine oil, stimulate respiratory secretions directly when their vapors are inhaled.

Many OTC human cold preparations that contain expectorants also contain decongestants, such as phenylephrine or phenylpropanolamine, for the relief of nasal congestion. **Decongestants** reduce congestion (vascular engorgement) of the mucous membranes (see Box 5-7).

BRONCHODILATORS

Bronchoconstriction is caused by the contraction of smooth muscles surrounding the small terminal bronchioles deep within the respiratory tree. Drugs that inhibit broncho-constriction are called **bronchodilators** (see Box 5-7). Terbutaline, albuterol, and clenbuterol are available in an oral dosage form and as an inhaler. The methylxanthines include bronchodilators such as theophylline and aminophylline. The difference between theophylline and aminophylline is that aminophylline is approximately 80% theophylline and 20% ethylenediamine salt. Because 100 mg of aminophylline contains only 80 mg of active theophylline, the dose of theophylline must be adjusted if the animal is switched to aminophylline or vice versa, based on the amount of active ingredient (theophylline) in the compound. Aminophylline is used more often in the clinical setting because it is available in injectable form.

DRUGS AFFECTING THE ENDOCRINE SYSTEM

DRUGS USED TO TREAT HYPOTHYROIDISM

Drugs used to treat hypothyroidism (insufficiency of thyroid hormone) include levothyroxine (T_4) and synthetic liothyronine (the L-isomer of triiodothyronine [T_3]; Box 5-8). Supplementing a hypothyroid animal with T_4 provides the

BOX 5-8	Commonly Used Drugs Affecting the Endocrine System

Thyroid Medications
Levothyroxine (Soloxine)
Methimazole (Tapazole)
Radioactive iodine (I-131)

Pancreatic Drugs
Injectable (Insulin)
Porcine origin lente (Vetsulin)
NPH (Humulin N, Novolin N)
Glargine (Lantus)
Protamine Zinc (PZI)

Oral Forms
Glipizide

Adrenal Gland Medications
Desoxycorticosterone pivalate (DOCP)
Fludrocortisones acetate (Florinef)
Prednisone, prednisolone
Mitotane (o,p'-DDD, lysodren)
L-Deprenyl (Anipryl)

Adapted from Sirois M: Principles and practice of veterinary technology, ed 3, St Louis, 2011, Mosby.

various organs and tissues with the appropriate amount of thyroid hormone because each organ or tissue converts T_4 to T_3. With T_3 supplementation, the local tissue regulation of thyroid hormone conversion is bypassed.

Another advantage of synthetic levothyroxine is its ability to trigger the natural negative feedback mechanism, thus emulating the normal regulatory mechanism for thyroid hormone production. Levothyroxine (e.g., Synthroid, Soloxine) is usually the drug of choice for treating hypothyroidism. Also, T_3 products (e.g., Cytomel) are generally more expensive than T_4 products and must be administered three times daily, rather than once daily.

DRUGS USED TO TREAT HYPERTHYROIDISM

Hyperthyroidism is an increase in thyroid hormone production. It is most common in cats and is associated with a hormone-secreting thyroid tumor. Hyperthyroidism is treated by surgical removal of the thyroid gland with drugs that decrease thyroid hormone production or drugs that destroy the thyroid tissue (antithyroid drugs).

Methimazole (Tapazole) and propylthiouracil have been used to control hyperthyroidism in cats by blocking the thyroid tumor's ability to produce T_3 and T_4. Of the two drugs, methimazole causes fewer complications and is preferred over propylthiouracil for decreasing thyroid hormone production. Methimazole can be compounded for topical application (onto the ear pinna) as well.

Radioactive iodine (I-131) is an alternative to the oral treatment of hyperthyroidism. I-131 is injected IV. The iodine, a normal component of thyroid hormone, is taken up and concentrated by the active thyroid tumor cells, which are then destroyed by the radioactivity.

ENDOCRINE PANCREATIC DRUGS

Insulin is responsible for the movement of glucose from the blood into tissue cells. Lack of insulin results in diabetes mellitus, a condition characterized by high blood glucose levels (hyperglycemia) and passage of glucose in the urine (glucosuria). Blood glucose levels can be controlled by one or two SC insulin injections daily (see Box 5-8). The insulins of choice for maintaining diabetic dogs are NPH insulin (Humilin N, Novolin N, PZI), which are of intermediate duration. Diabetic cats sometimes require the longer-acting insulin (Glargine), which is administered once or twice daily. ProZinc is a human recombinant long-acting PZI insulin also used in cats. Regular insulin is not commonly used to maintain diabetic cats or dogs because its short duration of activity requires multiple doses during a 24-hour period. However, because regular insulin is the only type that can be given IV, it is used initially to stabilize the glucose concentrations of animals with severe uncontrolled diabetes or diabetic ketoacidosis.

DRUGS USED TO TREAT HYPOADRENOCORTICISM

Hypoadrenocorticism (Addison's disease) is characterized by a lack of glucocorticoid and/or mineralocorticoid secretion from the adrenal cortex. It can be caused by the gland itself or by a hormone (adrenocorticotropic hormone [ACTH]) that helps tell the gland to secrete the corticoid. Hypoadrenocorticism is treated with corticoid supplementation (see Box 5-8). Mineralocorticoid supplementation is achieved with desoxycorticosterone pivalate (DOCP; Percorten-V), or fludrocortisone acetate (Florinef). Desoxycorticosterone is a long-acting mineralocorticoid that requires functioning kidneys to work properly. It is used only for dogs as an injection once every 23 to 25 days. Desoxycorticosterone may require the use of concurrent glucocorticoids. Fludrocortisone has mineral and glucocorticoid activity and is used in dogs and cats. It is given daily PO. Because fludrocortisone has some glucocorticoid activity, additional supplementation may not be necessary.

Glucocorticoid supplementation is achieved using a number of glucocorticoid agents, including betamethasone, dexamethasone, fludrocortisone, flumethasone, hydrocortisone, methylprednisolone, prednisolone, prednisone, or triamcinolone. Glucocorticoids vary in their duration of effectiveness, which is usually the determining factor for the choice of drug used.

DRUGS USED TO TREAT HYPERADRENOCORTICISM

Hyperadrenocorticism (Cushing's disease) is characterized by excess glucocorticoids in the system. This can be caused by bilateral adrenocortical hyperplasia, a pituitary microadenoma, functional adrenal tumors (benign or cancerous), or excessive or prolonged administration of oral, parenteral, or topical corticosteroids (termed *iatrogenic hyperadrenocorticism*).

The treatment of hyperadrenocorticism is based on suppressing the adrenal gland, by discontinuing corticosteroid use or by surgically removing the adrenal gland. Mitotane (o,p'-DDD, Lysodren) causes the selective necrosis of two sections of the adrenal gland, decreasing the release of corticosteroids. It is administered daily at first and eventually is tapered to twice-weekly dosing. Ketoconazole reversibly inhibits the development of corticosteroids by twice-daily administration but has fallen out of favor because of the lack of response by approximately 50% of patients on which it is used. L-Deprenyl (Anipryl) is a selective monoamine oxidase B (MAOB) inhibitor. MAOB causes dopamine depletion. In dogs with pituitary-based disease, this dopamine depletion causes an increase in the production of cortisol. In essence, L-deprenyl helps stop the dopamine depletion and therefore reduces the amount of cortisol produced. All forms of treatment can lead to hypoadrenocorticism.

DRUGS AFFECTING REPRODUCTION

Hormone drugs, natural or synthetic, are used primarily to prevent pregnancy or alter the state of the uterus (Box 5-9). Gonadotropin-releasing hormone (GnRH) drugs (e.g., Cystorelin) stimulate the release of luteinizing hormone (LH) and/or follicle-stimulating hormone (FSH) from the pituitary gland, causing the ovary to develop follicles. The FSH and

| BOX 5-9 | Commonly Used Drugs Affecting the Reproductive System |

Estradiol
Megestrol acetate (Ovaban)
Mibolerone (Cheque Drops)
Oxytocin

From Sirois M: Principles and practice of veterinary technology, ed 3, St Louis, 2011, Mosby.

LH produced by the pituitary gland are also called gonadotropins. In addition to pituitary gonadotropins, some species produce chorionic gonadotropins from the placenta. These can be used as drugs and include human chorionic gonadotropin (hCG), a hormone produced by pregnant women, and equine chorionic gonadotropin (eCG), formerly known as pregnant mare serum gonadotropin (PMSG). These agents are used occasionally in dogs and cats to induce estrus.

Pregnancy can be prevented (contraception) by suppressing the estrous cycle or by preventing implantation of the fertilized ova into the uterine wall. Megestrol acetate (Ovaban) is an oral progestin used for contraception in female dogs and cats. Megestrol use increases the risk of cystic hyperplasia of the endometrium, endometritis, or pyometra. Prolonged use of megestrol can result in mammary hyperplasia (proliferation of mammary tissue). Mibolerone (Cheque Drops) is another contraceptive used in female dogs. Because mibolerone is a testosterone analogue (similar structure), it produces effects similar to those of high levels of testosterone, including increased production of anal sac secretions, masculinization of developing female fetuses, and increased vulvar discharge.

Estradiol cypionate (ECP) is an injectable estrogen used after mismating in dogs. Estrogens prevent pregnancy by increasing the number and thickness of folds within the oviducts, preventing passage of the ova to the uterus. Because there are safer alternatives to estradiol therapy, such as ovariohysterectomy (spaying), many theriogenologists (specialists in animal reproduction) do not recommend the use of estradiol for dogs.

Oxytocin is commonly used to increase uterine contractions in animals with dystocia (difficult birth) related to a weakened or fatigued uterus. Anabolic steroids, such as testosterone and progesterone, have been used to increase the weight and conditioning of feedlot cattle. Progestins (e.g., megestrol acetate) have been used to modify behavior in cats.

DRUGS AFFECTING THE NERVOUS SYSTEM

ANESTHETICS

Barbiturates are used infrequently to produce short-term anesthesia and induce general anesthesia and are frequently used to control seizures and euthanize animals. Thiobarbiturates contain a sulfur molecule on the barbituric acid molecule; oxybarbiturates contain an oxygen molecule. Thiamylal and thiopental are thiobarbiturates; methohexital, pentobarbital, and phenobarbital are oxybarbiturates. Thiobarbiturates have a more rapid onset but shorter duration of action than oxybarbiturates.

Propofol is usually injected as an IV bolus and provides rapid induction of anesthesia and a short period of unconsciousness. It is relatively expensive and may cause pain when injected IV.

Ketamine and tiletamine are short-acting injectable anesthetics that produce a rather unique form of anesthesia in which the animal feels dissociated (apart) from its body. Retention of laryngeal, pharyngeal, and corneal reflexes, lack of muscular relaxation (often rigidity), and an increased heart rate characterize this dissociative effect.

The lack of muscular relaxation makes ketamine unsuitable as a sole anesthetic agent for major surgery. Ketamine and tiletamine produce good somatic (peripheral tissue) analgesia (pain relief) and are suitable for superficial surgery; however, they are much less effective in blocking visceral (internal organ) pain and should not be used alone as an anesthetic for internal procedures. Tiletamine is included with zolazepam, a benzodiazepine tranquilizer, in a product marketed as Telazol. Zolazepam reduces some of the CNS excitation and side effects produced by tiletamine.

Nitrous oxide, also referred to as laughing gas, is safe when used properly and has much weaker analgesic qualities than other inhalant anesthetics. The major role of nitrous oxide is to decrease the amount of the more potent inhalant anesthetics needed to achieve a surgical plane of anesthesia.

Isoflurane (Forane, AErrane) is an inhalant anesthetic that has gained popularity in veterinary practice because of its rapid, smooth induction of anesthesia and short recovery period. Other inhalant agents with properties similar to those of isoflurane include enflurane (Ethrane), desflurane (Suprane), and sevoflurane (Ultane; Box 5-10).

TRANQUILIZERS AND SEDATIVES

Acepromazine maleate is a phenothiazine tranquilizer that reduces anxiety and produces a mentally relaxed state. It is often used to calm animals for physical examination or transport. Unlike xylazine or detomidine, phenothiazine tranquilizers have no analgesic effect (do not relieve pain).

Droperidol is a butyrophenone with much more potent sedative effects than most phenothiazine tranquilizers. Droperidol has been combined with fentanyl, a strong narcotic analgesic with emetic activity, and marketed as a neuroleptanalgesic product called Innovar-Vet.

Diazepam (Valium), zolazepam (contained in Telazol), midazolam (Versed), and clonazepam (Klonopin) are benzodiazepine tranquilizers often used with other agents as part of a preanesthetic protocol for their calming and muscle relaxing effects.

Xylazine (Rompun, Anased), dexmedetomidine (Dexdomitor), and detomidine (Dormosedan) produce a calming effect and somewhat decrease an animal's ability to respond to stimuli. These drugs also have some analgesic activity. A disadvantage of xylazine is that sedative doses produce vomiting in about 90% of cats and 50% of dogs (see Box 5-10).

| BOX 5-10 | Commonly Used Drugs Affecting the Nervous System |

Anesthetics
Phenobarbital
Propofol
Ketamine-tiletamine
Isoflurane
Sevoflurane

Tranquilizers and Sedatives
Acepromazine
Fentanyl
Diazepam (Valium)
Zolazepam
Xylazine
Dexmedetomidine

Analgesics
Hydromorphone
Oxymorphone
Butorphanol (Torbugesic, Torbutrol)
Tramadol
Fentanyl
Buprenorphine (Buprenex)

Anticonvulsants
Phenobarbital
Diazepam (Valium)
Potassium bromide (KBr)
Methocarbamol (Robaxin-V)

Central Nervous System Stimulants
Doxapram (Dopram)
Yohimbine
Atipamezole

Adapted from Sirois M: Principles and practice of veterinary technology, ed 3, St Louis, 2011, Mosby.

ANALGESICS

Analgesics are drugs that reduce the perception of pain without loss of other sensations (see Box 5-10). Oxymorphone (Numorphan) and hydromorphone are commonly used for preanesthesia and anesthesia. Butorphanol (Torbutrol, Torbugesic) is used for cough control and GI-related pain in small animals. Tramadol is also used for generalized pain and cough control but has less sedating effects than butorphanol. Fentanyl has an analgesic effect 250 times greater than that of morphine. Meperidine (Demerol) is a fairly weak analgesic-sedative and is often injected SC to restrain cats. Pentazocine (Talwin) is a weak analgesic used for dogs recovering from painful surgery.

Buprenorphine (Buprenex) is commonly combined with sedatives or tranquilizers (e.g., acepromazine, xylazine, detomidine). It is also used alone for dogs and cats as an analgesic, both for its potency (30 times the analgesic potency of morphine) and its long duration of analgesia (6 to 8 hours). Etorphine (M-99) is an extremely potent narcotic (1000 times the analgesic potency of morphine) used to sedate and capture wildlife or zoo animals. Butorphanol, pentazocine, and buprenorphine are sometimes used for partial reversal of some of the respiratory depression and sedation caused by stronger narcotic agents. Nalorphine is another reversal agent.

Neuroleptanalgesia refers to a state of CNS depression (sedation or tranquilization) and analgesia induced by a combination of a sedative (e.g., xylazine) or tranquilizer (e.g., acepromazine) and an analgesic (oxymorphone). Phenothiazine tranquilizers or butyrophenone tranquilizers (e.g., droperidol) calm the animal and also decrease or block the emetic (vomiting) side effect of a narcotic analgesic.

ANTICONVULSANTS

Seizures are periods of altered brain function characterized by loss of consciousness, altered muscle tone or movement, altered sensations, or other neurologic changes. Drugs used to control seizures are called **anticonvulsants** (see Box 5-10). Phenobarbital is a drug of choice for long-term control of seizures in dogs and cats. This barbiturate is inexpensive and, because of its long half-life, may be given orally once or twice daily. The main side effect is increased blood levels of liver enzymes and possible liver damage. The dose of phenobarbital is often measured in grains (1 grain [gr] = approximately 60 mg). Although primidone has some anticonvulsant activity, most of its efficacy is attributable to phenobarbital, produced by the metabolism of primidone.

Phenytoin (Dilantin) is a human anticonvulsant that was once popular for use in treating epilepsy in animals. The major disadvantage of phenytoin is that it is difficult to maintain therapeutic plasma concentrations in dogs. Diazepam (Valium) is the drug of choice for emergency treatment of convulsing animals. Diazepam is effective when given IV but is poorly effective when given PO and is absorbed irregularly if injected SC or IM. Clonazepam is occasionally used with phenobarbital in animals in which plasma concentrations of barbiturate are in the therapeutic range, but the seizures are not adequately controlled.

Potassium bromide (KBr) is the other drug of choice for long-term seizure control in dogs. It can be used alone or in conjunction with phenobarbital. The exact mechanism is not fully understood, but it is thought that it has generalized depressant effects on neuronal excitability and activity. The bromide also competes for chloride transport, raising the seizure threshold. The main disadvantage of a bromide is the long half-life and consequent necessity to take it for at least 1 month before therapeutic effects occur. Bromides are commonly used for dogs but not cats.

Methocarbamol (Robaxin-V) is not an antiseizure medication but a muscle relaxant used to help seizurelike tremoring in dogs that have metaldehyde poisoning (active ingredient in slug and snail baits). It is also used for acute inflammatory and traumatic conditions of the skeletal muscle and to reduce muscle spasms (e.g., in a back injury) in dogs. The exact mechanism of how it relaxes the muscles is unknown.

CENTRAL NERVOUS SYSTEM STIMULANTS

CNS stimulants (see Box 5-10) are primarily used to stimulate respiration in anesthetized animals or to reverse CNS depression caused by anesthetic or sedative agents. Doxapram

(Dopram) is a CNS stimulant that increases respiration in animals with apnea (cessation of breathing) or bradypnea (slow breathing). Doxapram is most often used in animals that have received large amounts of respiratory depressant drugs. For example, doxapram is commonly used to stimulate respiration in neonates following cesarean section. It can be administered through the umbilical vein or sublingually. Yohimbine, tolazoline, and atipamezole increase respiration through reversal of CNS depression caused by such drugs as xylazine, detomidine, and dexmedetomidine.

ANTIMICROBIALS

Antimicrobials are drugs that kill or inhibit the growth of microorganisms or microbes, such as bacteria, protozoa, viruses, or fungi. The term *antibiotic* is often used interchangeably with the term *antimicrobial*. An antimicrobial can be classified by the type of microorganism against which it is effective and whether the antimicrobial kills the microorganism or prevents the microorganism from replicating and proliferating (Box 5-11).

The suffix *-cidal* generally describes drugs that kill the microorganism (e.g., *bactericidal*). The suffix *-static* usually describes drugs that inhibit replication but generally do not kill the microorganism outright (e.g., fungistatic). Examples include the following:

- **Bactericidal**: Kills bacteria
- **Bacteriostatic**: Inhibits bacterial replication
- **Virucidal**: Kills viruses
- Protozoastatic: Inhibits protozoal replication
- **Fungicidal**: Kills fungi

Antimicrobials work by different mechanisms to kill or inhibit bacteria and other microorganisms. Antimicrobials generally exert their effects on the cell wall, cell membrane, ribosomes, critical enzymes or metabolites, or nucleic acids of microorganisms.

Some microorganisms have developed the ability to survive in the presence of antimicrobial drugs. This ability to survive is referred to as resistance. Bacteria may become resistant to certain drugs because of genetic changes inherited from previous generations of bacteria, or they may acquire resistance by spontaneous mutations of chromosomes.

A **residue** is an accumulation of a drug, chemical, or its metabolites in animal tissues or food products resulting from drug administration to an animal or contamination of food products

PENICILLINS

Penicillins (see Box 5-11) are bactericidal and can usually be recognized by their *-cillin* suffix on the drug name. The most frequently used penicillins in veterinary medicine include the following: the natural penicillins, penicillin G and penicillin V; the broad-spectrum aminopenicillins, ampicillin, amoxicillin, and hetacillin; the penicillinase-resistant penicillins, cloxacillin, dicloxacillin, and oxacillin; and the extended-spectrum penicillins, carbenicillin, ticarcillin, piperacillin, and others. Penicillins are generally effective

| BOX 5-11 | Commonly Used Antimicrobials |

Penicillins
Ampicillin
Amoxicillin
Penicillin G
Amoxicillin-Clavulanate (Clavamox)

Cephalosporins
Cefadroxil
Cefazolin
Cephapirin
Ceftiofur
Cefovecin (Convenia)
Cefpodoxime (Simplicef)

Aminoglycosides
Gentamicin
Amikacin
Neomycin
Tobramycin

Fluoroquinolones
Enrofloxacin (Batyril)
Ciprofloxacin (Cipro)
Marbofloxacin (Zeniquin)
Ofloxacin (Ocuflox)

Tetracyclines
Tetracycline
Oxytetracycline
Doxycycline

Sulfonamides
Trimethoprim-sulfas (various types)
Sulfachloropyridazine
Sulfasalazine

Lincosamides
Lincomycin
Clindamycin (Antirobe)

Macrolide
Erythromycin

Antifungal Drugs
Amphotericin B
Nystatin
Flucytosine
Fluconazole
Ketoconazole
Griseofulvin

Adapted from Sirois M: Principles and practice of veterinary technology, ed 3, St Louis, 2011, Mosby.

against gram-positive bacteria and varying types of gram-negative bacteria. Penicillins are generally well absorbed from injection sites and the GI tract. A penicillin that should not be given PO is penicillin G. Penicillin G is inactivated by gastric acid and so is used only in injectable form.

Amoxicillin–clavulanate acid (Clavamox) is another bactericidal aminopenicillin with a beta-lactamase inhibitor, which expands its spectrum of coverage. It is most commonly used in dogs and cats for urinary tract, soft tissue, and skin infections by susceptible organisms.

CEPHALOSPORINS

Cephalosporins are bactericidal beta-lactam antimicrobials with a *ceph-* or *cef-* prefix in the drug name (see Box 5-11). Cephalosporins are classified by generations, according to when they were first developed. First-generation cephalosporins are primarily effective against gram-positive bacteria (e.g., *Streptococcus, Staphylococcus* spp.). They are less effective against gram-negative bacteria than the second- or third-generation cephalosporins. Veterinary products include cefadroxil (first generation, Cefa-Tabs), cefazolin (first generation, Kefzol, Ancef, Zolicef, cefazolin sodium), cephapirin (first generation, Cefa-Lak, Cefa-Dri intramammary infusions), ceftiofur (third generation, Naxcel injectable), cefovecin sodium (Convenia, 2-week injectable), and cefpodoxime proxetil (third generation, Simplicef). Human products used in veterinary medicine include cefixime (third generation, Suprax), cefoperazone (third generation,

Cefobid), cefpodoxime proxetil (third generation, Vantin), cefotetan disodium (second or third generation, Cefotan), cephalothin (first generation, Keflin), ceftriaxone (third generation, Rocephin), cephalexin (first generation, Keflex), cefoxitin (second generation, Mefoxin), and cefotaxime (third generation, Claforan). First-generation cephalosporins are well absorbed from the GI tract.

BACITRACINS

Bacitracins are a group of polypeptide antibiotics, of which bacitracin A is the major component. Bacitracin is a common ingredient in topical antibiotic creams or ointments. It is often combined with polymyxin B and neomycin to provide a broad spectrum of antimicrobial activity.

AMINOGLYCOSIDES

Aminoglycosides (see Box 5-11) used in veterinary medicine include gentamicin, amikacin, neomycin, streptomycin, dihydrostreptomycin, apramycin, kanamycin, and tobramycin. With the exception of amikacin, most aminoglycosides can be recognized by the -*micin* or -*mycin* suffix in the nonproprietary name. Aminoglycosides are bactericidal and are effective against many aerobic bacteria (bacteria that require oxygen to live) but are not effective against most anaerobic bacteria (those that do not require oxygen). Aminoglycosides are potentially nephrotoxic (toxic to the kidney) and ototoxic (toxic to the inner ear), even at normal dosages.

FLUOROQUINOLONES

Fluoroquinolones (quinolones) are bactericidal antimicrobials (see Box 5-11) used commonly for their effectiveness against a variety of pathogens. Quinolones are not effective against anaerobes. Enrofloxacin (Baytril) is approved for use in dogs, cats, cattle, horses, ferrets, reptiles, birds, and rodents. Ciprofloxacin (Cipro) is similar to enrofloxacin and mostly used when larger dosages are necessary. Orbifloxacin (Orbax) is also similar to enrofloxacin and is approved for use against susceptible infections in dogs and cats. Difloxacin (Dicural) and marbofloxacin (Zeniquin) are approved for use against susceptible infections in dogs only. Ofloxacin (Ocuflox) is used as an ophthalmic medication only. The quinolones are effective against common gram-negative and gram-positive bacteria found in skin, respiratory, and urinary infections. Quinolones can cause arthropathies in immature growing animals and therefore should not be used in these animals.

TETRACYCLINES

Tetracyclines (see Box 5-11) are bacteriostatic drugs with a nonproprietary name ending in -*cycline*. They work most effectively against mycoplasma, spirochetes (including *Borrelia*), chlamydia, and rickettsia. The gram-positive organisms against which they have been effective in the past are now becoming more resistant. Tetracycline and oxytetracycline have similar spectra of antibacterial activity and actions in the body. The newer and more lipophilic doxycycline and minocycline are human drugs that are being used more frequently in animals (unapproved use) because of their longer half-life (increased duration of activity), broader spectrum of antibacterial action, and better penetration of tissues than the older tetracyclines. After oral administration, doxycycline and minocycline are absorbed better than oxytetracycline or tetracycline. Oxytetracycline is the most commonly used injectable tetracycline because of its good absorption from IM injection sites. Chlortetracycline is used as a food or water treatment or as an ophthalmic agent.

SULFONAMIDES AND POTENTIATED SULFONAMIDES

Because sulfonamides (sulfa drugs) have been in use for many years, many strains of bacteria have become resistant to them. To increase the efficacy of sulfonamides and convert them from bacteriostatic to bactericidal drugs, they are sometimes combined with other compounds, such as trimethoprim and ormetoprim, to potentiate (increase) their antibacterial effects. Some of the more common sulfonamides used in veterinary medicine include sulfadimethoxine (combined with ormetoprim in Primor), sulfadiazine (combined with trimethoprim in Tribrissen), sulfamethoxazole (combined with trimethoprim in Septra), sulfachloropyridazine (used for livestock and poultry), and sulfasalazine (used for its anti-inflammatory effect in inflammatory bowel disease). Potentiated sulfas used in veterinary medicine have a fairly broad spectrum of antibacterial activity, including many gram-positive organisms (e.g., *Streptococcus, Staphylococcus, Nocardia* spp.). Although sulfas and potentiated sulfas are not effective against gram-negative organisms, they are the drugs of choice for treating some protozoal infections, including *Coccidia* and *Toxoplasma* spp. (see Box 5-11).

LINCOSAMIDES

Lincosamide antibiotics, including lincomycin and clindamycin (Antirobe), can be bacteriostatic or bactericidal, depending on the concentration attained at the site of infection (see Box 5-11). The lincosamides are generally effective against many gram-positive aerobic cocci. Lincomycin is approved for use in a variety of species (e.g., dogs, cats, swine, poultry), but clindamycin is approved for use only in dogs, cats, and ferrets.

MACROLIDES

The macrolide antibiotics used in dogs and cats include erythromycin and azithromycin. The drugs are bacteriostatic and share similar spectra of antibacterial activity and bacterial cross-resistance (see Box 5-11).

METRONIDAZOLE

Metronidazole (Flagyl) is a bactericidal antimicrobial that is also effective against protozoa that cause intestinal disease, such as *Giardia* (giardiasis), *Entamoeba histolytica* (amebiasis), *Trichomonas* (trichomoniasis), and *Balantidium coli* (balantidiasis).

NITROFURANS

The nitrofurans are a large group of antimicrobials; of these, nitrofurantoin (Furadantin) is most commonly used in veterinary medicine. Nitrofurantoin is bacteriostatic or bactericidal, depending on concentration attained at the site of infection. Because about half of the drug administered is secreted into the renal tubule, it is used to treat infections of the lower urinary tract (bladder, urethra) in dogs and cats.

CHLORAMPHENICOL AND FLUORFENICOL

Chloramphenicol is an antimicrobial that is bacteriostatic at a low concentration but may become bactericidal when used at higher dosages. Chloramphenicol has produced fatal aplastic anemia in humans. For this reason, chloramphenicol is totally banned from any use in food animals. Fluorfenicol is a new drug similar to chloramphenicol but without the risk of aplastic anemia.

RIFAMPIN

Rifampin is a bactericidal or bacteriostatic antimicrobial belonging to the rifamycin group. It is primarily used with or without erythromycin for the treatment of *Rhodococcus equi* infections in young foals and sometimes in conjunction with antifungal agents for the treatment of aspergillosis or histoplasmosis in dogs and cats.

ANTIFUNGALS

Box 5-11 contains a summary of commonly used antifungal drugs.

AMPHOTERICIN B AND NYSTATIN

Amphotericin B is an antifungal that is administered IV for the treatment of deep or systemic mycotic infections. Nystatin, because of its toxicity to tissues, is used only to treat *Candida* infections (candidiasis) on the skin, mucous membranes (e.g., mouth, vagina), and lining of the intestinal tract in dogs, cats, and birds.

FLUCYTOSINE

Flucytosine is an antifungal agent used mostly against *Cryptococcus* and *Candida*. It is often used in conjunction with amphotericin B because resistance is common when used alone.

FLUCONAZOLE, KETOCONAZOLE, AND ITRACONAZOLE

Fluconazole, ketoconazole, and itraconazole are imidazole antifungals with fewer side effects than amphotericin B. Of the imidazoles, fluconazole has the fewest side effects and is apparently safe for use in multiple species.

GRISEOFULVIN

Griseofulvin is a fungistatic drug used primarily to treat infections with *Trichophyton*, *Microsporum*, and *Epidermophyton* dermatophytes (superficial fungi) in dogs and cats. These fungi usually infect the skin, hair, nails, and claws, causing the condition known as ringworm.

ANTIPARASITICS

Anthelmintic is a general term used to describe compounds that kill various types of internal parasites (helminths, or worms; Box 5-12). A **vermicide** is an anthelmintic that kills the worm, as opposed to a vermifuge, which only paralyzes the worm and often results in the passage of live worms in the stool. Antinematodal compounds are used to treat infections with nematodes (roundworms). Nematodes include hookworms, ascarids, whipworms, and strongyles. Anticestodal compounds are used to treat infections with cestodes (tapeworms or segmented flatworms). Antitrematodal compounds are used to treat infection with trematodes (flukes or unsegmented flatworms), including *Paragonimus, Fasciola,* and *Dicrocoelium* spp. Antiprotozoal compounds are used to treat infection with protozoa (single-celled organisms), including *Coccidia, Giardia,* and *Toxoplasma* spp. Coccidiostats are drugs that specifically inhibit the growth of coccidia.

INTERNAL ANTIPARASITICS

Piperazine, a vermicide and vermifuge, is the active ingredient in most of the once-monthly dewormers sold in grocery stores and pet shops. Piperazine is safe but is effective only against ascarids. The benzimidazoles include fenbendazole (Panacur), mebendazole (Telmin, Telmintic), thiabendazole (Equizole, Tresaderm Otic), oxibendazole (Anthelcide EQ, Filaribits-Plus), albendazole, oxfendazole, and cambendazole.

Organophosphates are used as internal antiparasitics (Task, Combot) and in external antiparasitics to combat fleas, ticks, and flies. The organophosphates most commonly used internally are dichlorvos and trichlorfon. Ivermectin (Ivomec, Eqvalan, Heartgard-30) is an avermectin widely

---

BOX 5-12 | Commonly Used Antiparasitics

For Treatment of Internal Parasites
Piperazine
Fenbendazole
Ivermectin
Praziquantel (Droncit)
Epsiprantel (Cestex)
Pyrantel (Strongid, Nemex)
Febantel
Melarsomine (Immidicide)
Milbemycin (Interceptor, Sentinel, Capstar)
Sulfadimethoxine (Albon)

For Treatment of External Parasites
Pyrethrins
Permethrins (Advantix, Vetra, Virbac)
Amitraz (Mitoban, Preventic)
Imidacloprid (Advantage, Advantix)
Fipronil (Frontline)
Selamectin (Revolution)
Lufenuron (Program, Sentinel)
Spinosad (Comfortis)

Adapted from Sirois M: *Principles and practice of veterinary technology,* ed 3, St Louis, 2011, Mosby.

used in almost every species treated by veterinarians. Ivermectin can produce adverse reactions in collies and collie cross-breeds. Anticestodals used in animals include praziquantel (Droncit) and epsiprantel (Cestex).

Anthelmintics containing pyrantel (Strongid, Nemex, Banminth, Imathal) safely remove a variety of nematodes in domestic species. They are marketed as pyrantel pamoate and a more water-soluble salt, pyrantel tartrate. Morantel tartrate (Nematel) is similar to pyrantel and has similar uses. Febantel is marketed in combination with the anticestodal drug praziquantel (Vercom) for dogs and cats.

For years, thiacetarsamide sodium (Caparsolate), given by IV injection, had been the only drug approved for the treatment of adult heartworms. In 1996, melarsomine dihydrochloride (Immiticide) was approved as an adulticide; it is given by IM injection. After adulticide treatment a microfilaricide can be administered to eliminate circulating heartworm microfilariae. Ivermectin is the microfilaricide of choice. Milbemycin oxime (Interceptor, Sentinel), a drug similar to ivermectin, is also used as a microfilaricide. After microfilariae have been cleared from the blood, the animal can begin receiving a heartworm preventive to prevent reinfection. Diethylcarbamazine (DEC), marketed as Caricide, Nemacide, and Filarbits, is given daily during seasons when an animal could be bitten by a mosquito and for 2 months thereafter. Because they must be given only once a month, ivermectin (Heartgard-30) and milbemycin (Interceptor, Sentinel) have captured a significant percentage of the heartworm preventive market. Ivermectin is also available as a heartworm preventive for cats (Heartgard-30 for Cats).

Antiprotozoals are most commonly used against coccidia, *Giardia,* and other protozoa. They include sulfonamide antimicrobials such as sulfadimethoxine (Albon, Bactrovet), metronidazole, and amprolium (Corid).

EXTERNAL ANTIPARASITICS

Chlorinated hydrocarbons constitute one of the oldest groups of the synthetic insecticides. The only chlorinated hydrocarbon currently used in veterinary medicine is lindane, which is incorporated in some dog shampoos. Lindane is easily absorbed through the skin and can produce harmful side effects if absorbed in sufficient quantities.

Organophosphates and carbamates are usually grouped together because of their similar mechanisms of action, effects on insects, and toxic effects. Unlike the chlorinated hydrocarbons, organophosphates and carbamates decompose readily in the environment and do not pose a significant threat to wildlife. Included in this group are chlorpyrifos, carbaryl (Sevin), and propoxur (Baygon).

Pyrethrins and pyrethroids (synthetic pyrethrins) constitute the largest group of insecticides marketed for use against external parasites and as common household insect sprays. They are generally safe. Pyrethrins and pyrethroids produce a quick knockdown effect, but the immobilized flies or fleas may recover after several minutes. Pyrethroids include resmethrin, allethrin, permethrin, tetramethrin, bioallethrin, and fenvalerate.

Amitraz is a diamide insecticide that was one of the first effective agents available for the treatment of demodectic mange in dogs. Since its introduction, amitraz has been incorporated into other insecticidal products. It is toxic to cats and rabbits, so it should not be used in those species. The liquid form, available as a dip or sponge-on bath product (Mitaban), is used to treat demodectic mange in dogs. Amitraz is also available as Preventic, a tick collar for dogs.

Imidacloprid (Advantage) is a chloronicotinyl nitroguanidine insecticide used topically to kill adult fleas on dogs and cats. Imidacloprid is applied to the back of the neck in cats or between the shoulder blades in dogs (and over the rump area of large dogs) and kills adult fleas on contact. Fipronil (Frontline and Top Spot) and selamectin (Revolution) are once-monthly flea sprays and topical applications that are similar to ivermectin in their insecticidal activity.

Rotenone (Derris Powder) is a natural insecticide derived from derris root. It may be included with other insecticides in dips, pour-ons, and powders. D-Limonene, derived from citrus peel, purportedly has some slight insecticidal activity. When included in insecticidal products, it imparts a pleasant citrus smell to the hair coat. Sulfur is sometimes included in tar and sulfur shampoos to help reduce skin scaling and to treat sarcoptic mange. These products are usually recognized by their strong sulfur odor.

Insect growth regulators are compounds that affect the immature stages of insects and prevent maturation to adults. They are insecticidal, without toxic effects in mammals.

Methoprene (Siphotrol, Ovitrol) and fenoxycarb (e.g., Basus, Ectogard) were some of the first insect growth regulators incorporated into topical products or flea collars. These compounds are distributed over the animal's skin. Female fleas absorb the drug and it is incorporated into the flea eggs. The drug-impregnated eggs hatch and the larvae do not mature to adult fleas.

Lufenuron (Program, Sentinel) is an insect development inhibitor given once monthly in tablet form for dogs and cats and as an oral liquid for cats. It interferes with the development of the insect's chitin, which is essential for proper egg formation and development of the larval exoskeleton. If flea larvae survive within the egg, despite a defective shell, they will be unable to hatch. Because lufenuron is orally ingested and distributed throughout the animal's tissue fluids, a flea must bite the animal to be exposed to the drug.

Spinosad (Comfortis) is a neurotoxin that works on fleas only and, like lufenuron, is orally ingested and distributed throughout the animal's tissue. It should not be given to dogs and cats with epilepsy or those already on ivermectin.

Insect repellents are used to repel insects and keep them off animals. Butoxypolypropylene glycol (Butox PPG) has been incorporated into flea and tick spray products for use in dogs and cats. It is also used in equine fly repellents.

Diethyltoluamide (DEET) is a common ingredient in repellent products formulated for use in humans.

ANTI-INFLAMMATORIES

Drugs that relieve pain or discomfort by blocking or reducing the inflammatory process are called **anti-inflammatory drugs**. There are two general classes of anti-inflammatories, steroidal anti-inflammatory drugs (glucocorticoids) and nonsteroidal anti-inflammatory drugs (**NSAIDs**). Most of these drugs relieve pain indirectly by decreasing inflammation; however, some also have direct analgesic (pain-relieving) activity.

GLUCOCORTICOIDS

When veterinarians use the terms *cortisone* or **corticosteroid**, they are usually referring to glucocorticoids (Box 5-13). A glucocorticoid such as hydrocortisone, which exerts an anti-inflammatory effect for less than 12 hours, is considered a short-acting glucocorticoid. Many glucocorticoids used in veterinary medicine are classified as intermediate-acting glucocorticoids, with activity for 12 to 36 hours. These include prednisone, prednisolone, triamcinolone (Vetalog), methylprednisolone, and isoflupredone. Long-acting glucocorticoids, such as dexamethasone, betamethasone, and flumethasone, exert their effects for longer than 48 hours.

Glucocorticoids are generally available in three liquid forms—aqueous solutions, alcohol solutions, and suspensions. Glucocorticoids in aqueous (water) solution are usually combined with a salt to make them soluble in water. Dexamethasone sodium phosphate (Azium SP) and prednisolone sodium succinate (Solu-Delta-Cortef) are aqueous solutions of glucocorticoids. The advantage of aqueous forms is that they can be given IV in large doses with less risk than alcohol solutions and suspensions; suspensions should never be given IV. The aqueous forms are often used in emergency situations (e.g., shock, CNS trauma) because they can be delivered IV in large amounts and have a fairly rapid onset of action. If the label of a vial of dexamethasone specifies the active ingredient as dexamethasone, without mention of sodium phosphate, it is likely an alcohol solution. Suspensions of glucocorticoids contain the drug particles suspended in the liquid vehicle. Suspensions are characterized by their opaque appearance (after shaking), the need for shaking the vial before use, and the terms *acetate, diacetate, pivalate, acetonide,* or *valerate* appended to the glucocorticoid name. When injected into the body, the drug crystals dissolve over several days, releasing small amounts of glucocorticoid each day and providing prolonged action. Topical preparations of glucocorticoid suspensions using the acetate ester are used in topical ophthalmic medications. Oral tablets are available for prednisone and prednisolone.

Overuse of glucocorticoid drugs can produce Cushing's syndrome. The signs of Cushing's syndrome are related to the effects of glucocorticoids and include alopecia (hair loss), muscle wasting, pot-bellied appearance, slow healing of wounds, polyuria, polydipsia, and polyphagia. Physical changes (alopecia, muscle wasting) do not become apparent until the animal has been treated for weeks.

NONSTEROIDAL ANTI-INFLAMMATORY DRUGS

The advantage of NSAIDs (see Box 5-13) over glucocorticoids is that they have fewer side effects. Among the few adverse effects associated with NSAIDs are a decrease in protective prostaglandin levels in the stomach and kidney. In large doses or in sensitive animals, NSAIDs can also produce gastric ulcerations or decreased blood flow to the kidneys.

Aspirin (acetylsalicylic acid) is a fairly safe NSAID in most animal species. Like other NSAIDs, aspirin is metabolized by the liver. Aspirin is metabolized much more slowly in cats than in other species. It has a half-life of 1.5 hours in humans, approximately 8 hours in dogs, and 30 hours in cats. Thus, as with many other drugs, the aspirin dosage for cats is lower than dosages used for other species; it usually consists of one baby aspirin tablet (81 mg) every 2 or 3 days. If used prudently, however, aspirin is one of the safest and most effective NSAIDs for cats.

Ibuprofen and naproxen are available as OTC medications (ibuprofen is marketed as Advil; naproxen is marketed as Aleve). Naproxen is marketed as the veterinary product Naprosyn. Both dogs and cats are sensitive to these OTC medications and can develop liver and kidney failure with overdosing, so these are not generally recommended for clients to give to their pets. Carprofen (Rimadyl), deracoxib (Deramaxx), etodolac (Etogesic), meloxicam (Metacam), and firocoxib (Previcox) are all cyclooxygenase (COX)-inhibiting (coxib) class, non-narcotic NSAIDs with anti-inflammatory and analgesic properties. There are two main cyclooxygenase enzymes, COX-1 and COX-2, and a newly discovered third enzyme, COX-3, which has yet to be fully characterized. Cyclooxygenase-1 (COX-1) is the enzyme responsible for helping with physiologic processes, such as platelet aggregation, gastric mucosal protection, and renal perfusion. Cyclooxygenase-2 (COX-2) is responsible for the synthesis of inflammatory mediators. The effects of cyclooxygenase-3 (COX-3) are still undetermined. These coxib class NSAIDs therefore decrease the levels of prostaglandins associated with inflammation but do not significantly reduce

---

| **BOX 5-13** | Commonly Used Anti-Inflammatories |

Glucocorticoids
Prednisone
Prednisolone
Triamcinolone (Vetalog)
Methylprednisolone
Dexamethasone
Dexamethasone sodium phosphate
Prednisolone sodium succinate (Solu-Delta-Cortef)

NSAIDs
Carprofen (Rimadyl)
Deracoxib (Deramaxx)
Meloxicam (Metacam)
Firocoxib (Previcox)

Adapted from Sirois M: Principles and practice of veterinary technology, ed 3, St Louis, 2011, Mosby.

the levels of protective prostaglandins in the stomach and kidneys. Tepoxalin (Zubrin) is a coxib class NSAID but also has 5-lipoxygenase (LOX) inhibition that may be useful in allergic conditions.

OTHER ANTI-INFLAMMATORIES

Although acetaminophen is not an anti-inflammatory drug, it is included here because its analgesic and antipyretic (fever-reducing) properties often result in it being grouped with NSAIDs. Acetaminophen (e.g., Tylenol) does not cause the GI upset, ulcers, or interference with platelet clumping associated with NSAIDs. Unfortunately, the metabolites of acetaminophen can have other severe side effects, especially in cats. A single extra-strength acetaminophen tablet (500 mg) can kill an average-sized cat. In dogs a higher dosage (>150 mg/kg) is required before signs of hepatic necrosis, weight loss, and icterus (jaundice) become evident.

Phenacetin is a compound found in many cold preparations. This drug is metabolized to acetaminophen and thus can produce acetaminophen toxicity in susceptible species and individual animals. Gold salts, such as aurothioglucose, have been used to treat severe immune-mediated skin problems, such as the various forms of pemphigus. The anti-inflammatory activity of dipyrone is weak compared with its analgesic properties and its ability to decrease fever.

DISINFECTANTS AND ANTISEPTICS

Disinfection is the destruction of pathogenic microorganisms or their toxins. **Antiseptics** are chemical agents that kill or prevent the growth of microorganisms on living tissues. Disinfectants are chemical agents that kill or prevent the growth of microorganisms on inanimate objects (e.g., surgical equipment, floors, tabletops). Antiseptics and disinfectants may also be described as sanitizers or sterilizers. **Sanitizers** are chemical agents that reduce the number of microorganisms to a safe level, without completely eliminating all microorganisms. Sterilizers are chemicals or other agents that destroy all microorganisms completely. As with antimicrobials, it is important to know against which organisms the antiseptic or disinfectant is effective (Table 5-5).

PHENOLS

Phenols are used as scrub soaps and surface disinfectants. Phenols are also the main disinfecting agents found in many household disinfectants (e.g., Lysol, pine oil). They are effective against gram-positive bacteria but generally not effective against gram-negative bacteria, viruses, fungi, or spores. Hexachlorophene is a phenolic surgical scrub that has decreased in popularity because of its suspected neurotoxicity (damage to the nervous system) and teratogenic effects (birth defects) in pregnant nurses who performed hexachlorophene scrubs on a regular basis.

ALCOHOLS

Alcohols, such as ethyl alcohol or isopropyl alcohol, are among the most common antiseptics applied to the skin. Solutions of 70% alcohol are used to disinfect surgical sites, injection sites, and rectal thermometers. Nonenveloped viruses are not susceptible to the virucidal effects of alcohol. Alcohol is also ineffective against bacterial spores and must remain in contact with the site for several seconds to be effective against bacteria (several minutes for fungi). Therefore, a cursory swipe with an alcohol-soaked swab on an animal's skin, especially if the skin is encrusted with dirt or feces, does little to disinfect an injection site.

QUATERNARY AMMONIUM COMPOUNDS

Quaternary ammonium compounds are used to disinfect the surface of inanimate objects. One of the most commonly used quaternary ammonium compounds in veterinary medicine is benzalkonium chloride. Quaternary ammonium compounds are effective against a wide variety of gram-negative and gram-positive bacteria, but they are ineffective against bacterial spores and have poor efficacy against fungi. Although quaternary ammonium compounds can destroy enveloped viruses, they are ineffective against nonenveloped viruses, such as parvovirus. They act rapidly at the site of application and are not normally irritating to the skin or corrosive to metals.

CHLORINE COMPOUNDS

Chlorine compounds, such as sodium hypochlorite (Clorox, household bleach), can kill enveloped and nonenveloped

TABLE 5-5	Relative Efficacy of Disinfectants and Antiseptics*					
ACTION	CHLORHEXIDINE	QUATERNARY AMMONIUM COMPOUNDS	ALCOHOL	IODOPHOR	CHLORINE	PHENOLS
Bactericidal	3+†	2+	2+	3+	2+	2+
Lipid-enveloped virucidal	3+	2+	2+	2+	3+	1+
Nonenveloped virucidal	2+	1+	(−)‡	2+	3+	(−)
Sporicidal	(−)	(−)	(−)	1+	1+	(−)
Effective in presence of soap	1+	(−)	2+	2+	2+	2+
Effective in hard water	1+	1+	1+	2+	2+	1+
Effective in organic material	3+	1+	1+	(−)	(−)	(−)

*Ratings are relative indicators, and the effectiveness is dependent upon concentration of compound used.
†The higher the positive number, the greater the efficacy.
‡Minus signs (−) indicate lack of efficacy.
From Sirois M: Principles and practice of veterinary technology, ed 3, St Louis, 2011, Mosby.

viruses and are the disinfectants of choice against parvovirus. Chlorines are also effective against fungi, algae, and vegetative forms of bacteria. Like many other disinfectants, chlorine is not effective against bacterial spores.

IODOPHORS

Iodophors are used as topical antiseptics before surgical procedures or for the disinfection of tissue. An iodophor is a combination of iodine and a carrier molecule that releases the iodine over time, prolonging the antimicrobial activity. The most common iodophor is iodine combined with polyvinylpyrrolidone, more commonly known as povidone-iodine (e.g., Betadine). Iodophors are bactericidal, virucidal, protozoacidal, and fungicidal.

BIGUANIDES

Chlorhexidine, a biguanide antiseptic, is commonly used to clean cages and to treat various superficial infections in animals. Its wide variety of uses is likely related to its low tissue irritation and its virucidal, bactericidal (both gram-positive and gram-negative), and fungicidal activity. Because chlorhexidine binds to the outer surface of the skin, it is thought to have some residual activity for up to 24 hours if left in contact with the site.

RECOMMENDED READINGS

Bill RL: *Pharmacology for veterinary technicians*, ed 3, St Louis, 2006, Mosby.

Mosby: Mosby's drug consult, St Louis, 2007, Mosby.

Papich MG: *Saunders handbook of veterinary drugs*, ed 3, St Louis, 2011, Saunders.

Plumb DC: *Veterinary drug handbook*, ed 7, Ames, IA, 2012, Wiley-Blackwell.

Sirois M: *Principles and practice of veterinary technology*, ed 3, St Louis, 2011, Elsevier.

Wanamaker BP, Pettes CL: *Applied pharmacology for the veterinary technician*, ed 5, St Louis, 2014, Saunders.

6 Animal Behavior and Restraint[1]

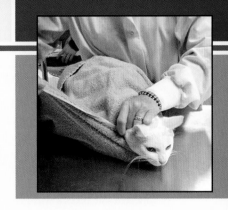

OUTLINE

Dog and Cat Breeds, *132*
What is Behavior and Where Does it Come From? *141*
Preventing Behavior Problems in Companion Animals, *142*
House Training, *142*
Preventing Destructive Behavior, *144*
Preventing Aggressive Behavior Problems, *147*
Puppy Tests, *147*
Castration, *147*
Socialization, *147*
Providing Services for Problems, *148*
Problem Prevention, *148*
Problem Resolution, *148*
Referring Cases to Behavior Specialists, *150*

Behavior Problems in Exotic Animals, *151*
Restraint and Handling of Dogs, *151*
Canine Body Language, *151*
Danger Potential, *151*
Restraint Devices, *151*
Special Handling, *155*
Restraint Techniques, *156*
Restraint and Handling of Cats, *160*
Feline Behavior, *160*
Danger Potential, *160*
Mechanical Devices, *160*
Distraction Techniques, *164*
Restraint Techniques, *164*

LEARNING OBJECTIVES

After reviewing this chapter, the reader will be able to:

1. Describe the processes by which behaviors develop.
2. Differentiate between positive and negative reinforcement and punishment.
3. List and describe types of aggressive behavior that may be seen in dogs and cats.
4. Describe the role of veterinary professionals in preventing behavior problems.
5. List the steps in house training a puppy.
6. Describe proper litter box care.
7. List the different options cats look for in scratching posts.
8. Describe the role of veterinary professionals in managing behavior problems.
9. List and give examples of various behavior modification techniques.
10. Describe the procedure for referring clients to professionals for resolution of behavior problems.
11. Describe the psychological principles underlying physical restraint techniques.
12. Explain and implement the safety precautions taken before and during physical restraint.
13. Restrain dogs and cats for routine procedures such as physical exams, nursing care, and sample collection.
14. Give examples of behavior responses of animals to physical restraint.
15. Correctly identify and use restraint equipment.

KEY TERMS

Aggression
Agonistic
Anthropomorphism
Behavior
Catchpole
Distraction technique

Dorsal recumbency
Elimination
Ethology
Gauntlet
Imprinting
Lateral recumbency

Muzzle
Operant conditioning
Pheromone
Punishment
Queen
Reinforcement

Selective breeding
Socialization
Sternal recumbency
Stimulus
Substrate
Veterinary behaviorist

[1]Elsevier and the author acknowledge and appreciate the original contributions from Sirois M: Principles and practice of veterinary technology, ed 3, St Louis, 2011, Mosby; and Sheldon CC, Sonsthagen T, Topel JA: Animal restraint for veterinary professionals, St Louis, 2006, Mosby, whose work forms the heart of this chapter.

DOG AND CAT BREEDS

Hundreds of breeds of dogs and cats are in existence. The development of different breeds of animals is primarily the result of **selective breeding,** in which humans bred specific individual animals in an effort to develop animals with certain desirable characteristics. Breeds of dogs have been developed for specific purposes, such as hunting and guarding. The development of different cat breeds was primarily the result of a desire for animals with a specific appearance. Some aspects of dog and cat behavior are based on instinctive behaviors common to all animals of the same species. Other traits are primarily the result of selective breeding that led to the breeds of dogs and cats we now have. For example, the Labrador retriever is a hunting dog bred to retrieve game, whereas the Boxer breed was developed to chase, capture, and hold large game until the hunter arrives. Although both are working dogs, the two breeds have significantly different appearances and natural abilities. A wide variety of mixed breed dogs are also common. In many cases, these have also been specifically bred from two purebred parents. The result of the breeding is a hybrid of the two breeds and generally has aspects of both parent breeds. These dogs are sometimes referred to as "designer dogs" (Fig. 6-1). It is possible now to have DNA testing performed to determine the ancestry of mixed-breed dogs.

The International Cat Association (http://www.tica.org) maintains a database of recognized cat breeds. Common cat breeds include the domestic short hair, Abyssinian (Fig. 6-2), Burmese (Fig. 6-3), Persian (Fig. 6-4), and Siamese (Fig. 6-5).

The American Kennel Club (AKC) (www.akc.org) maintains a database of dog breeds. Specific information on the origin of the breed, as well as the breed's physical characteristics and expected temperament, are in the database. The AKC organizes dogs into one of seven specific groups (Table 6-1). The groups have similar behavioral characteristics. An additional class, the Miscellaneous class, contains breeds that are being developed but are not yet recognized as belonging to one of the seven groups.

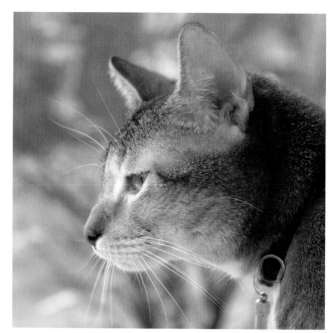

FIGURE 6-2 Abyssinian cat. (From Dyce KM, Sack WO, Wensing CJG: Textbook of veterinary anatomy, ed 4, St Louis, 2010, Saunders.)

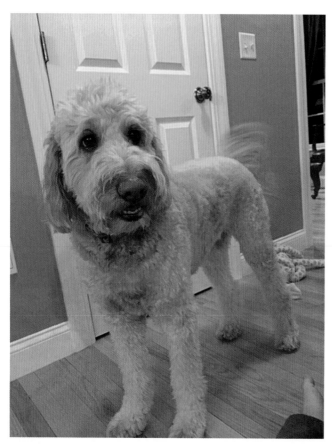

FIGURE 6-1 Goldendoodle. A hybrid between a purebred Golden Retriever and Standard Poodle. (Courtesy Rosie Fess.)

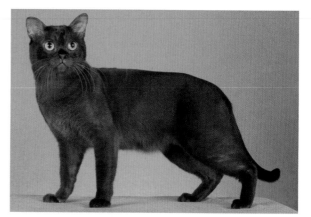

FIGURE 6-3 Burmese. (From Little S: The cat: Clinical medicine and management, St Louis, 2012, Saunders.)

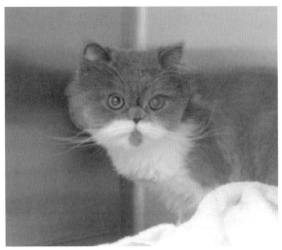

FIGURE 6-4 Persian cat. (From Little S: The cat: Clinical medicine and management, St Louis, 2012, Saunders.)

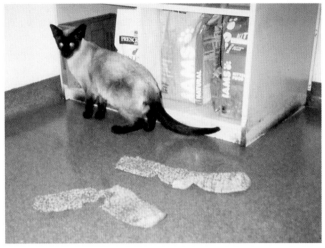

FIGURE 6-5 Siamese cat. (From Little S: The cat: Clinical medicine and management, St Louis, 2012, Saunders.)

TABLE 6-1	AKC Recognized Dog Breeds

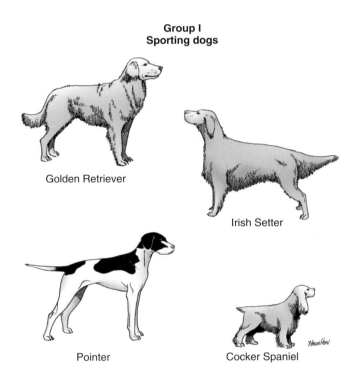

**Group I
Sporting dogs**

Golden Retriever

Irish Setter

Pointer

Cocker Spaniel

American Water Spaniel
Boykin Spaniel
Brittany Spaniel
Chesapeake Bay Retriever
Clumber Spaniel
Cocker Spaniel(Fig. 6-6)
Curly-Coated Retriever
English Cocker Spaniel
English Setter
English Springer Spaniel
Field Spaniel
Flat-Coated Retriever
German Shorthaired Pointer
German Wirehaired Pointer
Gordon Setter
Golden Retriever (Fig. 6-7)
Irish Red and White Setter
Irish Setter
Irish Water Spaniel
Labrador Retriever (Fig. 6-8)
Nova Scotia Duck Tolling Retriever
Pointer
Spinone Italiano
Sussex Spaniel
Vizsla
Weimaraner (Fig. 6-9)
Welsh Springer Spaniel
Wirehaired Pointing Griffon
Wirehaired Vizsla

Continued

TABLE 6-1   AKC Recognized Dog Breeds—cont'd

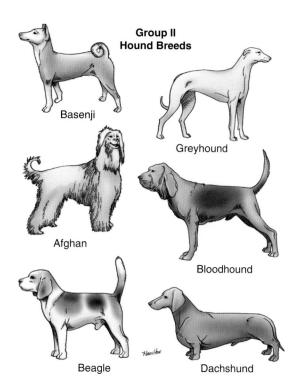

**Group II
Hound Breeds**

Basenji

Greyhound

Afghan

Bloodhound

Beagle

Dachshund

Afghan Hound
American English Coonhound
American Foxhound
Basenji
Basset Hound
Beagle (Fig. 6-10)
Black and Tan Coonhound
Bloodhound (Fig. 6-11)
Bluetick Coonhound
Borzoi
Cirneco dell'Etna
Dachshund (Fig. 6-12)
English Foxhound
Greyhound (Fig. 6-13)
Harrier
Ibizan Hound
Irish Wolfhound
Norwegian Elkhound
Otterhound
Petit Basset Griffon Vendeen
Pharaoh Hound
Plott
Portugese Podeno Pequeno
Redbone Coonhound
Rhodesian Ridgeback
Saluki
Scottish Deerhound
Treeing Walker Coonhound
Whippet

**Group III
Working Breeds**

Boxer

Alaskan Malamute

Saint Bernard

Akita

Standard Schnauzer

Doberman Pinscher

Akita
Alaskan Malamute
Anatolian Shepherd Dog
Bernese Mountain Dog
Black Russian Terrier
Boerboel
Boxer (Fig. 6-14)
Bullmastiff
Cane Corso
Doberman Pinscher (Fig. 6-15)
Dogue de Bordeaux
German Pinscher
Giant Schnauzer
Great Dane
Great Pyrenees
Greater Swiss Mountain Dog
Komondor
Kuvasz
Leonberger
Mastiff (Fig. 6-16)
Neapolitan Mastiff
Newfoundland
Portuguese Water Dog
Rottweiler
Saint Bernard
Samoyed
Siberian Husky
Standard Schnauzer
Tibetan Mastiff

TABLE 6-1	AKC Recognized Dog Breeds—cont'd

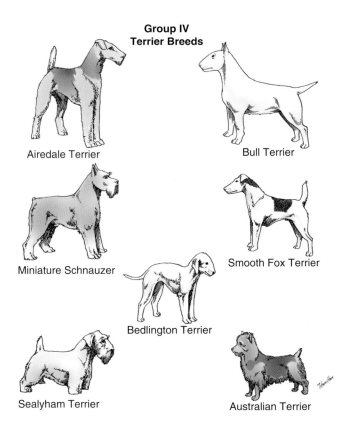

**Group IV
Terrier Breeds**

Airedale Terrier

Bull Terrier

Miniature Schnauzer

Smooth Fox Terrier

Bedlington Terrier

Sealyham Terrier

Australian Terrier

Airedale Terrier
American Staffordshire Terrier
Australian Terrier
Bedlington Terrier
Border Terrier
Bull Terrier
Cairn Terrier
Cesky Terrier
Dandie Dinmont Terrier
Glen of Imall Terrier
Irish Terrier
Kerry Blue Terrier
Lakeland Terrier
Manchester Terrier
Miniature Bull Terrier
Miniature Schnauzer
Norfolk Terrier
Norwich Terrier
Parson Russell Terrier
Rat Terrier
Russell Terrier
Scottish Terrier (Fig. 6-17)
Sealyham Terrier
Skye Terrier
Smooth Fox Terrier
Soft-Coated Wheaten Terrier
Staffordshire Bull Terrier
Welsh Terrier
West Highland White Terrier
Wire Fox Terrier

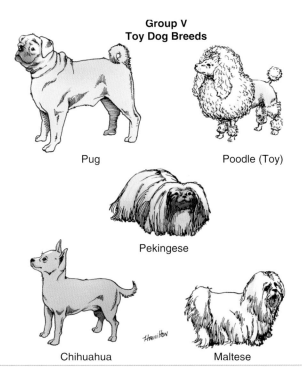

**Group V
Toy Dog Breeds**

Pug

Poodle (Toy)

Pekingese

Chihuahua

Maltese

Affenpinscher
Brussels Griffon
Cavalier King Charles Spaniel
Chihuahua (Fig. 6-18)
Chinese Crested
English Toy Spaniel
Havanese
Italian Greyhound
Japanese Chin
Maltese
Manchester Terrier (Toy)
Miniature Pinscher
Papillon (Fig. 6-19)
Pekingese
Pomeranian
Poodle (Toy)
Pug (Fig. 6-20)
Shih Tzu
Silky Terrier
Toy Fox Terrier
Yorkshire Terrier (Fig. 6-21)

Continued

TABLE 6-1 AKC Recognized Dog Breeds—cont'd

Group VI
Non-Sporting Breeds

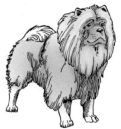

Chow Chow

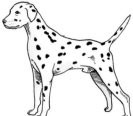

Dalmation

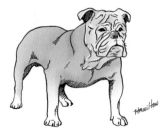

English Bulldog

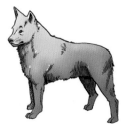

Schipperke

American Eskimo Dog
Bichon Frise
Boston Terrier (Fig. 6-22)
Bulldog
Chinese Shar-Pei (Fig. 6-23)
Chow-Chow
Coton de Tulear
Dalmatian
Finnish Spitz
French Bulldog (Fig. 6-24)
Keeshond
Lhasa Apso(Fig. 6-25)
Löwchen
Norwegian Lundehund
Poodle (Miniature and Standard)
Schipperke
Shiba Inu
Tibetan Spaniel
Tibetan Terrier
Xoloitzcuintli

Group VII
Herding Breeds

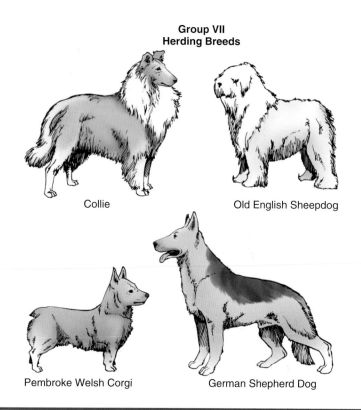

Collie

Old English Sheepdog

Pembroke Welsh Corgi

German Shepherd Dog

Australian Cattle Dog
Australian Shepherd (Fig. 6-26)
Bearded Collie
Beauceron
Belgian Malinois
Belgian Sheepdog
Belgian Tervuren
Bergamasco
Border Collie
Bouvier des Flandres (Fig. 6-27)
Briard
Canaan Dog
Cardigan Welsh Corgi
Collie
Entlebucher Mountain Dog
Finnish Lapphund
German Shepherd Dog (Fig. 6-28)
Icelandic Sheepdog
Norwegian Buhund
Old English Sheepdog
Pembroke Welsh Corgi
Polish Lowland Sheepdog
Puli
Pyrenean Shepherd
Shetland Sheepdog (Fig. 6-29)
Spanish Water Dog
Swedish Vallhund

Illustrations from Evans H, Lahunta A: Miller's anatomy of the dog, ed 4, St Louis, 2013, Saunders.

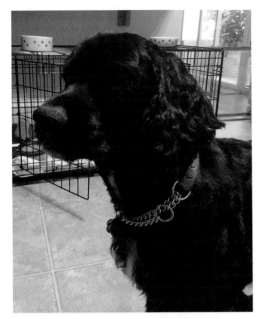

FIGURE 6-6 Cocker Spaniel. (Courtesy Brady Harris.)

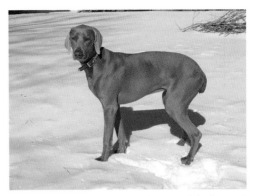

FIGURE 6-9 Weimaraner. (Courtesy Kobi Stearns.)

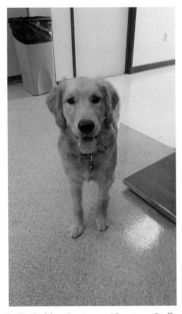

FIGURE 6-7 Golden Retriever. (Courtesy Daffodil Serling.)

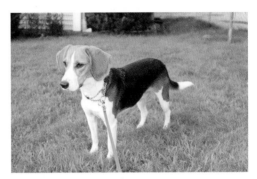

FIGURE 6-10 Beagle. (Courtesy Donna Harris.)

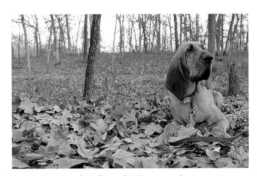

FIGURE 6-11 Bloodhound. (Courtesy Georgia Haywood.)

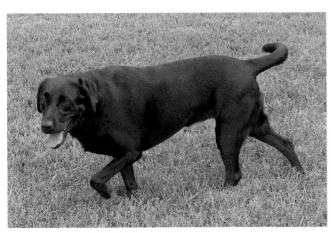

FIGURE 6-8 Labrador Retriever.

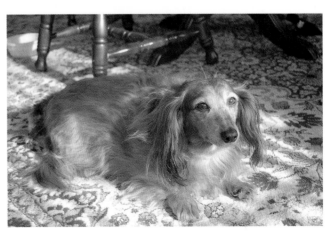

FIGURE 6-12 Dachshund. (Courtesy Dylan McWade.)

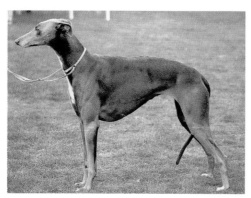

FIGURE 6-13 Greyhound. (From Dyce KM, Sack WO, Wensing CJG: Textbook of veterinary anatomy, ed 4, St Louis, 2010, Saunders.)

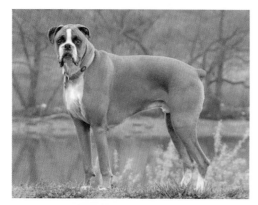

FIGURE 6-14 Boxer.

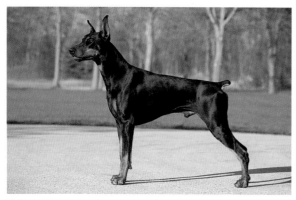

FIGURE 6-15 Doberman Pinscher. (©iStock.com/James Brey.)

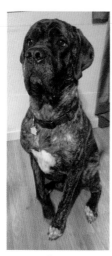

FIGURE 6-16 Mastiff . (Courtesy Gorgon Wirth.)

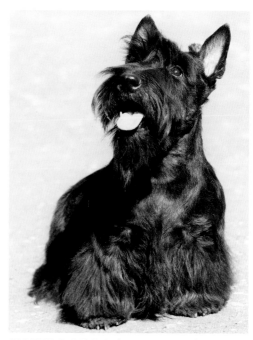

FIGURE 6-17 Scottish Terrier, (©iStock.com/vtls.)

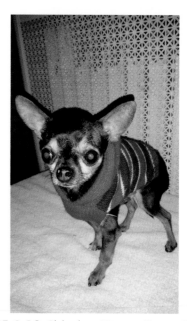

FIGURE 6-18 Chihuahua. (Courtesy Batman Evenhus.)

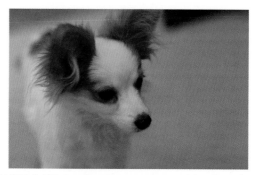

FIGURE 6-19 Papillon. (Courtesy Peanut Whipple Neibauer.)

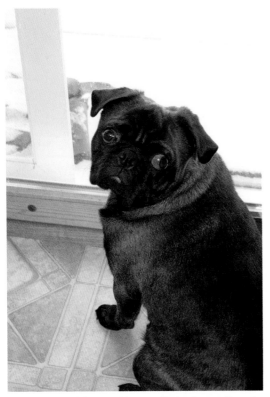

FIGURE 6-20 Pug. (Courtesy Pudge Lowery-Burns.)

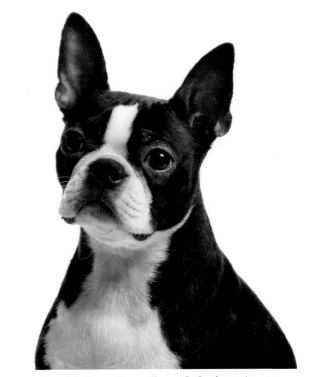

FIGURE 6-22 Boston Terrier. (Figure © iStock.com.)

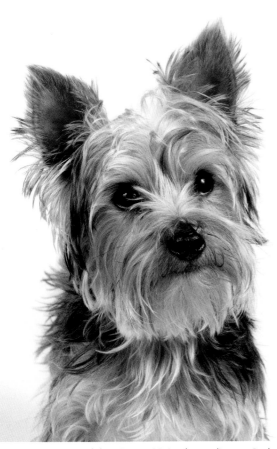

FIGURE 6-21 Yorkshire Terrier. (©iStock.com/Joanna Pecha.)

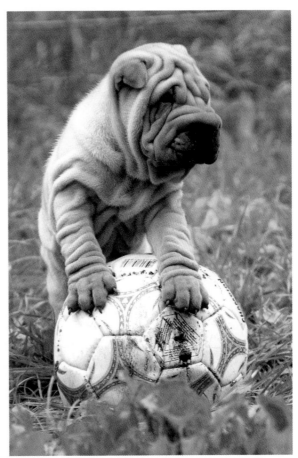

FIGURE 6-23 Shar-pei. (From Dyce KM, Sack WO, Wensing CJG: Textbook of veterinary anatomy, ed 4, St Louis, 2010, Saunders.)

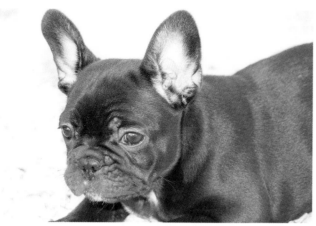

FIGURE 6-24 French Bulldog. (Courtesy Fribble Lowery-Burns.)

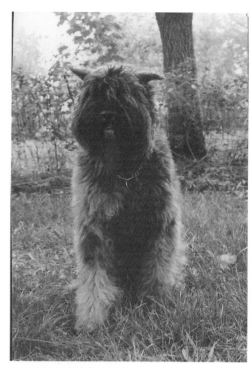

FIGURE 6-27 Bouvier des Flandres.

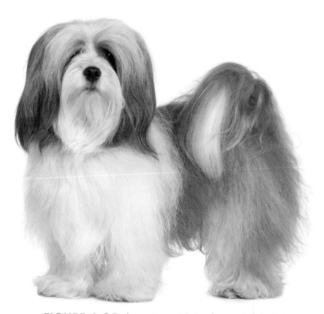

FIGURE 6-25 Lhasa Apso. (©iStock.com/GlobalP.)

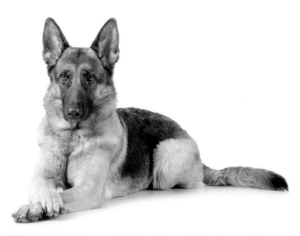

FIGURE 6-28 German Shepherd Dog. (©iStock.com/Alexia_Khrush-cheva.)

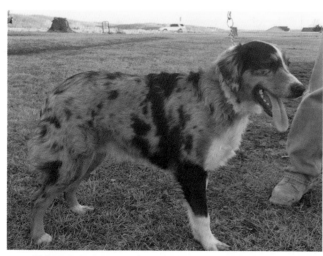

FIGURE 6-26 Australian Shepherd. (Courtesy Milo Berg.)

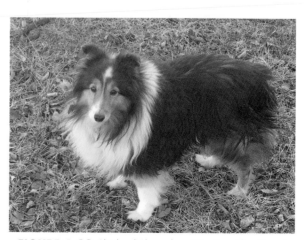

FIGURE 6-29 Shetland Sheepdog. (Courtesy Skye Berg.)

WHAT IS BEHAVIOR AND WHERE DOES IT COME FROM?

Behavior is any act done by an animal. An animal does not exhibit a behavioral act without a reason, although the reason may not be obvious to humans. For any behavior to occur, there must be a **stimulus**, some internal or external change that exceeds a threshold and causes stimulation of the nervous and/or endocrine systems. This receptor and cellular stimulation and integration of information requires a number of chemical messengers in the animal's body, including epinephrine, acetylcholine, dopamine, serotonin, and many others. Some problem behaviors are caused by increased or decreased amounts of these neurotransmitters. This has led to the development of veterinary psychopharmacology.

The study of animal behavior is referred to as **ethology**. Most ethologists agree that animal behavior is genetically programmed (instinctive) and learned (conditioned response). There are two general categories of conditioned responses, classical conditioning and operant conditioning. Classical conditioning refers to the association of stimuli that occur at approximately the same time or in roughly the same area. **Operant conditioning** refers to the association of a particular activity (the operant) with a **punishment** or reward.

The pattern of behaviors that bonds animals to their caretakers occurs in early life and is referred to as **imprinting**. In wild animals, this is the process that allows a newborn animal to recognize and follow its parents. In domestic animals, the imprinting process usually involves other animals and humans that the animal encounters during a specific period in early life. The most important period for behavior development in dogs and cats is from 3 to 12 weeks. At this young age, the animal learns about its environment, how to interact with others, and what not to fear. What occurs during this habituation or socialization period can affect the animal for the rest of its life. For example, animals that are not socialized during this period can develop lifelong phobias (Fig. 6-30).

Animals also must learn how to interact with one another. Many households have more than one dog or cat and often have both. Introducing young animals is usually easier than introducing adults. Being social animals, dogs have a hierarchy, or pecking order, that determines which one gets first access to coveted resources such as food, toys, owners, and resting spots (Fig. 6-31). These relationships can fluctuate and are not to be confused with the more structured hierarchy relationships among nondomestic species, such as wolves.

Operant conditioning can be used to reinforce a desired behavior or punish an undesirable one, although the latter is not recommended. Positive **reinforcement** refers to any immediate pleasant occurrence that follows a behavior. For example, if a dog receives a treat or immediate praise when it sits on command, that behavior is reinforced with a pleasant experience. Negative reinforcement refers to any immediate unpleasant occurrence used to create a desired behavior. An example of negative reinforcement is the use of an electric

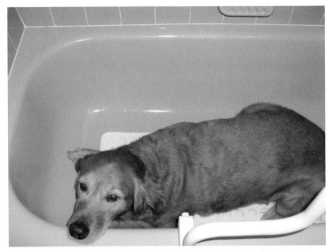

FIGURE 6-30 This dog was frightened by thunder when it was 10 weeks old and became afraid of thunder and then loud noises for the next 14 years. For years, it exhibited destructive behavior trying to escape the noise. The dog finally found refuge in the bathtub. (From Sirois M: Principles and practice of veterinary technology, ed 3, St Louis, 2011, Mosby.)

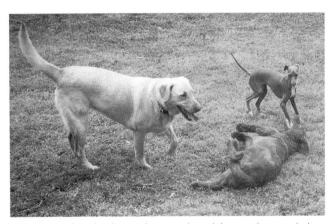

FIGURE 6-31 The dog on the ground is exhibiting submissive behavior to its sibling. It is important for owners to recognize and respect the canine hierarchy in the home, or interdog aggression may result. (From Beaver BV: Canine behavior: Insights and answers, ed 2, St Louis, 2009, Saunders.)

fence to help a dog learn the boundaries that it may navigate. This differs from punishment in that punishment is used to remove or decrease a behavior. For example, depending on how they are used, shock collars and citronella collars designed to reduce barking behaviors are forms of positive punishment (Fig. 6-32). Positive punishment involves adding an undesirable occurrence to decrease a behavior. Negative punishment involves removing a desirable occurrence to decrease a behavior. Withholding affection when a dog jumps up to greet you or not giving a treat when a dog is begging are examples of negative punishment. It is more difficult to use punishment to influence a dog's behavior and it may cause the dog to become fearful or aggressive. Many trainers and behaviorists use a combination of positive reinforcement and negative punishment.

Although veterinary professionals have little effect on genetics, other than to recommend that an animal not be bred or

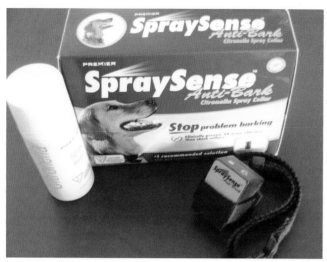

FIGURE 6-32 Citronella collars may be used to reduce barking behavior in dogs. (From Sirois M: Principles and practice of veterinary technology, ed 3, St Louis, 2011, Mosby.)

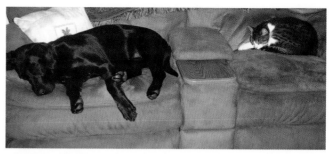

FIGURE 6-33 Owners need to decide whether a particular behavior is a problem, because the animal rarely recognizes it as such. For example, barking may be a desirable behavior for one owner, but a problem for another. (From Sirois M: Principles and practice of veterinary technology, ed 3, St Louis, 2011, Mosby.)

help a client choose a specific breed to adopt, they play an important role by educating clients about the correct way to raise and interact with their pets. It is important to remember that disease also plays a role in animal behavior problems, such as hypothyroidism in dogs, hyperthyroidism in cats, and cognitive dysfunction in older animals. Sometimes, **aggression** or even house soiling may be caused by a medical problem.

PREVENTING BEHAVIOR PROBLEMS IN COMPANION ANIMALS

Experts agree that behavior problems are common and a leading cause of death in dogs and cats. Often, the so-called problem is normal dog and cat behavior that the owner finds inappropriate and then makes worse when attempting to correct it (Fig. 6-33). This may start at an animal's young age with house training and continue with attention-seeking behaviors, destruction, barking, and aggression. Often, the pet owner does not know where to go for advice, and it is here that the veterinary staff can provide an important service to its clients and their pets.

Most behavior problems are easier to prevent than to correct. Aggression is the most common problem for which owners seek guidance, but many pet owners are annoyed when their animals damage household belongings and exhibit house-soiling behavior. Techniques based on scientifically valid ethologic and learning principles minimize such behaviors. However, much of the information to which owners have easy access does not always meet these criteria. Thus, the veterinary practice staff members are important sources of scientifically accurate information about preventing behavior problems.

Although many clients consider their pets to be part of the family, it is especially important that clients be provided with basic information on animal behavior to avoid the unrealistic expectations that develop when clients anthropomorphize their pets. **Anthropomorphism** refers to the attribution of human characteristics and emotions to animals. Pet owners often misinterpret their pet's behavior as spite, jealousy,

or guilt when the pet is in fact reacting based on learned behaviors. For example, a pet that an owner describes as looking guilty when the owner returns home to discover a house training accident is more likely to be exhibiting fear as a result of learning that the owner becomes angry in the presence of house soiling, not that the pet caused the anger by having an accident.

HOUSE TRAINING

House training is one of the most important and first behaviors that young pets are expected to learn. Many owners use outdated methods to attempt to house train their pets. These methods often interfere with success or damage the relationship with the pet. Problems related to house training may result in the animal being turned loose, isolated in a yard or tied, or relinquished to a shelter. Dogs and cats can be encouraged to eliminate reliably in locations that are acceptable to their human owners. Cats, dogs, pigs, ferrets, and rabbits can learn to use litter boxes. Other species of domestic companion animals are caged or kept outside because their **elimination** behavior is not restricted to specific locations.

DOGS

Humans have probably been training dogs not to eliminate in the house for almost as long as dogs have been domesticated. You might assume that thousands of years of practice have resulted in good house training techniques. Surprisingly, this is not always the case.

House training requires that the dog be taken out frequently, especially when it wakes up, after it eats, and whenever it appears to be sniffing around the house. When a puppy cannot be monitored, it should be confined to a crate (Fig. 6-34). Most accidents occur when the puppy is left alone. There are different types of crates, including collapsible ones and those made of wire, plastic, and wood. Crate training is also useful for preventing destructive behaviors such as chewing. The use of the crate should not be excessive because 8-week-old puppies cannot hold their bowels longer than 4 to 6 hours. Puppies will soil in the crate if they cannot get out when they need to eliminate or if the crate is too large. Crates can be purchased for the pet's adult size and many now come with partitions to subdivide it when the puppy is small.

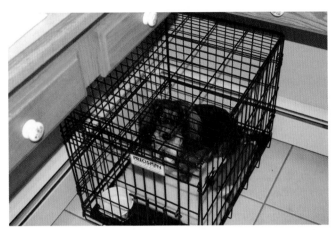

FIGURE 6-34 The crate is a useful tool to manage a puppy when it cannot be supervised in the home. This helps with house training as well as preventing destructive behavior. (From Sirois M: Principles and practice of veterinary technology, ed 3, St Louis, 2011, Mosby. Courtesy Donna Harris.)

> ### CRITICAL CONCEPT
> Help clients select a crate that is easy to clean and will be the correct size for the puppy when it is an adult.

Owners must be made aware of several important points when house training their dog. First, a dog's confinement to a crate must not exceed the time that the animal can control its bladder and bowels. For young puppies, this can be as little as 1 hour or sometimes as long as 2 or 3 hours at a time. In addition, many puppies need to eliminate at least once during the night.

Second, the dog must be actively taught, by reinforcing correct behavior, the desired location for elimination. Owners should reward elimination outside with verbal praise and petting, and possibly a special tidbit. The timing of this reward, however, is critical. Research in animal learning suggests that a delay of longer than 0.5 second between the behavior and subsequent reinforcement significantly decreases the effectiveness of the reinforcement. For example, if the owner waits by the door to reinforce the puppy at the door as it returns from eliminating in the yard, the behavior that has been reinforced is coming to the door. In these cases, owners often complain that all the puppy does when taken out is to attempt to go back in or to stand by the door. This should come as no surprise because going to the door is what the puppy has inadvertently been rewarded for doing. To reinforce the elimination behavior, the owner must go outside with the puppy and provide reinforcement immediately following elimination at the location where it occurs. Clicker training may also be useful for house training of puppies (Box 6-1).

Finally, use of physical punishment in regard to house training is never appropriate. Interactive punishment that involves the owner, even if delivered at the time of house soiling, may cause the dog to become reluctant to eliminate in the owner's presence at other times or may even result in the dog

| **BOX 6-1** | House Training Puppies: Clicker Method |

1. Use a collar and leash to take the puppy outside.
2. Go to the same spot in the yard each time.
3. Cue the puppy to "go potty."
4. Click and treat the puppy as the puppy passes urine or stool.

From Sirois M: Principles and practice of veterinary technology, ed 3, St Louis, 2011, Mosby.

becoming afraid of the owner. This interferes with the owner's attempts to appropriately reinforce elimination outside. Calmly saying "oops" or calling the puppy should be sufficient to interrupt the behavior temporarily. The dog can then be taken outside in a positive, nonthreatening manner and rewarded if it eliminates. The sound of aluminum cans containing pennies or other loud noises, even when not associated with humans, can startle the puppy and further inhibit learning.

In an ideal house training program, the dog's environment and behavior should be so well managed that correct behavior is reinforced with 100% consistency and opportunities for inappropriate behavior never occur. In reality, this ideal is seldom met, but if owners are made aware of it through your educational efforts, it may give them a much more accurate perspective on the time and effort required for house training.

Educating owners about house training dogs should be more detailed than simply telling the owner to get a crate and put the dog in it when the owner can't watch it. Handouts about this important process should also be provided.

CATS

One of the reasons people choose cats as pets instead of dogs is because they can be readily trained to use a litter box for elimination and do not need to be walked. The process of encouraging cats to use litter boxes consistently is based on different developmental events than house training dogs. It is normal instinctual behavior for kittens and cats to use a **substrate** for elimination. Kittens do not need to observe the **queen** eliminating or have the owner demonstrate part of the process by raking the cat's paws in the litter. Providing a clean, easily accessible litter box with an acceptable substrate is sufficient. However, the accessibility of the litter box and suitability of the substrate must be examined from the kitten's or cat's perspective. The major complaint of cat owners is that their cats stop or inconsistently use the litter box and choose to eliminate somewhere else in the house. If this problem is not corrected, these cats may be confined to the outdoors or relinquished to shelters. Because there are many reasons for a cat to stop using its litter box, a detailed history is needed to determine the cause.

Because kittens are physically and behaviorally immature, a litter box should be within easy access at all times. This may mean providing several litter boxes at strategic locations in the house or initially limiting the cat's access to only portions of the house. The litter box should be easily accessible but also should afford some privacy. High-traffic areas are not a good choice, but neither is locating the box in a basement with a cold cement floor. Proximity to appliances that make unexpected startling noises, such as the washer, furnace, or hot water heater, should also be avoided.

Studies have found that cats prefer the softer texture of fine-grained substrates. Thus, a cat is less likely to develop an aversion to a clumping litter composed of very small particles. However, cats develop idiosyncratic preferences for substrates and locations for elimination for reasons that are not well understood. These changing preferences are often the basis of many inappropriate elimination problems in cats. Sometimes, these preferences can be influenced by the condition of the litter material. Cats may avoid litter that is consistently dirty, too deep, or scented (Fig. 6-35). One study found that cats with elimination problems were more likely to be using scented than unscented litter as compared with cats without these problems.

Owners are sometimes under the impression that the more litter they put in the box, the less often they need to clean it. General guidelines are to keep the litter depth at no more than 2 inches, remove feces and urine clumps daily, change the litter frequently enough to prevent odors from developing, and ensure that most of the litter is always dry. **Veterinary behaviorists** recommend that the litter box be changed once a week. Changing the litter should include disposing of dirty litter and washing the box with warm soapy water.

CRITICAL CONCEPT

Covered litter boxes may appeal to owners but from a cat's point of view it is difficult to see who may be lurking outside. When collecting a history on an inappropriate elimination case, always ask for the type and location of litter box in addition to the substrate.

Another consideration influencing the cat's perception of litter box accessibility is the presence of other cats in the household. A litter box may be temporarily unavailable

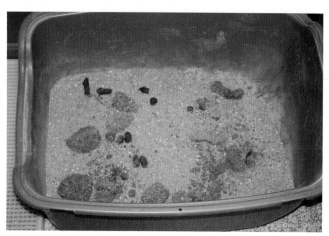

FIGURE 6-35 Cats are fastidious, and one reason they stop using a litter box is that it is too dirty for them. Litter boxes should be cleaned daily, and there should be one litter box per cat in the household, plus one. (From Sirois M: Principles and practice of veterinary technology, ed 3, St Louis, 2011, Mosby.)

because another cat is using it or guarding it. Thus, advise owners to provide one litter box per cat, plus one extra, and to keep the boxes in different locations so that a single cat cannot block another cat's access to the litter box area. In addition, the litter box location should allow the cat using it to be aware of the presence of other cats to prevent any surprise attacks that might occur during elimination. The owner must also understand that if the cat learns to associate the litter box with punishment, such as being caught and having medication administered, it may stop using it. Box 6-2 provides a checklist of important issues related to litter boxes.

PREVENTING DESTRUCTIVE BEHAVIOR BY CATS

Probably more owners recognize the need to provide their cats with litter boxes than to provide scratching posts. Because cats scratch for a variety of reasons, cats may want to scratch in different locations for different reasons. One of the most important motivations for cats scratching objects with their front claws is territorial marking. Scratching leaves a visual as well as an olfactory mark that serves as an indication of the cat's presence. In addition to marking, scratching also serves to stretch the muscles and tendons of the legs and remove the worn outer sheaths from the claws. It may also be used as a greeting or play behavior.

Scratching objects should be provided in locations in which the behavior is likely to be triggered. Even if the cat scratches objects when allowed outdoors, it still should have access to an acceptable object indoors. Merely providing a scratching object does not guarantee the cat will use it preferentially to carpet, drapes, or furniture. The scratching objects must match the cat's preferences for desirable locations and with regard to height, orientation, and texture (Fig. 6-36).

If a new cat is encouraged to use its own scratching post, it may avoid exercising its claws on furniture or drapes. Owners must understand that they should discourage cats from clawing their possessions. They can do this by distracting the cat caught in the act or preventing its access to the items. Many clients merely resort to having the cat declawed as a preventive measure or solution to the problem behavior. Veterinary staff members are in the best position to educate owner about all the options surrounding nail care and scratching behavior.

BOX 6-2 | Checklist for Litter Boxes

1. Place the box in a quiet location.
2. Make sure that the location is accessible from the cat's perspective.
3. Use fine-grained unscented litter.
4. The litter depth should be approximately 2 inches.
5. Scoop daily, empty, and wash the litter box once a week.

From Sirois M: Principles and practice of veterinary technology, ed 3, St Louis, 2011, Mosby.

SCRATCHING POSTS. Many scratching posts available commercially do not permit the cat to reach vertically to its full height to scratch, as many cats like to do (Fig. 6-37). Also, they are not sturdy enough to support the cat's weight and readily fall over, frightening the cat. For larger cats using relatively short posts, this means that they are scratching almost with their abdomen on the floor. It may be a good idea to talk to owners about the desirability of taller or even floor to ceiling scratching poles. If the back of the sofa allows the cat to reach to its full height to scratch but the scratching post does not, it is easy to guess which surface the cat will prefer.

ORIENTATION. Not all cats scratch vertically all of the time. Some cats may prefer to stretch their legs out in front and rake backward in a horizontal motion. If this is the case, the cat may be more likely to use a flat horizontal object (Fig. 6-38) than a vertical post. Some cats may use both, depending on where, when, and why they scratch. One unusual cat was reported only to scratch upside down by pulling herself along on her back as she scratched the underside of the sofa.

TEXTURE. This may be the most frequently overlooked aspect of providing an acceptable scratching object. As with other aspects of the behavioral pattern of scratching, cats vary in the textures that they prefer. Cats that like to rake their claws in long vertical motions may be more likely to use an object with a texture that permits this. If the cat scratches vertically and the texture is not conducive to those motions, the cat may not use the object. Other cats use more of a picking motion and may prefer items covered with sisal, wrapped horizontally. It has been proposed that an object that has been scratched repeatedly, with the result that the covering is somewhat shredded and holds the cat's scent, will be preferred over a new, unused object. This suggests that owners should not replace well-worn scratching posts, even if they appear unsightly.

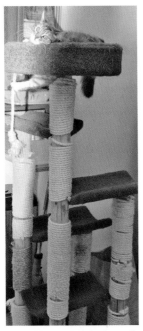

FIGURE 6-36 Cats normally exercise their claws, and it important to provide them with scratching posts that are large and sturdy enough to support their weight. The scratching posts must also be located in appropriate places in the home. (From Sirois M: Principles and practice of veterinary technology, ed 3, St Louis, 2011, Mosby. Courtesy Donna Harris.)

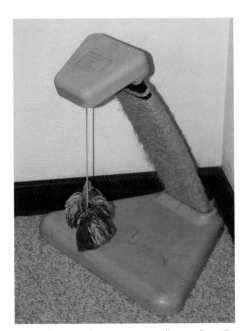

FIGURE 6-37 This scratching post is not tall enough to allow the cat to stretch to its full height while using it. This may result in the cat finding more suitable objects to use, such as the sofa or the curtains. (From Sirois M: Principles and practice of veterinary technology, ed 3, St Louis, 2011, Mosby. Courtesy Donna Harris.)

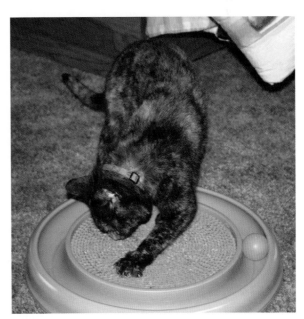

FIGURE 6-38 Horizontal scratching objects such as this pad scented with catnip may be preferred over vertical objects. (From Sirois M: Principles and practice of veterinary technology, ed 3, St Louis, 2011, Mosby. Courtesy Donna Harris.)

The scratching object should be placed in a location where the cat is likely to be motivated to scratch, or adjacent to an unacceptable item that the cat is already using. To encourage the cat to use the desirable object, it can be scented with catnip or a commercial **pheromone** (Feliway, CEVA Animal Health, St Louis), or a toy can be attached to the top to entice the cat to reach high up the post. Raking the cat's feet up and down the post is not necessary and may actually have adverse effects. The most reliable way to discourage scratching of inappropriate objects is to first provide an appropriate substitute and then change the texture of the off-limit items. Owners can change the texture by covering it with plastic, sandpaper, or another covering with an unpleasant (from the cat's perspective) texture.

BY DOGS

Destructive behavior is a classification of behavior based more on the owner's view of the result (destruction) than on the actual behavior that caused it. Digging, chewing, tearing, scratching, moving objects from one place to another, and removing the contents from the trash are all considered destructive behavior and are self-rewarding.

Dogs show these behaviors for a variety of reasons. Destructive behavior that is the symptomatic manifestation of other problems, such as separation anxiety or noise phobias, can be treated but may not be prevented. In these cases, the underlying problem must be resolved, rather than trying to treat the symptom. However, destructive behavior that occurs as the result of a normal developmental process, such as teething, play, and investigative behavior, can often be prevented or at least minimized.

Dogs vary in their need for physical activity and play. Some dogs are content to lead relatively inactive lives, whereas others seem to be on the move constantly. Just as with cats' scratching, the goal in minimizing problem destructive behavior resulting from teething, play, and investigative behavior is not to eliminate the behavior but to direct it toward acceptable objects by making acceptable toys more attractive than household items. This must be done on a consistent basis or some items may be destroyed.

APPEALING TOYS. Dogs should be exposed to suitable toys when they are young. The attractiveness of acceptable toys can be maximized by first rewarding the dog every time it plays with them. Toys should also elicit the play patterns that the dog is likely to exhibit. For example, dogs that like to shake toys may be more satisfied with one made of lambskin than with a tennis ball. Toys should be available for chewing and tearing, as well as for carrying and chasing, if the dog displays both patterns of play behavior. It may be helpful to establish a toy rotation so that different toys are available each day to make them more appealing.

If the dog is caught chewing an unacceptable item, the item should be taken away and replaced with one that is acceptable (Figs. 6-39 and 6-40). To decrease the dog's interest in household items, even when the owner is not present, attempts can be made to lessen their appeal. Commercial products such as Bitter Apple (Grannick's Pharmacy, Greenwich, CT) are available to give objects a bad taste. Motion detectors or a Snappy Trainer (modified mousetrap that does not harm the animal) can discourage animals from bothering specific items or areas, or items can be booby-trapped in other creative ways. Remind owners of the advisability of dog-proofing the house just as they would for a young child.

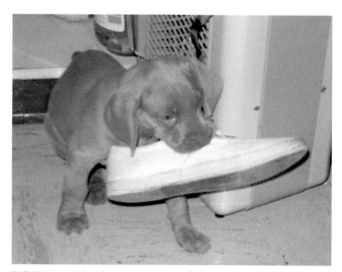

FIGURE 6-39 Chewing is normal dog behavior and needs to be directed to acceptable objects. Owners should remove their things from the dog's mouth and replace them with the dog's own toys. A dog cannot tell the difference between an old shoe and a new one. (From Beaver BV: Canine behavior: Insights and answers, ed 2, St Louis, 2009, Saunders.)

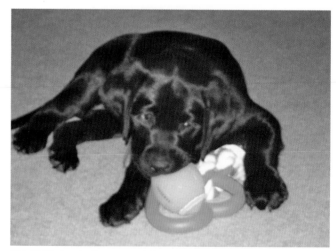

FIGURE 6-40 This puppy did not even notice that a different item had been placed in its mouth. It is best to introduce puppies to suitable toys when they are young and encourage them to play with the toys. (From Sirois M: Principles and practice of veterinary technology, ed 3, St Louis, 2011, Mosby.)

Dogs that insist on digging outside can be provided with their own area in which to do so. This area should consist of loose soil or sand to facilitate digging. Owners can bury enticing items shallowly in this area to attract the dog.

PREVENTING AGGRESSIVE BEHAVIOR PROBLEMS

Aggression is the most common type of behavior problem reported in dogs and occurs in cats as well. Aggressive behavior is normal behavior for most species of animals, including companion animals. Aggression, defined as behavior that is intended to harm another individual, is an aspect of **agonistic** behavior. Agonistic behaviors are behaviors that animals show in situations involving social conflict. Submission, avoidance, escaping, offensive and defensive threats, and offensive and defensive aggression are all part of the agonistic behavior system. There are many different types of aggression displayed by dogs and cats (Table 6-2). Aggression may be directed against people, family members or strangers, children, or other dogs and species. Different types of aggression include fearful, territorial, maternal, intermale, interfemale, predatory, play-related, and redirected aggression. It is important to determine which type is present so it can be treated. The most common complaint from dog owners is aggression toward people, whereas the most common complaint from cat owners is aggression toward other cats. Because the factors that determine when and where an animal will display aggressive or threatening behavior are not fully understood, it is unlikely that preventing problems will be a simple process. In some cases, owners inadvertently reinforce aggressive behavior by withdrawing from the pet when it acts aggressively.

Aggression directed at children is considered the primary public health problem in children. The statistical group reporting the highest number of bites is young boys, 5 to 9 years of age. More than 50% of children have sustained a bite injury before the age of 18. Dogs must be socialized to children when they are young, and children must be taught how to behave around dogs, particularly strange ones. Parents also often worry about dog aggression toward infants. It is important to advise new parents about how to introduce their new baby to their dog.

> **CRITICAL CONCEPT**
> Aggression is the most common type of behavior problem reported in dogs.

PUPPY TESTS

One way to prevent aggression problems in animals is to select pets that are unlikely to develop such problems. Popular literature describes of a variety of puppy tests that supposedly predict a puppy's likelihood for dominant behavior or aggression problems as an adult. This information can be used to suggest behavioral tendencies and match puppies and new owners. Current research suggests that temperament testing may be too subjective to aid in matching puppies with owners reliably. When selecting a new pet, it is more advisable to match activity and lifestyle. An active puppy living in a small apartment with a sedentary family is more likely to develop behavior problems than a puppy with an active family who receives daily exercise.

CASTRATION

Castrating male animals clearly reduces some forms of aggressive behavior in many species, including dogs, cats, and horses. Postpubertal castration seems to be as effective as prepubertal castration. Reports on dog bite statistics show that intact male dogs are more often involved in dog bites (70% to 76% of dog bite incidents reported). The gender of dogs in unreported dog bite incidents is not known. Therefore, selection of female animals as pets may reduce problems with aggressive behavior. All male dogs should be castrated unless they are purebreds that are to be used in a breeding program. In addition to aggression, castration prevents other potential problems such as roaming, urine marking, and prostate problems.

SOCIALIZATION

Many species of mammals and birds have sensitive periods of development of normal species-typical social behavior. This sensitive period has been well studied in dogs and to a lesser degree in cats and horses. The sensitive **socialization** period usually occurs fairly early in life. For example, in dogs, it is from 3 to 12 weeks of age and, in cats, from 2 to 7 weeks.

Companion animals must have a variety of pleasant experiences with different types of people, other animals, and environments during these sensitive periods so that they are able to accept humans as their social peers later in life. Poorly socialized animals are typically fearful of people or may attach strongly to one or two individuals

TABLE 6-2	Common Type of Aggressive Behavior in Dogs and Cats	
TYPE OF AGGRESSION	**COMMENTS**
Conflict related	Result of unpredictable environment or inconsistent or inappropriate use of punishment
Fear induced	Fearful situations (e.g., noises, being in the veterinary office)
Predatory	Instinctual stalking and pouncing with no warning growl
Pain induced	Protective instinct
Intermale	Natural instinct usually eliminated by castration
Territorial	Dogs—usually directed toward humans that are not members of their household Cats—usually directed toward other cats
Maternal	Normal protective instinct

From Sirois M: Principles and practice of veterinary technology, ed 3, St Louis, 2011, Mosby.

but are unable to generalize this acceptance to unfamiliar individuals. It is also important to habituate the puppy and kitten to a variety of environmental situations (Fig. 6-41). Fear of people or specific situations can sometimes develop into defensive aggression problems (Fig. 6-42). Because many young animals are seen in the veterinary

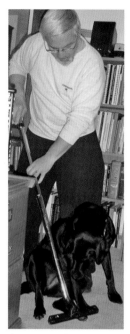

FIGURE 6-41 This dog was well socialized to loud noises during the sensitive socialization period and shows no fear of the vacuum cleaner. (From Sirois M: Principles and practice of veterinary technology, ed 3, St Louis, 2011, Mosby.)

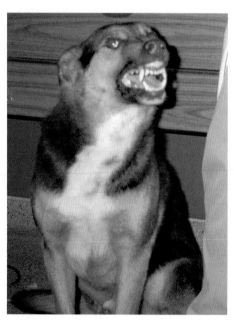

FIGURE 6-42 Aggression is a common owner complaint. Sometimes the aggression occurs only in the veterinary hospital and is related to fear. Veterinary health professionals should strive to prevent this from occurring and attempt to find ways to alleviate this behavior in hospitalized animals. (From Beaver BV: Canine behavior: Insights and answers, ed 2, St Louis, 2009, Saunders.)

hospital, it is important that these experiences be pleasant to avoid fear and aggression problems. Veterinary staff members should encourage dog owners to enroll puppies in puppy classes and expose puppies and kittens to a variety of gentle handling and play sessions with people outside the family.

> **CRITICAL CONCEPT**
>
> Training and educational materials on running puppy or kitten kindergarten classes are widely available.

PROVIDING SERVICES FOR PROBLEMS

PROBLEM PREVENTION

Knowing what to tell clients to prevent problems is a separate issue from finding sufficient time to do so. It may not be realistic to expect the veterinary professional to address these issues during a 15-minute office visit when the time is allocated to addressing the presenting medical concern, or in a brief telephone call while greeting clients at the front desk or searching for a client record. Veterinarians and staff members must purposely decide how the valuable information regarding problem prevention can be disseminated. One obvious way is to make it a policy to schedule extra time for appointments involving new animal examination and to charge accordingly. These are often new puppy and kitten appointments, but not always. The fee structure for new animal appointments can include an extra 15 to 20 minutes of staff time, even if the problem prevention discussion takes place separately from the medication examination and vaccination time. Talking to clients about these issues is preferable to relying on videos and written materials alone. However, written materials can be of value because they reinforce what was said and allow clients to read them as often as needed, and at their convenience. It can also be argued that the expenses for the time required for problem prevention, even if not charged directly as a fee, may be recouped indirectly. Problem prevention sessions can improve the chances that the animal will remain in the home and thus continue being a patient. Also, the owner's perception of the clinic is enhanced, making word of mouth referral of new clients more likely.

PROBLEM RESOLUTION

Problem resolution is almost always a more complex process than problem prevention. It requires first arriving at a behavioral diagnosis for the type of problem. The presenting complaint, whether excessive barking, house soiling, or aggression, can be thought of as behavioral signs similar to medical signs, such as vomiting, limping, or a poor hair coat. Each of these signs might be related to a variety of problems. In the case of behavior problems, medical conditions that could account for the behavioral signs should be evaluated first. This is especially important with aggression and house soiling. Once this is done, arriving at a behavioral diagnosis requires obtaining a complete behavioral history and, ideally, observing the animal and its environment.

For some types of problems, such as feline elimination problems, seeing the animal in its home environment may make it possible to identify physical features of the environment that are contributing to the problem. Behavioral diagnosis sometimes requires several hours to interview the owner and observe the animal. In some cases, the owner may need to return home and maintain a log or even videotape the behavior.

Once the type of problem has been narrowed down to one or more possibilities, a behavior modification plan must be devised. The type of problem dictates the specific procedures used. A variety of methods are used to treat behavior problems (Table 6-3). Time is required to explain these procedures to the owner, provide written handouts, demonstrate them if necessary, and have the owner practice them, if appropriate. Keep in mind that severe behavior disorders that involve aggression or intense fear often require referral to a behavior specialist. Once treatment begins, the case must be followed up with additional in-home or clinic visits or regularly scheduled telephone calls. These follow-up contacts may be relatively brief, sometimes less than 15 minutes, or longer in more complex cases.

A number of pharmacologic agents are used to treat animal behavior problems such as aggression, house soiling, and various phobias. Medications used to treat behavioral problems may be U.S. Food and Drug Administration (FDA)–approved or have an off-label use (Fig. 6-43). Often, the purpose of drug therapy is to relieve symptoms and allow the patient to learn new behaviors. There are many different human tranquilizers and antianxiety drugs that have shown promise as adjuncts for treating problem behaviors. A variety of nutritional and herbal remedies also have been used for certain behavioral problems (Fig. 6-44). Clients must be aware of the limitations of these products in behavioral therapy, including the fact that the problem may return when the drug therapy is stopped, the dosages may need to be adjusted to obtain the desired effect, and

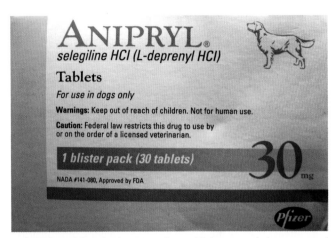

FIGURE 6-43 Selegiline (Anipryl) is an FDA-approved pharmaceutical product used to treat behavioral changes related to canine cognitive dysfunction. (From Sirois M: Principles and practice of veterinary technology, ed 3, St Louis, 2011, Mosby.)

TABLE 6-3	Types of Behavioral Modification Programs	
METHOD	**DESCRIPTION**	**EXAMPLE(S) AND POSSIBLE USES**
Command-response-reward	Involves giving a command and immediately rewarding the desired response every time it is performed	Giving the command to sit and providing praise and/or treats as soon as the pet sits
Clicker training	Use of a sound to signal to the animal that it performed the right behavior and will receive a reward	Clicking when a puppy eliminates outside and immediately giving a treat
Extinction	Elimination of a problem behavior by completely removing the reinforcement for the behavior	Not providing food when a pet is begging
Aversion therapy	Associating an unpleasant stimulus with an object	Spraying an object with something that has a foul odor or taste to keep a pet from chewing it
Avoidance therapy	Associating an unpleasant stimulus with a behavior	Using a citronella collar to minimize barking behavior
Habituation	Involves surrounding the animal with the stimulus at low levels until the animal becomes acclimated to the stimulus and is no longer afraid of it	Playing recordings of thunderstorms or vacuum cleaners to a litter of puppies so that they become accustomed to the sound
Counterconditioning	Replacing an undesirable behavior with a desirable one	Using rewards to teach a pet to pull a bell on a string rather than scratching at the door to be let inside
Desensitization	Often used in combination with counterconditioning; involves diminishing a particular behavior by gradually exposing the animal to the stimulus that produces the inappropriate response	Exposing a pet that is afraid of children to children using longer periods of time and decreasing distance
Environmental modification	Changing one or more environmental parameters	Placing pet in crate when unsupervised; changing the location of a litter box
Surgery	Anatomic alteration	Castration of male pets to decrease aggressiveness and territorial urine marking
Medication	Sedatives, hormonal agents, herbal remedies	Canine cognitive dysfunction; as an adjunct to other behavioral therapies in aggressive or extremely fearful animals

From Sirois M: Principles and practice of veterinary technology, ed 3, St Louis, 2011, Mosby.

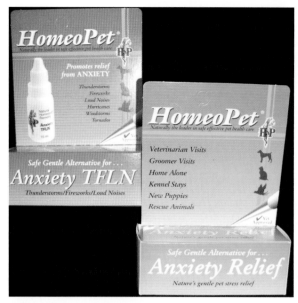

FIGURE 6-44 Various homeopathic remedies may be used to calm an animal experiencing shock, trauma, or panic. (From Sirois M: Principles and practice of veterinary technology, ed 3, St Louis, 2011, Mosby.)

side effects may occur. Some form of behavior modification is needed to accompany drug therapy to increase the chances of a successful resolution of the problem. The ultimate goal is to wean the animal from the drug(s) and correct the problem.

The process of problem resolution cannot be collapsed into a simple solution. An oversimplified approach to problem solving trivializes the importance of the problem and omits the scientific knowledge required to modify behavior successfully. Because veterinary staff members often have the opportunity to solve behavior problems but may not have the time or expertise to do so, it is important to be aware of the veterinary practice's policies regarding referrals and become proficient in referring cases to behavior specialists.

REFERRING CASES TO BEHAVIOR SPECIALISTS

Before referral of an animal to a behavior specialist, evaluate medical conditions that could contribute to the problem behavior. Behavior referrals should be based on the same model of professionalism as medical case referrals (Box 6-3). This includes determining the qualifications of the referral resource, learning the preferred method of referral, facilitating contact between client and specialist, and informing the client about what type of services to expect from the referral.

EVALUATING REFERRAL RESOURCES

Many types of professionals offer to assist pet owners with animal behavior problems. These can range from self-taught dog trainers to academically trained, degreed, and certified behavior specialists. Veterinarians who meet the established criteria may become board certified by the American College of Veterinary Behavior and are considered to be vet-

Treat behavior cases just like a surgical or medical case. Include the following:
1. Physical examination
2. CBC, profile, urinalysis, and fecal results
3. Past and current medical history

From Sirois M: Principles and practice of veterinary technology, ed 3, St Louis, 2011, Mosby.

erinary behavior specialists. The Animal Behavior Society, the largest organization in North America dedicated to the study of animal behavior, offers two levels of certification to individuals holding a master's or doctoral degree in the behavioral sciences and who meet educational, experiential, and ethical criteria. Although veterinary behaviorists can be board certified and applied behaviorists can be certified by the Animal Behavior Society, anyone, regardless of academic training, can legally use the professional title of animal behaviorist.

The National Association of Dog Obedience Instructors (NADOI) and the Association of Pet Dog Trainers (APDT) are two professional organizations that dog trainers can join. NADOI membership is open only to trainers who meet the organization's qualifications. APDT, which recently developed its own certification program, encourages and promotes the use of positive reinforcement in training, but its membership is open to anyone who trains dogs.

It is the referring professional's responsibility to evaluate the credentials, knowledge, competence, and philosophy of individuals considered as potential referral resources for the clinic. This is because certification does not guarantee competence, and professionally trained and other qualified people may not be certified. The evaluation may include interviewing these individuals and also observing their classes and/or behavior consulting sessions. Gathering information about these individuals from others who offer behavioral assistance can be a valuable service that the assistant can perform for the clinic.

When choosing a referral resource for behavior cases, be aware that obedience or command training does not resolve behavior problems. Teaching a dog sit, down, and/or stay does not address aggression, separation anxiety problems, house-soiling problems, or other types of problems unrelated to obedience performance. However, training classes can be a useful tool in helping dog owners establish a more consistent relationship with their dogs. You may want to identify referral resources for dog training classes and for behavior counseling for whatever species of animal for which the clinic provides medical care. You may need to select several individuals. Certified behavior specialists consult only on those species with which they have experience. Thus, a behaviorist may work with cats and dogs but not birds or horses. Every veterinary hospital should refer all their puppy owners to an educated trainer. Some practices offer training classes in the hospitals, which may even be taught by staff members.

MAKING THE REFERRAL

Handle behavior referral cases as you would medical referrals. When referring a client to a veterinary medical specialist, such as a cardiologist or oncologist, a veterinary professional probably would not instruct the client to call the specialist for tips or advice. Unfortunately, all too often this is how clients are referred to behavior specialists. Find out whether the behavior specialist prefers the initial contact to be from the client or veterinary medical professional. If contact from the veterinary professional is preferred, be prepared to provide a pertinent medical and behavioral history during the initial conversation.

Give the client a reasonable set of expectations about the referral. Discuss information about the fee structure, where the consultation will take place, how to schedule the appointment, and how much time will be required. You can also encourage the client to seek behavioral help without giving false expectations. Although most animal behavior problems can benefit from professional assistance, not all problems can be completely and permanently resolved.

Dealing with behavior referrals in a professional manner may help clients to view the behavior consulting process as a legitimate aspect of health care and overcome some of their embarrassment about seeking psychological help for their pets. It may also help them to understand better why behavior specialists charge fees for professional services, just as veterinarians do. The veterinary clinic can facilitate referrals by having business cards, brochures, and other information about the behavior specialist available to give to clients at the clinic.

BEHAVIOR PROBLEMS IN EXOTIC ANIMALS

Avian and small mammal species are commonly seen in companion veterinary practice. The basic mechanisms for behavioral development are similar in these species to those described for dogs and cats. The sensitive periods for socialization vary considerably among different species. The most common problem behavior seen in pet birds and small mammals is biting. Often, this is aggression directed toward humans as a result of fear. Additional information on avian and exotic animal behavior can be found in Chapter 12.

RESTRAINT AND HANDLING OF DOGS

Most dogs brought to veterinary facilities are friendly and require minimal restraint. However, it is best to be cautious with every dog. All animals can become startled or anxious in a medical facility. The proper way to approach an unknown dog is to extend your hand palm down, with fingers bent slightly, allowing the dog to sniff the back of your hand. Watch the dog's reaction and avoid direct eye contact. A friendly dog's body will be relaxed, and the animal will actively sniff your hand, wag its tail, and eventually lose interest in the offered hand. You can then begin gently scratching below the dog's ear, advancing to its chest, neck, shoulders, and the top of its hips. At this point, a friendly dog trusts you enough to allow restraint holds.

A cardinal rule is never to have a client restrain his or her own animal. This is important for several reasons. First, clients usually do not know the restraint techniques necessary for various procedures. The second, more important reason is that the veterinarian is liable if the owner is bitten.

CANINE BODY LANGUAGE

Dogs exhibit a number of personalities that can be identified by their body language. This is important to note before attempting to restrain them. Most dogs are happy to be with people and enjoy interacting with others. The body language can be straightforward or somewhat submissive. They greet you with a wagging tail and a slightly lowered and cocked head and initiate affection. These dogs rarely bite but can retaliate if handled too harshly or cornered. A second common personality is the nervous or fearful dog. They exhibit a fearful expression by having their ears drawn down and back, showing white around the pupils of their eyes, not making any eye contact, and cowering. If cornered, they feel threatened and often bite. The last personality type is the aggressive dog. Aggressive dog body language is head lowered between the shoulders, a level stare, tail straight out (possibly wagging), and perhaps a grimace or growl. These dogs take offense at anyone's improper body language, such as a direct look into their eyes or a frontal approach. Aggressive dogs and nervous or fearful dogs should be handled with the knowledge that they will bite, and appropriate steps, such as a muzzle and sedation, should be considered before working with this type of dog. Figures 6-45 and 6-46 summarize common canine postures.

> **CRITICAL CONCEPT**
> Study the body language of every dog you meet to enable you to identify its personality at a glance.

DANGER POTENTIAL

A dog's main means of defense is retreat, but it will fight if cornered. Dogs are equipped with formidable teeth that are designed to crush and tear. Regardless of personality, if a dog is curling its lips, showing its teeth, growling, or raising its hackles, it is imperative to control its muzzle to avoid being bitten.

A lesser weapon is a dog's toenails. They rarely cause severe injuries but can inflict painful scratches that can become infected.

RESTRAINT DEVICES
MECHANICAL DEVICES

LEASH. The rope leash is a standard tool for restraining dogs. It can be made of a rolled or flat nylon rope with a

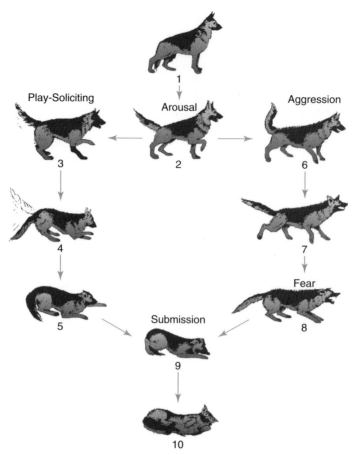

FIGURE 6-45 General body postures of dogs. Dog 1 shows a relaxed dog. Dog 2 is alert. Dog 3 shows playful behavior. Dogs 4 and 5 show increasing fear and submission. Dog 6 displays offensive aggression. Dog 7 shows mixed motivations of offensive and defensive aggression. Dog 8 shows defensive aggression. Dogs 9 and 10 show fear and/or submission. (From Millis D, Levine: Canine rehabilitation and physical therapy, ed 2, St Louis, 2014, Saunders.)

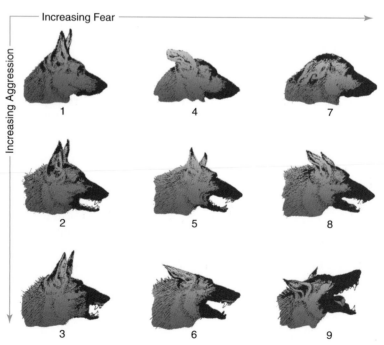

FIGURE 6-46 Facial postures of dogs. Figures from left to right show increasing fear. Figures from top to bottom show increasing aggressive motivation. Dog 1 is an alert dog. Dog 3 is offensively aggressive. Dog 7 is fearful and/or submissive. Dog 9 is defensively aggressive. All others are intermediate in fear and/or aggression (From Millis D, Levine: Canine rehabilitation and physical therapy, ed 2, St Louis, 2014, Saunders.)

handle at one end and a slip ring to form a sliding loop at the other. The loop is easy to keep open and can be flipped over the head and/or body of a dog to bring it out of a cage or run (Fig. 6-47). It is easy to remove by allowing the loop to loosen and the dog to slip its head out. It fits easily into a pocket and can be used on cats just as effectively as dogs.

GAUNTLET. **Gauntlets** are heavy leather gloves designed to protect the hands and forearms (Fig. 6-48). Even though they are made of thick leather, most dogs, cats, and birds can pinch or actually bite through them. However, the leather slows them down enough that you can usually escape the worst of it. One way to use them is to place one partially on your nondominant hand and hold it in front of the animal as a distraction. The animal will usually bite the empty fingers of the glove, allowing you to reach in and scruff or leash it with

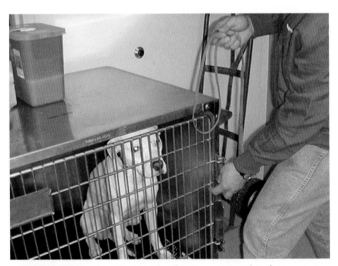

FIGURE 6-47 Using a rope leash to remove a dog from a cage. (From Sheldon CC, Sonsthagen T, Topel JA: Animal restraint for veterinary professionals, St Louis, 2006, Mosby.)

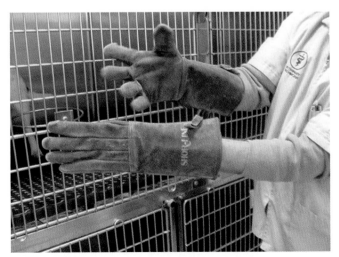

FIGURE 6-48 Gauntlets or restraint gloves. (From Sirois M: Principles and practice of veterinary technology, ed 3, St Louis, 2011, Mosby.)

the other hand. If you restrain an animal with the gloves on, take care not to exert too much pressure because the gloves reduce your sense of touch and strength. Once the animal is out of the kennel and placed on a table, another person can grasp the animal, or you can wrap your hand and arm around the animal's neck or head, get rid of a glove, or switch hands and get rid of the gloves. This allows you to restrain the animal with your bare hands. If this is not possible because the animal is too aggressive, keep the gloves on and monitor the animal to ensure it is not turning blue from the pressure that you are exerting.

MUZZLE. Many commercially manufactured **muzzles** are available and should be fitted to the dog by the owner. Before coming to the clinic, the client should muzzle an aggressive or nervous dog. A muzzle can also be made with a length of roll gauze, nylon sock, or length of rope (Procedure 6-1).

To remove the gauze muzzle, untie the bow knot and gently pull the ends back and forth and forward. Often, the dog will help with a paw. Be careful that the dog does not bite as the muzzle is removed; have people cleared out or have the head restrained carefully. Also, note that this muzzle is used only for short-term procedures because the dog cannot pant and will overheat if the muzzle is left on for extended periods. Keep scissors close by in case the muzzle must be cut off quickly.

CATCHPOLE. Many types of catchpoles are available commercially. A **catchpole** is used to move an aggressive or fearful dog to or from a run or cage. The rigid pole separates the restrainer and dog, and a quick-release handle is used to prevent strangulation. The loop at the end of the pole is placed around the dog's neck and tightened (Fig. 6-49). This allows the restrainer to move the dog in and out of a run or cage. Care should be taken not to choke the dog while ensuring that the loop is tight enough that the dog's head does not slip out. Often, another person can approach the rear of the dog and administer a sedative or vaccination without fear of being bitten.

VOICE. Dogs often respond to voice commands and tones. The voice can be a useful tool to comfort and soothe or direct an animal to obey. When using it to direct an animal, make the tone of your voice deep and commanding. Avoid the uplift inflection of a question because, to them, it is similar to puppy talk, the high-pitched yelping and barking that is used for play or attention. For example, a sit command is given as a command, not a question. However, almost all animals respond to a soothing croon or shushing noise as a distraction, so do not be afraid of sounding silly when comforting an animal.

MOBILITY-LIMITING DEVICES
Movement-limiting devices are designed to prevent a dog from chewing on itself or its bandages, or generally to restrict movement.

PROCEDURE 6-1 APPLYING A GAUZE MUZZLE

1. Tear off a 4-foot-long piece of gauze.
2. Make a loop by tying an overhand knot that is not tightened down (Fig. 1).

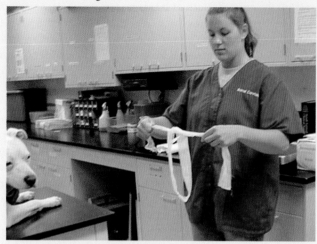

FIGURE 1

3. Have the dog either restrained by the scruff of the neck or a capture pole.
4. Stand slightly to the left or right of the dog's head, just out of its reach, and slide the loop around the dog's muzzle (Fig. 2).

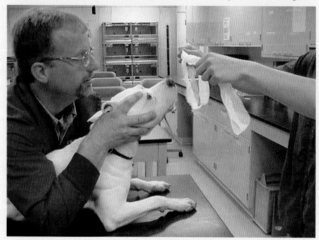

FIGURE 2

5. Quickly tighten the gauze down around the muzzle by pulling on the ends of the knot (Fig. 3).

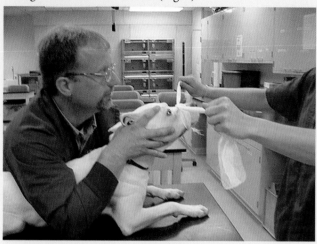

FIGURE 3

6. Bring the ends under the muzzle and tie another overhand knot under the chin (Fig. 4).

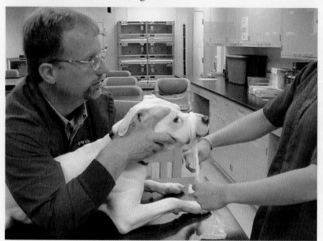

FIGURE 4

7. Move in closer, pass the ends behind the ears, and tie a bow knot (Fig. 5).

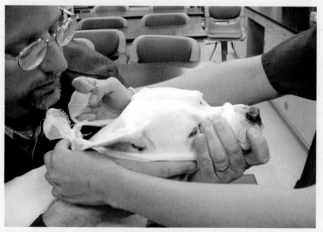

FIGURE 5

From Sirois M: Principles and practice of veterinary technology, ed 3, St Louis, 2011, Mosby.

Elizabethan collars are cone-shaped collars that fit around a dog's neck (Fig. 6-50). They can be attached to the dog's collar or secured around its neck. These collars are available commercially or can be made from plastic buckets, x-ray film, cardboard (short term), or large plastic bottles. Any material can be used that is sturdy enough to withstand being knocked about or bent, thus keeping the dog from chewing or licking other areas of its body.

Some precautions must be taken when using Elizabethan collars. With a commercially available collar, the main considerations are its length and tightness. The collar should extend past the end of the nose and be snug but not constrictive around the neck. Homemade collars can present problems because many of them have sharp edges that could injure the dog's neck. With both types, you may have to show the dog how to eat with the collar in place, elevate the food and water dishes, or take the collar off for the dog to eat or drink.

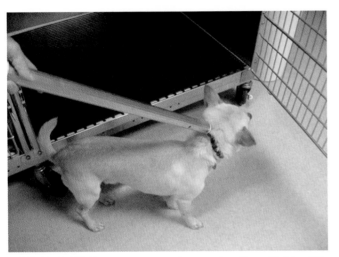

FIGURE 6-49 Using a capture pole on a dog. (From Sheldon CC, Sonsthagen T, Topel JA: Animal restraint for veterinary professionals, St Louis, 2006, Mosby.)

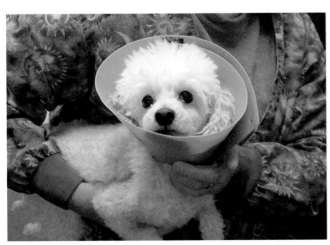

FIGURE 6-50 Elizabethan collars are cone-shaped collars that fit around a dog's neck. (From Sheldon CC, Sonsthagen T, Topel JA: Animal restraint for veterinary professionals, St Louis, 2006, Mosby.)

Dogs also often run into walls, door frames, and the back of your legs when wearing an Elizabethan collar because their peripheral vision is impaired.

No-bite collars are designed to fit snugly around the dog's neck, much like a cervical collar for humans (Fig. 6-51). The dog is able to eat and drink normally and has full peripheral vision, so you do not have to worry about it bumping into things.

SPECIAL HANDLING

It would be wonderful if all dogs could be treated and handled the same way. However, considerations must be given to their size, shape, condition, and personality. Puppies, pregnant bitches, and old animals, as well as nervous, aggressive, and injured dogs, all require special handling, not only for the safety of the animal but also for the safety of the handler.

PUPPIES

Puppies are full of energy and must be watched constantly. Never place them on an examination table or countertop without making sure that your hand is always in contact with them, because they are likely to fall and injure themselves.

When procedures are performed on puppies of any breed, most sit calmly and offer no resistance. If they do squirm or try to get free, lift them up and hold them snugly and close to your body.

PREGNANT BITCHES

In the advanced stages of pregnancy, applying excessive pressure on the dog's abdominal organs during restraint can have severe repercussions. When restraining a pregnant bitch, always be aware of where your hands are and how much pressure you are applying to the dog's abdomen.

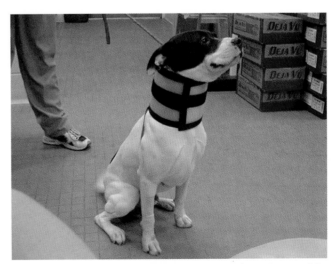

FIGURE 6-51 Restrictive collars are designed to fit snugly around the dog's neck, much like a cervical collar for humans. (From Sheldon CC, Sonsthagen T, Topel JA: Animal restraint for veterinary professionals, St Louis, 2006, Mosby.)

OLD DOGS

Old dogs often are pampered pets accustomed to being treated gently. Their joints can be arthritic and should not be maneuvered into awkward positions. Gentle handling is the key to working with these old-timers.

NERVOUS DOGS

Nervous dogs must be handled with great caution because they can be easily provoked to bite. You can recognize a nervous dog by its shivering, anxious expression, rapid head and ear movements, and ducking of its head. The animal may cower in a corner.

These animals often try to flee from the situation. If a cornered dog attempts to escape, never grab at it as it goes by because its instinctive reaction is to bite at the hand preventing it from reaching freedom. You might calm some of these fear biters by moving slowly, kneeling down to the dog's level, and softly talking it out of its fears. Offer your hand for sniffing. If the dog pulls its lips back in a grimace or growls, it is best to retreat and handle it as an aggressive dog.

AGGRESSIVE DOGS

Occasionally, animals do not accept your friendly advances and warn you off with a growl or some other form of body language. Signs of aggression, however, may be difficult to perceive. Some dogs bite with little or no warning. Signs of impending aggression include a head held low, either below or level with the dog's shoulders, a gaze that is averted to the side, raised hair along the back, ears down, and tail straight out, and an ominous growl or snarl. Dogs showing any of these signs should be handled with extreme caution and must always be considered dangerous.

When you must handle an aggressive dog, two or more people should be involved. If one person gets into trouble, the other can help or bring help. Some handlers do not look directly at an aggressive dog and stand sideways instead of facing the dog straight on. Both these signals are considered nonchallenging in canine body language. Aggressive dogs may answer a challenge if you inadvertently exhibit challenging body language. If you are attacked by a dog, you should remain still, curl into a fetal position if pulled down or hold on firmly to a solid object if standing, raise your opposite arm to protect your face and throat, and scream for help.

INJURED DOGS

Injured dogs must always be treated with extreme caution and care. As a rule, an injured dog should be muzzled before being moved or handled. The exception to this rule is if the dog has an injury to the head or is vomiting. Care must be taken not to jar or twist broken bones when transporting these animals. The best way to transport an injured animal is on a stretcher or flat board. If neither of these is available, a towel or blanket can work well, depending on the animal's size.

To use a blanket or towel for transportation, move the animal onto the blanket by supporting all portions of its body. Two or more people may be required to lift and shift the body. Once the animal is on the blanket, you can move it by lifting up on the corner of the blanket. Be careful to keep the blanket as level as possible so that the animal does not roll off.

RESTRAINT TECHNIQUES
REMOVING DOGS FROM CAGES OR RUNS

Because many dogs bolt out from kennels if given the opportunity, make certain that all escape routes are closed before opening any kennel door. To prevent this, the handler should block the door with a knee or forearm in the door opening (Fig. 6-52).

> **CRITICAL CONCEPT**
>
> To keep a dog from bolting out of the cage, place your knee or body in the open space between the door and door frame.

NONAGGRESSIVE, NONFEARFUL DOGS. Small dogs usually can be grasped gently by the scruff or under the chin and then lifted out of the cage, with one hand around and under the dog's thorax. Hold its body snugly, close to yours, or place a leash around its neck and place the dog on the floor. Medium-sized to large dogs are usually led out with a leash from a floor-level cage (Fig. 6-53).

Never pull a dog out of a cage, allowing it to jump to the floor. Most are not ready for the jump, and the height of the cage can cause injury to its legs and joints as well as the neck if it is jerked.

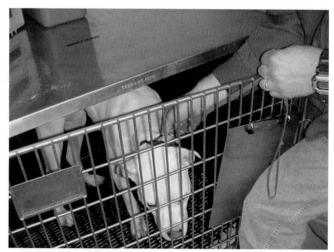

FIGURE 6-52 Blocking a dog from bolting out of a cage. (From Sheldon CC, Sonsthagen T, Topel JA: Animal restraint for veterinary professionals, St Louis, 2006, Mosby.)

FEARFUL AND AGGRESSIVE DOGS. It takes practice and good sense to remove fearful or aggressive dogs safely from cages or runs (Procedure 6-2). Ideally, dogs that are likely to bite should be muzzled, sedated, or both before placed in a cage or run. If this is not possible, proceed with caution. Do not corner the dog by stepping into the run or leaning into a cage. Calmly encourage the dog verbally with praise and comfort.

An alternative with a dog in a run or floor-level cage is to open the door narrowly, stepping behind the door to allow the dog to exit. As the dog's head comes through the doorway, quickly flip a leash over its head and move out with it. Most dogs actually calm down once they are out of their territory and will come along willingly. Remain on

guard, however, because these animals can turn nasty without much notice.

If a dog is attacking the leash or the front of the kennel, the use of a capture pole is warranted, regardless of whether the dog is small, medium, or large.

LIFTING A DOG

Small dogs are draped over a forearm, with the other hand holding onto the head just below the mandible. Medium-sized dogs are held around the neck with one arm and around its rear end or under the abdomen with the other. Carry both sizes of dogs close to your body until they can be placed in a kennel or on an examination table (Fig. 6-54).

Large dogs should be lifted by two people, one with an arm around the neck and thorax and the other with an arm around the abdomen and rear quarters. A count or signal should be given to lift in concert. Most large dogs get nervous on a table; procedures should be done on the floor, if possible. If this is not possible, be sure to have enough people to hold the dog securely on the table.

STANDING RESTRAINT

Wrap one arm around the dog's neck to control its head and keep it pressed close to your shoulder. Place the other arm under its abdomen to maintain the dog in a standing position and close to your body (Fig. 6-55). Keeping the dog close to your body and at the edge of the table closest to you gives you maximum control over the dog. If held at arm's length away from you, there is little chance of keeping the dog under control. If you have a very small dog, lift it into your arms and snug it close. This hold is used for physical examinations, including tests of temperature, pulse, and respiration (Fig. 6-56). You can also use this hold when subcutaneous (SC) and intramuscular (IM) injections

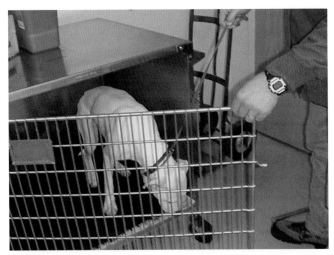

FIGURE 6-53 Slip the leash around a dog's head and allow it to step out of the cage. (From Sheldon CC, Sonsthagen T, Topel JA: Animal restraint for veterinary professionals, St Louis, 2006, Mosby.)

> ### 📋 PROCEDURE 6-2 REMOVING A DOG FROM A CAGE
>
> 1. Open the kennel door and slip a leash over the dog's head, if possible.
> 2. Walk the dog out of the run or floor-level kennel if it is a medium-sized dog.
> 3. With a small dog, capture it with the leash and then pull it to the edge of the kennel, retaining a steady pressure on the neck with the leash.
> 4. Reach in with a gloved hand and grasp a hindquarter.
> 5. Quickly lower it to the ground or place it on a table, holding the leash tight around the neck and the leg with the other hand.
> 6. Never pull a dog out and let it drop to the floor. You can cause severe injury to its legs, joints, back, and neck.

From Sirois M: Principles and practice of veterinary technology, ed 3, St Louis, 2011, Mosby.

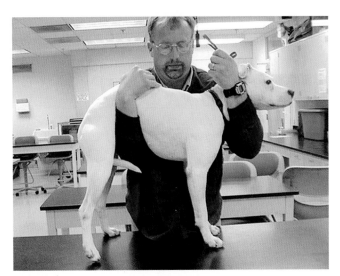

FIGURE 6-54 Lift and hold a medium-sized to large dog. (From Sheldon CC, Sonsthagen T, Topel JA: Animal restraint for veterinary professionals, St Louis, 2006, Mosby.)

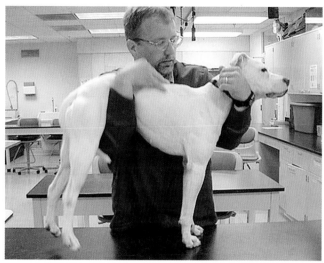

FIGURE 6-55 Wrap one arm around the dog's neck to control its head and keep it pressed close to your shoulder. Place your other arm under its abdomen to maintain the dog in a standing position and close to your body. (From Sheldon CC, Sonsthagen T, Topel JA: Animal restraint for veterinary professionals, St Louis, 2006, Mosby.)

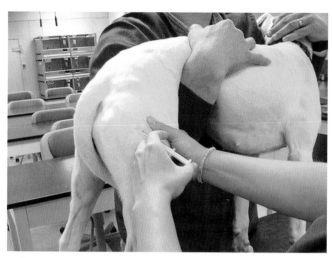

FIGURE 6-57 It is also used for administering SC and IM injections. (From Sheldon CC, Sonsthagen T, Topel JA: Animal restraint for veterinary professionals, St Louis, 2006, Mosby.)

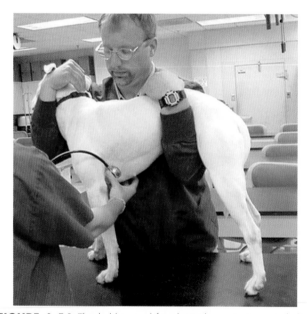

FIGURE 6-56 This hold is used for physical examinations, including those used to test temperature, pulse, and respiration. (From Sheldon CC, Sonsthagen T, Topel JA: Animal restraint for veterinary professionals, St Louis, 2006, Mosby.)

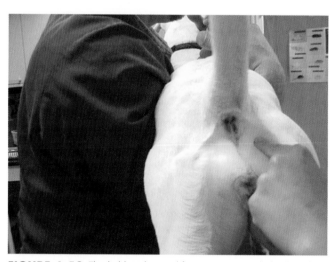

FIGURE 6-58 This hold is also used for expressing anal glands, administering enemas, and examining the limbs. (From Sheldon CC, Sonsthagen T, Topel JA: Animal restraint for veterinary professionals, St Louis, 2006, Mosby.)

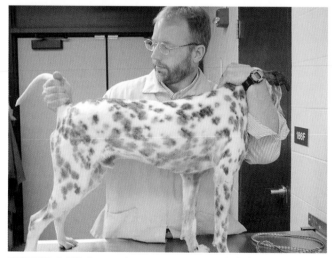

FIGURE 6-59 For rectal examinations, instead of placing your hands between the dog's back legs, grasp the dog's tail near its base and hold it up out of the way. (From Sheldon CC, Sonsthagen T, Topel JA: Animal restraint for veterinary professionals, St Louis, 2006, Mosby.)

must be administered (Fig. 6-57), as well as to express anal glands, administer enemas, and examine the animal's limbs (Fig. 6-58).

For rectal examinations, instead of placing your hands between the dog's back legs, grasp the tail near its base and hold it up out of the way (Fig. 6-59). With dogs of normal weight, you can support some of their weight with the tail as long as you do not fully lift the dog's rear end by its tail. Be prepared to adjust your grasp on the tail, because the veterinarian may want to hold it during the rectal examination. You can then support the hindquarters, as noted.

CROWDING

This technique may be used with very large dogs. Place the dog in a sitting position close to a corner of the room. Gently slide the dog's rear into the corner so it cannot back away. Then straddle the dog and restrain its head with both hands, gripping the mandibles, or kneel to the side and wrap an arm around the neck and steady the front legs with the other hand. Do not make it appear that you are cornering the dog; otherwise, it may become frightened and retaliate.

SITTING OR STERNAL RECUMBENCY

Sternal recumbency is usually used on the examination table and sometimes on the floor with large dogs (Procedure 6-3). This technique is useful for blood collection from the cephalic or jugular vein, IV injection, nail trimming, oral and ophthalmic examination or medication, and some radiographs.

One difficulty with this hold is keeping the dog from scratching you with its front paws. Instead of holding on to its rear, move your arm into the same position as you would for a venipuncture procedure, but grasp both legs, with a finger in between the legs, just above the carpals (Procedure 6-4). This will keep the dog from scratching you or the person performing the procedure.

PROCEDURE 6-3 RESTRAINING A DOG IN SITTING POSITION

1. Ask the dog to sit or place the dog in a sitting position (Fig. 1).
2. Place one arm around the dog's neck or hold onto the muzzle and put the other arm around the rear of the dog. This will prevent it from biting and backing away.
3. Pull the dog close to your body to provide added security. Lean your body onto the dog's body to keep it from backing up.
4. If you need to abduct one of the dog's forelegs for venipuncture, move the arm that normally holds on to the rear across the shoulders and grasp the leg opposite from your body.
5. Hold the leg by placing the elbow into the palm of that hand and push the leg forward. To occlude the vein, place your thumb on top of the leg, squeeze, and rotate laterally. This occludes and helps stabilize the vein.

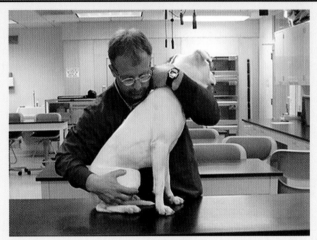

FIGURE 1

From Sirois M: Principles and practice of veterinary technology, ed 3, St Louis, 2011, Mosby.

PROCEDURE 6-4 STERNAL RESTRAINT FOR A CEPHALIC VENIPUNCTURE

1. For sternal recumbency restraint, say "down" or gently pull the front legs out until the dog rests on its sternum.
2. Hold the neck or muzzle as described in Procedure 6-3 and use your free hand either to steady the rear or hold the foreleg out for venipuncture (Fig. 1).
3. Lean some of your body weight on top of the dog to keep it in the down position.
4. This technique can also be used for jugular venipuncture. One hand reaches over the shoulders under the chin and wraps around the muzzle, raising the head to expose the neck.
5. The other hand grasps both front legs and stretches them over the edge of the table.
6. Put a finger between the legs and grasp around the carpal area, which will allow you to hold on better. Again, lean your body on top of the dog.
7. This is a very uncomfortable position for you and the dog. Do not apply this hold until the phlebotomist is ready to begin.

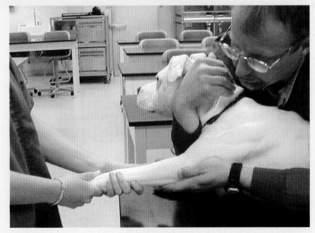

FIGURE 1

From Sirois M: Principles and practice of veterinary technology, ed 3, St Louis, 2011, Mosby.

LATERAL RECUMBENCY

Lateral recumbency is usually used on the examination table but also can be used on the floor. It is useful for urinary catheterization, radiographs, suture removal, electrocardiography, access to the lateral saphenous vein, nail trims, and other short procedures (Procedure 6-5).

DORSAL RECUMBENCY

Dorsal recumbency is used for procedures such as radiography, cystocentesis, and blood collection from the jugular vein. It sometimes requires two persons, depending on how restless and how wide the dog is. Place the dog in lateral recumbency and then roll it onto its back. If it is a very deep-chested dog, a V trough or foam wedges may be necessary to keep the dog from rolling. The forepaws are stretched cranially and the back paws are stretched caudally, exposing the thorax and abdomen.

SNUBBING

Snubbing can be used to administer an IM injection if you are alone; it can be used to prevent an aggressive dog from getting too close to the restrainer. In one variation one end of the leash is run through the wires on a kennel door. The leash is then pulled so the restrainer is on one side of the door and the dog on the other, again tying with a quick-release knot. This allows another staff member to vaccinate or give an injection to the dog.

RESTRAINT AND HANDLING OF CATS

FELINE BEHAVIOR

When restraining a cat, start with a minimum amount of restraint and perform the procedure as quickly as possible. Many procedures can be accomplished by barely holding on, but you need to be ready to tighten the hold as necessary. If the cat begins to resist, tighten your grip so no one gets hurt. However,

if the cat vigorously resists the restraint, release it and consider using a chemical restraint after it has calmed down. Before releasing the cat, make sure that the person doing the procedure knows that you are going to let go. Rough handling, extreme physical restraint, and a hot temper are counterproductive and have no place in cat restraint. Keep in mind that it is a good idea to make friends before placing a cat in any restraint hold. Relax the cat by petting it, speaking to it gently, and finding its favorite spot where it likes to be scratched.

> **CRITICAL CONCEPT**
>
> Cats do not like to be held tightly or for very long. Start with a gentle hold, but be ready to tighten your hold, if necessary.

DANGER POTENTIAL

Cats will also try to get away from a scary or painful procedure; most of the time, a cat will try to scare you off by batting at you with its front feet and/or hissing. If you are foolish enough to keep coming, it will resort to bringing out its formidable weapons. Their canine teeth are sharp but small in diameter. If you are bitten, the result is a deep puncture wound that often becomes infected. They also defend themselves with very sharp claws. Hanging onto a cat is difficult because they are agile and strong enough to bring into use all four feet as well as their teeth in defense. Remember, the idea is to not push a cat into fighting for its life.

MECHANICAL DEVICES
TOWEL AND BLANKET

A large towel is one of the best tools to keep around to assist in restraining a cat. It can be used to wrap the cat's body snugly, thus controlling the feet and body. A front or back leg can be pulled out for a cephalic or femoral vein exposure or,

---

📋 PROCEDURE 6-5 RESTRAINING A DOG IN LATERAL RECUMBENCY

1. Place the dog on its left or right side by reaching over the dog, grasp the legs closest to you, and pull them out from under the dog.
2. Hold on to the legs touching the table (left legs in left recumbency, right legs in right recumbency), lifting them slightly.
3. Put one wrist or arm across the dog's neck and the other across the flank. This prevents the dog from getting up (Fig. 1).
4. If you need one hand free, the only hand available is the one holding the rear legs. Lift the front legs slightly so that the dog's weight is shifted onto its shoulder; then you can release the rear legs. Maintain pressure on the dog's neck with your forearm.
5. For a more secure hold on the legs, place a finger between them above the carpal joint on the front legs and the tarsal joint on the back.

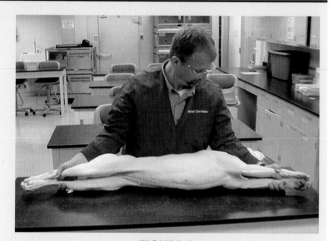

FIGURE 1

From Sirois M: Principles and practice of veterinary technology, ed 3, St Louis, 2011, Mosby.

for an IM injection, the cat can be rolled onto its back for a jugular venipuncture, and oral or ophthalmic medicines can be given without fear of being scratched. Also, covering the head with a towel often calms the cat down. Procedures 6-6 and 6-7 provide details on two techniques that can be used to wrap a cat. Both methods are useful if you have to give an oral or ophthalmic medication by yourself or they can be used for a jugular, cephalic, femoral, or saphenous venipuncture.

📋 PROCEDURE 6-6 BURRITO TECHNIQUE FOR WRAPPING A CAT FOR RESTRAINT

1. The towel is placed flat on the table, and the cat is placed approximately one third of the way from one end of the towel.
2. Taking the short end or the end closest to the cat, wrap it very snugly around its body.
   Once that is in place, quickly wrap the long end around and around its body.
3. This covers everything but the head, and a front or back leg can be extracted or the cat rolled onto its back and the head extended for a jugular venipuncture (Fig. 1).

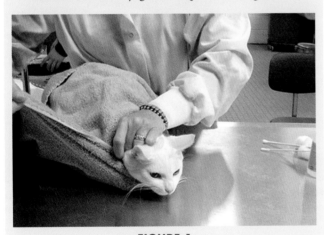

FIGURE 1

From Sirois M: Principles and practice of veterinary technology, ed 3, St Louis, 2011, Mosby.

📋 PROCEDURE 6-7 TACO TECHNIQUE FOR WRAPPING A CAT FOR RESTRAINT

1. Drape a towel over the cat so that the middle of the towel is directly over the cat's back.
2. Quickly sweep the sides of the towel together and lay the cat on its side.
3. Continue to wrap the two ends of the towel completely and snugly around the cat.
4. As with the burrito wrap, it completely encircles the legs but allows access to the head and rear.
5. This technique is especially useful for getting angry cats out of a cage.

From Sirois M: Principles and practice of veterinary technology, ed 3, St Louis, 2011, Mosby.

FELINE RESTRAINT BAGS

This manufactured nylon or canvas bag secures a cat's legs and body and has a number of strategically placed zippered openings (Procedure 6-8). The key to getting a cat into the bag is speed. Choose a properly sized bag. If the cat bag is too small, you will never get the cat into it; if it is too large, the cat will still be able to squirm around. Start by laying the bag open wide on the table, scruff the cat with your right hand, and lift, placing it into sternal recumbency on top of the open bag (Fig. 6-60). Use your body and scruffing hand to keep the cat down. If it stands up, it will scramble to its feet and bunch the bag up. With your left hand, bring one side of the neck strap up and scruff the cat while holding onto the neck band (Fig. 6-61). Quickly grasp the other band and bring it under the cat's neck, securely fastening the bag. Be careful to keep your fingers out of the cat's bite range (Fig. 6-62). Switch control of the scruff back to your right hand and maintain a downward pressure over the cat's shoulders.

Quickly slide your left hand in between the cat's back legs and move them up and toward the thorax, curling the cat's body into the bag. This prevents the cat from standing up and stepping out of the bag (Fig. 6-63). Bring the sides

---

📋 PROCEDURE 6-8 RESTRAINING A CAT USING A CAT BAG

1. To insert a cat into a cat bag, you must have the bag laid out and open wide.
2. Place the cat in the middle of the bag and quickly wrap the neck strap around the neck, fastening it snugly but not so much that it occludes the airway.
3. Then, with a hand on its back or over its shoulders and hip, have another person zip the zipper, being careful not to zip the cat's hair or skin.
4. The legs can be brought through zippered openings for injections or venipunctures (Fig. 1).

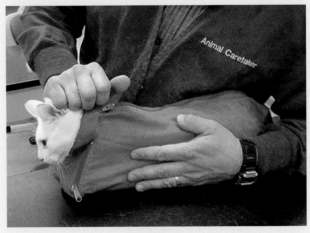

FIGURE 1

From Sirois M: Principles and practice of veterinary technology, ed 3, St Louis, 2011, Mosby.

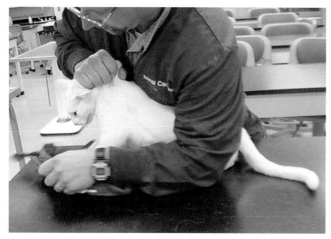

FIGURE 6-60 *Start by laying the bag open wide on the table, scruff the cat with your right hand, and lift the cat, placing it into sternal recumbency on top of the open bag. (From Sheldon CC, Sonsthagen T, Topel JA: Animal restraint for veterinary professionals, St Louis, 2006, Mosby.)*

up and, if the bag has a hair guard, smooth that into place. Tuck the cat's head tightly between your body and elbow and zip the bag. Be careful not to zip the cat's hair, tail, or legs into the bag (Fig. 6-64). If the bag does not have a hair guard, grasp the zipper and pull it with your thumb and index finger while sliding your fingers underneath it. As you move your fingers along, push the cat's hair out of the way (Fig. 6-65). Once you have zipped the bag, quickly gain control of the cat's head (Fig. 6-66). The cat can still bite. This bag is wonderful to use for cephalic, femoral, and saphenous venipunctures, IM injections, administering medications, and applying treatments to the head (Fig. 6-67). Note that you should never leave a cat unattended in a bag! It can roll off the table and be severely injured.

To remove a cat from a bag, close all the auxiliary zippers, scruff the cat with your right hand, and unzip the bag with your left. Be careful not to zip the cat's hair, tail,

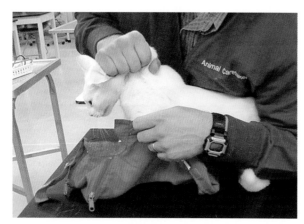

FIGURE 6-61 *With the left hand, bring one side of the neck strap up and scruff the cat while holding onto the neck. (From Sheldon CC, Sonsthagen T, Topel JA: Animal restraint for veterinary professionals, St Louis, 2006, Mosby.)*

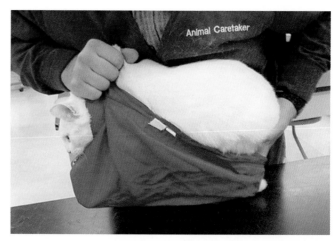

FIGURE 6-63 *Quickly slide your left hand in between the back legs and move them up and toward the cat's thorax, curling the cat's body into the bag. (From Sheldon CC, Sonsthagen T, Topel JA: Animal restraint for veterinary professionals, St Louis, 2006, Mosby.)*

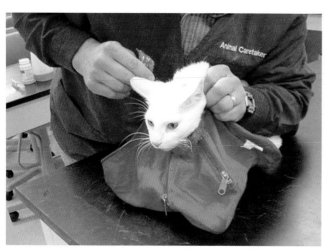

FIGURE 6-62 *Quickly grasp the other band, bring it under the cat's neck, and securely fasten the bag around the cat's neck. (From Sheldon CC, Sonsthagen T, Topel JA: Animal restraint for veterinary professionals, St Louis, 2006, Mosby.)*

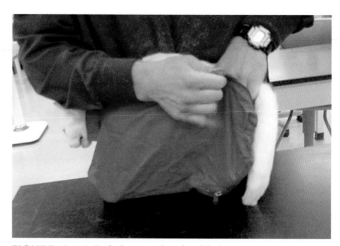

FIGURE 6-64 *Tuck the cat's head tightly between your body and your elbow, and zip the bag. (From Sheldon CC, Sonsthagen T, Topel JA: Animal restraint for veterinary professionals, St Louis, 2006, Mosby.)*

or legs as you open the zipper. Next, working quickly, release the neck strap and allow the cat to step forward out of the bag. If the cat is wise to the restraint bag, you may need someone else to help you keep the cat's body pushed down until you zip the bag.

MUZZLES

Muzzles are of dubious worth on cats. They must be wide enough to cover the cat's entire face, including the eyes, but have an opening positioned so that the cat can still breathe through its nose. It is difficult to secure them behind the cat's ears because its head is so rounded and there is not much ledge there to keep the strap from moving forward. The restrainer may inadvertently pull the muzzle off if the cat moves its head or body violently.

Choose the properly sized muzzle. Be sure you know which side goes up. Cats give you only one chance to get

the muzzle in place. Place the cat in sternal recumbency. Hold one tab of the muzzle in your hand as you scruff the cat, with your thumb pointing toward the cat's head. Use your forearm to hold the cat snugly, close to your body (Fig. 6-68). With your other hand, grasp the end of the other tab and swing wide to avoid the cat's mouth; then bring the muzzle over the cat's face (Fig. 6-69). Secure the

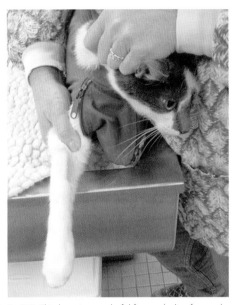

FIGURE 6-67 This bag is wonderful for cephalic, femoral, and saphenous venipunctures, IM injections, administering medications, and treatments to the head. (From Sheldon CC, Sonsthagen T, Topel JA: Animal restraint for veterinary professionals, St Louis, 2006, Mosby.)

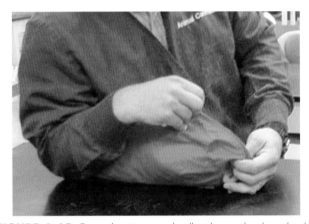

FIGURE 6-65 Grasp the zipper and pull with your thumb and index finger while sliding your fingers underneath the zipper. As you move your fingers along, push the cat's hair out of the way. (From Sheldon CC, Sonsthagen T, Topel JA: Animal restraint for veterinary professionals, St Louis, 2006, Mosby.)

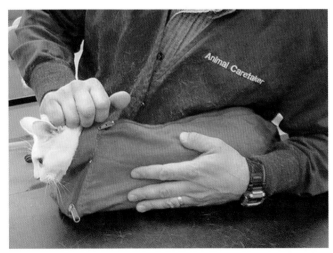

FIGURE 6-66 Once the bag is zipped, quickly gain control of the cat's head. (From Sheldon CC, Sonsthagen T, Topel JA: Animal restraint for veterinary professionals, St Louis, 2006, Mosby.)

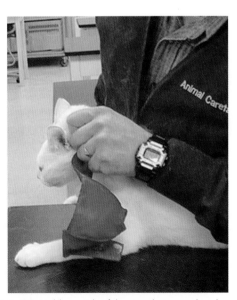

FIGURE 6-68 Hold one tab of the muzzle in your hand as you scruff the cat, with your thumb pointing toward the cat's head. Hold the cat snugly against your body by using your forearm to slide it close. (From Sheldon CC, Sonsthagen T, Topel JA: Animal restraint for veterinary professionals, St Louis, 2006, Mosby.)

muzzle tabs behind the ears as low and tight as they will go (Fig. 6-70).

Check that the muzzle does not cover the cat's nares. If they are covered, the cat will panic because it cannot breathe and will struggle to be free of the muzzle.

To remove the muzzle, scruff the cat, quickly release the tabs, and pull the muzzle away from the cat's face. It is important to move your hand quickly away from the cat's mouth so that the cat does not bite you.

GAUNTLETS

Refer to the dog restraint section; these gauntlets are used in the same manner. The only difference is that you may use them more for cats than for dogs.

DISTRACTION TECHNIQUES

Cats can often be distracted from procedures by the restrainer. The following are some **distraction techniques** that work well with cats.

CAVEMAN PATS

Caveman pats are exaggerated heavy but gentle pats or rubbing on the head. They can be rapid or slow and steady, or somewhere in between. The idea is to get the cat to concentrate on what you are doing and ignore the procedure being performed. Varying the pressure and stroke is usually more successful than a continuous pattern. Some people tap a cat's nose with their finger. This is not recommended, because the cat may not be able to resist biting such a tempting target.

PUFFS OF AIR

Blowing or puffing air into a cat's face is another way to redirect its interest. Again, vary the speed and force of the puff of air to obtain better results.

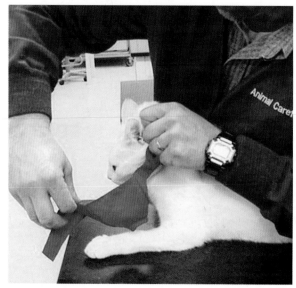

FIGURE 6-69 With your other hand, grasp the end of the other tab, swing wide to avoid the mouth, and then bring the muzzle over the cat's face. (From Sheldon CC, Sonsthagen T, Topel JA: Animal restraint for veterinary professionals, St Louis, 2006, Mosby.)

RESTRAINT TECHNIQUES
REMOVAL FROM A CARRIER

Be sure that all routes of escape are closed before restraining. Most cats will not willingly walk out of a carrier on demand. Therefore, it is a good idea to open the carrier door as soon as the client is escorted into the examination room. While you are talking to the client, the cat may decide to walk out and explore. If not, you can assess the temperament of the cat. If the cat is friendly, reach in, gently grasp the scruff, and bring it forward until you can get a hand around its midsection. Most cats do not object to this; however, most clients do not understand this and may think you are hurting their cat. Always explain that scruffing is a natural hold for them because it is how their mother carried them.

If the cat resists, elevate the rear of the carrier and allow the cat to slide out. Do not raise it so high that the cat drops from the carrier. If you are not successful, you can dismantle most carriers quickly. This is much safer than reaching into its territory and trying to grab it.

REMOVAL FROM A CAGE

If the cat is friendly, reach in across its shoulders, grasp the front feet, quickly lift it out of the cage, and hold its body snugly against yours. Your elbow can gently pin the cat's body against yours, thereby controlling the back legs. Cradle the chin or encircle the neck with the other hand.

If the cat is upset, you can try a number of things. Throwing a large beach towel or small blanket over the cat and then scooping it up works well to get it out of the cage. Once out of its territory, it will usually calm down and allow you to work with it. It is also recommended that you wear gauntlets while getting it out of the cage. You can also try lassoing a cat with a rope leash; you usually end up getting the leash around its chest, which is not all that bad. If that does occur, you can pull the cat to the front of the cage and, with a gloved hand, reach in for a back leg and quickly transport the cat to an examination table. If it is terribly upset, there are devices

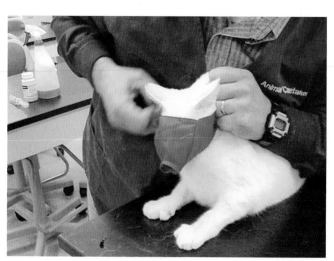

FIGURE 6-70 Secure the muzzle tabs behind the ears as low and tight as they will go. (From Sheldon CC, Sonsthagen T, Topel JA: Animal restraint for veterinary professionals, St Louis, 2006, Mosby.)

designed to trap and/or pin it to the floor of a cage or inside a device so a sedative can be administered (Fig. 6-71). A dose of ketamine can be given by squirting it into the cat's eyes or open mouth if it is hissing. It is absorbed through the mucous membranes, and the cat will quickly become sedated.

SITTING OR STERNAL RECUMBENCY

This procedure can be used for physical examinations, oral and ophthalmic examinations and medications, and cephalic or jugular venipuncture. For a routine physical examination, have the cat sit and place one hand in front of its chest while the other hand steadies its back. Gently talk to and stroke the animal as it is being examined. When it is time to examine the head or perform a more invasive procedure, encircle the

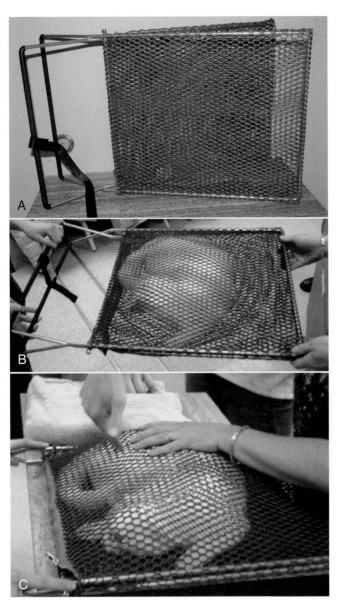

FIGURE 6-71 **A,** A device such as the easy nabber tool works well in subduing an aggressive cat. **B,** You can transport the cat to an examination table or wherever you need to take it. **C,** The cat is encircled inside the nabber and cannot move much, so IM or SC injections can be given through the netting. (From Sheldon CC, Sonsthagen T, Topel JA: Animal restraint for veterinary professionals, St Louis, 2006, Mosby.)

neck, holding its mandibles with one hand (Fig. 6-72); with the other hand, reach across the back and grasp its front feet. Hold the cat snugly up against your body. If necessary, lean over the cat a little to keep its back legs in place.

A gentle grip is a must to keep the cat from getting worried and struggling. If the procedure is almost finished and the cat starts to struggle, it is a simple matter to tighten your grip and hang on until the procedure is completed. If at all possible, do not let go. However, if you are losing your grip and the cat is trying to bite and/or scratch, alert the person performing the procedure and let go when she or he steps away. This works well, and most cats do not object unless they are being held too tightly.

Cats often respond negatively to being poked. This usually makes the new restrainer nervous, who then holds the cat with a death grip. It has already been discussed how cats respond to being held too tightly and for too long. Do not put the cat into these holds until the person performing the venipuncture has the syringe assembled, cap on the needle loosened, cotton ball soaked, and the tube ready to go.

RESTRAINT FOR CEPHALIC VENIPUNCTURES. Cephalic venipuncture requires the cat to be in sternal recumbency. Scruff the cat with your right hand, with your thumb pointing toward the cat's back end. Slide the cat to the edge of the table and then bring your left hand around the side of the cat's body and hold it snugly against your body (Fig. 6-73). Turn the cat's head away from your partner and toward your body. With your left hand cradling the cat's left elbow, wrap your thumb across the proximal part of the forearm as you extend its left leg forward, toward your partner (Fig. 6-74). Your partner will grasp the cat's foot, which frees your hand to occlude the vessel. To occlude the vessel, keep your thumb in place but roll it laterally so that it ends up perpendicular to the vessel. This causes the vessel to stand up and rolls it to

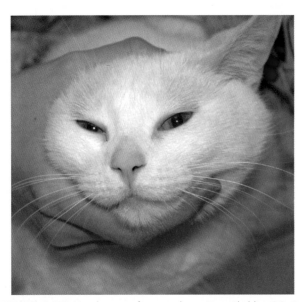

FIGURE 6-72 Head restraint for procedures. (From Sheldon CC, Sonsthagen T, Topel JA: Animal restraint for veterinary professionals, St Louis, 2006, Mosby.)

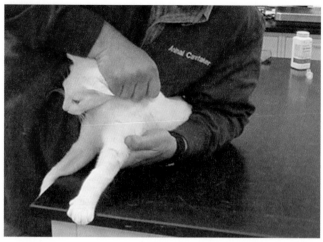

FIGURE 6-73 Scruff the cat with your right hand, with your thumb pointing toward the cat's back end. Slide the cat to the edge of the table, bring your left hand around the side of the cat's body, and hold it snugly up against your body. (From Sheldon CC, Sonsthagen T, Topel JA: Animal restraint for veterinary professionals, St Louis, 2006, Mosby.)

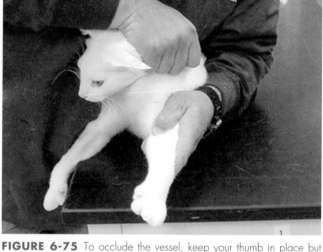

FIGURE 6-75 To occlude the vessel, keep your thumb in place but roll it laterally so that your thumb ends up perpendicular to the vessel. (From Sheldon CC, Sonsthagen T, Topel JA: Animal restraint for veterinary professionals, St Louis, 2006, Mosby.)

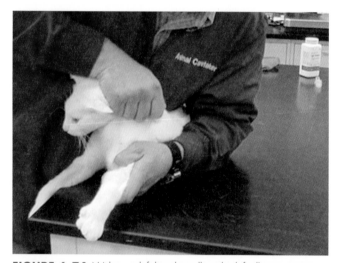

FIGURE 6-74 With your left hand cradling the left elbow, wrap your thumb across the proximal part of the forearm as you extend the left leg forward, toward your partner. (From Sheldon CC, Sonsthagen T, Topel JA: Animal restraint for veterinary professionals, St Louis, 2006, Mosby.)

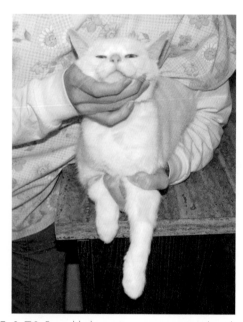

FIGURE 6-76 For added security, you can grasp the other leg and pin it between your little finger and palm. (From Sheldon CC, Sonsthagen T, Topel JA: Animal restraint for veterinary professionals, St Louis, 2006, Mosby.)

the top of the cat's leg for easier access. Continue to hold the cat's elbow securely in the palm of your hand (Fig. 6-75). For added security, grasp the cat's other leg and pin it between your little finger and palm. This prevents the cat from using it to scratch you or your partner while performing the venipuncture (Fig. 6-76). Be able to switch hands and hold the scruff with the left hand and the front leg with the right (Fig. 6-77).

Applying a Tourniquet for Cephalic Venipuncture. Place the cat in sternal recumbency using the same technique as you would for a cephalic venipuncture. The restrainer extends the limb to be used by cradling the elbow in the palm of the left hand without laying the thumb across the vessel. The phlebotomist slips the tourniquet over the paw (Fig. 6-78). The tourniquet goes proximal to the cat's elbow, and the tails and clip are on the caudolateral aspect of the elbow.

Pull the ends of the tourniquet to tighten it. The restrainer reestablishes the hold on the cat's leg so that the cat does not pull it back (Fig. 6-79). To release the tourniquet, grab both sides (top and bottom) of the clip and pull it away from the base as you pull the entire locking mechanism away from the leg (Fig. 6-80). Use this same technique to place a tourniquet on a dog's limb.

RESTRAINT FOR JUGULAR VENIPUNCTURE. There are two holds to use for jugular venipuncture. The first method involves starting just as you would for the cephalic hold. Once to the edge of the table, shift your left hand to a cupping technique with your fingers under the mandible and the thumb

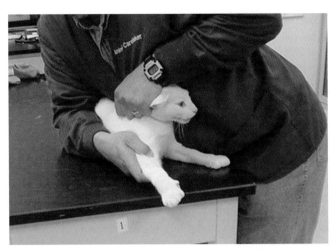

FIGURE 6-77 Be able to switch hands and hold the scruff with the left hand and the front leg with the right. (From Sheldon CC, Sonsthagen T, Topel JA: Animal restraint for veterinary professionals, St Louis, 2006, Mosby.)

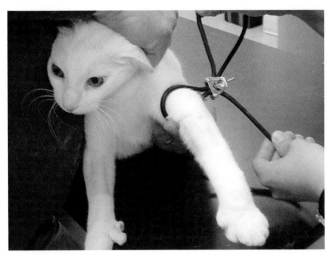

FIGURE 6-79 Pull the ends of the tourniquet to tighten it. (From Sheldon CC, Sonsthagen T, Topel JA: Animal restraint for veterinary professionals, St Louis, 2006, Mosby.)

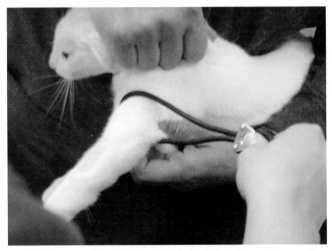

FIGURE 6-78 The restrainer extends the limb to be used by cradling the elbow in the palm of his or her left hand without laying the thumb across the vessel. The phlebotomist slips the tourniquet over the paw. (From Sheldon CC, Sonsthagen T, Topel JA: Animal restraint for veterinary professionals, St Louis, 2006, Mosby.)

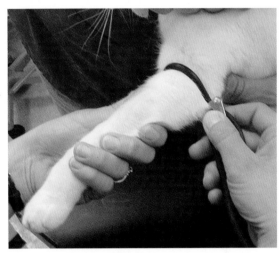

FIGURE 6-80 To release the tourniquet, grab both sides (top and bottom) of the clip and pull it away from the base as you pull the entire locking mechanism away from the leg. (From Sheldon CC, Sonsthagen T, Topel JA: Animal restraint for veterinary professionals, St Louis, 2006, Mosby.)

on top of the cat's head. Note how the left arm is snuggling the cat's body up against the restrainer's chest. Gently move your right hand under the cat and grasp both front legs above the elbows, with your finger in between the legs for added gripping power. Extend its head upward while extending its legs down so that you can see the jugular vessel (Fig. 6-81). Be prepared to switch hands and start the hold with the right hand (Fig. 6-82). The difficult part of this hold is getting your fingers out of the way while maintaining control of the cat's head. Only two fingers are used to hold the head up securely. It takes a lot of practice to develop the strength to hold a cat like this.

Cats do not tolerate this hold for long. The phlebotomist should have everything ready to go before the restrainer puts the cat into position. This includes wetting the cotton ball, having the needle cover loose, and breaking the seal on the plunger.

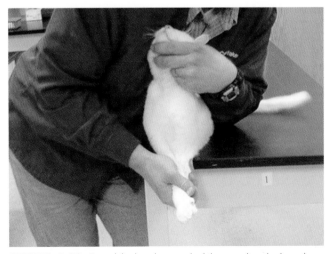

FIGURE 6-81 Extend the head upward while extending the legs down so that you can see the jugular vessel. (From Sheldon CC, Sonsthagen T, Topel JA: Animal restraint for veterinary professionals, St Louis, 2006, Mosby.)

The other method is to hold the cat on its back. It is easier to do this if the cat is wrapped in a towel or placed in a cat bag. Once the cat is wrapped up in the towel, roll it over so that it is lying on its back. The restrainer uses one hand to grasp the head from the back and holds the cat's front feet under the towel and down toward its chest. When ready, the phlebotomist takes the cat's head and the restrainer occludes the vessels. The phlebotomist cups the back of the head in the palm of one hand and lays a thumb across its mandibles (Fig. 6-83). The phlebotomist has to be careful when holding the head. If the cat should struggle and the phlebotomist's thumb slips down over the trachea, the cat could actually suffocate. Most cats do not object to this hold and seem to stay still a bit longer than they do for the previous technique.

LATERAL RECUMBENCY

Cats can be restrained in lateral recumbency, just as for a dog. However, they are agile and can often maneuver their heads around and bite. This method should be reserved for very placid cats and noninvasive procedures. If you need them in lateral recumbency for a femoral venipuncture, placing them in a cat bag or burrito towel wrap is the safest way to accomplish the task.

A fetal hold or scruffing technique is more useful for giving subcutaneous or intramuscular injections or placing a rectal thermometer (Procedure 6-9).

Small cats can be lifted off the table and a back leg can be moved up toward the neck and be hooked by the thumb of the hand holding the scruff. This presents the biceps femoris muscle into which an IM injection can be given by the restrainer with the other hand (Fig. 6-84).

Do not use this on cats weighing more than 7 pounds because it can cause a lot of damage to tissues and vertebrae. Another precaution when using this technique is to have the injection ready to go and the cotton ball full of alcohol before placing the cat into position. The cat should not be held in this position longer than 5 to 6 seconds; otherwise,

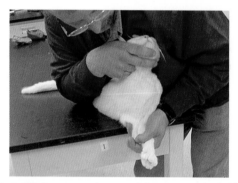

FIGURE 6-82 Be prepared to switch hands; start the hold with the right hand. (From Sheldon CC, Sonsthagen T, Topel JA: Animal restraint for veterinary professionals, St Louis, 2006, Mosby.)

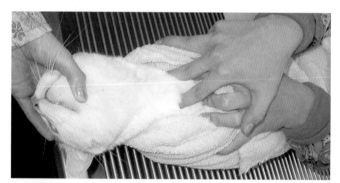

FIGURE 6-83 The phlebotomist holds the head by cupping the back of the head in the palm of his her hand and laying the thumb across the mandibles. (From Sheldon CC, Sonsthagen T, Topel JA: Animal restraint for veterinary professionals, St Louis, 2006, Mosby.)

📋 PROCEDURE 6-9 RESTRAINING A CAT IN LATERAL RECUMBENCY

1. As the cat sits, grasp the scruff of its neck, gathering as much of the skin as possible in one hand.
2. Lift the cat slightly off the table and grasp both back legs with the other hand.
3. Stretch the cat's back against the forearm, holding the scruff.
4. If the cat is stretched out fully, a reflex causes the cat's tail to curl ventrally toward its abdomen and the legs tend to be relaxed (Fig. 1).
5. The person doing the IM injection can take the top back leg or both back legs, which then allows the restrainer to grasp the front legs.

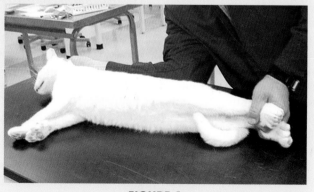

FIGURE 1

From Sirois M: Principles and practice of veterinary technology, ed 3, St Louis, 2011, Mosby.

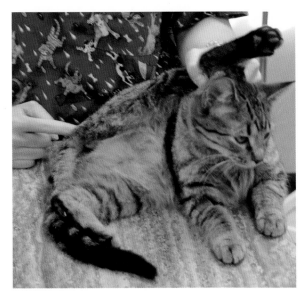

FIGURE 6-84 Restraint for IM injections when alone. (From Sheldon CC, Sonsthagen T, Topel JA: Animal restraint for veterinary professionals, St Louis, 2006, Mosby.)

even a small cat can suffer some injury. However, it is a real timesaver if you are alone and an injection must be given.

DORSAL RECUMBENCY

This technique is used for blood collection from the jugular vein, radiography, and cystocentesis. It sometimes requires two persons. However, with practice one person can usually accomplish the hold alone (Procedure 6-10).

CHEMICAL RESTRAINT

An inhalation chamber is a great tool that can be used for cats that will not surrender, no matter what you do. You can place them in the chamber and use isoflurane or sevoflurane to anesthetize them. The only drawback to using this technique is that the animal does not stay asleep for very long, so you either have to work fast or insert an endotracheal tube and keep the cat on the inhalant gas until the procedure is completed.

Another chemical restraint technique is to squirt ketamine into the cat's mouth. It is absorbed by the mucous membranes and the cat is sedated. However, it is easier to do than it sounds. Load a dose of ketamine into a syringe with a Tom Cat catheter attached and, as the cat hisses, squirt it into the cat's mouth. You may have to do this once or twice to get the entire dose into the cat, but it works well. This is much easier than trying to give the cat a sedative by an IM injection.

CAT LASSO

The cat lasso is really a tool of last resort (Fig. 6-85). The pole has a noose at one end that draws tight when placed around the cat's body. If the noose can be placed around the cat's shoulders, you avoid choking it. If you capture it around the neck, the cat will often react violently because it feels threatened by this hold. If the cat is so wild that you have to use the

PROCEDURE 6-10 RESTRAINING A CAT IN DORSAL RECUMBENCY

1. Scruff the cat, grasp the rear legs with the other hand, and roll it on its back.
2. Coming from the rear with the other hand, palm up, gather the back legs and then the front legs between the fingers of that hand.
3. Try to grasp the back legs above the hocks and the front legs above the carpals. This gives you more purchase on the legs.
4. Continue to scruff the head, or switch your hold so that you are hanging on to the mandibles from the back of the head.
5. The phlebotomist can hold off the jugular vein with one hand and insert the needle with the other.
6. Often, it is easier to insert the needle pointing toward the chest versus the traditional insertion point.
7. If the procedure is for a radiograph or cystocentesis, you will most likely need two people.

From Sirois M: Principles and practice of veterinary technology, ed 3, St Louis, 2011, Mosby.

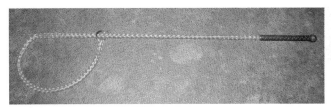

FIGURE 6-85 The cat lasso is really the last resort for restraining cats. The pole has a noose at one end that draws tight when placed around the cat's body. (From Sheldon CC, Sonsthagen T, Topel JA: Animal restraint for veterinary professionals, St Louis, 2006, Mosby.)

cat lasso, it is best to put the cat directly into the inhalation chamber or quickly give it a sedative.

RECOMMENDED READINGS

Beaver BV: *Canine behavior: Insights and answers*, St Louis, 2009, Saunders.
Beaver BV: *Feline behavior: A guide for veterinarians*, ed 2, St Louis, 2003, Saunders.
Horwitz D, Neilson J: *Blackwell's five-minute veterinary consult clinical companion: Canine and feline behavior*, Indianapolis, 2007, Wiley-Blackwell.
Landsberg G, Hunthausen W, Ackerman L: *The handbook of behavior problems in the dog and cat*, ed 2, Philadelphia, 2003, Saunders.
Miklosi A: *Dog behaviour, evolution, and cognition*, Oxford, England, 2009, Oxford University Press.
Shaw J: *Companion animal behavior for veterinary technicians and nurses*, Indianapolis, 2010, Wiley-Blackwell.
Sheldon CC, Sonsthagen T, Topel JA: *Animal restraint for veterinary professionals*, St Louis, 2006, Mosby.
Sirois M: *Principles and practice of veterinary technology*, ed 3, St Louis, 2011, Elsevier.
Tully T, Mitchell M: *A technician's guide to exotic animal care*, Lakewood, CO, 2001, AAHA Press.
Turner D, Bateson P: *The domestic cat: The biology of its behaviour*, ed 2, Cambridge, England, 2000, Cambridge University Press.

Yin S: *Low stress handling*, Davis, CA, 2009, Cattle Dog Publications.

Behavior Organizations

Academy of Veterinary Behavior Technicians Academy of Veterinary Behavior Technicians (http://www.AVBT.net)

American College of Veterinary Behaviorists American College of Veterinary Behaviorists, (http://www.veterinarybehaviorists.org)

American Veterinary Animal Behavior Society American Veterinary Animal Behavior Society (http://www.avsabonline.org)

Animal Behavior Society Animal Behavior Society (http://www.animalbehavior.org)

Society of Veterinary Behavior Technicians Society of Veterinary Behavior Technicians (http://www.SVBT.org)

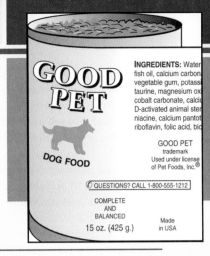

INGREDIENTS: Water
fish oil, calcium carbon
vegetable gum, potass
taurine, magnesium ox
cobalt carbonate, calci
D-activated animal ster
niacine, calcium pantot
riboflavin, folic acid, bio

GOOD PET
trademark
Used under license
of Pet Foods, Inc.®

ⓒ QUESTIONS? CALL 1-800-555-1212

COMPLETE
AND
BALANCED

15 oz. (425 g.)   Made
in USA

7 Animal Husbandry and Nutrition[1]

OUTLINE

Husbandry, *172*
Temperature, Light, and Ventilation, *172*
Housing, *172*
Animal Identification, *173*
Housekeeping, *173*
Disinfection and Sanitation, *174*
Attending to the Psychological Needs of Dogs and
   Cats, *174*
Animal Nutrition, *174*
Energy-Producing Nutrients, *175*
Non–Energy-Producing Nutrients, *175*
Feeding Considerations for Dogs, *176*

Feeding Considerations for Cats, *178*
Pet Food Considerations, *181*
Nutritional Support, *183*
Common Diseases, *190*
Terminology, *191*
Pathogens, *192*
Nonpathogens, *192*
Immune Response, *192*
Zoonotic Diseases, *193*
Vaccination and Preventive Medications, *195*
Factors Predisposing to Disease, *202*

LEARNING OBJECTIVES

After reviewing this chapter, the reader will be able to:

1. Discuss general housekeeping concerns in the veterinary practice.
2. List basic energy-producing and non–energy-producing nutrients.
3. Describe considerations for feeding young and adult dogs.
4. Describe considerations for feeding young and adult cats.
5. Discuss the fundamentals of exotic pet diet considerations.
6. Discuss basic differences in the digestive tracts of ruminants and monogastric animals.
7. List and describe common diseases and ways in which they can affect people.
8. Discuss methods used to control spread of zoonotic diseases.
9. Explain the general principles underlying disease prevention.
10. Discuss features of appropriate housing and nutrition for animals.
11. List and discuss types of vaccinations and schedules of vaccinations for domestic animal species.
12. Explain the principles of sanitation that relate to disease prevention.
13. Describe factors that predispose to disease.

KEY TERMS

Ad libitum
Body condition scoring
Capsid
Concussion
Contusion
Disinfection
Essential amino acids

Etiology
Fibrosis
Granulation tissue
Laceration
Necropsy
Nonessential amino acids
Nosocomial infection

Nutrient
Pathology
Public health
Pyrogen
Reservoir
Sanitizer
Toxoid

Vaccine
Virus
Vitamins
Wound
Zoonoses

---

[1]Elsevier and the author acknowledge and appreciate the original contributions from Sirois M: Principles and practice of veterinary technology, ed 3, St Louis, 2011, Mosby, whose work forms the heart of this chapter.

Veterinary preventive medicine is the science of preventing disease in animals. The three major components of a preventive medicine program include husbandry, vaccination or prevention through medication, and sanitation. Husbandry involves the housing, diet, and environment of animals. Vaccination involves the use of **vaccines** or bacterins to prevent diseases such as rabies or canine distemper; medication can be given regularly to prevent diseases such as heartworm infections or flea infestations. Sanitation focuses on cleanliness and the use of disinfectants to prevent infection or disease transmission. All three components are interrelated; disease is prevented only by attention to all components. For example, poor husbandry practices cannot be accommodated by overvaccination and rigorous sanitation. Failure to vaccinate an animal properly may well result in disease, even if the husbandry is the best and sanitation is impeccable. Poor sanitation frequently results in animal and human disease.

The goal of any preventive medicine program is the lowest possible incidence of disease in animals under the care of the veterinary practice. The mutual goal of veterinary professionals and animal owners should be to preserve animal health using preventive practices. Such efforts save money that otherwise would be spent for the treatment of disease. Preventive medicine also prolongs the life span, improves the well-being of animals, and fosters a good client-veterinarian relationship.

Unfortunately, some clients cannot see the benefit of spending a few dollars for preventive care, such as for vaccination. These clients then complain about the large sums of money they must spend to correct problems that could have been avoided through preventive methods. The challenge for the veterinary health care team is to empathize and work with these clients for the benefit of the patient. By educating animal owners about the benefits of proper preventive medicine, you will be given the opportunity to provide the best veterinary care possible.

HUSBANDRY

TEMPERATURE, LIGHT, AND VENTILATION

For small animals, such as dogs, cats, birds, and small mammals, the ambient (room) temperature should ideally be 65° to 84° F (18° to 29° C). Birds, very young pets, old pets, and those with a sparse hair coat should be maintained at the higher end of this temperature range. Those that are well-furred or overweight should be kept at the lower end of this range. Smaller animals of any species generally require warmer temperatures, whereas larger animals, with their greater body mass, generally require cooler temperatures.

Light sufficient for a human is adequate for most animals. Too little light makes sanitation difficult. All species do better when there is a definite difference between day and night. Animals should never be kept in direct sunlight without access to shade because they may become sunburned and overheated. Such environmental stress can also predispose to disease.

Ventilation is extremely important in maintaining good health. Inadequate air exchange in an enclosure increases urine odors, ammonia levels, and the numbers of airborne bacteria and **viruses**. These conditions irritate the respiratory tract and predispose to respiratory disease. Drafty conditions or excessive ventilation can be dangerous. Excessive cool airflow can cause chilling. In a low-humidity environment, as with air conditioning, high airflow can dehydrate an animal. Small pets caged indoors must be kept away from air-conditioning drafts or heater vents. It is usually best to place a cage along an interior wall, away from ventilation or heating ducts.

HOUSING

An important aspect of husbandry is housing, such as cages, pens, or stalls. It is important to keep in mind the following considerations. Housing should do the following:

- Prevent contamination of the animal with feces or urine.
- Provide for the psychosocial comfort of companion animals.
- Be appropriate for the species.
- Be structurally sound.
- Be free of dangerous surfaces.
- Be constructed so that the animal cannot escape and vermin are not allowed access.
- Be easy for the owner to clean.

Housed animals should be dry, clean, and protected from environmental extremes. Walls and roofing should be sufficient to protect animals from the sun, wind, rain, and snow. Attention should be paid to escape-proofing cages. Accommodation must also be made for species-specific behavior. For example, cats need scratching posts and resting boards (Fig. 7-1).

A major failure of many animal enclosures is that they do not allow sufficient room for normal movement or even

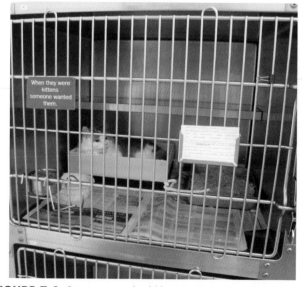

FIGURE 7-1 Cats in cages should be provided with resting boards or boxes elevated above the cage floor. (From August JR: Consultations in feline internal medicine, vol 6, ed 6, St Louis, 2009, Saunders.)

postural changes. Cages, pens, and stalls that are too small increase the risk of disease and may predispose to abnormal behavior, such as pacing or excessive barking. Pets may be kept in close confinement for short periods, such as a dog kept for a few hours in a portable kennel or carrier; however, these enclosures should have sufficient room for normal postural movements and stretching. A general rule for holding enclosures is that they be a minimum of 10 times the body size of the animal. This recommendation assumes that the animal will be given opportunity to exercise routinely outside the primary enclosure. Also, housing too many animals in a single primary enclosure of insufficient size can increase the risk of stress, aggression, and disease transmission.

Animals of different species should be housed separately or, in some cases, at least in separate rooms. Do not house natural predators and prey animals in the same room, such as cats with mice or birds, because this leads to stress and possible attack. There are also medical reasons for housing different species separately. A disease considered inconsequential in one species can be deadly in another species.

ANIMAL IDENTIFICATION

An often-overlooked aspect of preventive medicine is animal identification. The method of identification depends on the species. For pets allowed outdoors, an implanted microchip or tattoo is preferred to a collar with a name tag. Collars may be removed or fall off and tags may be lost. Permanent identification ensures that a lost pet can be identified for return to its owner. When hospitalized, each animal should be adequately identified with cage cards and paper ID neck bands (Fig. 7-2).

HOUSEKEEPING

General maintenance of the veterinary practice is an ongoing challenge. The floors, flat surfaces, walls, cages, runs, and stalls must be kept sparkling clean and odor-free. The counters, magazine racks, and pictures need to be organized and dusted frequently. The reception room, examination rooms, and public bathrooms must be inspected and cleaned regularly throughout each day. Some of this general maintenance needs to be scheduled on a regular basis. Everyone in the practice must assume some of the cleaning responsibility. An old adage for new graduates is that "veterinary medicine is 90% cleanup and 10% medical practice." No one should look for someone else to clean up a fresh urine or fecal deposit. It is usually quicker and easier to clean it up yourself.

One of the reasons cleanup in a veterinary practice is so challenging is the large quantity of hair shed by animals. Hair is such a major problem that a vacuum system needs to be available and used before general mopping; otherwise, there is a buildup of hair that is simply moved around the facility. Some practices have been built with a central vacuum system to improve the efficiency of hair reduction from the floors. The removal of hair from the environment is extremely important for the proper care of electronic equipment and computers.

Clients notice hospital cleanliness. The lack of it can result in complaints or **nosocomial** (hospital-acquired) **infections**. When one client actually complains, there are probably many other clients quietly forming a negative impression about the practice. If the veterinary hospital is to be considered a modern and progressive medical facility, all personnel must monitor odors and sanitation. Whenever a pet soils an area or cage, it must be cleaned quickly and thoroughly. Appropriate disinfectants need to be used to prevent odor buildup. Deodorizers may be of benefit to help clean the area but should not be used to cover up a sanitation problem. The ventilation system should be capable of exhausting all air within the building within 15 to 20 minutes to facilitate odor control. In addition to exhaust fans in the wards, fans can also be useful in the examination rooms and laboratory areas.

It is imperative that the practice stay in immaculate condition at all times. Odors travel quickly through the practice; therefore, urine, feces, anal gland secretions, and other unpleasant odors must be removed immediately. Odors are also absorbed into the walls, baseboards, and tile grout; once the odors have permeated, they may be impossible to remove.

	Owner		Name												
	Date in:		Ph #1												
	Est. date out:		Ph #2												
	Sunday		Monday		Tuesday		Wednesday		Thursday		Friday		Saturday	
	am	pm	am	pm	am	pm	am	pm	am	pm	am	pm	am	pm
Fed															
Ate															
Water															
Urine															
Stool															
Meds															
Walked															

FIGURE 7-2 Stable hospitalized patients require minimally a daily weight and record of eating, drinking, and elimination. This example of a cage card is conveniently graphed for recording this information. This type is also a sticker that can be applied to the permanent medical record after use. (From Sirois M: Principles and practice of veterinary technology, ed 3, St Louis, 2011, Mosby.)

Cages, runs, and other enclosures should be cleaned and sanitized frequently. Few pet owners clean their pets' cages or pens too often. Small cages can be sanitized by hand or even in a dishwasher. Generally speaking, any good dishwashing detergent will effectively clean holding areas. Additional sanitation can be obtained with a dilute solution of laundry bleach, using one part bleach to 20 parts of water. All surfaces should be rinsed thoroughly after cleaning and disinfecting. Wet items should be left to dry completely before returning the animal to the cage.

DISINFECTION AND SANITATION

Disinfection is the destruction of pathogenic microorganisms or their toxins. Disinfectants are chemical agents that kill or prevent the growth of microorganisms on inanimate objects, such as surgical equipment, floors, and tabletops. **Sanitizers** are chemical agents that reduce the number of microorganisms to a safe level, without completely eliminating all microorganisms. Sterilizers are chemicals or other agents that completely destroy all microorganisms. As with antimicrobials, it is important to know against which organisms the antiseptic or disinfectant is effective. See Chapter 5 for more information about the types of disinfectants used in veterinary practice.

Chemicals used to clean floors should never be mixed. The label on bleach notes that it should be diluted to a 10% or 20% solution and not be mixed with other products. Caustic vapors may result, causing harm to patients and team members. Labels must be read clearly to dilute the product to the correct strength to have a solution that kills viruses, fungi, or bacteria.

Trash should be emptied several times a day. Trash cans absorb odors that can also travel through the practice. Rooms must be cleaned after every patient, preventing the transmission of odors and diseases.

Walls should be cleaned weekly, if not more often. Blood, hair, and dirt collect on walls and cabinets and must be cleaned off as soon as they are spotted.

Potted plants that sit on the floor must be cleaned frequently because animals often urinate on them. The entire pot must be cleaned. It should be moved each night while cleaning the practice, removing hair and dirt that has collected under the plant.

Blinds, fans, vents, baseboards, and door frames must be dusted weekly. Dirt collects in these locations quickly, and clients notice the dirt while waiting in the examination room.

The outside of the practice must remain clean as well (Fig. 7-3). Feces must be removed daily, and common urination areas must be scrubbed with a dilute Clorox solution. Urine stains walls and sidewalks and produces a terrible smell. Trash, including cigarette butts and cans, must be removed from the parking lot. Windows should be washed weekly and dirt swept away from the entrance and exit areas. The outside of the building must be as presentable as the inside of the practice.

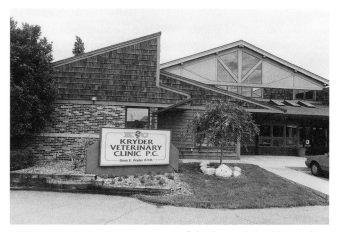

FIGURE 7-3 Exterior appearance of the hospital should provide a positive image. (From Bassert JM, McCurnin DM: McCurnin's clinical textbook for veterinary technicians, ed 7, St Louis, 2010, Saunders.)

ATTENDING TO THE PSYCHOLOGICAL NEEDS OF DOGS AND CATS

An often-overlooked aspect of nursing care includes petting and simply touching or praising the patient verbally. The hospitalized pet can be afraid and uncomfortable in a new environment, which can have a negative effect on appetite, temperature, and mentation. Make friends with the patient by always talking gently and quietly. When interacting with the patient, place yourself on the patient's level by sitting on the cage edge or squatting down to pet the chest or chin. Repeat this at every opportunity. Establish a rapport with the patient. At treatment times, double the amount of positive interaction, especially when the procedure or treatment involves pain or discomfort. Patients respond positively to gentle reassurance and support. If the patient's condition permits, provide special snacks or food. Each patient has individual needs, and it requires observation and often owner input to help make the patient's hospitalization as positive as possible.

ANIMAL NUTRITION

Animals must have free access to fresh potable water. Water in containers should be changed frequently enough to prevent accumulation of slime, algae, or dirt. Bowls should be kept clean and sanitized in a dishwasher (180° F [82° C]) at least once monthly. Animals should be fed a wholesome, palatable diet on a regular schedule and in sufficient quantity. Feeding devices must be designed to prevent contamination by wastes. As with water containers, feeding devices should be sanitized routinely.

The diet fed should be formulated for that species. Cats should not be fed food formulated for dogs. The most common question in veterinary practices today is, "What should I feed my pet?" This common inquiry compels all members of the veterinary health care team to maintain a high level of current knowledge about the best feeding recommendations for pets. Veterinary clinical practice continues to integrate

BOX 7-1	Nutrients

Energy-Producing
- Fats
- Carbohydrates
- Proteins

Non–Energy-Producing
- Water
- Vitamins
- Minerals

From Sirois M: Principles and practice of veterinary technology, ed 3, St Louis, 2011, Mosby.

BOX 7-2	Essential Amino Acids

- Arginine
- Histidine
- Isoleucine
- Leucine
- Lysine
- Methionine
- Phenylalanine
- Threonine
- Tryptophan
- Valine
- Taurine (for cats, conditionally essential)

From Sirois M: Principles and practice of veterinary technology, ed 3, St Louis, 2011, Mosby.

BOX 7-3	Essential Fatty Acids

Dogs
- Linolenic
- Linoleic

Cats
- Linolenic
- Linoleic
- Arachidonic

From Sirois M: Principles and practice of veterinary technology, ed 3, St Louis, 2011, Mosby.

the application of nutrition successfully to include both the healthy and ill patient. The quality of a pet's life can be dramatically influenced by the intake of nutrients balanced to its lifestyle and state of health.

A **nutrient** is any constituent of food that is ingested to support life. The six basic nutrients are proteins, fats, carbohydrates, water, **vitamins**, and minerals. Energy-producing nutrients have a hydrocarbon structure that produces energy through digestion, metabolism, or transformation. Energy is used for all metabolism, cell rejuvenation, maintenance of homeostasis, and production of new cells. Non–energy-producing nutrients play an important role throughout the body system and are often called the gatekeepers of metabolism (Box 7-1).

ENERGY-PRODUCING NUTRIENTS
PROTEINS

Dietary protein is used to build body tissues. Amino acids, the building blocks of protein, are categorized as either essential or nonessential. **Essential amino acids** cannot be synthesized in the body and so must be supplied by the diet (Box 7-2). **Nonessential amino acids** are synthesized in the body. The proportion of essential and nonessential amino acids largely determines the quality, or biologic value, of a particular protein source. A protein's biologic value represents the amount that is retained by the body after ingestion. A protein with a 100% biologic value is entirely retained by the body after ingestion. A protein of very low biologic value, such as 5%, is almost entirely excreted by the body after ingestion.

FATS

Vegetable and animal fats, oils, and lipids are composed of fatty acids and contain more energy per unit of weight than any other nutrient. There is a direct correlation between fat content and caloric density in a diet; the more fat there is in a diet, the more calories it contains. Cats require three essential fatty acids in their diet, whereas only two are essential in dogs (Box 7-3).

> **CRITICAL CONCEPT**
> Fat has more energy per gram than all other nutrients.

CARBOHYDRATES

Carbohydrates are classified as soluble or insoluble, based on their digestibility. Mammals cannot digest insoluble carbohydrates, such as fiber, although bacteria can degrade fiber in the stomach of herbivores. Fiber decreases a diet's digestibility and caloric density. Soluble carbohydrates, such as sugar and starches, can be readily digested and are metabolized for energy needs.

> **CRITICAL CONCEPT**
> Fiber is added to a diet for the treatment of obesity or management of gastrointestinal (GI) disorders.

NON–ENERGY-PRODUCING NUTRIENTS
WATER

Water provides the foundation for the metabolism of all nutrients in the body. Minor alterations in the body's water content and distribution can result in dramatic alterations in nutritional requirements. Water balance in the system affects the ability to excrete waste into the urine by the kidneys. Water is also essential for absorption and metabolism of water-soluble vitamins B and C. Access to fresh, clean water is imperative for all animals. An animal's water needs may not be met if the water source freezes during inclement weather or if the water container is tipped over. It is important to educate clients on providing access to fresh, clean water in all seasons.

BOX 7-4	Vitamins

Water-Soluble
- Thiamin
- Riboflavin
- Niacin
- Pyridoxine
- Pantothenic acid
- Folic acid
- Cobalamin
- Vitamin C
- Choline
- L-Carnitine

Fat-Soluble
- A
- D
- E
- K

From Sirois M: Principles and practice of veterinary technology, ed 3, St Louis, 2011, Mosby.

BOX 7-5	Minerals

- Calcium
- Phosphorus
- Potassium
- Sodium
- Chloride
- Magnesium
- Iron
- Zinc
- Copper
- Manganese
- Selenium
- Iodine
- Boron

From Sirois M: Principles and practice of veterinary technology, ed 3, St Louis, 2011, Mosby.

VITAMINS

Vitamins play a very important role in maintaining normal physiologic functions. These organic molecules are required only in minute amounts to exert their function as coenzymes, enzymes, or precursors in metabolism. Water-soluble vitamins are passively absorbed from the small intestine, and excess amounts are excreted in the urine. Fat-soluble vitamins are metabolized in a manner similar to that of fats and stored in the liver. Because of this storage mechanism, toxicity from excessive intake of fat-soluble vitamins can occur. A deficiency of fat-soluble vitamins is not as common as with water-soluble vitamins (Box 7-4).

MINERALS

Within the body, minerals are often distributed in ionized form as a cation or anion electrolyte. In this form, they are involved with acid-base balance, clotting factors, osmolality, nerve conduction, muscle contraction, and other cellular activities.

Deficiencies or excesses in mineral intake can lead to problems through imbalances. Minerals are closely interrelated, and an imbalance in one mineral can affect several others. Dietary minerals include calcium, phosphorus, potassium, sodium, chloride, magnesium, iron, zinc, copper, manganese, selenium, iodine, and boron (Box 7-5).

FEEDING CONSIDERATIONS FOR DOGS

Contrary to popular belief, domestic dogs do not need variety in their diet. Frequent changes in diet have few positive effects, encourage finicky eating, and can cause digestive disorders. It is best consistently to feed a diet formulated to meet the animal's needs at each stage of its life. Regular assessment of weight can help determine the amount to feed. Weight loss or gain indicates a need to reevaluate the amount being fed or diet selection. **Body condition scoring** is a valuable way to assess the appropriate amount of food; a review

of one type of body condition scoring system can be found in Figure 7-4.

FEEDING METHODS

PORTION CONTROL. Portion control is currently the most popular way to feed dogs. After determining the animal's nutritional requirements, the daily portion is offered to the animal in a single feeding or divided into several portions offered several times per day. The animal is then allowed to consume the food throughout the day or during 5 to 10 minutes for each divided portion.

FREE CHOICE. In free-choice feeding, also referred to as **ad libitum** (ad lib), the animal is allowed access to food 24 hours per day. The food supply is replenished as needed. It may be difficult to detect subtle changes in food intake with this method. Free-choice feeding is not recommended for puppies and obese dogs, but it works well for cats.

TIME CONTROL. In time-controlled feeding, a portion of food is offered and the animal is allowed access for only 5 to 10 minutes. Any remaining food is taken away after that time. Puppies are commonly fed in this manner.

FEEDING THE GESTATING OR LACTATING DOG

The daily energy requirement during gestation in the bitch increases during the length of the pregnancy. Although clients may have the impulse to increase food consumption dramatically, it is important to educate them about how to feed an appropriate amount. Excessive weight gain in the gestating bitch can make parturition more difficult and affect the overall health of the dog. The goal is to increase food intake gradually, assessing weight gain carefully during the pregnancy. In the lactation phase, many dogs will require free feeding because they will need to eat smaller meals more frequently to reduce their absence from the puppies during this critical growth phase. Figure 7-5 shows the relationship between body weight and food intake during lactation and gestation in the dog.

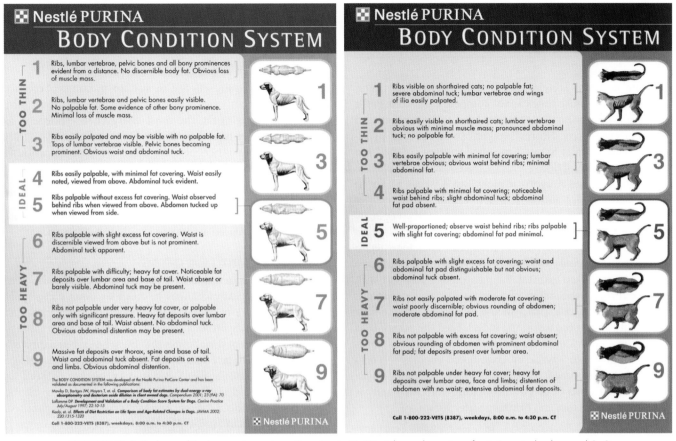

FIGURE 7-4 Body conditioning scoring system. (From Sirois M: Principles and practice of veterinary technology, ed 3, St Louis, 2011, Mosby.)

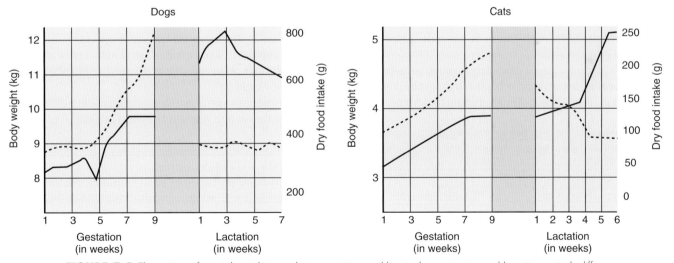

FIGURE 7-5 The pattern of normal weight gain during gestation and loss in the postpartum and lactation periods differs between cats and dogs. *Solid line* indicates food intake. *Dashed line* indicates body weight. (Courtesy Hill's Pet Nutrition, Topeka, KS.)

FEEDING PUPPIES

With puppies born by cesarean section, or if the bitch has no milk, the veterinary staff must intervene and provide nutritional support to neonatal puppies. Fortunately, puppies can be raised successfully on canine milk replacer. Cow's milk is not an acceptable substitute because it contains inappropriate levels of protein and lactose. Initially, it may be necessary to use orogastric intubation or a feeding syringe and then gradually adopt a regular small animal feeding bottle as the puppies begin to thrive.

Daily or twice-daily weighing and physical examination of the puppies help identify problems early enough to adjust feeding protocols or begin other therapeutic measures to avoid mortality. Puppies typically gain 2 to 4 g/kg of anticipated adult weight each day.

Some neonatal puppies fail to gain weight when nursing the bitch because they cannot compete with siblings for a nipple. Puppies in this situation tend to be restless and whimper excessively. Normal weight can be restored by allowing these puppies to nurse the bitch without competition three to four times daily.

Weaning begins at approximately 3 to 4 weeks of age in large-breed puppies and at 4 to 5 weeks of age in smaller breeds. To facilitate the transition to solid foods, begin by making a gruel or slurry of a growth type of diet. Gruel is created by mixing equal parts of food and water together to form a homogeneous consistency. The mixture should have the texture of cooked oatmeal. Puppies initially may play with or walk through the slurry, but eventually they consume it in increasing amounts. Gruel should be offered three to four times daily during the weaning process. Feed the puppy with increasing amounts until the puppy can be maintained without nursing, at 5 to 7 weeks in large-breed puppies and 6 to 7 weeks in smaller breeds. Once weaning is complete, decrease the volume of water added to the mixture until the puppy is eating the desired diet and drinking water voluntarily.

FEEDING ADULT DOGS

As a dog matures, be sure to monitor activity level and predisposition to obesity to preserve a neutral energy equilibrium. Reassess feeding methods because inappropriate techniques commonly result in excessive nutrient intake and obesity. Review feeding habits with clients to preclude future problems (Box 7-6).

Most dogs are managed efficiently through time-restricted meal feeding. Some dogs nibble throughout the day when offered food free choice. Daily energy requirements are

| BOX 7-6 | Recommended Feeding Practices for Dogs and Cats |

- Match the diet to the animal's stage of life.
- Feed for the ideal body weight.
- Measure the amount of food fed.
- Adjust the amount fed to the animal's body condition.
- Don't feed table scraps.
- Don't overfeed.
- Don't change the diet frequently.
- If the diet is to be changed, do so gradually, over 3 to 5 days.
- Don't feed multiple animals from a single bowl.
- Treats should not comprise more than 10% of the diet.
- Use dry food (kibble), ice chips, and vegetables as treats.
- Deduct the amount fed as a treat from the total amount fed daily.

From Sirois M: Principles and practice of veterinary technology, ed 3, St Louis, 2011, Mosby.

outlined in Figure 7-6. Care should be taken in these situations to ensure that optimal body condition is maintained, with weight neither lost nor gained.

FEEDING ACTIVE DOGS

Active dogs require energy to sustain hunting, obedience trial, or other activities. The diets for active dogs must have enhanced levels of fat, the most energy-dense nutrient, as well as increased total digestibility. Dogs that are only slightly more active than others need slightly more food, but working dogs with significant energy demands require a substantial increase in food portions. Any increase in food portions to condition a dog for work should be gradually instituted over a 7- to 10-day period. Hunting dogs should be fed just before a period of increased activity to avoid hypoglycemia.

FEEDING GERIATRIC DOGS

Older dogs are less able to adjust to prolonged periods of poor nutrition. Any changes in an older dog's diet should be based on careful patient assessment and not solely on the dog's age. Dietary protein should be of high biologic value to reduce the level of metabolites that must be excreted through the kidneys. Dietary fats must be sufficiently digestible to provide adequate levels of essential fatty acids without an excess that could lead to obesity. Because of its detrimental effects on the kidneys, dietary phosphorus should be limited. Increased levels of zinc, copper, and vitamins A, B complex, and E may be required in the diet of older dogs.

FEEDING OVERWEIGHT DOGS

Obesity is the most common nutritional disorder of pets. Obesity places significant stress on the body system and may predispose to diabetes mellitus, cardiovascular disease, and skeletal problems. Early counseling of owners can alert them to weight gain. Educate clients about the potential adverse effects of weight gain.

A review of nutritional considerations for different life stages in the cat and dog can be found in Table 7-1.

FEEDING CONSIDERATIONS FOR CATS
FEEDING KITTENS

Kittens that are orphaned or born to queens unable to nurse must be hand fed. Weaning should not commence until 7 weeks of age. Kittens can be gradually introduced to a diet by first offering a slurry of canned food mixed with kitten milk replacer. As with puppies, the amount of liquid is gradually reduced. Later, they can be offered a dry diet, if desired.

FEEDING ADULT CATS

Adult cats typically eat several small meals throughout a 24-hour period. Unfortunately, many clients provide food to their cats in unlimited amounts, filling the food dish each time their cat empties it. Such free-choice feeding predisposes to obesity. Overfeeding can be prevented by offering limited amounts of food throughout the day. This gives the cat the opportunity to nibble throughout the day while avoiding excessive caloric intake.

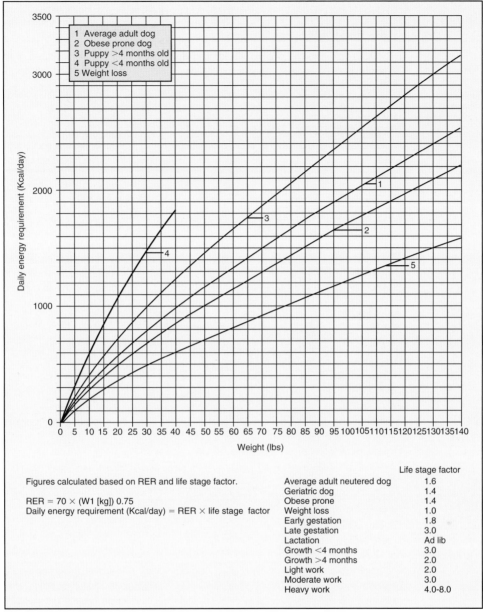

FIGURE 7-6 Canine daily energy requirements. (Courtesy Hill's Pet Nutrition, Topeka, KS.)

TABLE 7-1	Nutrient Considerations for Different Life Stages in Cats and Dogs	
LIFE STAGE	FOOD CHARACTERISTICS	COMMENTS
Cats		
Kittens 8 wk-1 yr; gestation, lactation	Metabolizable energy, 4.5 kcal/g dry matter Digestibility ≤ 80% Protein, 35%-50% Fat, 17%-30% Fiber ≥ 5% Calcium-to-phosphorus ratio, 1.0-1.8 to 0.8-1.5 Magnesium ≤ 20 mg/100 kcal	Transition queen to growth diet at 3 wk of gestation.
Adult cat	Metabolizable energy, 3.75 kcal/g dry matter Digestibility > 78% Protein, 0%-45% Fat, 9%-25% Magnesium < 20 mg/100 kcal	Ad lib feeding acceptable to kittens and queens. Free-feeding adults may result in overnutrition.

Continued

TABLE 7-1	Nutrient Considerations for Different Life Stages in Cats and Dogs—cont'd	
LIFE STAGE	FOOD CHARACTERISTICS	COMMENTS
Obese-prone cat	Metabolizable energy, 3.50-3.75 kcal/g dry matter Digestibility > 75% Protein, 30%-45% Fiber, 7%-12% Fat, 9%-25% Magnesium < 20 mg/100 kcal	Feed multiple (three or four) times daily. Fiber provides satiety and decreased caloric density.
Geriatric cat	Metabolizable energy, 3.75 kcal/g dry matter Digestibility > 80% Protein, 35%-45% Fiber, 7%-12% Fat, 9%-25% Magnesium < 20 mg/100 kcal	Watch excess sodium and energy intake. Increased palatability may be needed.
Dogs		
Puppies; gestation, lactation	Metabolizable energy > 3.9 kcal/g of diet Digestibility > 80% Protein, 27%-30% Fiber < 4% Fat, 8%-20% Calcium-to-phosphorus ratio, 1.0-1.8 to 0.8-1.6	Avoid excessive weight during pregnancy. Puppies reach skeletal maturity at approximately 12 mo of age.
Adult dog	Metabolizable energy > 3.5 kcal/g of diet Digestibility > 75% Protein, 15%-25% Fiber ≥ 5% Fat, 7%-15%	Food and feeding consistency encouraged.
Obesity-prone dog	Metabolizable energy < 3.5 kcal/g of diet Digestibility > 80% Protein, 15%-25% Fiber > 5% Fat, 6%-10%	Free feeding can contribute to obesity.
Increased activity or stressed dog	Metabolizable energy > 4.2 kcal/g of diet Digestibility > 82% Protein, 25%-32% Fiber < 4% Fat, 23%-27%	
Geriatric dog	Metabolizable energy = 3.75 kcal/g of diet Digestibility > 80% Protein, 14%-21% Fiber > 4% Fat, 10%-12% Control sodium	The average small-medium breed dog is considered geriatric after 7 yr. Giant and large breeds are geriatric at 5 yr of age.

From Sirois M: Principles and practice of veterinary technology, ed 3, St Louis, 2011, Mosby.

Caution owners against offering a constantly changing diet, such as various brands and types of commercial diets, because this can result in undesirable eating behavior.

FEEDING CATS WITH LOWER URINARY TRACT DISEASE

Feline urinary tract disease is a complex disease characterized by bouts of frequent painful urination, bloody urine, and, in males, possible urethral obstruction. It tends to occur more often in obese, sedentary cats. Factors other than diet are involved in lower urinary tract disease, but careful attention to the diet of affected cats can help prevent future episodes.

Depending on the type of uroliths (small stones composed of cellular debris and mineral crystals) present in the urinary tract (struvite or calcium oxalate), prevention involves manipulation of dietary mineral, fiber, and water intake. Special commercial diets are available for the dietary management of feline urinary tract disease.

FEEDING GERIATRIC CATS

Because aging can diminish the senses of smell and taste, it is sometimes necessary to enhance the aroma and taste of foods to improve their palatability for aged cats. Successful techniques include warming canned food to body temperature in the microwave to improve the aroma, applying garlic powder to canned food before it is warmed, and adding aromatic foodstuffs, such as clam juice or bits of canned fish.

FEEDING THE GESTATING AND LACTATING CAT

Food intake for the gestating queen is not as dramatic as that found in the canine. Allow the queen to have free access to food during the last 30 days of gestation. Assess weight gain and body condition on a weekly basis to reduce the occurrence of excess weight gain. Free food should be available to the queen throughout lactation to ensure ample milk availability to the kittens. Figure 7-5 shows the relationship between food intake and body weight during lactation and gestation in the cat. Feline daily energy requirements have been calculated in Figure 7-7.

PET FOOD CONSIDERATIONS

When a nutritional assessment is made for a pet, the need of fulfilling dietary requirements is only partially met by the veterinary health care team. To gratify all the dietary needs fully, it is also necessary to understand the broad assortment of types, classifications, and varieties of diets available commercially today. Often, questions arise regarding effective techniques when comparing diets. The effective veterinary health care team member must be able to answer these questions with insight and full understanding of the pet's nutritional need. To evaluate commercial diets for dogs and cats accurately, it is necessary to obtain accurate information about the common pet foods that clients consider feeding and that are recommended by the veterinary practice.

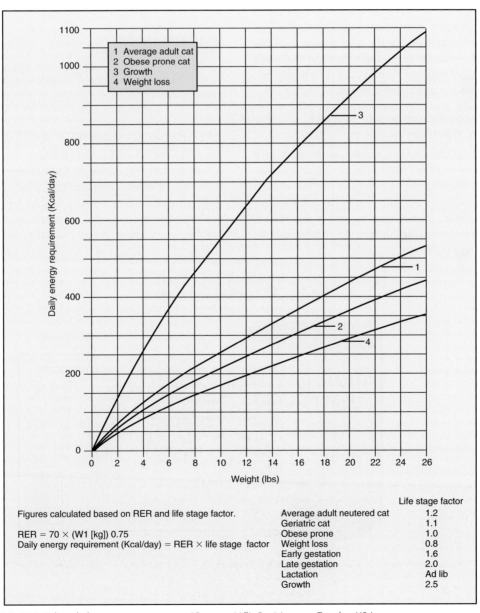

Figures calculated based on RER and life stage factor.

$RER = 70 \times (W1 \, [kg]) \, 0.75$
Daily energy requirement (Kcal/day) = RER × life stage factor

	Life stage factor
Average adult neutered cat	1.2
Geriatric cat	1.1
Obese prone	1.0
Weight loss	0.8
Early gestation	1.6
Late gestation	2.0
Lactation	Ad lib
Growth	2.5

FIGURE 7-7 Feline daily energy requirements. (Courtesy Hill's Pet Nutrition, Topeka, KS.)

Occasionally, clients inquire regarding their potential to produce a homemade diet. This presents a multifaceted dilemma because of the difficulty in maintaining balance from batch to batch. Most homemade diet recipes have not been analyzed for adequacy, possess ingredients that are often hard to come by, and are hard to reproduce consistently. Clients should be alerted to these concerns and be reminded of the reliability and convenience of many commercial pet foods available today.

Assessing pet food begins with making an overview of general considerations and then progressing to more specific evaluations as the diet continues to meet nutritional expectations. The following section is a review of common questions to assist in making effective comparisons and determinations of pet foods. It is essential to review the information available on a pet food label to determine its ability to meet the needs of pets during different stages of their lives. A review of information available on a pet food label is shown in Figure 7-8.

DETERMINING WHETHER A PET FOOD PRODUCES THE DESIRED RESULTS

Questions about fecal consistency, quality of product, and physiologic response to a diet from previous recommendations, which must be answered by assessment of clinical trials and experience, should also become part of the information retained at the veterinary clinic regarding diet comparisons. Keeping records of this valuable information is important so it can be referred to in the future.

Pet foods should also be tested by the AAFCO (Association of American Feed Control Officials; http://www.aafco.org). AAFCO provides a resource to formulate uniform and equitable regulations and policies. These laws apply to ingredient definitions, labeling, and feeding trials. Diets to be considered for veterinary clinic recommendation should be tested by AAFCO with approved feeding trials to substantiate adequacy regarding actual application of the diet to a particular species and life stage as it is intended to be fed.

HOW TO CHOOSE WHICH PET FOOD TO FEED

Decisions on feeding for pets must be based on activity level, breed, age, health status, and reproductive condition (spayed or neutered). Considerations must be made about what will provide the pet with a consistent, high-quality, balanced diet that produces the best results in the pet. Periodically a diet should be reevaluated to verify it's appropriateness for the pet and that the right amount is being fed.

DETERMINING WHETHER A PET SHOULD BE ALLOWED FREE FEEDING

Allowing pets free access to food at any time increases the incidence of excess caloric intake, which leads to obesity. In most situations, free feeding should be discouraged. Free feeding may be acceptable for cats that are able to maintain their weight without obesity, lactating females, and particularly fussy pets. The goal is to maintain optimal weight.

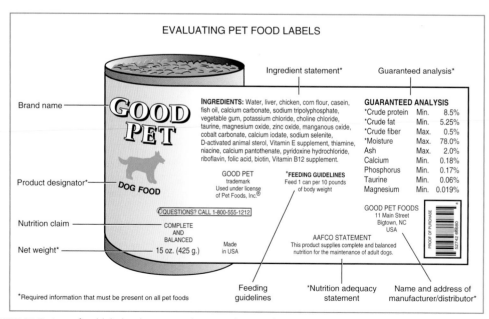

EVALUATING PET FOOD LABELS

Ingredient statement*   Guaranteed analysis*

Brand name

GOOD PET

DOG FOOD

Product designator*

INGREDIENTS: Water, liver, chicken, corn flour, casein, fish oil, calcium carbonate, sodium tripolyphosphate, vegetable gum, potassium chloride, choline chloride, taurine, magnesium oxide, zinc oxide, manganous oxide, cobalt carbonate, calcium iodate, sodium selenite, D-activated animal sterol, Vitamin E supplement, thiamine, niacine, calcium pantothenate, pyridoxine hydrochloride, riboflavin, folic acid, biotin, Vitamin B12 supplement.

GOOD PET
trademark
Used under license
of Pet Foods, Inc.®

*FEEDING GUIDELINES
Feed 1 can per 10 pounds
of body weight

GUARANTEED ANALYSIS		
*Crude protein	Min.	8.5%
*Crude fat	Min.	5.25%
*Crude fiber	Max.	0.5%
*Moisture	Max.	78.0%
Ash	Max.	2.0%
Calcium	Min.	0.18%
Phosphorus	Min.	0.17%
Taurine	Min.	0.06%
Magnesium	Min.	0.019%

©QUESTIONS? CALL 1-800-555-1212

Nutrition claim

COMPLETE
AND
BALANCED

Net weight*

15 oz. (425 g.)

Made
in USA

AAFCO STATEMENT
This product supplies complete and balanced
nutrition for the maintenance of adult dogs.

GOOD PET FOODS
11 Main Street
Bigtown, NC
USA

PROOF OF PURCHASE

Feeding
guidelines

*Nutrition adequacy
statement

Name and address of
manufacturer/distributor*

*Required information that must be present on all pet foods

FIGURE 7-8 A pet food label is the contract between the manufacturer and consumer. A label provides information required by law and may have optional information, such as a statement of calorie content, the universal product code, batch information, and/or a freshness date. (Courtesy Hill's Pet Nutrition, Topeka, KS.)

DETERMINING WHETHER IT IS BETTER TO FEED CANNED OR DRY FOOD

Although canned food has greater palatability, there are some concerns regarding dental health. For that purpose, dry food may be a better choice. Some pets that are finicky may find canned food to be their preference over dry food. If caloric intake falls in a pet, increasing palatability can assist in rectifying the situation. It is also important to rule out the presence of disease if a pet's feeding habits change. Palatability of a diet can be enhanced by warming canned food to body temperature or by adding warm water to dry food, as well as by using a small amount of fat or oil as a top dressing for dogs. Additional palatability factors are given in Box 7-7.

NUTRITIONAL SUPPORT
FOR ILL OR DEBILITATED PATIENTS

Proper nutritional support is an important aspect of therapy for hospitalized patients. Sick or injured patients need good nutritional support to counteract the immunosuppressive effects of sepsis, neoplasia, chemotherapy, anesthesia, and surgery. This support enhances wound healing and minimizes the length of hospitalization without significant weight loss and muscle atrophy. Initiation of nutritional support early in the course of hospitalization is crucial for a successful outcome.

Nutritional status should be assessed when the patient is admitted to the hospital and daily during hospitalization. During the physical examination, the patient's weight is recorded and compared with that of previous visits. A history from the owner regarding type of food, quantity fed, and frequency of feeding is helpful. During hospitalization, the patient is a candidate for nutritional support if the following occurs:

- The patient loses more than 10% of body weight.
- The patient has a decreased appetite or anorexia.
- The patient loses body condition from vomiting, diarrhea, trauma, or wounds.
- The patient has increased needs because of fever, sepsis, wounds, surgery, low serum albumin level, organ dysfunction, or chronic disease.

Unfortunately, nutritional support in hospitalized patients is often delayed because the patient is not reassessed daily for nutritional needs, the amount of food a patient consumes is not recorded, the patient is not weighed daily, and dextrose and electrolyte solutions are erroneously thought to provide

BOX 7-7	Palatability Factors

- Texture
- Odor
- Temperature
- Fat and protein levels
- Moisture content
- Shape of dry food (cats)
- Acidity (cats)

From Sirois M: Principles and practice of veterinary technology, ed 3, St Louis, 2011, Mosby.

adequate nutritional support. Most previously healthy dogs can go approximately 1 week without nutritional support and suffer few ill effects. Cats, however, especially overweight cats, can only go a few days without nutritional support before ill effects develop, such as hepatic lipidosis.

Nutritional support is often the last consideration when evaluating a patient's daily treatment regimen until the patient does not recover as quickly as expected. The goal of nutritional support is to provide the patient's nutritional requirements while it is recovering from its disease process and/or anorexia, trauma, or surgery until the patient is able to eat enough on a regular basis to accommodate any ongoing losses. With nutritional support, patients can gain weight and have an improved response to medical or surgical therapy.

> ### CRITICAL CONCEPT
> Parenteral nutritional support is used with patients that are unable to digest or absorb nutrients via the GI tract or have uncontrolled vomiting.

The route of nutritional support administration can be enteral, parenteral, or a combination of both. Enteral feeding may be accomplished with orogastric, nasogastric, nasoesophageal, pharyngostomy, gastrostomy, and jejunostomy tubes. Parenteral nutrition is administered via a catheter placed in the cranial or caudal vena cava.

The route selected depends on factors such as function of the GI tract, disease process, duration of support, equipment and personnel available to provide the necessary support, and cost of the chosen method. Enteral support is chosen most often because it is physiologically sound, easy, relatively free of complications, and inexpensive. If the GI tract is functional and the patient can swallow, use as much as possible. Parenteral support should be used if the patient has a medical or surgical condition that prevents ingestion or digestion of nutrients (e.g., vomiting, diarrhea, ileus, pancreatitis, malabsorption, reconstructive surgery, coma), and as adjunctive therapy for patients with organ failure or when malnutrition is severe.

ENTERAL NUTRITIONAL SUPPORT

Hand feeding favorite foods and tempting with warm, odoriferous foods in multiple, small meals can be used in conjunction with other methods of nutritional support. Forced feeding can be stressful to the patient and may deliver only a portion of the nutrition required for recovery.

Orogastric intubation is excellent for rapid administration but can cause aspiration and trauma and is stressful for patients other than neonates. This method is for short-term use only.

Placement of a nasoesophageal or nasogastric tube is an easy, simple, and relatively inexpensive procedure that allows liquid nutritional support for an extended time. It can be easily administered by the owner at home for continued convalescence (Box 7-8).

A nasoesophageal or nasogastric tube is placed through the nasal cavity into the distal esophagus or stomach to

BOX 7-8	Methods of Enteral Feeding

- Oral feeding (increased palatability)
- Oral feeding (forced feeding)
- Orogastric tube feeding
- Nasogastric tube feeding
- Pharyngostomy tube feeding
- Esophagostomy tube feeding
- Gastrostomy tube feeding
- Jejunostomy tube feeding

From Sirois M: Principles and practice of veterinary technology, ed 3, St Louis, 2011, Mosby.

bypass the oral cavity (Fig. 7-9). Placement is contraindicated in patients with nasal masses, esophageal disorders (e.g., megaesophagus), or no gag reflex. A nasoesophageal or nasogastric tube can usually be placed without chemical restraint, ideal for animals unable to tolerate general anesthesia. It is tolerated by most patients and used when the animal is anorexic, too stressed for forced feeding, and not receiving enough nutrition through hand feeding. The tube can remain in place for 1 week or longer until the patient's appetite increases or the oral cavity can be used again. Feedings through the tube can start immediately after placement, unlike pharyngostomy or gastrostomy tubes. Have the patient in a sitting position when tube feeding. Common problems with nasoesophageal or nasogastric tubes include epistaxis (nosebleed) when the tube is first placed, accidental placement in the trachea, patient intolerance of the tube, and tube obstruction by medications or diet.

Soft, flexible pediatric feeding tubes, red rubber tubes, and seamless polyurethane tubes in a variety of lengths and diameters are used for cats and dogs. Animals weighing less than 5 kg require a 5-Fr feeding tube, whereas some cats and all dogs weighing 5 to 15 kg can accept an 8-Fr tube. In larger dogs, the larger diameter feeding tubes require a guidewire for placement in the esophagus or stomach.

For nasoesophageal placement with the tube tip at the level of the midthoracic esophagus, measure from the tip of the nose to the eighth or ninth rib. For nasogastric placement, measure from the tip of the nose to the 13th rib to ensure safety in its position. Occasionally, tubes placed in the stomach may cause gastroesophageal reflux and irritation, but this is usually not a problem with a small-diameter tube. Mark the premeasured length on the tube with a permanent marker.

For nasoesophageal tube feeding, aspirate the tube before each feeding. If air is aspirated, do not feed. During aspiration, there should be negative pressure on the syringe if the tube is correctly placed. Accidental tracheal intubation can cause aspiration pneumonia. Before each feeding, also assess tube location by injecting 3 mL of sterile water through the tube and listening for coughing or gagging. If this occurs, do not administer the feeding; remove the tube.

A pharyngostomy tube is placed through the wall of the pharynx into the esophagus or stomach, bypassing the oral cavity. Placement requires general anesthesia and surgery. The many possible complications (e.g., esophagitis, pharyngitis, laryngitis,

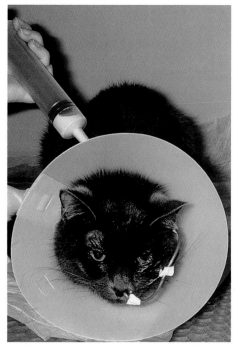

FIGURE 7-9 Nasoesophageal tube in place in a cat being fed a liquid enteral diet. (From Nelson RW, Couto G: Small animal internal medicine, ed 4, St Louis, 2009, Mosby.)

vomiting, regurgitation, aspiration pneumonia) and the difficulty of pharyngostomy tube placement outweigh the benefits.

A jejunostomy tube is a feeding tube surgically placed in the mid to distal duodenum or proximal jejunum, bypassing the stomach. Continuous feeding of easily digestible diets through the jejunostomy tube requires prolonged hospitalization, without the benefits of home care. This procedure is rarely used because of the cost of placement and maintenance and possible complications.

A gastrostomy or percutaneous endoscopic gastrostomy (PEG) tube is placed through the body wall into the lumen of the stomach, bypassing the mouth and esophagus. A gastrostomy tube is used for patients requiring long-term nutritional supplementation because of orofacial neoplasia, surgery or trauma, esophageal disorders, or liver disease. The diet can be easily prepared and administered by the owner, increasing owner compliance. The tube's bulb or mushroom tip helps retain the tube in the desired location (Fig. 7-10). Gastrostomy tubes can be placed with the use of endoscopic equipment (e.g., percutaneous endoscopic gastrostomy) or without endoscopic equipment (e.g., blind percutaneous gastrostomy). Placement requires general anesthesia and trained personnel.

ENTERAL NUTRITION DAILY CALORIC REQUIREMENTS. Diet selection is based on caloric density, diameter of the feeding tube, and daily caloric needs of the patient. Each illness is assigned a factor to increase the calculated estimate of the patient's basal energy requirements by 25% to 75%. The volume and consistency of the diet are limited by the size of the animal's stomach and diameter of the feeding tube, but total caloric requirements can usually be delivered when using a calorically dense diet. Stomach volume is approximately

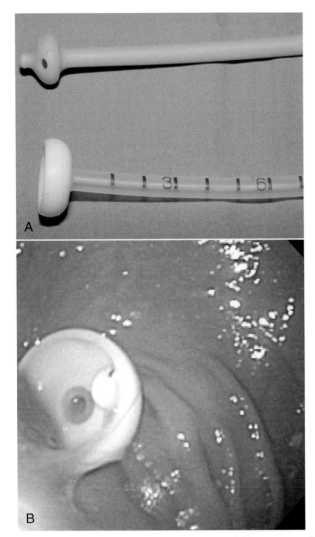

FIGURE 7-10 A, Typical gastrostomy tube available commercially. B, Endoscopic view of the PEG tube in place in the stomach wall. (From August J: Consultations in feline internal medicine, vol 5, St Louis, 2006, Saunders.)

BOX 7-9 | Enteral Feeding Calculation

- Calculate resting energy requirement (RER):

$$RER = 70 \times BW \text{ (body weight in kg)}$$

- Calculate illness/infection/injury energy requirements (IER):

$$Factor = 1.2 - 1.5$$

- Multiply chosen factor by RER to equal IER.
- Choose a veterinary-specific critical care formula.
- Calculate the volume of diet required and identify amount of kcal/mL:

$$\frac{IER}{\frac{kcal}{mL}} = mL \text{ of diet/day}$$

- Calculate the number and volume of feedings:

$$(mL \text{ of diet/day}) / (\text{number of feedings/day}) = mL \text{ diet/feeding}$$

From Sirois M: Principles and practice of veterinary technology, ed 3, St Louis, 2011, Mosby.

20 mL/kg body weight. Daily water requirement is 12 mL/kg body weight.

Patients with a nasoesophageal or nasogastric tube require a liquid diet because of the small tube diameter. Human enteral feeding products are easily administered through these tubes but are not developed for veterinary patients and may need supplementation with additional nutrients. Hyperosmolar diets can cause diarrhea. Liquid veterinary products are available. Canned diets, such as Hill's a/d and Eukanuba Nutritional Recovery Formula, can also be delivered through a feeding tube as small as 8-Fr.

Select the appropriate diet of canned food, and calculate the caloric density (kcal/mL) of the diet based on information on the label or supplied by the manufacturer. The total volume (mL) to be delivered daily is calculated by using the maintenance energy requirement (MER) and caloric density (Box 7-9).

For anorexic patients, after placement of the tube, the volume fed is gradually increased over 3 days, with 5 mL of water administered through the tube every 2 hours for 12 hours. Change to the selected diet and double the volume to

10 mL every 2 hours for 12 to 24 hours. Gradually increase the volume to achieve full caloric intake, divided into four to six feedings daily, by the third day. For patients with delayed or inadequate gastric emptying, a meal may need to be skipped or smaller, more frequent feedings administered if too much food remains in the stomach. If the patient vomits, skip the next scheduled feeding and adjust the amount, rate, and frequency of the feeding.

To prepare the diet using canned food, place one can of food in a blender and add enough water to achieve a consistency that will pass through a large-bore nasogastric tube or gastrostomy tube. You can also use dry food by allowing the food to soak thoroughly in water before blending. The mixture must be blended well and then strained twice to remove any large chunks that would occlude the feeding tube. All food should be able to pass through a syringe without occluding the tip. For example, one can of Hill's Feline p/d mixed with 340 mL of warm water is the proper consistency to pass through the feeding tube; it has a caloric density of 0.8 kcal/mL.

The volume of water added to the canned food when blended is usually adequate for the patient's water requirement. All feedings should be administered slowly, at room temperature. Hill's a/d and Iams Eukanuba Nutritional Recovery Formula can be given straight out of the can through an 8-Fr feeding tube, at room temperature or slightly warmed, with no premixing with water. Hill's a/d provides 1.2 kcal/mL, and the Nutritional Recovery Formula provides 2.1 kcal/mL. If a smaller-diameter tube is used, mixing two 5.5-oz. cans of Hill's a/d with 50 mL of water provides a caloric density of 1.0 kcal/mL. Flush the tube with 5 or 10 mL of water after each feeding to prevent tube occlusion.

Animals with feeding tubes in place should be offered fresh food before each feeding once the oral cavity and esophagus can be used. Most animals begin to eat with the feeding tube still in place. When the animal begins voluntarily to eat at least half of its maintenance energy requirement daily, the amount of food given through the feeding tube can be decreased until the patient is consuming its full caloric intake PO. The change from enteral feedings to the normal diet should be gradual, over 3 to 5 days, if the patient's normal diet is not used for enteral feedings.

Clients can be instructed on how to feed their animal through the tube at home, if necessary. Ease of administration, minimal maintenance, and owner compliance makes this method of nutritional support a viable alternative for patient care in a nonhospital situation.

PARENTERAL NUTRITIONAL SUPPORT

Patients that cannot receive enteral nutrients must be supported by total parenteral nutrition (TPN), which involves IV infusion of nutrient solutions. This is a practical alternative for patients that cannot absorb nutrients through the GI tract (e.g., malabsorption), require rest of the GI tract (e.g., vomiting because of severe pancreatitis), cannot swallow (e.g., comatose patients), or are so debilitated that additional nutrition must be administered by another route.

Carbohydrates are administered in the form of dextrose. The most common concentration used is 50% dextrose, which provides 1.7 kcal/mL. Dextrose and lipids each provide 50% of the canine patient's daily MER. Dextrose and lipids are used in a 1:1 ratio to meet the MER.

Gradual introduction of dextrose is necessary to avoid hyperglycemia. On the first day of TPN, only half the calculated amount of dextrose is administered. If the patient's urine glucose remains negative and the blood glucose level is below 200 mg/dL, the entire calculated dose of dextrose can be administered on day 2. Occasionally, a patient requires the addition of insulin to the TPN solution. This should be added immediately, before administration of the parenteral nutrition.

Lipids, including essential fatty acids, provide the fat required by the patient. These are available in 10% and 20% solutions, with 20% used more commonly. Made of soybean or safflower oil, egg yolk phospholipids, and glycerol, they provide a concentrated energy source that supplies 50% of the patient's energy requirements. Visually checking the patient's plasma for lipemia on a daily basis can help decrease hyperlipidemia. Patients with hepatic, pancreatic, or endocrine disease may develop hyperlipidemia. For patients with severe hyperlipidemia, decrease the rate of infusion or the concentration of the lipids, or discontinue the use of lipids altogether.

Proteins are supplied in the form of crystalline amino acids, made of essential and nonessential amino acids, available in a variety of concentrations, with or without electrolytes. The most common concentration used is 8.5% with electrolytes. The basic solutions of amino acids contain all the essential amino acids required by dogs and cats, except taurine. If TPN is to be continued for longer than 1 week, supplementation of taurine is essential in cats. For patients with renal or hepatic insufficiency, reduced amounts of amino acids or specially formulated amino acid products should be administered.

Electrolytes can be included in the amino acid solutions. This is usually sufficient to maintain a normal electrolyte balance. Hypokalemia is the most common electrolyte abnormality. For patients with ongoing potassium losses (e.g., because of vomiting), additional supplementation may be necessary. If the patient is in renal failure, amino acids are administered without electrolytes.

Vitamins are administered as a multivitamin supplement. B complex vitamins should be added daily to the feeding solution. Vitamin K is incompatible with parenteral solutions and should be administered by subcutaneous or intramuscular injection only if parenteral nutrition is continued longer than 1 week.

Trace elements only need to be supplemented if long-term (>1 week) parenteral nutritional support is needed. Zinc may need to be supplemented after 1 week in patients with GI disease. Phosphorus may be added for diabetics.

The total daily fluid volume for maintenance TPN is 30 mL/lb of body weight. If the total volume of TPN is less than the calculated required amount, add an additional amount of balanced electrolyte solution or sterile water to equal the calculated fluid requirements. If the patient is experiencing ongoing fluid losses, a second catheter, or an additional lumen on a central catheter, can be used to deliver the fluids.

When mixing the appropriate solutions, strict asepsis is essential. Using a laminar flow hood, an automatic mixing pump, or a so-called all-in-one bag will help keep contamination to a minimum. Add the dextrose and amino acids before the lipids to prevent lipid destabilization. Add the water or electrolyte solutions next, and any vitamins last.

Parenteral nutrition is administered via a catheter in the cranial or caudal vena cava. A double-lumen catheter is of benefit if additional medication, fluids, blood products, or blood sampling is needed. Administration by a fluid pump is the most accurate method of delivering parenteral nutrition.

Many complications of parenteral nutrition involve problems with the catheter. Sepsis is another complication of parenteral nutrition. Nutrient solutions are an excellent growth medium for bacteria. Contamination of the solutions, lines, or catheters can cause fever, depression, and pain or swelling at the catheter insertion site. Daily patient monitoring can help eliminate or minimize this complication. Administering TPN through a dedicated IV line can decrease the likelihood of sepsis. The catheter should be used for parenteral nutrition only and not for blood sampling, medication administration, or central venous pressure (CVP) monitoring. New bags of TPN solution should be made daily for the patient and hung for a maximum of 24 hours at room temperature before changing to another bag. All administration lines should be changed every 48 hours when the bag is changed. The catheter bandage should be replaced whenever it is soiled, as well as every 48 hours, when the administration lines are changed.

Gradually tapering of TPN can prevent hypoglycemia. If TPN must be discontinued abruptly, use a 5% dextrose solution to maintain blood glucose levels. Patients on TPN longer than 1 week may develop intestinal villous atrophy. Partial parenteral nutrition in conjunction with enteral nutrition may be advised when parenteral nutrition is being withdrawn. Care must be taken when changing from one diet to another; the transition should be gradual. Table 7-2

TABLE 7-2 | Summary of Small Animal Clinical Nutrition*

OBJECTIVES	CONSIDERATIONS	PRODUCT†	COMMENTS
Allergy, Food			
Dogs			
Reduce antigen ingestion.	Novel highly digestible protein source or protein hydrolysate Reduce total protein content. Simplify food. Distilled H_2O	Hill's Prescription Diet—Canine d/d or Canine z/d	8- to 10-wk trial period Avoid treats, snacks, access to other food sources, chewable medications, supplements.
Cats			
Reduce antigen ingestion.	Same as dog except control Mg^{2+} intake. Provide taurine. Control urine pH.	Hill's Prescription Diet—Feline d/d or Feline z/d	
Anemia			
Support RBC production.	↑ Iron, cobalt, and copper ↑ B complex vitamins ↑ Protein	Hill's Prescription Diet—Canine p/d Feline p/d	
Anorexia			
Prevent protein and caloric malnutrition. Stimulate appetite.	Establish fluid-electrolyte balance and acid-base balance. ↑ Protein and fat ↑ Micronutrients	Hill's Prescription Diet—Feline, Canine a/d, Canine p/d, Feline p/d	Cat foods are suitable for dogs in acute care settings.
Ascites			
Reduce fluid retention.	Restrict sodium chloride. Maintain hydration.	Hill's Prescription Diet—Canine h/d, k/d; Feline h/d, k/d	h/d = marked salt restriction k/d = moderate salt restriction
Bone Loss And Fracture Healing			
Correct deficiency of energy and protein.	↑ Protein ↑ Energy Avoid supplementation.	Hill's Prescription Diet—Canine p/d, Feline p/d	Extra dietary calcium does not increase rate of fracture healing.
Cancer			
Increase longevity and quality of life.	↓ Soluble carbohydrate ↑ Fat and n-3 fatty acids ↑ Arginine	Hill's Prescription Diet—Canine n/d, Canine/Feline a/d	Use in conjunction with chemotherapy or other forms of cancer therapy.
Colitis			
Normalize gastrointestinal motility. Rebalance microflora. Provide local healing factors.	Feed small meals three to six times/day. Control dietary antigens. Vary levels of dietary fiber.	Hill's Prescription Diet—Canine w/d, i/d, d/d; Feline w/d, d/d	
Constipation			
Normalize gastrointestinal motility. Maintain stool water. Maintain stool bulk.	>10% fiber	Hill's Prescription Diet—Canine w/d, Feline w/d	No table scraps or bones Increase exercise. Encourage water intake. Cats: keep litter box clean.
Copper Storage Disease			
Restrict copper intake.	<1.2 mg copper/100 g dry diet	Hill's Prescription Diet—Canine l/d	No table scraps or treats
Debilitation			
Restore tissue, plasma, and nutrients.	↑ Protein ↑ Fat ↑ Macronutrients and micronutrients	Hill's Prescription Diet—Canine a/d, Feline a/d	Assist feed if needed.

Continued

TABLE 7-2	Summary of Small Animal Clinical Nutrition*—cont'd		
OBJECTIVES	**CONSIDERATIONS**	**PRODUCT†**	**COMMENTS**
Developmental Orthopedic Disease			
Reduce rapid growth.	↓ Fat and energy density ↓ Calcium	Hill's Prescription Diet—Canine p/d, large breed	Avoid calcium-phosphorus supplements.
Diabetes Mellitus			
Even rate of glucose absorption. Provide consistent caloric intake.	>10% fiber ↓ Soluble carbohydrates	Hill's Prescription Diet—Canine w/d, Feline w/d	Weigh animal frequently and note in medical record.
Diarrhea, Acute			
Normalize GI tract motility and secretion.	Withhold food for 1-2 days. Feed small amounts three to six times/day. ↓ Fiber ↓ Sugar ↑ Digestibility	Hill's Prescription Diet—Canine i/d Feline i/d	Electrolyte disturbances and dehydration are common.
Eclampsia			
Provide Ca and P in correct quantity and ratio prepartum.	High digestibility of diet Balanced minerals, vitamins	Hill's Prescription Diet—Canine p/d Feline p/d	Avoid supplementation.
Flatulence			
Decrease aerophagia. Avoid food fermentation.	Avoid milk or milk products. Feed small meals three to six times/day. ↑ Caloric density	Hill's Prescription Diet—Canine i/d, Feline i/d	Feed in a flat, open dish. Avoid vitamin or fatty acid supplementation. Separate competitive eaters.
Gastric Dilation and Bloat (Postoperative)			
Prevent gastric distention.	Avoid exercise before and after feeding. ↑ Digestibility of diet Small frequent feedings	Hill's Prescription Diet—Canine i/d	Diet form or type is *not* related to risk of occurrence or recurrence.
Heart Failure			
Dogs			
Control Na⁺ retention.	↓ Na⁺ intake Maintain energy and protein intake. ↑ B-complex vitamins ↓ Na⁺ intake	Hill's Prescription Diet—Canine h/d, Canine k/d	Hill's Prescription Diet—k/d has moderate Na⁺ restriction.
Cats			
Control Na⁺ retention.	↑ Taurine Control Mg²⁺ levels.	Hill's Prescription Diet—Feline h/d, Feline k/d	Avoid high-Na⁺ treats and water.
Hyperlipidemia			
Control fat intake.	↑ Fiber intake ↓ Fat intake	Hill's Prescription Diet—Canine w/d, Feline w/d	Common in Schnauzers Consider fat in treats, table foods, and supplements.
Hyperthyroidism (Cats)			
Support increased energy need.	↑ Energy intake ↑ Vitamins and minerals ↑ Protein	Hill's Prescription Diet—Feline a/d	Monitor for evidence of concurrent renal disease.

TABLE 7-2	Summary of Small Animal Clinical Nutrition*—cont'd		
OBJECTIVES	CONSIDERATIONS	PRODUCT†	COMMENTS
Liver Disease (Fat-Tolerant)			
Reduce protein metabolism. Maintain liver glycogen. Prevent ammonia toxicity.	↑ Digestible energy Protein restriction High–biologic value proteins Control Na^+ intake.	Hill's Prescription Diet—Canine l/d, Feline l/d	May feed small meals (four to six times/day)
Lymphangiectasia			
Decrease dietary fat.	↓ Intake of long-chain triglycerides Control protein levels. Consider medium-chain triglycerides.	Hill's Prescription Diet—Canine w/d or r/d	Medium-chain triglyceride oils and powder can increase caloric density.
Obesity			
Maintain intake of all nutrients except energy.	↓ Energy digestibility Replace digestible calories with indigestible fiber. Increase bulk to control hunger. Add carnitine.	Hill's Prescription Diet—Canine r/d, Feline r/d	Requires professional advice and teamwork with veterinary technician and client.
Oral Disease: Gingivitis (Gum Inflammation), Periodontitis (Loss of Tooth Attachment)			
Control accumulation of plaque, stains, and calculus. Maintain gingival health.	Provide food that promotes chewing and mechanical cleansing of teeth.	Hill's Prescription Diet—Canine t/d, Feline t/d	Many treats make dental claims but are not effective.
Pancreatitis, Acute (Recovery Phase)			
Control pancreatic secretions.	↓ Fat ↑ Digestibility Feed small meals three to six times/day	Hill's Prescription Diet—Canine i/d, Feline i/d	Frequent, small meals
Pancreatic Exocrine Insufficiency			
Reduce requirements for digestive enzymes.	↓ Fiber ↓ Fat Highly digestible carbohydrates ↑ Caloric density	Hill's Prescription Diet—Canine i/d, Feline i/d	Pancreatic enzymes complement highly digestible food.
Renal Failure			
Reduce signs of uremia. Slow progression of disease.	↓ Protein (↑ biologic value of protein) ↑ Nonprotein calories ↓ Phosphorus and sodium ↑ B complex vitamins	Hill's Prescription Diet—Canine k/d, Canine g/d, Canine u/d Hill's Prescription Diet—Feline k/d, Feline g/d	Small meals four to six times/day Conversion to a protein-restricted diet may take 7-10 days. Water available at all times
Canine Urolithiasis (Struvite)			
Treatment			
Urine volume Urine pH Restrict Mg^{2+}, NH_4^+, and PO_4.	↓ Protein ↓ PO_4, Mg^{2+} ↑ $Na+$ ↓ Urine pH (5.9-6.1)	Hill's Prescription Diet—Canine s/d	Evaluate and treat urinary tract infection. Average duration of stone dissolution is 36 days; follow up via radiography.
Prevention			
Maintain physiologic level of urinary solutes and urine pH.	Control protein excess. ↓ Ca^{2+}, P, Ma^{2+} ↓ Sodium mildly ↓ Urine pH (6.2-6.4)	Hill's Prescription Diet—Canine c/d	Monitor urine sediment for crystalluria and infection.

Continued

TABLE 7-2	Summary of Small Animal Clinical Nutrition*—cont'd		
OBJECTIVES	**CONSIDERATIONS**	**PRODUCT**[†]	**COMMENTS**
Canine Urolithiasis (Ammonium Urate)			
Prevention			
	↓ Protein ↑ Nonprotein calories ↓ Nucleic acids ↓ Ca^{2+}, P, Mg^{2+}, Na^+ Urine pH (6.7-7.0)	Hill's Prescription Diet—Canine u/d	Drugs plus diet may be successful treatment. Monitor urinary crystalluria. Prevention may require long-term drug treatment.
Canine Urolithiasis (Calcium Oxalate and Cystine)			
Prevention			
↓ Urinary concentration of calcium oxalate or cystine	↓ Protein ↑ Nonprotein calories ↓ Ca^{2+}, P, Na^+, Mg $^{2+}$ ↑ Urine pH (6.1-7.0)	Hill's Prescription Diet—Canine u/d	Treat by surgical removal. Prevent by dietary management ± drugs.
Feline Urolithiasis (Struvite)			
Treatment			
↑ Urine volume ↓ Urine pH (5.9-6.1) Restrict Mg^{2+}, Ca^{2+}, and PO_4.	↑ Caloric density ↓ P and Ca^{2+} Mg^{2+} > 20 mg/100 kcal ↑ Na^+ Urine pH (6.2-6.4)	Hill's Prescription Diet—Feline s/d	Dissolution is complete 1 mo after negative x-rays. Recurrence is high if prevention is not implemented.
Prevention			
Maintain physiologic levels of urinary solutes and urine pH.	Mg^{2+} > 20 mg/100 kcal (0.1% DMB) ↓ P ↑ Caloric density Urine pH (6.2-6.4)	Hill's Prescription Diet—Feline c/d-s	For obesity, use calorie-restricted diets that maintain urine pH at 6.2-6.4 (Hill's Prescription Diet w/d is suggested).
Feline Urolithiasis (Calcium Oxalate)			
Prevention			
↑ Urine volume ↓ Urinary Ca^{2+}, oxalate ↑ Urine pH	↓ Protein ↑ Nonprotein calories ↓ P, Ca^{2+}, Na^+ Mg^{2+} < 20 mg/100 kcal	Hill's Prescription Diet—Feline c/d-oxl	Monitor urinary crystalluria.
Vomiting			
Minimize gastric secretion. Provide GI rest.	↑ Digestibility ↑ Caloric density	Hill's Prescription Diet—Canine i/d, Feline i/d	Frequent, small meals

Ca, Calcium; *DMB*, dry matter basis; *Mg*, magnesium; *Na*, sodium; NH_4, ammonium; *P*, phosphorus; PO_4, phosphate; *RBC*, red blood cells.
*Nutrients in table are expressed on a dry weight basis.
[†]Other North American therapeutic brands with wide distribution include the following CNM (Purina); VMD, Medi-Cal, and IVD Select Care (Heinz); Eukanuba Veterinary Diets (Iams); and Waltham Veterinary Diets (Mars).
From Sirois M: Principles and practice of veterinary technology, ed 3, St Louis, 2011, Mosby.

summarizes the nutritional requirements of pets with various diseases.

COMMON DISEASES

Disease is any alteration from the normal state of health. Disease may range from a superficial skin laceration to widely disseminated metastatic neoplasia—malignant tumors spread to many different organs. A pathologist is one who studies diseases and often is responsible for accurate diagnosis, as well as determining the cause of those diseases.

Pathologists are trained in different areas of expertise, including anatomic **pathology** or clinical pathology. A veterinary pathologist is a specialist who, after receiving an advanced degree in veterinary pathology, works in a veterinary school, state diagnostic laboratory, or pharmaceutical company.

The primary responsibility of a veterinary anatomic pathologist is the prosection (dissection) of cadavers (carcasses) presented for **necropsy**, which is analogous to an autopsy in humans. During necropsy, the pathologist collects tissue sections from lesions, which are grossly observable diseased tissues, and examines them with a microscope. Evaluating tissues with a microscope is termed histopathology. The study of causes of disease, or sometimes the causes themselves, is referred to as the **etiology**. Histopathology may allow the pathologist insight into the cause and prognosis of the disease. The prognosis is the expected outcome of the patient affected by the disease and is usually stated as good, guarded, or poor. Veterinary anatomic pathologists also evaluate tissues that have been surgically removed by the veterinarian. Thus, these tissues are often referred to as surgical biopsies.

Veterinary clinical pathologists evaluate components of the blood as well as types of body fluids, such as transudates and exudates. These provide valuable information regarding the causes and prognoses of diseases.

TERMINOLOGY

Pathologists use specific terms to describe the lesions observed at necropsy and with the microscope. Gross lesions are described by stating the location, color, size, texture, and appearance of the altered tissue. The diagnosis may be a morphologic (anatomic) diagnosis or an etiologic (causative) diagnosis. The morphologic diagnosis is usually limited to describing the lesion within that organ system. An example of a morphologic diagnosis is "acute necrotizing enteritis," which states that the intestine is inflamed and necrotic and that it occurred very suddenly. The corresponding etiologic diagnosis may be "enteric salmonellosis," which means that the animal had the intestinal form of infection with *Salmonella* bacteria. Other bacterial and viral agents may also cause the lesions described in the morphologic diagnosis, so acute necrotizing enteritis does not always indicate a specific diagnosis of enteric salmonellosis.

FEVER, INFLAMMATION, AND RESPONSE TO INJURY

Fever and inflammation are protective responses of the animal's body to fight infection resulting from pathogens (disease-causing agents). Pathogens include viruses, bacteria, parasites, fungi, and molds. Pathogens are described in more detail later in the chapter.

> **CRITICAL CONCEPT**
> Pyrogens are agents that cause an abnormal increase in body temperature.

Fever, also called pyrexia, is an abnormal increase in body temperature caused by the release of agents, called **pyrogens**, within the body. Pyrogens can be thought of as substances that cause the body to adjust its biologic thermostat to a higher setting. This differs from hyperthermia, in which the body temperature increases above the body's thermostat setting because of such things as drugs, toxins, or external temperatures, as in heat stroke. Many pyrogens are released by the body's own immune cells when they encounter pathogens; however, some pathogens also produce substances that act as pyrogens.

BOX 7-10	Signs of Inflammation

Heat
Swelling
Pain
Redness
Loss of function

SIGNS OF INFLAMMATION

The five cardinal signs of inflammation are heat, redness, swelling, pain, and loss of function (Box 7-10). These signs result from complex interactions between the cells and fluids in the involved area. The cells involved in the inflammatory process are the leukocytes (white blood cells). Blood vessels are highly dynamic structures that respond rapidly during inflammation. The first response of the blood vessel to vascular injury is dilation, which means the diameter of the blood vessel increases, allowing more blood to flow into the affected area. Next, there is increased vascular permeability, which means that the blood vessels become slightly leaky. Increased vascular permeability allows a wide array of proteins to pass through the vessel walls to the site of inflammation. Immediately after vascular permeability increases, the process of exudation allows an influx of leukocytes and red blood cells to the inflammatory site. Congestion of the blood vessels occurs in the next step, which means stasis or sludging of blood flow in the vessels from fluid loss through exudation.

All these events work in concert with the cells associated with inflammation so that the host is able to repair the injured site and defend itself against infection. The entire process occurs rapidly, beginning with vascular dilation, which occurs within minutes of the initial insult, and ending with the initiation of congestion within 8 hours of the initial vascular dilation.

HEALING AND REPAIR OF DAMAGED TISSUES

The repair process really starts as soon as injury occurs, but healing is the last event to be completed in the inflammatory process. In almost every organ system, the end result of tissue repair is **fibrosis**, or scarring. The exception to this is in the central nervous system, which includes the brain and spinal cord. Fibrosis does not occur in the central nervous system because it would be detrimental to the functioning of these vital tissues. Repair can take place by first- or second-intention healing of a wound. A **wound** is an injury caused by physical means, with disruption of normal structures.

> **CRITICAL CONCEPT**
> The end result of tissue repair is usually fibrosis or scarring.

First-intention healing occurs when the edges of the wound surfaces close together with no discernible scarring. This type of healing generally occurs when the edges of a fresh wound are evenly opposed with the aid of a bandage, sutures, or skin staples. Second-intention healing repairs wounds involving much greater tissue damage. Second-intention healing produces much more granulation tissue. **Granulation tissue** is a highly vascularized connective tissue that is only produced after extensive tissue damage (Fig. 7-11).

PATHOGENS

Pathogens are infectious organisms that can cause disease in a host. Pathogenic agents include multicelled and single-celled parasites, protozoans, bacteria, fungi, rickettsiae, mycoplasmas, chlamydiae, and viruses. Many of these organisms are specific in their ability to cause disease, affecting only certain animal species. In some cases, they affect specific organs or organ systems of the body.

PARASITES

Parasites are organisms that have adapted to live on or within a host organism, deriving all their nutrients from that host, ideally without killing the host. Nomenclature can be confusing because all the pathogens described in the preceding section may live on or in a host organism, from which they derive a benefit whereas the host may experience disease. However, we generally use the word parasite only in conjunction with multicelled organisms such as worms, flukes, and arthropods, or single-celled protozoans; we tend to classify bacteria, fungi, rickettsiae, mycoplasmas, chlamydiae, and viruses separately.

BACTERIA

Bacteria make up another group of pathogens that cause disease in animals. Bacteria are single-celled organisms referred to as prokaryotes because they lack a nucleus and organelles and their DNA consists of one double-stranded chromosome. Most bacteria have a cell wall outside their cell membrane, as do plant and fungal eukaryotic cells, although composed of different materials. It is the staining characteristics of this cell wall that form two major classifications

of bacteria. Bacteria are classified as gram positive or gram negative, depending on the staining characteristics of their cell walls with Gram stain. Gram-positive organisms stain purple, and gram-negative organisms stain red.

VIRUSES

Viruses are extremely small infectious agents that can cause disease in a wide variety of animals. For viruses to cause disease, they must enter the animal's body, bind to the surface of a host cell, enter the cell, and destroy it. Viruses are technically nonliving agents, which consist of genetic material in the form of DNA or RNA surrounded by a protein coat, called a **capsid**. Some viruses may have an envelope, derived in part from the host cell membrane, which surrounds the protein coat. After the virus enters a host cell, it uses the host cell's machinery to transcribe, translate, and replicate the viral genetic material, thereby creating new viral proteins and new viruses. Viruses can destroy the cells by suppressing the cells' metabolic activity or causing them to lyse, releasing the newly formed viruses. In some cases, viruses may cause no immediate damage and may remain latent in cells for years.

As is the case with parasites and bacteria, a large number of viruses can infect animals.

NONPATHOGENS

Disease can also be produced in animals by nonpathogens. Nonpathogenic causes of disease include trauma associated with mechanical, sonic, thermal, and electrical injuries, temperature extremes, and irradiation.

The primary effects of trauma, regardless of the initiating cause, are tissue necrosis and hemorrhage. Trauma is a physical wound or injury. Internal, localized mechanical injury can be associated, for example, with intestinal foreign bodies, which can cause necrosis by strangulating blood supply to the intestines. An abrasion is an injury whereby the epithelium is removed from the tissue surface. A **contusion** is a bruise or injury with no break in the surface of the tissue. A **laceration** is a tear or jagged wound. A **concussion** is a violent shock or jarring of the tissue, a common injury to the brain after blunt trauma to the head. In all these cases, the inflammatory process occurs as described earlier, with the exception of the destruction and removal of the pathogen.

IMMUNE RESPONSE

The immune system is another inherent protective mechanism of the body. This highly complex and complicated system has many components that, along with the inflammatory process, prevent pathogens from causing disease. The immune system consists of nonspecific and specific defenses. Nonspecific defenses include the body's defenses against pathogens in general, regardless of pathogen type. These include mechanical barriers to infection such as skin and mucous membranes, chemical barriers such as lysozymes in tears, salt in sweat, antiviral substances such as interferon in blood, and acid in the stomach. Fever and inflammation,

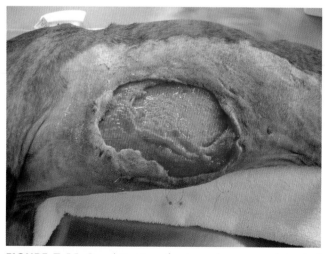

FIGURE 7-11 Granulation tissue forming under an area of sloughed skin on a dog's abdomen. (From Sirois M: *Principles and practice of veterinary technology*, ed 3, St Louis, 2011, Mosby.)

discussed earlier, are also part of the nonspecific defenses. Specific defenses comprise what is normally thought of as immunity, the body's protection against specific pathogens. Specific defenses include antibodies and a number of other cells and biochemicals that work together to protect an animal from disease.

ZOONOTIC DISEASES

Zoonoses are the major area of involvement for veterinarians in **public health**. Zoonoses are diseases transmitted between animals and people; however, this definition is not always clear-cut. Some diseases are indirect zoonoses and can be transmitted to animals and humans, and between species, by arthropods such as ticks or mosquitoes. Still other infectious diseases are common to but not transmitted between animals and people; these can be caused by similar exposures to the same infectious organism. More than 150 zoonoses have been reported, and diseases not previously thought to be zoonotic are frequently added to the list. For example, *Bordetella bronchiseptica,* one of the pathogens associated with the canine infectious respiratory disease (CIRD) complex, also known as kennel cough, was previously not though to be zoonotic; however, it has recently been discovered to be transmissible to humans. Zoonoses are a significant cause of human disability, hospitalization, death, and high economic cost in the United States and underdeveloped countries. Table 7-3 lists the causative organism, hosts, and mode of transmission for some common zoonoses.

DISEASE TRANSMISSION

For an infectious disease to survive in a population, the agent causing the disease must be transmitted. The mode of transmission is an important epidemiologic clue for understanding the disease. It is important for the veterinary profession to be aware of how specific diseases are transmitted so that preventive measures can be taken and the public educated. Reservoirs and hosts of a specific disease are important to identify because these are essential for the transmission of a disease and its maintenance in the population. Control programs for a disease are often aimed at the **reservoirs**, or hosts of the disease. For example, spraying programs aimed at controlling mosquito populations are initiated when there is an outbreak of encephalitis.

> ### CRITICAL CONCEPT
> Diseases can be transmitted via the direct or indirect route.

Reservoirs can be inanimate (e.g., soil) or animate (e.g., animals, people, birds). Reservoirs are essential and necessary for the survival and reproduction of the organism. Hosts are living beings that offer an environment for maintenance of the organism, but they are not necessary for the organism's survival. Depending on the disease, the infectious organism may be transmitted through several hosts of different species. Direct transmission of disease requires close association or contact between a reservoir of the disease and a susceptible host. Contact with infected skin, mucous membranes, or droplets from an infected human or animal can cause disease. Examples of disease that are transmitted directly are rabies transmitted by a bite, leptospirosis by contact with contaminated urine, and brucellosis by contact with infected tissues.

Animal bites can be a source of infections, trauma, and even zoonotic disease. *Pasteurella* is responsible for 50% of dog bite infections and 90% of cat bite infections. Cat bites are 10 times more likely to become infected than dog bites. Soil or vegetation contaminated with parasites, bacteria, or spores may be another source of direct transmission. Visceral larval migrans is transmitted when children eat soil or vegetables that have been contaminated with feces that contain *Toxocara canis* or *T. cati* (roundworm) eggs. The eggs hatch in the individual's gastrointestinal system, and the larvae migrate through the organs. A similar disease occurs with *Ancylostoma* spp. (hookworm). The signs of cutaneous larval migrans are those of dermatitis, which is caused by the hookworm larvae migrating in the skin.

Indirect transmission of disease is more complicated and involves intermediaries that carry the agent of disease from one source to another. The intermediary may be airborne, vector-borne (an arthropod), or vehicle-borne through water, food, blood, or an inanimate object. A vector is a living organism that transports the infectious agent. A vehicle is simply the mode of transmission of an infectious agent from the reservoir to the host. Indirect airborne transmission involves spread of the agent through tiny dust or droplet particles over long distances. Droplet spread is differentiated from airborne transmission by the fact that the droplets travel only a short distance (i.e., a few feet) and involve larger particles that often are removed by mechanisms in the upper respiratory passages. Various types of arthropods may serve as vectors of disease; these may include mosquitoes, ticks, and fleas. Each type of arthropod has its own life cycle, which is often reflected by seasonal and geographic patterns in transmission of disease. Arthropods may carry the agent mechanically to a susceptible host or may be involved biologically in multiplication of the organism or stage of development.

Food and water are also vehicles of indirect transmission of disease. Both are sources of bacterial, viral, and parasitic diseases. Foodborne diseases are acquired by consumption of contaminated food or water and include foodborne intoxications and foodborne infections. Foodborne intoxications are caused by toxins produced by certain bacteria that may contaminate food, such as *Staphylococcus aureus*. The toxins may be present in the food or may be formed in the intestinal tract after the contaminated food is eaten. Foodborne infections are caused by bacterial or viral organisms that cause infection. These include *Salmonella* spp., *Campylobacter* spp., hepatitis virus, and *Vibrio* spp. Each organism also causes certain clinical signs, such as diarrhea, vomiting, or nausea. These specific incubation periods and particular clinical signs help epidemiologists determine the organism's identity and source.

TABLE 7-3 Causative Organisms, Animal Hosts, and Modes of Transmission for Selected Common Zoonoses

| | | HOSTS | | |
DISEASE	CAUSATIVE ORGANISM	SMALL ANIMALS	WILDLIFE	MODES OF TRANSMISSION
Viral Diseases				
Rabies	Rhabdovirus	Most	Most	Animal bite
Encephalitis (eastern equine encephalitis [EEE], western equine encephalitis [WEE])	Togavirus		Birds, rodents	Mosquito bite
Lymphocytic choriomeningitis	Arenavirus	Mice		Varied
Contagious ecthyma (orf)	Poxvirus	Sometimes dogs		Contact
Simian herpes (B virus)	*Herpesvirus simiae*		Primates	Animal bite, direct contact
Newcastle disease	Paramyxovirus	Domestic birds	Wild fowl	Contact, inhalation
Yellow fever	Togavirus		Primates	Mosquito bite
Hantavirus infection	Hantavirus		Rodents	Contact
Rickettsial Diseases				
Q fever	*Coxiella burnetii*		Birds, rabbits, rodents	Inhalation, milk ingestion, contact
Rocky Mountain spotted fever	*Rickettsia rickettsii*	Dogs	Rodents, rabbits	Tick bite
Psittacosis	*Chlamydia psittaci*	Psittacine birds	Birds	Inhalation
Mycoses				
Ringworm	*Trichophyton* spp., *Microsporum* spp.	Cats, dogs	Rodents	Contact
Parasitic Diseases				
Trichinosis	*Trichinella spiralis*		Rats, bears, carnivores	Ingestion
Scabies	*Sarcoptes scabiei*	Dogs, rodents, cats	Primates	Contact
Taeniasis, cysticercosis	*Taenia* spp., *Cysticercus*		Boars	Ingestion
Hydatid disease	*Echinococcus* spp.	Dogs	Wolves	Ingestion
Schistosomiasis	*Schistosoma* spp.	Dogs, cats	Rodents	Contact
Larva migrans	*Toxocara, Ancylostoma, Strongyloides*	Dogs, cats	Raccoons	Ingestion
Bacterial Diseases				
Anthrax	*Bacillus anthracis*	Dogs	Most, except primates	Contact
Brucellosis	*Brucella* spp.	Dogs	All, except primates	Contact, inhalation, ingestion
Plague	*Yersinia pestis*	Cats	Rodents, rabbits	Flea bite
Campylobacteriosis	*Campylobacter fetus*	Dogs, cats	Rodents, birds	Ingestion, contact
Cat scratch disease	*Bartonella henselae*	Cats	Cats	Cat bite, scratch
Leptospirosis	*Leptospira* spp.	All, especially dogs	Rats, raccoons	Contact with urine
Salmonellosis	*Salmonella* spp.	All, especially dogs, cats	Rodents, reptiles	Ingestion
Tuberculosis	*Mycobacteria* spp.	Dogs, cats	All except rodents, monkeys	Ingestion, inhalation
Tularemia	*Francisella tularensis*	All	Rodents, rabbits	Tick bites, contact with tissue
Erysipelas	*Erysipelothrix rhusiopathiae*		Rodents	Contact
Tetanus	*Clostridium tetani*		Reptiles	Wound
Lyme disease	*Borrelia burgdorferi*	Dogs, cats	Deer, birds, rodents	Tick bite

TABLE 7-3	Causative Organisms, Animal Hosts, and Modes of Transmission for Selected Common Zoonoses—cont'd				
		HOSTS		
DISEASE	**CAUSATIVE ORGANISM**	**SMALL ANIMALS**	**WILDLIFE**	**MODES OF TRANSMISSION**
Protozoal Diseases				
Cryptosporidiosis	*Cryptosporidium* spp.	Most	Birds	Ingestion
Toxoplasmosis	*Toxoplasma gondii*	Cats, rabbits, guinea pigs	Cats	Ingestion
Balantidiasis	*Balantidium coli*		Rats, primates	Ingestion
Sarcocystosis	*Sarcocystis* spp.	Dogs, cats		Ingestion
Giardiasis	*Giardia lamblia*	Dogs, cats	Beavers, zoo monkeys	Ingestion

From Sirois M: Principles and practice of veterinary technology, ed 3, St Louis, 2011, Mosby.

Parasitic diseases are also transmitted through food and water. Nematode and trematode infections are usually transmitted through the ingestion of eggs or undercooked meat that contains cysts. *Giardia* is a protozoan that causes gastrointestinal disease in people; giardiasis can be serious in immunosuppressed individuals. Although *Giardia* is usually transmitted from person to person, it is also a source of waterborne outbreaks when people use mountain streams as community water sources without proper filtration techniques or drink the water during outdoor activities.

Animals admitted to the veterinary clinic for hospitalization and treatment of any disease caused by a transmissible pathogen must be kept in isolation to avoid infecting other animals in the clinic. Personnel working with these animals must take appropriate protective measures, such as wearing disposable gowns and gloves, while treating these patients. In general, patients in isolation are treated after all other patients have been treated. Careful attention to proper disinfection of food and water bowls is also needed to minimize the possibility of transmitting disease from isolated patients to those elsewhere in the veterinary facility.

CONTROL OF ZOONOTIC DISEASES

Because of their regular contact with animals, animal tissues, animal environments, and pet owners, veterinarians and veterinary staff members are often the first to notice a zoonotic disease or the potential for one.

CRITICAL CONCEPT

Veterinary professionals are at risk of contracting zoonotic diseases and must have knowledge about the ways diseases are transmitted to aid in their prevention and control.

Knowledge of the ways in which zoonotic diseases are transmitted and maintained in a population is important for preventing the spread of disease and infection in veterinarians and veterinary technicians. Because of their close working contact with animals, veterinary professionals are at risk of contracting zoonotic diseases. It is important to determine which diseases are most common in certain animal species so that the risk of contracting a particular disease can be estimated. Certain groups of people are more susceptible to zoonotic diseases and suffer more serious effects. Children and older adults are more susceptible because their immune systems function at a lower level than those of normal healthy adults. Children are also more likely to put contaminated soil or materials in their mouth. Pregnant women are also highly susceptible.

Control of zoonotic diseases is aimed at the reservoir of disease or the intermediaries that transmit the disease. Control measures include spraying for mosquitoes, use of tick repellent, pasteurization of milk, adequate water filtration, and proper cooking and handling of food. Control programs also include the treatment of infected animals in the reservoir population and decreased contact with infected animals in the reservoir to prevent further transmission. Prevention programs require a thorough knowledge of the disease and how it is maintained and transmitted to help break the cycle of disease in the population and/or prevent disease transmission. Prevention programs include vaccination of animals in the reservoir population, potential hosts, and people, if vaccines against that disease are available. Prevention of human infection is possible by the treatment of infected animals that may transmit the disease to humans. For example, treating puppies and kittens for roundworms and hookworms can prevent contamination of soil by feces containing infective eggs.

VACCINATION AND PREVENTIVE MEDICATIONS

There are two basic ways that an animal can acquire the immunity that it needs, passively and actively. Passive immunity occurs when the animal acquires preformed antibodies to various pathogens. This can take place naturally, such as when maternal antibodies cross the placenta into the fetus or neonates ingest the dam's colostrum. It can also occur artificially, such as when antibodies are administered exogenously. An example of artificially acquired passive immunity is through the administration of rattlesnake antivenin. Antivenin contains antibodies harvested from the serum of horses that have developed immunity to the rattlesnake venom. Active immunity is when an animal develops its own antibodies to pathogens. This can also occur naturally, through infection or exposure to the pathogen, or artificially through vaccination. Students sometimes become confused between artificially acquired passive and artificially acquired active immunity, especially when both exist for the same disease. For example, the tetanus antitoxin is an example of artificially acquired passive immunity. It consists of preformed antibodies to the toxin produced by the bacterium *Clostridium tetani,* the causative agent of tetanus. There is also a tetanus **toxoid**, which consists of inactivated antigenic toxin molecules that stimulate the development of the animal's own antibodies. Because the preformed antibodies persist for only a few weeks, the antitoxin is usually given in a situation when the animal may have been exposed to the toxin or has developed tetanus. The tetanus toxoid is administered as a preventive because it provides long-lasting immunity.

Animals can be vaccinated against a wide variety of diseases. These vaccines are commonly administered by injection and are critical for disease prevention. After injection, the vaccine does not cause disease but stimulates the cells of the immune system to develop antibodies against the portion of the pathogen that is antigenic. On the next exposure to the pathogen, a vaccinated animal will not become infected because it has been immunized.

A vaccine consists of a particular antigen unique to a pathogen, such as the cell wall of the causative bacterium or a small unit of the virus. The pathogen can be in several forms, including modified live, inactivated, or recombinant. A modified live vaccine consists of a weakened version of the pathogen, which will induce an immune response but is attenuated enough so that it will not cause disease. An inactivated or noninfectious vaccine consists of whole killed pathogens or selected antigenic subunits, enough to induce immunity. A recombinant vaccine consists of a live nonpathogenic virus into which the gene for a pathogen-related antigen has been inserted. When the virus is injected into the animal, viral genes, including the inserted gene for the antigen of interest, will be expressed. This will cause the animal to produce antibodies to the antigen without ever having been exposed to the pathogen.

Certain diseases are readily prevented by vaccination. Domestic animals should be routinely vaccinated against prevalent diseases. Serious diseases such as parvovirus infection and distemper in dogs and panleukopenia and feline leukemia virus infection in cats can be prevented by vaccination. In some cases, vaccination is beneficial to humans as well as animals. For example, animals at risk of developing rabies from the bite of rabid animals should receive regular rabies prophylaxis.

The decision as to whether to vaccinate an animal is influenced by the risk of contracting the disease, effects of the disease, and benefits and cost of vaccination. Vaccination may not be warranted if the disease is unlikely to develop or causes only mild illness. For example, veterinarians do not routinely vaccinate dogs or cats against tetanus because they are unlikely to contract the disease. Vaccination against a very rare disease may not be necessary. However, vaccination is worthwhile if the disease poses a substantial threat to human and animal health, such as rabies. Vaccination also benefits the offspring of vaccinated females; for example, a vaccinated female will develop antibodies to the disease and then transfer maternal immunity through her colostrum.

A growing number of practitioners are concerned about the apparent association between vaccines and a particular type of cancer (sarcoma) at the injection site in cats. The American Association of Feline Practitioners (AAFP) currently recommends using different vaccines at different locations on the body. It is recommended that feline leukemia virus (FeLV) vaccine be given in the left rear limb as distally as possible and rabies vaccine be given in the right rear limb as distally as possible.

Animal vaccines are available in many combinations. For example, Duramune DAP (Boehringer Ingelheim Vetmedica St. Joseph MO) is a canine vaccine against three viruses. Duramune DAP+C protects against four viruses. Duramune DAP + C4L protect against four viruses and four *Leptospira* spp. There are many such products available with multiple combinations of pathogens to accommodate different animal needs based on their lifestyles. It is also because some vaccines are considered core vaccines and others are noncore vaccines. Core vaccines are recommended for all dogs, whereas noncore vaccines are recommended based on a dog's lifestyle. For example, the vaccine against *Borrelia burgdorferi*, the causative agent of Lyme disease, is a noncore vaccine; it is recommended for dogs that have a likelihood of contact with ticks that transmit *B. burgdorferi.*

VACCINATION
VACCINATION OF DOGS. The following vaccines are available for dogs:
- Rabies
- Distemper
- Parvovirus
- Coronavirus
- Canine adenovirus (CAV-1 or CAV-2)
- *Bordetella bronchiseptica*
- Parainfluenza
- Leptospirosis
- *Borrelia burgdorferi*

Puppies are usually immunized with one to three doses in the first few months of life and then annually as adults (Table 7-4). The American Animal Hospital Association (AAHA) vaccination guidelines for dogs offer specific recommendations about which vaccines are core and noncore and when vaccinations should be administered.

Newer or less common vaccines available for dogs include the *Crotalus atrox* toxoid, which protects against rattlesnake venom, and canine influenza vaccine. There is limited information available regarding their efficacy. There is also a vaccine against *Giardia,* but this is not recommended for most pets.

VACCINATION OF CATS. The following vaccines are available for cats:
- Rabies
- Panleukopenia (feline distemper)

TABLE 7-4 | 2011 AAHA Canine Vaccination Guidelines* for the General Veterinary Practice

VACCINE†	INITIAL VACCINATION (<16 WK OF AGE)	INITIAL VACCINATION (>16 WK OF AGE)	REVACCINATION (BOOSTER) RECOMMENDATION	COMMENTS AND RECOMMENDATIONS
CDV (MLV) or rCDV	Puppies should be vaccinated every 3-4 wk between the ages of 6 and 16 wk (e.g., at 6, 10, and 14 wk, or 8, 12, and 16 wk). To minimize the risk of maternal antibody interference with vaccination, the final dose of the initial series should be administered between 14 and 16 wk of age, regardless of the product used.	One dose is considered protective and acceptable. Revaccination is recommended every ≥3 yr after completion of the initial vaccination, regardless of the product used.	Dogs (puppies) completing the initial vaccination series by 16 wk of age or younger should receive a single booster vaccination no later than 1 yr after completion of the initial series and be revaccinated every ≥3 yr thereafter, regardless of the product used.	Core • Among healthy dogs, all commercially available distemper vaccines are expected to induce a sustained protective immune response lasting at least 5 yr. • Among healthy dogs, the rCDV vaccine has been shown to induce a protective immune response lasting at least 5 yr. • Although rare, some dogs are genetically predisposed "nonresponders" and are incapable of developing protective immunity subsequent to CDV vaccination. • The rCDV vaccine can be used interchangeably with MLV-CDV vaccine. • It is recommended that all CDV vaccines be administered within 1 hr after reconstitution; vaccine held >1 hr should be discarded. MLV-CDV vaccine is particularly vulnerable to inactivation after reconstitution (rehydration).
MV (MLV–an aid in the prevention of CDV infection in puppies only) (Note: measles antigen is currently available in a 4-way combined MLV vaccine: CDV + measles + CAV-2 + CPiV) and a 2-way combined MLV vaccine: CDV + Measles IM route only	A single dose is recommended for administration to healthy dogs between the ages of 6 and 12 wk.	Not recommended	Not recommended	Noncore • Measles vaccine is only intended to provide temporary immunization of young puppies against CDV. MV has been shown to cross-protect puppies against CDV in presence of MDA to CDV. • These vaccines should not be administered to dog <6 wk or female dogs >12 wk of age that will be used for breeding because these puppies may have maternally derived measles antibody and will block MV-induced immunity. • After administration of a single dose of measles virus–containing vaccine, subsequent vaccination with a CDV vaccine that does not contain MV is recommended at 2-4 wk intervals until the patient is 14-16 wk of age. • Vaccine that contains MV must be administered by the IM route. • It is recommended that MV-containing vaccine be administered within 1 hr after reconstitution; vaccine held >1 hr should be discarded.

Continued

TABLE 7-4	2011 AAHA Canine Vaccination Guidelines* for the General Veterinary Practice—cont'd			
VACCINE†	INITIAL VACCINATION (<16 WK OF AGE)	INITIAL VACCINATION (>16 WK OF AGE)	REVACCINATION (BOOSTER) RECOMMENDATION	COMMENTS AND RECOMMENDATIONS
CPV-2 (MLV)	Puppies should be vaccinated every 3-4 wk between the ages of 6 and 16 wk (e.g., at 6, 10, and 14 wk, or 8, 12, and 16 wk). To minimize the risk of maternal antibody interference with vaccination, the final dose of the initial series should be administered between 14 and 16 wk of age, regardless of the product used.	One dose is considered protective and acceptable. Revaccination is recommended every ≥3 yr after completion of the initial vaccination, regardless of the product used.	Dogs (puppies) completing the initial vaccination series by ≤16 wk of age should receive a single booster vaccination not later than 1 yr after completion of the initial series and be revaccinated every ≥3 yr thereafter, regardless of the product used.	**Core** • All MLV-CPV-2 vaccines available today are expected to provide immunity from disease caused by any field variant recognized today (CPV-2a, -2b, and -2c). • As new variants of CPV-2 occur, those variants will need to be evaluated, as the previous ones have, to ensure vaccines in use at the time are protective. • Among healthy dogs, all commercially available MLV-CPV-2 vaccines are expected to induce a sustained protective immune response lasting at least 5 yr. • Although rare, some dogs are genetic nonresponders and are incapable of developing protective immunity subsequent to CPV-2 vaccination no matter how often vaccine is administered. • Today, specific-breed susceptibility to CPV-2 nonresponsiveness is not recognized. There is no value in extending initial CPV-2 vaccination series beyond 16 wk of age. • It is recommended that CPV-2 vaccine, especially when administered in combination with CDV vaccine, be administered within 1 hr after reconstitution; vaccine held >1 hr should be discarded.
CAV-2 (MLV parenteral)	Puppies should be vaccinated every 3-4 wk between the ages of 6 and 16 wk (e.g., at 6, 10, and 14 wk, or 8, 12, and 16 wk). To minimize the risk of maternal antibody interference with vaccination, the final dose of the initial series should be administered between 14 and 16 wk of age, regardless of the product used.	One dose is considered protective and acceptable. Revaccination is recommended every ≥3 yr after completion of the initial vaccination, regardless of the product used.	Dogs (puppies) completing the initial vaccination series by ≤16 wk of age should receive a single booster vaccination not later than 1 yr after completion of the initial series and be revaccinated every ≥3 yr thereafter, regardless of the product used.	**Core** • CAV-2 induces protection against CAV-1 (canine hepatitis virus) as well as CAV-2 (one of the agents known to be associated with canine infectious respiratory disease). • Among healthy dogs, all commercially available MLV-CAV-2 vaccines are expected to induce a sustained protective immune response lasting at least 7 yr. • It is recommended that CAV-2 vaccine, especially when administered in combination with CDV vaccine, be administered within 1 hr after reconstitution; vaccine held >1 hr should be discarded.
Rabies 1 yr (killed)	Administer a single dose not earlier than 12 wk of age or as required by state, provincial, and/ or local requirements.	Administer a single dose of a "1yr" rabies vaccine.	Administer a single dose of a "1-yr" rabies vaccine annually. State, provincial, and/or local laws apply.	**Core** • State, provincial, and local statutes govern the frequency of administration for products labeled as "1-yr" rabies vaccine. • Route of administration may not be optional; see product literature for details.

Vaccine	Initial	Revaccination	Booster	Core/Noncore and Comments
Rabies 3 yr (killed)	Administer a single dose of a "3-yr" rabies vaccine not earlier than 12 wk of age or as required by state, provincial, and/or local requirements.	Administer a single dose of a "3-yr" rabies vaccine or as required by state, provincial, and/or local requirements.	Administer a single dose of a "3-yr" rabies vaccine within 1 yr after administration of the initial dose, regardless of the animal's age at the time the initial dose was administered. Subsequently, revaccination with a "3-yr" rabies vaccine should be administered every 3 yr thereafter, unless state, provincial, and/or local requirements stipulate otherwise.	Core • State, provincial, and local statutes govern the frequency of administration for products labeled as "3-yr rabies" vaccines. • Use of rabies vaccine multidose ("tank") vials in companion animals is not recommended. • Route of administration may not be optional; see product literature for details.
CPiV (MLV) For parenteral administration only. (Available only as a combined product for parenteral administration)	Parenteral CPiV vaccine is only available in combination with core vaccines (CDV-CPV-2 and CAV-2). Therefore, veterinarians who elect to administer parenteral CPiV vaccine should follow the same administration recommendations as outlined above for the core vaccines.	Veterinarians who elect to administer parenteral CPiV vaccine should follow the same administration recommendations as outlined above for the core vaccines.		Noncore • Parenterally administered CPiV vaccine does prevent clinical signs but has not been shown to prevent infection and shedding. • Use of the parenteral vaccine is recommended for those patients that aggressively resist IN vaccination.
Bb (inactivated-cellular antigen extract) For parenteral administration only.	Administer first dose at 8 wk of age and second dose at 12 wk of age (see comments).	Two doses, 2-4 wk apart are required.	Annually	Noncore • There is no known advantage to administering parenteral and IN Bb vaccines simultaneously. • On initial vaccination, administration should be scheduled such that the second dose can be administered at least 1 wk before exposure (kennel, dog show, daycare, etc). • The parenteral vaccine is not immunogenic if administered by the IN route.
Bb (live avirulent bacteria) For IN administration only.	A single dose should be administered in conjunction with 1 of the core vaccine doses. Note: The initial IN dose may be administered to dogs as young as 3-4 wk of age (depending on manufacturer) when exposure risk is considered to be high (see comments).	A single dose is recommended.	Annually or more often in high-risk animals.	Noncore • Transient (3-10 days) coughing, sneezing, or nasal discharge may occur in a small percentage of vaccinates. • IN Bb vaccine must not be administered parenterally.
CPiV (MLV) For IN administration only. (IN CPiV vaccine is only available in combination with IN Bb vaccine or Bb + CAV-2)	A single dose should be administered in conjunction with 1 of the core vaccine doses. Note: The initial IN dose may be administered to dogs as young as 3-4 wk of age (depending on manufacturer) when exposure risk is considered to be high (see comments).	A single dose is recommended.	Annually or more often in high-risk animals.	Noncore • When feasible, IN vaccination is recommended over parenteral vaccination. Parenterally administered CPiV vaccine does prevent clinical signs, but has not been shown to prevent infection and shedding. IN CPiV vaccine prevents not only clinical disease but also infection and viral replication (shedding).

Continued

TABLE 7-4 | 2011 AAHA Canine Vaccination Guidelines* for the General Veterinary Practice—cont'd

VACCINE†	INITIAL VACCINATION (<16 WK OF AGE)	INITIAL VACCINATION (>16 WK OF AGE)	REVACCINATION (BOOSTER) RECOMMENDATION	COMMENTS AND RECOMMENDATIONS
CAV-2 (MLV) (for IN administration only) (Available only in combination with IN Bb and CPiV vaccine)	A single dose should be administered in conjunction with 1 of the core vaccine doses. Note: The initial IN dose may be administered to dogs as young as 3-4 wk of age (depending on manufacturer) when exposure risk is considered to be high (see comments).	A single dose is recommended.	Annually or more often in high-risk animals.	Noncore • Administration of IN CAV-2 vaccine is recommended for use in dogs considered at risk for respiratory infection caused by the CAV-2 virus. • IN CAV-2 vaccine may not provide protective immunity against CAV-1 (canine hepatitis virus) infection and should not be considered a replacement for parenteral MLV-CAV-2 vaccination.
Canine influenza vaccine (killed virus)	Administer 1 dose not earlier than 6 wk of age and a second dose 2-4 wk later.	Two doses, 2-4 wk apart are required. A single initial dose will not immunize a seronegative dog.	Annually	Noncore
Borrelia burgdorferi (Lyme disease) (killed whole cell bacterin) or Borrelia burgdorferi (rLyme: rOspA)	Administer 1 dose not earlier than 12 wk of age and a second dose 2-4 wk later. For optimal response, do not administer to dogs <12 wk of age.	Two doses, 2-4 wk apart. A single initial dose will not immunize a seronegative dog.	Annually. Alternatively, it has been recommended that initial vaccination or revaccination (booster) be administered before the beginning of tick season, as determined regionally.	Noncore • Generally recommended only for use in dogs with a known risk of exposure, living in or visiting regions where the risk of vector tick exposure is considered to be high, or where disease is known to be endemic. • In addition to vaccination, prevention of canine Lyme borreliosis includes regular utilization of tick control products.
Leptospira interrogans (4-way killed whole cell or subunit bacterin) Contains serovars canicola + icterohemorrhagiae + grippotyphosa + pomona	Administer 1 dose not earlier than 12 wk of age and a second dose 2-4 wk later. For optimal response, do not administer to dogs <12 wk of age.	Two doses, 2-4 wk apart. A single initial dose will not immunize a seronegative dog.	Annually. Administration of booster vaccines should be restricted to dogs with a reasonable risk of exposure.	Noncore • Specific vaccination recommendations vary on the basis: (1) known geographic occurrence/prevalence, and (2) exposure risk in the individual patient. • It is recommended that the first dose of leptospira vaccine be delayed until 12 wk of age. • DOI based on challenge studies has been shown to be approximately 1 yr.
Leptospira interrogans (2-way killed bacterin) Contains serovars canicola + icterohemorrhagiae only	Intentionally left blank	Intentionally left blank	Intentionally left blank	Not recommended

Canine oral melanoma (plasmid DNA vaccine-expresses human tyrosinase). Availability is currently limited to practicing oncologists and selected specialists.	Not applicable. See Manufacturer's indications for use.	See Manufacturer's indications for use.	Use of this vaccine is limited to the treatment of dogs with malignant melanoma. • This vaccine aids in extending survival times of dogs with Stage II or III oral melanoma and for which local disease control has been achieved (negative local lymph nodes or positive lymph nodes that were surgically removed or irradiated). The human tyrosinase protein will stimulate an immune response that is effective against canine melanoma cells that overexpress tyrosinase. • Vaccination is not indicated for the prevention of canine melanoma.
Crotalus atrox (Western Diamondback rattlesnake vaccine) (toxoid)	Initial vaccination recommendation may depend on size of the individual dog. Refer to manufacturer's label. Current recommendations are to administer 2 doses, 1 mo apart, to dogs as young as 4 mo.	Refer to manufacturer's label. Annual revaccination requirements vary depending on prior exposure, size of dog, and risk of exposure. Refer to manufacturer's label.	• Field efficacy and experimental challenge data in dogs are not available at this time. • Intended to protect dogs against the venom associated with the bite of the Western Diamondback rattlesnake. Some cross-protection may exist against the venom of the Eastern Diamondback rattlesnake. There is currently no evidence of cross-protection against the venom (neurotoxin) of the Mojave rattlesnake. • Vaccine efficacy and dose recommendations are based on toxin neutralization studies conducted in mice. Conventional challenge studies in dogs have not been conducted. Neither experimental nor field data are currently available on this product. Note: Veterinarians should advise clientele of vaccinated dogs that vaccination does not eliminate the need to treat individual dogs subsequent to envenomation.
Canine coronavirus (CCoV) (killed and MLV)	Intentionally left blank	Intentionally left blank	Not recommended • Neither the MLV vaccine nor the killed CCoV vaccines have been shown to significantly reduce disease caused by a combination of CCoV and CPV-2. Only CPV-2 vaccines have been shown to protect dogs against a dual-virus challenge. • DOI has never been established. In controlled challenge studies, neither vaccinates nor control dogs developed clinical evidence of disease after experimental virus challenge.

Bb, *Bordetella bronchiseptica;* CAV-1, canine adenovirus, type 1 (cause of canine viral hepatitis); protection from CAV-1 infection is provided by parenterally administered CAV-2 vaccine; CAV-2, canine adenovirus, type 2; CCoV, canine coronavirus cause of enteric coronavirus infection (antigenically distinct from the canine respiratory coronavirus [CRCoV]); CDV, canine distemper virus; CIV, canine influenza virus—H3N8; CPIV, canine parainfluenza virus; CPV-2, canine parvovirus, type 2; DOI, duration of immunity; IN, intranasal; MLV, modified live virus, attenuated virus vaccine; MV, measles virus; OspA outer surface protein A (antigen) of Borrelia burgdorferi; RV, rabies virus.

*The AAHA 2011 Canine Vaccine Guidelines are provided to assist veterinarians in developing a vaccination protocol for use in clinical practice. They are not intended to represent vaccination standards for all dogs nor are they intended to represent a universal vaccination protocol applicable for all dogs.

†Route of administration is SQ (subcutaneous) or IM (intramuscular) unless otherwise noted by the manufacturer.

- *Chlamydophila felis*
- Feline leukemia virus
- Rhinotracheitis
- Calicivirus
- Feline immunodeficiency virus (FIV)
- *Bordetella bronchiseptica*

Most cats begin receiving vaccines as kittens, usually at approximately 6 weeks of age. Kittens require boosters after an original series of vaccines. Adult cats may require annual boosters against each of these diseases (Table 7-5).

The AAFP vaccination guidelines for cats offer specific recommendations about which vaccines are core and non-core and when vaccinations should be administered. Other vaccines available for cats include vaccines against feline infectious peritonitis, *Giardia,* and *Microsporum* spp. (ringworm), but these are not recommended.

ANTIBODY TITERS INSTEAD OF VACCINATION

Although mostly safe, annual vaccinations are a source of controversy because of risks that may be associated with vaccine use. Reactions to vaccine administration ranging from localized swelling to anaphylaxis and sarcoma formation (especially in cats) have been reported. Also, although there are recommendations for appropriate vaccination protocols, optimal intervals have not been established for many vaccines. It is likely that the vaccinations currently in use provide long-term immunity; however, some patients at risk for contracting common diseases may still need vaccination. In particular, pets exposed to other dogs or cats on a routine basis or are ill with some other disease (e.g., FIV, FeLV) may still need routine vaccinations.

Some veterinarians are now recommending the measurement of antibody titers to diseases normally vaccinated against as an alternative to routine annual vaccination. An antibody titer may help determine whether a patient is likely to need booster vaccinations. Although this is a promising alternative to vaccination, there is still much uncertainty surrounding titer use. Different outside laboratories have different measurement standards. Also, there is disagreement and inconsistency about the level of antibodies that constitutes protection against a disease if the animal were infected or challenged with the pathogen. Finally, antibody titers are also more costly than vaccines.

USE OF PREVENTIVE MEDICATION

Certain diseases can be prevented by the regular administration of preventive medication. This is best exemplified by the use of anthelmintics and other parasiticides to prevent heartworm infection and control internal and external parasites in dogs and cats.

FACTORS PREDISPOSING TO DISEASE

Some factors that predispose to disease can be controlled, but others cannot. Although some factors are beyond our control, we can often establish conditions so that even uncontrollable factors have only minimal impact on our animals. Table 7-6 lists some common diseases of dogs and cats. Animals are predisposed to disease by genetic, dietary, environmental, and metabolic factors.

GENETIC FACTORS

Genetic factors are largely not controllable, although their effects can be reduced to some extent by selective breeding. These include, for example, gender predisposition, inherited mutations, immunodeficiencies, and the effect of inbreeding. Most male tricolored cats are sterile, whereas tricolored female cats are usually fertile. Inherited malocclusions can interfere with chewing. Immunodeficiencies may be noted by an increased incidence of infections. Inbreeding can lead to physical abnormalities or diminished mental (intellectual) capacities.

DIETARY FACTORS

Dietary factors are generally controllable. Animal owners determine most aspects of an animal's diet, such as feed type, quality, amount, and regimen. A high-quality balanced ration is of little value if the feeder is inaccessible. This is occasionally seen with young bunnies, which are too short to reach the feeder. Limited feeding can prevent obesity but can lead to malnutrition if not applied properly. A diet formulated for one type or age of animal may not be healthful for another group of the same species. For example, hard pellets may not be chewable by aged animals, or kitten diets may have some nutrients in excess of that required by an adult cat, etc. The diet must change as the needs of the animal change.

> **CRITICAL CONCEPT**
> Genetic, dietary, environmental, and metabolic factors may predispose an animal to specific diseases.

ENVIRONMENTAL FACTORS

Environmental factors also require consideration in the preventive health plan. Climatic extremes or sudden climatic changes can clearly cause distress or even death. Although we cannot change the weather, we can adjust the animal's housing to reduce environmental stress. Additional bedding improves the insulation around animals housed in extremely cold conditions. Overhead cover is needed to prevent sunburn and heat prostration and shield animals from precipitation.

Inadequate ventilation increases the incidence of respiratory diseases through increased ammonia levels and large numbers of microorganisms in the air. Inadequate ventilation also impairs cooling in animals that use respiration to regulate body temperature (e.g., dogs) and prevents radiation of body heat. Inadequate ventilation inhibits the drying of bedding, favoring proliferation of bacteria or parasites. At the other end of the spectrum, excessive ventilation is also stressful. Drafts or excessive ventilation can cause chilling, dehydration, or inflamed ocular tissues.

TABLE 7-5 American Association of Feline Practitioners 2006 Feline Vaccination Guidelines. Summary: Vaccination in General Practice

VACCINE	PRIMARY SERIES-KITTENS (≤16 WK)	PRIMARY SERIES-ADOLESCENT, ADULT (>16 WK)	BOOSTER	COMMENTS
Panleukopenia virus (FPV), feline herpesvirus-1 and feline calicivirus (FHV-1, FCV) Injectable: MLV, nonadjuvanted killed, adjuvanted killed, nonadjuvanted Intranasal: MLV, nonadjuvanted	Begin as early as 6 wk of age, then every 3-4 wk until 16 wk of age.	Two doses, 3-4 wk apart	A single dose is given 1 yr following the last dose of the initial series, then no more frequently than every 3 yr.	*Core:* Killed vaccines are preferred for use in pregnant cats (only if absolutely necessary) and in FeLV- and/or FIV-infected cats, especially those showing evidence of immunosuppression. Killed panleukopenia vaccines should be used in kittens < 4 wk of age. All kittens and cats should receive at least one injectable panleukopenia injection.
Rabies injectable: canarypox virus–vectored recombinant (rRabies), nonadjuvanted 1-yr killed, adjuvanted; 3-yr killed, adjuvanted	Administer a single dose as early as 8 or 12 wk of age depending on product label. Revaccinate 1 yr later.	Administer two doses, 12 mo apart.	Annual booster is required, or every 3 yr or as required by state or local ordinance for 3 yr.	*Core:* In states and municipalities in which feline rabies vaccination is required, veterinarians must follow applicable statutes. Booster vaccination with a 1-yr rabies vaccine is only appropriate in states and municipalities where permitted by law. Any rabies vaccine can be used for revaccination, even if the product is not the same brand or type of product previously administered. No laboratory or epidemiologic data exist to support the annual or biennial administration of 3-yr vaccines following the initial series.
Feline leukemia virus (FeLV) transdermal: canarypox virus–vectored recombinant (rFeLV), nonadjuvanted Injectable or killed, adjuvanted	Administer an initial dose as early as 8-12 wk of age, depending on product; a second dose should be administered 3-4 wk later.	Two doses, 3-4 wk apart	When indicated, a single dose is given 1 yr following the last dose of the initial series, then annually in cats determined to have sustained risk of exposure.	*Noncore:* FeLV vaccination is highly recommended for all kittens. Booster inoculation is recommended only for cats considered to be at risk of exposure. In the United States, the 0.25-mL rFeLV vaccine dose may only be administered via the manufacturer's transdermal administration system. Only FeLV-negative cats should be vaccinated; FeLV testing prior to vaccine administration is recommended. Cats should be tested for FeLV infection before their initial vaccination and when there is a possibility that they have been exposed to FeLV since they were last vaccinated.
Feline immunodeficiency virus (FIV) Injectable: killed, adjuvanted	When indicated, three doses are required. The initial dose is administered as early as 8 wk of age; two subsequent doses should be administered at an interval of 2-3 wk.	When indicated, three doses are required. Each dose is administered 2-3 wk apart.	When indicated, a single dose is given 1 yr following the last dose of the initial series, then annually in cats determined to have sustained risk of exposure.	*Noncore:* FIV vaccine should be restricted to cats at high risk of infection. Vaccination induces production of antibodies indistinguishable from those developed in response to FIV infection, and interferes with all antibody-based FIV diagnostic tests for at least 1 yr following vaccination. Cats with positive FIV antibody assay results may have antibodies as a result of vaccination, infection, or both. FIV antibodies are passed from vaccinated queens to their kittens in colostrum. Colostrum-derived antibodies interfere with FIV diagnosis past the age of weaning in most kittens, but this interference appears to wane by 12 wk of age. Cats should test FIV-antibody negative immediately prior to vaccination. Permanent identification of vaccinated cats (e.g., using a microchip) will help clarify vaccination status, but will not indicate that such cats are free of infection. This vaccine has been shown to provide protection from some, but not all, strains of FIV.

Continued

TABLE 7-5	American Association of Feline Practitioners 2006 Feline Vaccination Guidelines. Summary: Vaccination in General Practice—cont'd			
VACCINE	**PRIMARY SERIES-KITTENS (≤16 WK)**	**PRIMARY SERIES-ADOLESCENT, ADULT (>16 WK)**	**BOOSTER**	**COMMENTS**
Feline infectious peritonitis (FIP) MLV, nonadjuvanted Intranasal	If administered, give a single dose as early as 16 wk of age and a second dose 3-4 wk later.	If administered, give two doses, 3-4 wk apart.	Annual booster is recommended by the manufacturer.	*Not generally recommended:* According to the limited studies available, only cats known to be feline coronavirus antibody–negative at the time of vaccination are likely to develop some level of protection. Vaccination of cats living in households in which FIP is known to exist or cats that are known to be feline coronavirus antibody–positive is not recommended.
Chlamydophila felis avirulent live, nonadjuvanted or killed, adjuvanted Injectable	Administer the initial dose as early as 9 wk of age; a second dose is administered 3-4 wk later.	Administer two doses, 3-4 wk apart.	Annual booster is indicated for cats with sustained exposure risk.	*Noncore:* Vaccination reserved as part of a control regimen for cats in multiple-cat environments in which infections associated with clinical disease have been confirmed. Inadvertent conjunctival inoculation of vaccine has been reported to cause clinical signs of infection.
Bordetella bronchiseptica avirulent, live, nonadjuvanted Intranasal	Administer a single dose intranasally as early as 8 wk of age.	Administer a single dose intranasally.	Annual booster is indicated for cats with sustained risk.	*Noncore:* Vaccination may be considered in cases in which cats are likely to be at specific risk of infection (e.g., rescue shelters, boarding facilities, catteries).
Feline *Giardia* killed, adjuvanted Injectable	Administer a single dose at 8 wk of age; a second dose is administered 2-4 wk later.	Two doses, 2-4 wk apart.	Annual booster is recommended by the manufacturer.	*Not generally recommended:* There are insufficient studies available to support the role of *Giardia* vaccination in preventing clinical disease in cats. Whether the *Giardia* vaccine is an effective therapeutic agent in naturally infected cats is currently unknown.

From Sirois M: Principles and practice of veterinary technology, ed 3, St Louis, 2011, Mosby.

TABLE 7-6 | Common Diseases of Dogs and Cats

DISEASE	CAUSE(S)	COMMON SIGNS AND SYMPTOMS
Anal sacculitis	Impaction, inflammation, or infection of anal glands	Scooting, tail chewing, malodorous perianal discharge
Anemia	Hemorrhage, iron deficiency, toxins, immune disorders	Anorexia, weakness, depression, tachycardia, tachypnea, pale mucous membranes
Arthritis	Acute—sepsis, trauma, immune-mediated Osteoarthritis—progressive degeneration of hyaline cartilage	Lameness, swelling, crepitus
Asthma (feline)	Inflammation of airways, bronchoconstriction	Dyspnea (acute onset), coughing, lethargy
Atopy	Allergic reaction to inhaled substances	Pruritus, alopecia, dermatitis
Aural hematoma	Trauma causing buildup of blood beneath skin surface	Head shaking, scratching at ear
Brachycephalic respiratory distress syndrome	Congenital airway obstruction	Coughing, exercise intolerance, cyanosis, dyspnea
Calicivirus (feline)	Viral infection of upper respiratory tract	Anorexia, lethargy, fever ulcerative stomatitis, nasal discharge
Cataracts	Inherited or secondary to diabetes and other diseases	Opaque pupillary opening, progressive vision loss
Congestive heart failure	Valvular insufficiency, myocarditis, hypertension, dilated cardiomyopathy	Anorexia, syncope, pulmonary edema
Corona virus	Viral infection of GI system	Asymptomatic or anorexia, dehydration, V, D
Cushing's disease	Hyperadrenocorticism	Bilateral, symmetrical alopecia
Cystitis	Inflammation or bacterial infection of urinary bladder	Hematuria, dysuria, inappropriate urination, pollakiuria, polyuria
Demodex	Infestation of hair follicles with *Demodex* mites	Alopecia, erythema, secondary pyoderma, pruritus
Dermatophytosis	*Microsporum canis, M. gypseum,* or *Trichophyton mentagrophytes* infection	Circular area of alopecia; lesion may be raised, red, crusty
Diabetes mellitus	Deficient or defective production of insulin	PU, PD, weight loss, polyphagia
Dilated cardiomyopathy	Dilation of all chambers of the heart	Ascites, hepatomegaly, weight loss, abdominal distension, dyspnea
Distemper (canine)	Paramyxoviral infection	Fever, cough, mucopurulent ocular and nasal discharge, V, D, hyperkeratosis of foot pads, ataxia
Dystocia	Primary uterine inertia, fetal obstruction	Active prolonged straining with no fetus produced, green, purulent, or hemorrhagic vaginal discharge, pain
Feline fibrosarcoma	Vaccine-induced	Swelling and rapidly growing firm mass at site of recent vaccination
Flea allergy dermatitis	Hypersensitivity to *Ctenocephalides* infestation	Pruritus, licking, chewing, erythema, alopecia
Fungal infection (systemic)	*Blastomyces dermatitidis*	Anorexia, depression, fever, dyspnea
	Coccidioides immitis	Cough, fever, anorexia, weight loss
	Histoplasma capsulatum	Weight loss, fever, anorexia
Geriatric vestibular syndrome	Otitis media	Head tilt, circling, disorientation, ataxia, nystagmus
Glaucoma	Increased intraocular fluid production	Ocular pain, corneal edema, buphthalmus, blindness
Heartworm disease	*Dirofilaria immitis* parasite	Exercise intolerance (dogs), dyspnea, coughing, ascites (dogs), vomiting (cats)
Hemobartonellosis	Mycoplasma, rickettsial infection	Pale or icteric mucous membranes, fever, tachypnea, tachycardia
Hip dysplasia	Laxity and subluxation of the hip joint	Lameness, gait abnormality, muscle atrophy
Histiocytoma	Benign skin tumor	Fast-growing dome or button-like nodules; may be ulcerated
Hyperthyroidism	Overproduction of thyroid hormone	Weight loss, polyphagia, vomiting, enlarged thyroid
Hypothyroidism	Underproduction of thyroid hormone	Weight gain, bilateral, symmetrical alopecia, cold intolerance
Hepatic lipidosis	Accumulation of triglycerides in liver	Prolonged anorexia, V, D, lethargy

Continued

TABLE 7-6	Common Diseases of Dogs and Cats—cont'd	
DISEASE	**CAUSE(S)**	**COMMON SIGNS AND SYMPTOMS**
Immune-mediated hemolytic anemia	Accelerated red blood cell destruction	Anorexia, depression, tachycardia, tachypnea, pale mucous membranes
Immunodeficiency virus (feline)	Lentivirus infection	Chronic infections (e.g., of oral cavity, skin, respiratory tract); chronic fever, cachexia
Infectious canine tracheobronchitis (kennel cough)	Bacterial and viral infection of lower respiratory tract (e.g., *Bordetella bronchiseptica*, canine adenovirus)	Dry, hacking, paroxysmal cough
Inflammatory bowel disease	Inflammation of intestinal mucosa	Diarrhea, increased frequency and volume of defecation
Intestinal parasitism	Infection with parasites including nematodes (e.g., ascarids, hookworms, whipworms), coccidia, protozoa (e.g., *Giardia*), cestodes	Depending on species of parasite; diarrhea, weight loss, anemia, unthriftiness
Lipoma	Benign fatty tumor	Soft, round or oval subcuticular mass
Liver disease	Drugs, toxins, bile duct inflammation	Anorexia, V, D, PU, PD, jaundice
Lyme disease	*Borrelia burgdorferi*	Fever, anorexia, lameness, lymphadenopathy
Sarcoptic mange	*Sarcoptes scabiei canis* mite infestation	Red, crusty lesions, intense pruritis
Osteochondrosis dissecans	Degeneration and reossification of bone and cartilage	
Otitis externa	Primary or secondary parasitic, bacterial or yeast infection of the soft tissues of the ear	Head shaking, head tilt, pain, foul odor
Panleukopenia (feline)	Parvoviral infection	Anorexia, fever, V, D, abdominal pain
Panosteitis	Possible viral infection, metabolic disease, allergic reaction, hormonal excesses	Intermittent lameness, anorexia, fever, weight loss
Pancreatitis	Inflammation of the pancreas caused by obesity, overingestion of fats, other diseases	Depression, anorexia, V, D, dehydration
Parvovirus (canine)	Viral infection of GI tract	Bloody diarrhea, lethargy, vomiting, dehydration, fever
Patella luxation	Genetic predisposition, trauma,	Abnormal gait with rotation of limbs
Periodontal disease	Bacterial infection of tissues surrounding teeth that leads to plaque accumulation and causes calculus buildup	Increased depth of periodontal pockets, increased tooth mobility, foul oral odor, pain
Peritonitis	Inflammatory process	Abdominal pain, reluctance to move, tachycardia, tachypnea, fever, V, D, dehydration
Pyoderma (deep)	Bacterial infection of the skin usually caused by *Staphylococcus intermedius*	Papules, pustules, draining fistulous tracts
Pyometra	Bacterial infection (e.g., *Escherichia coli*, *Staphylococcus*, *Pasteurella*)	Vulvar discharge, abdominal enlargement, PU, PD, dehydration
Renal failure	Damage to nephron causing reduction in glomerular filtration	Oliguria, polyuria, V, D, anorexia, dehydration
Skin tumors (sebaceous cysts, adenoma, adenocarcinoma, melanoma)	Unknown; possible genetic causes	Usually round masses, may be encapsulated or ulcerated
Thrombocytopenia	Numerous viral, bacterial, immune-mediated, and other noninfectious causes	Petechial hemorrhage, ecchymosis, epistaxis, lethargy
Tick-borne rickettsial disease	*Rickettsia rickettsii* (Rocky Mountain spotted fever)	Fever, anorexia, mucopurulent ocular discharge, coughing, tachypnea, V, D
	Ehrlichia canis, E. ewingi, E. equi (ehrlichiosis)	Lymphadenopathy, anemia, depression, anorexia, fever lethargy, lameness, muscular stiffness
Ulcerative keratitis (corneal ulcers)	Trauma, bacterial infection, feline herpesvirus	Ocular pain, corneal edema, photophobia
Urolithiasis	Precipitation of mineral substances in urine	Dysuria, hematuria
Viral rhinotracheitis (feline)	Herpesvirus infection	Acute onset of sneezing, conjunctivitis, purulent rhinitis, fever
Von Willebrand disease	Decreased or deficient production of von Willebrand factor	Purpura, prolonged bleeding from venipuncture or surgical sites
Viral enteritis	Parvovirus, coronavirus, rotavirus	Bloody diarrhea, lethargy, vomiting, dehydration, fever

D, Diarrhea; *PD*, polydipsia; *PU*, polyuria; *V*, vomiting.

METABOLIC FACTORS

Metabolic factors also must be considered in preventive health programs. Factors beyond our control include the age of the animal and reproductive status; concurrent disease; and nonspecific stressors. Young, old, pregnant, and lactating animals have different physiologic needs than other animals. These needs may require alteration of the animal's diet and housing.

A common metabolic problem that influences the health of many companion animals, and that can be effectively managed by the animal owner, is obesity from overfeeding and lack of exercise. We often focus on the animal's age group and manage health problems as they relate to age; however, a more effective preventive approach is to address factors under the client's control. Veterinary professionals should discuss proper nutrition and exercise programs with clients so that their animals can benefit from that knowledge.

RECOMMENDED READINGS

AVMA: *Zoonoses update*, ed 2, Schaumberg, IL, 1996, American Veterinary Medical Association.

Birchard SJ, Sherding RG: *Saunders manual of small animal practice*, ed 3, St Louis, 2006, Saunders.

Bonagura JD: *Kirk's current veterinary therapy XIV: Small animal practice*, St Louis, 2009, Saunders.

Case LP, et al.: *Canine and feline nutrition*, ed 3, St Louis, 2011, Mosby.

Cheville NF: *Introduction to veterinary pathology*, ed 3, Ames, IA, 2006, Wiley Blackwell.

Colville JL, Berryhill DL: *Handbook of zoonoses*, St Louis, 2007, Mosby.

Kumar V, et al.: *Robbins and Cotran pathologic basis of disease*, ed 8, Philadelphia, 2010, Saunders.

Maxie MG, et al.: *Jubb, Kennedy & Palmer's pathology of domestic animals*, ed 5, San Diego, 2008, Academic Press.

Morris ML, et al.: *Small animal clinical nutrition III*, Topeka, KS, 1987, Mark Morris.

Prendergast H: *Front office management for the veterinary team*, St Louis, 2010, Saunders.

Smith B: *Large animal internal medicine*, ed 4, St Louis, 2009, Mosby.

Summers A: *Common diseases of companion animals*, ed 2, St Louis, 2007, Mosby.

Tizard IR: *Veterinary immunology: An introduction*, ed 8, St Louis, 2008, Saunders.

Zachary JF, McGavin MD: *Pathologic basis of veterinary disease*, ed 5, St Louis, 2012, Mosby.

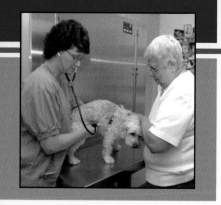

8 Animal Care and Nursing[1]

OUTLINE

Patient History and Client Interaction, *209*
Communicating With Clients, *209*
Obtaining a History, *210*
Physical Examination, *211*
Monitoring Vital Signs, *213*
Gastrointestinal Monitoring, *217*
Nutritional Support, *219*
Grooming and Skin Care, *219*
Bathing, *219*
Skin Care, *219*
Nail Trimming, *220*
Anal Sac Care, *221*
Ear Care, *222*
Administering Medications, *223*
Topical Administration, *223*
Oral Administration, *223*
Rectal Administration, *224*
Nasal Administration, *225*
Ophthalmic Application, *225*
Otic Application, *226*
Parenteral Administration, *226*
Intradermal Administration, *227*
Subcutaneous Administration, *227*
Intramuscular Administration, *228*

Intravenous Administration, *228*
Intraosseous and Intraperitoneal Administration, *229*
Intravenous Catheterization, *229*
Urinary Tract Catheterization, *231*
Gastric Intubation, *232*
Fluid Therapy, *232*
Wound Care and Bandaging, *232*
Wound Contamination and Infection, *232*
Wound Categories, *232*
Use of Antibacterials, *233*
First Aid, *233*
Wound Assessment, *233*
Lavage, *234*
Anesthesia and Analgesia, *235*
Débridement, *235*
Drainage, *236*
Wound Closure, *236*
Nonclosure, *236*
Covering Wounds, *237*
Nursing Care for Recumbent Patients, *240*
Turning, *240*
Padding, *240*
Euthanasia Methods, *241*

LEARNING OBJECTIVES

After reviewing this chapter, the reader will be able to:

1. Describe techniques used in the general nursing care of dogs and cats.
2. Discuss techniques used in the recording of patient care.
3. Describe procedures used in grooming and skin, nail, and ear care.
4. List common routes of administration of medication and describe procedures used for the administration of medications.

5. List and describe methods of enteral and parenteral administration.
6. List and describe methods of intravenous catheterization.
7. Explain the principles of first aid treatment of wounds.
8. Explain the principles of wound closure.
9. Give examples of the types and application of bandages.

[1]Elsevier and the author acknowledge and appreciate the original contributions from Sirois M: Principles and practice of veterinary technology, ed 3, St Louis, 2011, Mosby; Bassert JM, McCurnin DM: Clinical textbook for veterinary technicians, ed 8, St Louis, 2011, Saunders; and Thomas JT, Lerche P: Anesthesia and analgesia for veterinary technicians, ed 4, St Louis, 2011, Mosby, whose work forms the heart of this chapter.

KEY TERMS

Analgesia	Closed-suction drain	Hypothermia	Penrose drain
Arrhythmia	Débridement	Intraosseous	Percussion
Atelectasis	Decubital ulcer	Lavage	Phlebitis
Auscultation	Dyspnea	Mentation	Presenting complaint
Bradycardia	Eschar	Normothermia	Tachycardia
Capillary refill time	Euthanasia	Nystagmus	Tenesmus
Central catheter	Hyperthermia	Orthopnea	

PATIENT HISTORY AND CLIENT INTERACTION

A patient's history and physical examination are the foundations on which sound medical and nursing interventions are based. Animal patients cannot verbally communicate the ailments or discomforts caused by disease. Therefore, you must pay meticulous attention to the observations and concerns voiced by the client, who provides information from which you may formulate the patient's history. Astute observations from the veterinarian and the veterinary staff are crucial when performing the physical examination.

COMMUNICATING WITH CLIENTS

Communication is the key to successful history taking. The interviewer must be able to ask questions that are easily understood and are geared toward the animal's owner. If necessary, slang words describing certain conditions may be used to facilitate communication and avoid misunderstanding.

The interview is most successfully conducted when the veterinary staff member is professional but cheerful, friendly, and genuinely concerned about the patient (Fig. 8-1). A dry, inquisitional approach, consisting of rapid-fire questions, is typically less effective in unearthing important details of the history.

The best clinical interview focuses on the patient. When speaking with the client, determine the primary medical problem (presenting or chief complaint), as well as how the specific signs of illness are observed by the client. An important interviewing technique uses reflective listening methods that incorporate active listening, infrequent interruption, limited speaking, and asking for clarification when needed. Interrupting an animal owner may disrupt his or her train of thought and prevent the client from reporting important facts (Box 8-1).

Allow the client to control the interview, at least in part. Once the client has reported the facts, repeat important information, indicating that you have heard him or her and understand the concern. If the history given is vague, use direct questioning. Asking about how, where, and when is generally more effective than asking about why.

Obtaining a thorough history by a medical interview depends on the technical knowledge and communication skills of the interviewer. The interview should be flexible and spontaneous, not interrogative. The major goal of the interview is to sort through the reported signs associated with the illness. Although the novice may have limited knowledge of the signs associated with various diseases, with experience and education one can learn to recognize the history and signs as they relate to various injuries and illnesses.

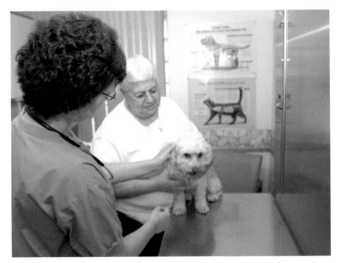

FIGURE 8-1 The interview should be conducted in a professional yet friendly manner while displaying genuine concern for the patient and client. The appearance, attire, and attitude of the veterinary staff set the tone of the visit and convey an impression of the quality of veterinary services being rendered. (From Sirois M: Principles and practice of veterinary technology, ed 3, St Louis, 2011, Mosby.)

BOX 8-1	Five Vowels of a Good Interview

1. **A**udition—listening carefully to the client's story
2. **E**valuation—sorting data to determine which is important and which is irrelevant
3. **I**nquiry—probing into the significant areas requiring more clarification
4. **O**bservation—observing nonverbal communication, body language, and facial expressions, regardless of what is said
5. **U**nderstanding the client's concerns and apprehensions; enables interviewer to play more empathic role

Adapted from Sirois M: Principles and practice of veterinary technology, ed 3, St Louis, 2011, Mosby.

OBTAINING A HISTORY

The information gathered when obtaining a history should alert the veterinary team to potential problems. Diseases tend to be characterized by a certain group of signs. With only one isolated clinical sign, do not jump to conclusions or allow premature assumptions or preconceptions to affect your objectivity when making additional assessments.

INTRODUCTORY STATEMENT

Open the interview by introducing yourself and explaining what you will be doing. For example, you might say, "Good morning, Mrs. Schwartz. My name is Joe Smith. I'm a veterinary assistant and I'll be obtaining a history and performing a preliminary examination on Buffy. Can you please tell me the reason for Buffy's visit today?" You can then validate the preliminary data, if needed, and go on to obtain the history for the presenting complaint (Box 8-2).

PATIENT CHARACTERISTICS

The receptionist can obtain certain preliminary data, such as patient characteristics (e.g., age, breed, gender, reproductive status). The technician or assistant should verify that the patient's age, breed, gender, and reproductive status have been correctly recorded and note any changes since the patient's last visit (e.g., if the patient has been spayed or castrated).

Pay close attention to the patient's age. Congenital and infectious diseases, parasitism, ingestion of foreign bodies, and intussusceptions are usually predominant in young animals. Degenerative diseases and neoplasia are more common in adult animals. Certain species or breeds are predisposed to particular problems. For example, toy breeds of dogs (e.g., Chihuahuas, Pomeranians) are predisposed to patellar luxation and hydrocephalus. Brachycephalic (short-nosed) dogs are predisposed to respiratory problems. Combined immunodeficiency affects Arabian horses. These predispositions are considered when the veterinarian formulates a list of differential diagnoses (diagnostic possibilities).

> **CRITICAL CONCEPT**
>
> The initial medical history often helps guide the diagnostic plan.

BOX 8-2 | Introduction to the Client

- Review the preliminary data (e.g., animal's name and gender) before introducing yourself to the client.
- If the patient is a new animal to the household or farm or a geriatric patient not seen recently, or if the owner is a new client, note the medical record.
- Greet the client by name, make eye contact, shake hands firmly, and smile.
- Always address the client by an honorific title (e.g., Mrs., Mr.) and his or her last name.

Adapted from Sirois M: Principles and practice of veterinary technology, ed 3, St Louis, 2011, Mosby.

The patient's gender and reproductive status are important because certain conditions are gender-specific and determine which areas should be given special attention in the patient evaluation. For example, in a 10-year-old intact (not spayed) female dog with a history of excessive water consumption and urination, vomiting, and lethargy, pyometra (uterine infection) would be an important differential diagnosis. In a 5-year-old spayed female with the same history, however, diabetes mellitus would be an important differential diagnosis. The incidence of some diseases decreases markedly as a result of ovariohysterectomy (spay) or castration. Dogs spayed at an early age are less likely to develop mammary tumors and castrated male dogs are at a lower risk of developing perianal adenomas.

ORIGIN, PRIOR OWNERSHIP, AND CURRENT ENVIRONMENT

Questions concerning geographic origin and prior ownership may indicate exposure to infectious or parasitic diseases. Information on the pet's current environment, including information about the patient's diet, is also needed to help identify risk factors for specific diseases. For example, free-roaming or pastured animals are at higher risk of exposure to toxins or trauma and multiple-cat households and catteries have a higher prevalence of infectious respiratory diseases and feline leukemia virus infection. Box 8-3 lists some common questions used to obtain this information from the client.

PAST MEDICAL HISTORY

Past medical history provides information about the patient's health before the current illness. Carefully inquire about and record the dates of previous illnesses and treatment, hospitalization, and surgeries, followed by a brief description of

---

BOX 8-3 | Questions for Obtaining Patient Environmental Information

Geographic Origin and Prior Ownership
1. Where the patient originated (e.g., home, breeder, pet shop, animal shelter, neighboring farm, livestock auction)
2. Where it has recently traveled
3. Whether it was recently boarded or shown

Environment and Activities
1. Is it an indoor or outdoor animal?
2. Is the pet free-roaming or confined to a yard or house?
3. Is the animal housed in a pasture or stable?
4. Does the patient share the environment with other animals?

Dietary Questions
1. Can you describe the pet's appetite?
2. Has there been any noticeable weight loss or gain?
3. What type of diet is fed? (e.g., dry, moist, or table food)
4. Does the pet receive any dietary supplements?
5. What is the brand name of food that is fed?
6. How often is the pet fed (free choice or individual meals)?
7. How much food is consumed daily?

Adapted from Sirois M: Principles and practice of veterinary technology, ed 3, St Louis, 2011, Mosby.

each problem, how it was managed, and how the patient responded to treatment. Ask the client to describe any allergies (e.g., environmental, ingestible, drug-related) and how these were diagnosed. Note any medications that the patient is currently receiving. It is important to determine whether the client is giving medications as prescribed.

VACCINATION STATUS

Question the client about the patient's vaccination status and when any vaccinations were given. Some clients are not familiar with vaccination schedules and may simply report that their animal has been vaccinated. It is easy to presume that the patient is up to date on vaccinations, when in fact the vaccinations may have been given several years ago. Be aware of recommended intervals for vaccinations and diagnostic tests. For example, inquire when a cat was last assessed for exposure to feline leukemia virus and feline immunodeficiency virus. Ask whether a dog has been checked for heartworm infection in the past year and whether heartworm preventive medication is being used and, if so, what type of preventive medication is being used.

PRESENTING COMPLAINT

The **presenting complaint** is why the client has sought veterinary care for the animal. For example, the client may say that a cat has had diarrhea for 3 days, is not eating, and is depressed. It is important to remember that the presenting complaint is what the client perceives the patient's problem to be. Pay attention to these concerns, even though the client's fears or anxieties may influence your observations of the animal. Allow the client to communicate these observations and then continue with the interview. This tends to relieve a client's anxieties about the animal.

Another important interviewing skill is the ability to assess the source and reliability of the information obtained. A history obtained from second parties presenting the animal for evaluation (e.g., friends, neighbors, children) may lack important information that only the client can provide.

It is also important to determine whether the client understands the meaning of the medical terms that he or she uses to describe the problem. Ask the client to define these terms. For example, "What do you mean when you say the cat regurgitated?" A client may bring in a dog and say that it "just had a stroke." To an experienced veterinary professional, the patient's ataxia, incoordination, head tilt, and horizontal **nystagmus** may indicate vestibular disease rather than a cerebrovascular accident (stroke). It is important to record the clinical signs observed and not the client's presumptive diagnosis. Be aware that the client's comments, observations, and conclusions are based on her or his experience. We must interpret the client's comments, observations, and conclusions in light of our professional experience.

Once the presenting complaint is listed, record the information gathered in chronologic order to clarify areas of possible confusion. Separate the client's observations from his or her conclusions and amplify certain portions of the complaint that may be important.

HISTORY OF PRESENTING COMPLAINT. The history is best recorded by chronology (i.e., in the order in which events occurred). This provides a better understanding of the sequence and development of the problem (Box 8-4). Begin with the first sign of illness observed by the client and follow its progression to the present time.

It is important to determine when the client first noticed the presenting complaint, apart from any other health problems. Some patients might have other ongoing health problems (e.g., flea bite dermatitis, food allergies) unrelated to the current complaint. Ask for specific information that describes the signs observed (e.g., color, odor, consistency, and volume of vomitus or diarrhea). When the client uses terms such as somewhat, a little, sometimes, or rarely, ask for clarification. Remember, precise communication is important.

Some clients simply cannot remember when the signs first developed. You may be able to help the client relate the onset of signs to some event. For example, ask, "Was the dog's lameness evident around the Thanksgiving or Christmas holiday?" When obtaining information about the presenting complaint, use open-ended questions that allow the client to describe the problem, rather than simple yes or no questions. Table 8-1 illustrates a series of open-ended questions that elucidate the sequence of events and nature of the problem.

CONCLUDING THE HISTORY

If any part of the history needs further clarification, it should be done after all the initial information has been gathered. At this point, you may wish to summarize the most important parts of the history for the client. Encourage the client to correct any misinterpretations and discuss any additional concerns. Allow the client the final say. At the conclusion of the interview, thank the client and say that you will now perform a physical examination of the patient.

PHYSICAL EXAMINATION

The physical examination assesses the animal's current state of health and is generally performed by the veterinary technician or veterinarian, with the veterinary assistant providing restraint and record-keeping support. It is crucial that all observations be recorded accurately, using standardized terminology. Figure 8-2 shows an example of a properly recorded comprehensive physical examination. Patients are evaluated using a combination of methods. These include

BOX 8-4	History of Presenting Complaint

The history of the current complaint helps determine the following:
- When the animal was last normal
- Whether the condition is acute or chronic
- What medications and dosages were used previously
- How the patient responded to previous therapy
- Duration and progression of clinical signs

Adapted from Sirois M: Principles and practice of veterinary technology, ed 3, St Louis, 2011, Mosby.

TABLE 8-1	Examples of Open-Ended Questions	
QUESTIONS	**PURPOSE**
Why is Buffy being presented?	Identifies the presenting complaint
When did you first notice the problem?	Determines the onset of the problem
What was the first sign that you observed? What did you notice after that initial sign?	Helps establish progression of the problem
Can you describe in detail the signs you observed?	Helps identify clinical signs observed, rather than the client's diagnosis
Was there any change in routine or anything new, unusual, or different in Buffy's routine at the time of onset?	Helps determine precipitating events
Has Buffy been treated for this problem before? How did she respond?	Determines the response to previous treatment

Adapted from Sirois M: Principles and practice of veterinary technology, ed 3, St Louis, 2011, Mosby.

REPORT OF PHYSICAL EXAMINATION

ABC Animal Clinic
South Beach Street
Sunshine FL

Patient Name ___Gandalf Abbott___
Description _brown_
Microchip ID__183469__
Date___12/12/09___
Gender _M_ Breed_Boxer_ Age _3yrs_

(1) General ☑ WNL ☐ Abn ☐ NE	(2) Integument ☐ WNL ☑ Abn ☐ NE	(3) M/S ☑ WNL ☐ Abn ☐ NE	(4) Circulatory ☑ WNL ☐ Abn ☐ NE	(5) Respiratory ☑ WNL ☐ Abn ☐ NE	(6) Digestive ☑ WNL ☐ Abn ☐ NE
(7) Genitourinary ☑ WNL ☐ Abn ☐ NE	(8) Eyes ☑ WNL ☐ Abn ☐ NE	(9) Ears ☑ WNL ☐ Abn ☐ NE	(10) NS ☑ WNL ☐ Abn ☐ NE	(11) Lymphatic ☑ WNL ☐ Abn ☐ NE	(12) Mucosa ☑ WNL ☐ Abn ☐ NE

Temp (F) 102	Pulse 140	Resp 18	Weight 41kg	WNL = no abnormalition; Abn = abnormalition; noted; NE= not examined

Temperament / Behavioral Assessment

Playful; curious; doesn't walk well on leash

Describe Examination Findings Below:

1. BAR; very playful

2. No evidence of alopecia, rashes, lesions; skin turgor reveals adequate hydration; s1 flea dirt at base of tail

3. No evidence of joint swelling; full range of motion on manipulation of limbs; no evidence of pain, limping, guarding, or tenderness; overall muscular symmetrical/ well fleshed

4. No evidence of arrhythmia on cardiac auscultation; No pulse deficit detected; CRT < 2 secs.

5. No evidence of crackles or wheezes on auscultation; no postural signs of dyspnea; no evidence of nasal discharge

6. No evidence of diarrhea on or around rectum, no evidence of vomitus in/around oral cavity, s1 tenderness on palpation-caudal 1/3 of abdomen

7. Kidneys palpate firm; bladder palpates full; no evidence of penile discharge; testicles present in scrotal sacs

8. Characteristic pupillary light response; no evidence of ocular abrasions or discharge

9. Characteristic odor; moderate cerumen; no evidence of parasites or tenderness

10. No evidence of head tilt or tremors; characteristic gait

11. Lymph nodes not palpable

12. Mucosa-pink; no evidence of periodontal disease

FIGURE 8-2 Completed physical examination form. (From Sirois M: Principles and practice of veterinary technology, ed 3, St Louis, 2011, Mosby.)

BOX 8-5	Systematic Method of Physical Examination

1. Record temperature, pulse, and respiration.
2. Evaluate and record animal's general condition (e.g., disposition, activity level, overall body condition).
3. Evaluate and record condition of each body system, including the following:
   - **Integumentary:** Note overall condition of hair coat, presence or absence of alopecia, parasites, lumps, wounds, rashes. Note hydration status with skin turgor test.
   - **Respiratory:** Evaluate respiratory rate and rhythm; record presence or absence of rales, rhonchi, crepitus, dyspnea, nasal discharge.
   - **Cardiovascular:** Evaluate cardiac rate and rhythm, CRT, presence or absence of pulse (e.g., deficit).
   - **Gastrointestinal:** Record presence or absence of diarrhea, vomiting (note character, if present). Palpate abdomen and record presence or absence of signs such as tenderness or impaction.
   - **Genitourinary:** Palpate kidneys and bladder. Note presence of characteristic urine volume; note any abnormalities in urine (e.g., blood). In male, check for presence or absence of testicles in scrotum; penile discharge. In female, record evidence of pregnancy, lactation, vaginal discharge (note character, if present).
   - **Musculoskeletal:** Evaluate presence or absence of swelling (particularly in joints); manipulate limbs; record any abnormal gait, limping, guarding, tenderness; note overall musculature.
   - **Nervous:** Record presence or absence of head tilt, tremors. Evaluate pupillary light reflexes. Evaluate and record triceps, patellar, and gastrocnemius reflexes.
   - **Eyes:** Evaluate and record presence or absence of abrasions, ulcers, discharge (note character, if present).
   - **Ears:** Evaluate and record presence or absence of tenderness, parasites, odor, ulcers, discharge (note character, if present).
   - **Mucosa:** Note color of mucous membranes, evaluate odor of mouth, evaluate periodontal tissues.
   - **Lymphatic:** Palpate peripheral lymph nodes, evaluate characteristic size and location of lymph nodes.

Adapted from Sirois M: Principles and practice of veterinary technology, ed 3, St Louis, 2011, Mosby.

inspection, palpation, auscultation, and **percussion**. A visual examination is performed on first contact with the patient, paying close attention to deviations or abnormalities. Box 8-5 provides an overview of physical examination procedures.

MONITORING VITAL SIGNS

Vital signs include the body temperature, respiratory rate and effort, heart rate and rhythm, and indications of perfusion. These reflect overall patient status; changes in any vital sign can warn the medical team of impending complications. Veterinary assistants generally can perform these assessments. Vital signs are monitored at regular intervals. The initial findings are used as the baseline, and subsequent findings help establish trends indicating improvement or deterioration. To identify abnormalities, you must know the normal ranges for each species, age group, and sometimes breed (Table 8-2).

> **CRITICAL CONCEPT**
> Respiratory rate and effort, heart rate and rhythm, and evaluation of perfusion are assessed and recorded at regular intervals.

AUSCULTATION

Listening to sounds produced by the body is termed **auscultation.** Auscultation may be direct (with the ear and no instrument) or indirect (using a stethoscope to amplify sounds). The stethoscope allows auscultation of specific areas within a body cavity for assessment of the cardiovascular, respiratory, and gastrointestinal systems (Fig. 8-3).

Abnormal sounds can be recognized only after one has learned to identify the types of sounds normally arising from each body structure and the location in which they are usually heard. Proficiency at auscultation requires good hearing, a good-quality stethoscope, and knowledge of how to use a stethoscope correctly.

The stethoscope's chest piece should have a stiff, flat diaphragm and a bell (Fig. 8-4). The diaphragm is the flat, circular portion of the chest piece covered by a thin, resilient membrane. It transmits high-pitched sounds, such as those produced by the bowel, lungs, and heart. The bell is not

TABLE 8-2	Normal Ranges of Heart Rate, Respiratory Rate, and Rectal Temperature in Adults of Some Domestic Species		
ANIMAL	**HEART RATE (BEATS/MIN)**	**RESPIRATORY RATE (BREATHS/MIN)**	**RECTAL TEMPERATURE**
Dogs	70-160	8-20	37.5°-39° C (99.5°-102.2° F)
Cats	150-210	8-30	38°-39° C (100.4°-102.2° F)
Hamsters	250-500	35-135	37°-38° C (98.6°-100.4° F)
Guinea pigs	230-280	42-104	37.2°-39.5° C (99°-103.1° F)
Rabbits	130-325	30-60	38.5°-40° C (101.3°-104° F)

Adapted from Sirois M: Principles and practice of veterinary technology, ed 3, St Louis, 2011, Mosby.

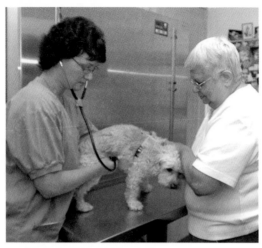

FIGURE 8-3 Thoracic auscultation is used to evaluate the lungs and heart. The abdomen can also be auscultated to evaluate gastrointestinal sounds. (From Sirois M: Principles and practice of veterinary technology, ed 3, St Louis, 2011, Mosby.)

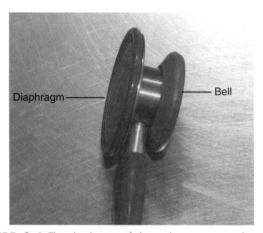

FIGURE 8-4 The diaphragm of the stethoscope is used to detect high-pitched sounds, such as heart, bowel, and lung sounds. The bell is used to detect lower-frequency sounds, such as the third and fourth heart sounds. (From Sirois M: Principles and practice of veterinary technology, ed 3, St Louis, 2011, Mosby.)

covered by a membrane. It facilitates auscultation of lower-frequency sounds, such as third and fourth sounds of the heart, or what is most commonly termed a gallop rhythm.

CRITICAL CONCEPT

Evaluation of perfusion involves assessment of mucous membrane color, capillary refill time, pulse strength and quality, and body temperature.

WEIGHT

Weigh each patient daily, at the same time and on the same scale, to help monitor hydration and nutrition status. Daily weighing is of particular importance in neonatal animals and in patients on high IV fluid rates (e.g., renal failure). All animals seen on appointment should also have their body weight recorded, regardless of the reason for the visit. Large walk-on scales or hydraulic lift tables are used to obtain the

weight of medium-sized to large dogs. A feline or pediatric scale can be used for small dogs and cats. The animal must be still to obtain an accurate weight (Fig. 8-5).

BODY TEMPERATURE

Get a baseline temperature on every patient immediately on admittance to the hospital and during every routine appointment. Body temperature can be monitored rectally with a standard mercury thermometer, digital thermometer (battery operated), or electronic probe for continuous monitoring rectally. Leave the thermometer in the rectum for 2 or 3 minutes—count the pulse and respiratory rates while waiting—and record the temperature. Disposable thermometer covers should be used to prevent nosocomial infection (Fig. 8-6).

Temperature change can be an early sign of a illness; for example, temperature can decrease in renal failure and increase in bacterial infection. Monitoring temperature can be an important indicator and early sign of a patient's condition improving or deteriorating. Monitoring temperature is critical for any patient undergoing surgery or anesthesia.

Maintenance of normal body temperature (**normothermia**) involves regulating the external environment and internal environment of the patient. **Hypothermia** (subnormal body temperature) can occur with shock, severe sepsis, severe cardiac insufficiency, multiple organ failure, poor perfusion secondary to anesthesia or surgery, or low environmental temperatures. Hypothermia can be combated with circulating warm water blankets (not electric heating pads), forced-air warming

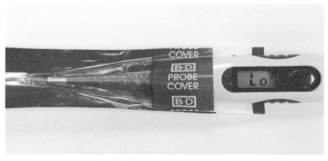

FIGURE 8-5 Pediatric scale used to obtain weight on cats and small dogs.

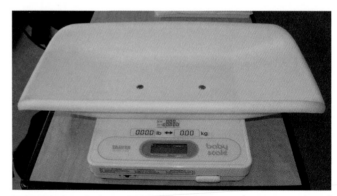

FIGURE 8-6 When taking a patient's temperature, use disposable thermometer covers to prevent nosocomial infection. (From Sirois M: Principles and practice of veterinary technology, ed 3, St Louis, 2011, Mosby.)

devices, warm water bottles, warmed towels or blankets, warm bath, blow dryer, heat lamp, or incubator. For patients with severely low temperatures, IV fluids can help increase perfusion and subsequently increase core body temperature. Fluids may be warmed to 37° C (98.6° F) with a fluid warmer, or the IV line can be run through a bowl of warm water.

Monitor the rectal temperature at least every 30 minutes in patients with marked hypothermia (<97° F [36° C]). Discontinue warming when the rectal temperature approaches the normal range (99° F [37° C]). Do not overheat the patient. Most water blankets can be adjusted (lowered) to normal body temperature to maintain normothermia and not overheat patients. Always have a towel or pad between the water blanket and patient. Electric heating pads are not recommended because of the possibility of electric shock, overheating, and burns. If a heat lamp is used, the patient must be able to move away from the heat source. When using an incubator or oxygen cage, extreme care must be taken to avoid overheating the patient; temperatures should be monitored and recorded frequently.

Hyperthermia (abnormally high body temperature) may occur with infection, sepsis, toxicity, inflammation, brain lesions or tumors (loss of thermoregulation), heat stroke, seizures, stress, and excitation. Patients with extreme and persistent hyperthermia (>104.5° F [40° C]) require constant monitoring. Hyperthermia can be controlled with ice wrapped in towels, fans, alcohol application, and cool drinking water. Cold water and/or ice applied to the jugular and femoral arteries will cool the patient more quickly. Discontinue cooling when the rectal temperature reaches 103° F (39.5° C). Do not overcool the patient; vasoconstriction may occur, which could impair perfusion.

> ### CRITICAL CONCEPT
> For severe hyperthermia, apply isopropyl alcohol to the foot pads in addition to spraying cold water on the patient and placing a fan nearby for convection.

PULSE

Determination of the heart rate is the first diagnostic clue about the cardiovascular status of the patient. Normal heart rate for the dog ranges from 70 beats/min in larger dogs to as high as 220 beats/min in puppies. Normal heart rates for cats and kittens range from 120 to 240 beats/min. A slower-than-normal heart rate is termed **bradycardia,** and a faster-than-normal rate is termed **tachycardia**. Abnormalities in heart rate or rhythm must be identified and characterized by performing electrocardiography to determine the precise nature of the rate and/or rhythm abnormality. Assessment of the pulse quality, heart rate, and heart rhythm can also help determine the patient's hemodynamic status and guide the course of treatment.

Auscultate the heart while palpating the pulse. A pulse deficit (a difference in the number of heartbeats and pulse beats) may indicate an **arrhythmia** (Fig. 8-7). Pulses can be described as absent, weak and thready, normal, bounding, or irregular. Pulse quality should be assessed in the dorsal pedal and femoral regions of the dog and cat; differences in pulse strength may indicate a perfusion abnormality.

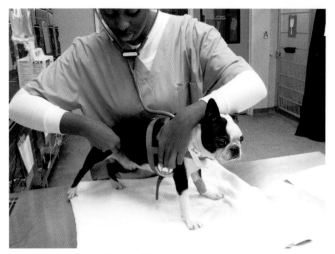

FIGURE 8-7 Auscultation of heart rate and rhythm in conjunction with the palpation of an arterial pulse will detect presence of "dropped beats" or arrhythmias. (From Sirois M: Principles and practice of veterinary technology, ed 3, St Louis, 2011, Mosby.)

There are two normal rhythm variations in the dog. Normal sinus rhythm has a regular beat with a normal rate. A normal respiratory sinus arrhythmia has a normal-to-slow heart rate and is characterized by an increase in heart rate during inspiration and a decrease in heart rate during expiration. Respiratory sinus arrhythmia is common in dogs but uncommon in the cat. Other common rhythm abnormalities include beats that occur prematurely and may be associated with pulse deficits. Arrhythmias that are characterized by intermittent prolonged periods of asystole are termed bradyarrhythmias.

Presence of a cardiac murmur should also be noted during cardiac auscultation. In general, the patient should be in a sternal or standing position during auscultation because a murmur can be positional. Characterization of murmurs is based on several criteria, of which timing in the cycle, location, or point of maximal intensity (PMI) of the murmur and intensity (loudness) are the most important.

Note that murmurs can often be heard in young puppies and kittens. These are generally soft systolic murmurs heard best at the mitral or aortic valves. Termed innocent murmurs, they are often transient and disappear by 3 to 4 months of age. Their cause is not known. Physiologic murmurs are categorized as those that occur in anemic animals and result from changes in blood viscosity, which results in disruption of normal blood flow. These are soft murmurs that resolve with resolution of the underlying disease.

RESPIRATION

Observe the patient's respiratory effort when it is relaxed and breathing normally, if possible. Check the rate and depth of respiration. Normal respiratory rates in small animals are approximately 18 to 30 breaths/min. The patient should be in sternal recumbency and allowed to inhale oxygen during the examination, if stressed, to facilitate lung expansion and accurate auscultation. It is recommended that the pediatric head of the stethoscope be used for smaller patients to avoid referred sounds. The auscultation should include both sides of the chest, ventrally and

BOX 8-6	Significance of Common Respiratory Sounds

Harsh or Static Sounds
- Trauma
- Lung parenchymal disease
- Early fluid overload
- Asthma

Crackles or Popping Sounds
- Lung parenchymal disease
- Severe fluid overload
- Asthma

Wheezes or Musical Sounds
- Asthma
- Chronic bronchitis

Upper Airway (Referred) Sounds
- Stenosis
- Elongated soft palate
- Tracheal collapse
- Tracheal constriction

Muffled or Absent Lung Sounds
- Pneumothorax
- Hemothorax
- Chylothorax
- Diaphragmatic hernia

Noisy Breathing (Inspiratory Stridor)
- Upper airway obstruction
- Laryngeal paralysis

From Sirois M: Principles and practice of veterinary technology, ed 3, St Louis, 2011, Mosby.

dorsally, while paying close attention to the respiratory pattern. Respiratory effort should be noted in conjunction with the respiratory component.

In general, respiratory patterns and lung sounds are subtler in cats than in dogs. Respiratory patterns should be assessed before restraint or manipulation, when possible. Chest expansion should be assessed in any respiratory movement, paying close attention to inhalation and exhalation sounds during auscultation.

Identifying the type of respiratory sounds in ill or injured patients can be difficult. Common respiratory sounds include harsh- or static-sounding lungs, crackles or popping sounds, wheezes or musical sounds, or upper airway sounds (Box 8-6). It is important to combine lung sounds with other physical examination findings such as patient **mentation**, respiratory rate, respiratory effort, respiratory pattern, heart rate, pulse quality, temperature, and mucous membrane color. Monitoring the trends of these examination findings is critical in providing good nursing care. Note that respiratory sounds in pediatric patients may fluctuate more easily than those in adults because of their more fragile, immature immune system.

Other respiratory sounds include inspiratory **dyspnea**, characterized by a prolonged, labored inspiratory effort and a quicker, easier expiratory phase. Stertors and/or stridors frequently accompany inspiratory dyspnea. Stertor is

defined as a low-pitched snoring noise, whereas stridor is a high-pitched, harsh, wheezy noise. Expiratory dyspnea is often characterized by a prolonged, labored expiratory effort.

Patient posture is noted as part of the respiratory evaluation. Dyspnea may be manifested as a refusal to lie down. Note the quality of the animal's breathing. Is there difficulty on inspiration or expiration? Is the breathing abdominal? **Orthopnea** is a term applied to respiratory distress that is exacerbated by recumbency. Animals showing orthopnea assume a standing or sitting position with elbows abducted and neck extended. Movement of the abdominal muscles that assist ventilation is often exaggerated. Such animals vigorously resist being placed in lateral recumbency. Finally, note any coughing, muscle wasting, or abdominal distention. Presence of a cough may indicate bronchial diseases in cats, causing abnormal airway sounds.

MUCOUS MEMBRANE COLOR

The mucous membrane color can also supply a wealth of information in assessing the respiratory system. Keep in mind that pink membranes may not necessarily indicate a stable, well-perfused patient. Combine pulse quality with the mucous membrane analysis to determine hemodynamic stability better. Note differences between pedal and femoral pulse quality; femoral pulses may be difficult to find in the cat versus the dog, particularly if overweight. Pale or white mucous membranes may not indicate respiratory dysfunction but rather hypothermia, pain, decreased cardiac output, anemia, or peripheral vasoconstriction. In addition, brick red membranes may indicate a hyperemic, hypercapnic state, indicating poor ventilation. Cyanotic mucous membranes (blue colored) may indicate an increase in the concentration of deoxygenated hemoglobin (Fig. 8-8).

CAPILLARY REFILL TIME

The **capillary refill time** (CRT) is the rate of return of color to oral mucous membranes after the application of gentle digital pressure (Fig. 8-9) and is indicative of the perfusion of the peripheral tissues with blood. The pressure applied to the mucous membranes compresses the small capillaries and temporarily blocks blood flow to that area. When the pressure is released, the capillaries rapidly refill with blood and the color returns, provided perfusion is adequate. A prolonged CRT (>2 seconds) indicates that tissues in the area tested have reduced blood perfusion. Poor perfusion will also result in reduced temperature of the affected part.

CRITICAL CONCEPT

Careful examination of the respiratory rate, effort, body posture, and respiratory pattern can help locate the source of respiratory distress. Pay close attention to each inspiratory and expiratory phase of respiration.

URINE PRODUCTION

Urination frequency should be recorded on all hospitalized patients, particularly critical pets. Walk dogs regularly and record any urination. Evaluate frequency of urination on cats

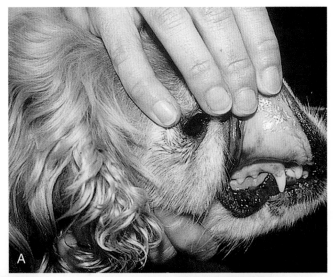

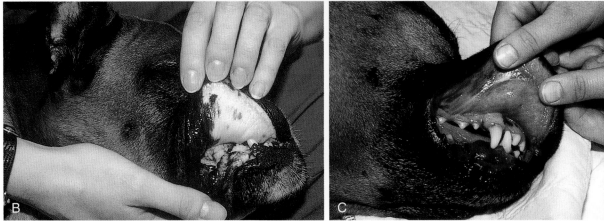

FIGURE 8-8 **A,** Icterus mucous membrane color in a cocker spaniel with liver disease. **B,** Pale mucous membrane in a boxer with a packed cell volume of 13%. **C,** Brick-red mucous membrane in a mongrel with septic shock. (From Battaglia A: *Small animal emergency and critical care,* ed 2, St Louis, 2007, Elsevier.)

by cleaning out the litter box often, also making sure to check bedding and underneath cage mats for possible eliminations. Patients on IV fluids may have an increased amount of urine production and may need to be walked more frequently.

Dogs can be taken outside to urinate if no urinary catheter is in place to collect and measure urine. Walk ambulatory canine patients outside every 4 hours during the day to eliminate. A bedpan works well for catching the urine; then pour the urine into a graduated container to measure. Disposable pads or diapers can be used in recumbent patients to facilitate cleaning and measure urine output by weight. After a patient urinates on the diapers, remove and weigh them. Subtract the initial weight of the paper or diaper; the remainder is the weight of the urine. Convert that into milliliters to determine the approximate urine output. Normal urine output is 1 to 2 mL/kg/hr. Recumbent animals can be placed on trampolines or cots; urine can be measured by placing paper, diapers, or even a bowl underneath the cot (Fig. 8-10).

Urinary catheterization permits accurate measurement of urine output, facilitates collection of urine for analysis, promotes cleanliness of recumbent patients, and reduces exposure of other patients or personnel to contaminated urine.

A urinary catheter and collection system also keeps the bladder empty in patients with bladder dysfunction or patients on high fluid administration rates. Indwelling urinary catheters should be placed and handled with sterile technique.

> ### CRITICAL CONCEPT
> Always wear gloves when handling animal urine. This is of particular importance in dogs that may have leptospirosis.

In cats with lower urinary tract disease, urinary catheters prevent reobstruction. Cats without urinary catheters can have their urine output quantitated by using an empty litter pan, paper litter, plastic beads, or diapers. The paper litter and litter pan should be weighed before placing in the cage. Plastic beads can be used as litter; urine can be collected by use of a strainer and bowl.

GASTROINTESTINAL MONITORING

Monitor all excretions (e.g., urine, feces, vomit, saliva) from the patient and record a description, including estimated quantity, on the patient's chart. Characterizing the color and

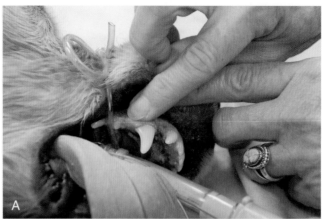

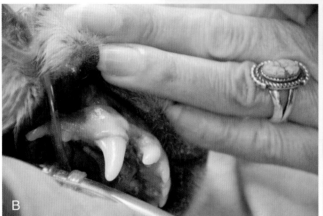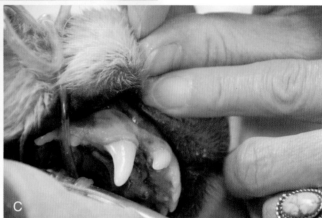

FIGURE 8-9 Capillary refill time. **A,** Application of digital pressure. **B,** Blanching of the mucous membranes. **C,** Return of color, which in a normal patient should occur in 2 seconds or less. (From Thomas JA, Lerche P: Anesthesia and analgesia for veterinary technicians, ed 4, St Louis, 2011, Mosby.)

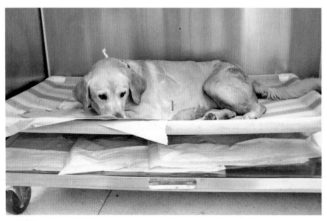

FIGURE 8-10 Trampolines will prevent decubital ulcers and urine scalding in the recumbent patient. (From Sirois M: Principles and practice of veterinary technology, ed 3, St Louis, 2011, Mosby.)

content of the vomitus (e.g., yellow or bile-like, green, coffee ground, partially or undigested food, watery, or foul-smelling) and the feces (e.g., black, red with frank blood, mucoid, watery) can help aid the diagnosis. Regurgitation must be differentiated from vomiting. Vomiting is typically active and projectile; regurgitation is typically passive, quiet, and often associated with movement. In patients that do not or

cannot drink water, calculated fluid losses should be replaced with IV fluids.

The patient's body must be kept clean and free of body waste and excretions. Cleaning and flushing the oral cavity with saline, water, or a weak tea solution can help prevent or heal oral ulcers. Flushing or suctioning any vomitus out of the mouth also makes the patient feel better. The mouth of patients that cannot take food or water per os (PO, by mouth) may be moistened with a gauze sponge and water. The skin around the mouth should be kept clean of vomitus and saliva to prevent scalding and secondary bacterial infections. In comatose patients, or patients intubated for extended periods, the tongue should be kept moist by frequent water application or kept wrapped with moist gauze.

Patients with diarrhea must be kept as clean and dry as possible. Clean the cage or run thoroughly and replace any soiled bedding. Frequent walks outside to eliminate help the patient feel better and reduce cage cleanup. Any abnormal stool should be characterized in the medical record; include the color, amount, and general composition. Large, watery stools are more typical of small bowel diarrhea, whereas bloody or tarry stools can indicate a potentially life-threatening condition such as gastrointestinal (GI) bleeding or ulceration. The veterinary assistant should help question the owner concerning diet history. The dietary history is paramount because in small animals diarrhea is often diet induced. Recent dietary changes to a moist high-fat or meat-based diet, more frequent feeding of table scraps, or access to garbage or dead animals can be responsible.

Patients that have not had a bowel movement in the past 2 days but are still eating should be closely monitored and encouraged to eliminate (e.g., taken outside on a long leash, placed in an outdoor run, provided a larger litterbox or different litter). Diet changes may be necessary (e.g., canned food, addition of fiber). Enemas may be indicated if constipation is diagnosed. Patients with certain neurologic abnormalities or patients in a drug-induced coma should have their colon evacuated manually. Any **tenesmus** (straining to defecate) should be reported to the veterinarian. Gut sounds should be monitored by auscultation at least twice daily as part of the physical examination.

> ### CRITICAL CONCEPT
> Gut sounds are important to monitor in any patient with a history of vomiting, diarrhea, inappetence, or recumbency. Place a stethoscope ventral to the last rib and monitor for gaseous, gurgling stomach sounds.

NUTRITIONAL SUPPORT

The primary goal of nutritional assessment is to identify whether a patient is at risk for malnutrition. Because altered nutritional status is associated with adverse clinical outcomes, it is important to address the nutritional needs early in the critically ill patient. Although clinical status alone may dictate the need for nutritional intervention, a thorough nutritional assessment consists of evaluating clinical and biochemical data, including patient history, and performing a thorough physical examination, including body weight and body condition scoring. A baseline nutritional assessment should be followed by serial assessments throughout the course of hospitalization. Nutritional intervention is crucial to recovery and survival, particularly with the critical patient, and appropriate consideration about the type and route of nutrition should be given based on the underlying disease process or diagnosis. Refer to Chapter 7 for detailed information on nutritional support for hospitalized patients.

GROOMING AND SKIN CARE

BATHING

The basic technique for bathing dogs and cats is to wet the coat thoroughly and then apply small amounts of shampoo, starting at the head and working back to the tail. Rubbing the shampoo into the coat until a lather is produced, again starting from the head and working back to the tail, is a generally accepted bathing method. The eyes should be protected from chemical injury by instilling a drop of mineral oil or a small amount of boric acid ophthalmic ointment in each eye before the bath. Care should be taken to prevent water from

entering the external ear canal; this can be accomplished by placing a small piece of cotton in each ear. Remember to remove the cotton when the bath has been completed. Thermal injury from excessively hot water can be prevented by monitoring the water temperature constantly. Thorough rinsing with clean water prevents irritation of the skin from residual shampoo. The axillary and scrotal regions of long-haired dogs are particularly vulnerable to residual shampoo irritation. If a cage dryer is used, caution must be exercised to prevent overheating (hyperthermia). Some states are taking steps to ban the use of cage dryers. Shampoos containing insecticides should be used only with the approval of the attending veterinarian because of the possibility of cumulative toxicity or drug interactions with medications or other topically applied insecticides. If insecticidal dips are used, correct dilutions are necessary to prevent toxic reactions. If a complete immersion bath is contraindicated, localized soiling of the animal may be handled with a sponge bath. Orthopedic or neurologic patients may not be able to stand steady in the bath tub; therefore, a rubber mat should be placed in the tub to help reduce the risk of injury.

> ### CRITICAL CONCEPT
> Always protect the eyes and ears of patients while bathing them.

Some hospitalized patients develop skin problems (e.g., decubital ulcers, pyoderma, urine scald, dry scaly skin) because of recumbency, urinary or fecal incontinence, stress, electrolyte imbalances, poor hydration, and general lack of appropriate care. Others have been healthy until admitted for trauma. Regardless of the reason for admittance to the hospital, all patients require routine grooming and skin care. Patients also feel better when kept clean and dry.

When a patient is admitted and its condition has been stabilized, any vomit, diarrhea, urine, or blood should be removed from the skin to prevent secondary infections. Skin care of the hospitalized patient involves bathing to remove body fluids, skin oil, or exudates, brushing to prevent mat formation, padding to prevent decubital ulcer formation, and medicating affected areas of skin. Surgical patients with diarrhea should be cleaned frequently to prevent incisional infections. Before the patient is discharged from the hospital, routine procedures such as toenail trimming, anal sac expression, and ear cleaning should be performed before a final bath.

SKIN CARE

Many critically ill patients are too weak or unable to get up to relieve themselves. Urine and fecal scalding develops if these patients are not cleaned after each incident. However, use good judgment before partially or completely bathing a critically ill patient. For example, if a dyspneic animal in an oxygen cage urinates on itself, remove the soiled bedding and spot-clean the patient. Do not jeopardize the patient's overall health to bathe the animal completely. Also, do not let the patient continue to lie in body waste without attempting to clean it. Sick pediatric patients should be dried thoroughly and kept warm if bathing is necessary.

Any long hair should be trimmed to prevent moisture from being trapped and causing a secondary infection. Carefully shave the hair around the perianal and inguinal areas for ease of cleaning. Avoid nicking or cutting the patient with the clippers. Apply a light tail wrap on long-haired patients with diarrhea to help keep the tail clean and prevent scalding. Wrap the tail loosely and incorporate some of the hair to keep the wrap in place. Change the wrap after each episode of diarrhea.

Patients with minor soiling can be spot-cleaned with mild solutions (e.g., Peri-Wash, Sween). Continuous diarrhea can cause perineal irritation and ulceration and may cause ascending urinary tract infection. A complete bath is recommended when large areas are soiled. Clean contaminated incision areas gently with water and a washcloth. Soak off any dried organic material. Pat the incision dry. Remove as much organic material from the patient as possible before placing in a bathtub and bathing. Apply a light layer of triple antibiotic ointment to the incision to prevent contact with water and shampoo.

If the patient is large and not able to walk, transfer the patient on a gurney to a tub with a grate placed over it, or slide the patient out of the cage onto a rack elevated above a floor drain. Have shampoo, several buckets of warm water, and towels ready before starting. If the patient does not have a urinary catheter, encourage urination before bathing. If the patient has not defecated in days, enemas or digital removal of feces may be necessary. Use this opportunity to make the patient more comfortable before bathing. Cover any clean and dry bandages with plastic to reduce the need for bandaging after the bath. Change any contaminated bandages. Patients with indwelling urinary catheters should have prepucial or vaginal areas free of any fecal material to prevent ascending urinary tract infections.

Wet the patient on the exposed side, apply shampoo, and scrub gently with your hands. Rinse thoroughly and turn the patient to the other side. Repeat the shampooing. Remove all wet and soiled bandages at this time. Clean and completely dry the areas under the bandages before replacing. Squeeze excess water from the hair and towel dry. Use a blow dryer to dry the exposed side; then turn the patient over and repeat on the other side. Completely dry the patient with a handheld dryer. Monitor patients frequently during drying, particularly obese or brachycephalic breeds.

A comb or brush may be used while drying the patient to decrease drying time. Use care when brushing thin-skinned patients with a slicker brush. The wire bristles can scratch the skin easily. Remove mats with scissors or electric clippers while the hair is dry, preferably before bathing. Before placing the patient back in the cage, make sure that the patient is completely dry and all irritated areas on the skin are examined, shaved if necessary, cleaned, and treated appropriately. Ointments, creams, lotions, drying solutions, or powders can be reapplied at this time. For recumbent patients, place clean towels or padding between the patient's legs to aerate the skin, make the patient more comfortable, and prevent scrotal edema. Roll a stockinette into a donut shape to pad any decubital ulcers, which typically form on bony prominences such as the scapula or femur (Fig. 8-11).

NAIL TRIMMING

Nail trimming (pedicure) is an important general care technique. Excessive nail length results in altered gait and the potential accentuation of lameness problems. Excessively long nails are more likely to split or to be traumatically avulsed. Finally, untrimmed nails can become ingrown (usually into the footpads), resulting in cellulite or abscess formation.

There are two common types of nail trimmers available (Whites, Resco; Fig. 8-12). To avoid cutting pigmented (black) nails too short in the dog, the cutting surface of the nail trimmer should be held parallel to the palmar or plantar

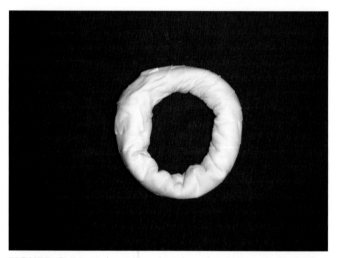

FIGURE 8-11 A donut-shaped pad used to help treat decubital ulcers. (From Sirois M: Principles and practice of veterinary technology, ed 3, St Louis, 2011, Mosby.)

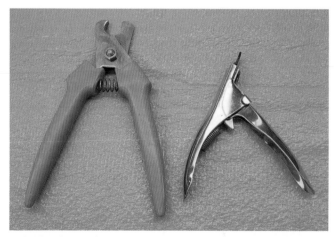

FIGURE 8-12 The two common types of nail trimmers, Whites (left) and Resco (right). The Whites nail trimmer is useful for very long nails that have curled back toward the footpad. (From McCurnin DM, Bassert JM: Clinical textbook for veterinary technicians, ed 6, St Louis, 2006, Saunders.)

surface of the digital footpads and the nail cut in this plane. In cats, the nails can be exposed by grasping the paw between the thumb and index finger and sliding the skin on the dorsum of the paw away from the nails (Fig. 8-13). Once exposed, the nails can be trimmed as described for the dog. It should be noted that nails that have not been trimmed regularly have a quick or nail vein that extends further out into the claw than that of regularly trimmed nails. In this situation, one should be conservative with regard to how much nail is trimmed. The center of the nail takes on a fleshy, shining appearance in the region next to the quick (Fig. 8-14). This is an indicator to trim no farther. Because some animals vehemently resent handling of their feet for nail trimming, it is a good practice to give a pedicure routinely to any animal anesthetized or tranquilized for any procedure.

> **CRITICAL CONCEPT**
>
> A Dremel tool may be used to ensure that the nail bed is trimmed down to the shortest possible length without eliciting trauma or bleeding.

The nail should be cut cleanly, with no frayed edges; smooth off any rough edges with nail file or Dremel tool (Fig. 8-15). After trimming, examine each nail for bleeding before going on to the next nail. Examine each foot to ensure that all nails, including the dewclaws, have been trimmed cleanly and are not frayed.

If the quick is accidentally cut, apply a cauterizing agent, such as silver nitrate applicators or Quick Stop powder (Fig. 8-16). Place the tip of the applicator directly on the quick and apply pressure. If no cauterizing agent is available, apply pressure with a cotton ball or gauze sponge directly on the quick to stop the bleeding gradually. Silver nitrate application may cause some discomfort in patients, so be prepared for the patient to attempt to withdraw the foot.

> **CRITICAL CONCEPT**
>
> Silver nitrate may permanently stain countertops or examination tables; place a towel under the patient before application.

ANAL SAC CARE

The anal sacs are paired sacs located beneath the skin on either side of the anus at the 4 and 8 o'clock positions, each with a duct opening directly into the terminal rectum (Fig. 8-17). The anal sacs normally empty their malodorous secretions during defecation. Occasionally, animals (rarely, cats) may not be able to empty their anal sacs naturally and develop painful distention or impaction of the anal sacs. Signs include scooting on the hindquarters and licking of the anal area. The anal sacs of dogs can be expressed (emptied manually) as a routine part of grooming, as part of the physical examination, and before bathing. The anal sacs are emptied with the dog restrained in the standing position.

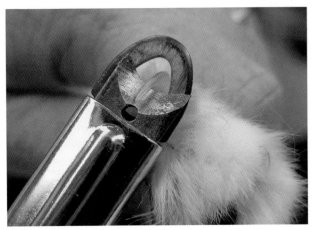

FIGURE 8-13 To trim the nails in cats, extend the claw by compressing the caudal part of the nail just in front of the footpad with the thumb and forefinger. At this point, one can visualize the vein, or quick (pink area in claw), and the nail trimmer can be placed in front of the vein for trimming. (From McCurnin DM, Bassert JM: Clinical textbook for veterinary technicians, ed 6, St Louis, 2006, Saunders.)

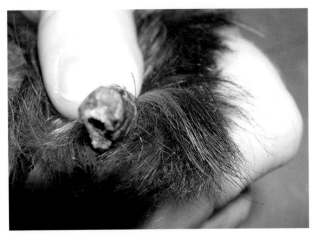

FIGURE 8-14 When trimming black nails, always trim a small amount at a time. Once you get close to the quick, you will note that the center of the nail begins to have a shiny, fleshy appearance. Once you see this, no further trimming is necessary. (From McCurnin DM, Bassert JM: Clinical textbook for veterinary technicians, ed 6, St Louis, 2006, Saunders.)

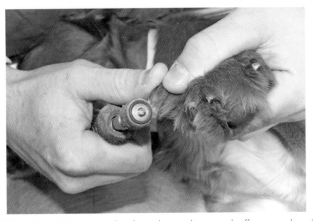

FIGURE 8-15 A Dremel tool may be used to smooth off any rough nail edges. (From Sirois M: Principles and practice of veterinary technology, ed 3, St Louis, 2011, Mosby.)

Anal sac expression may cause discomfort and a muzzle may be necessary.

The veterinarian or veterinary technician performs internal anal sac expression by first donning examination gloves that are well lubricated with a water-soluble lubricant or 2% lidocaine jelly. With the veterinary assistant holding the tail dorsally or laterally, the veterinarian or veterinary technician inserts the first joint of the index finger into the rectum and gently palpates the anal sac between the thumb (externally) and forefinger. Gentle massage with light to moderate pressure milks the secretions medially into the anal opening. The procedure is then repeated on the other side. Note the presence of any unusual secretions, such as thick, yellow mu-

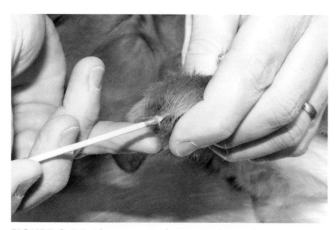

FIGURE 8-16 Silver nitrate applicators can be used as a cauterizing agent on a bleeding nail. (From Sirois M: Principles and practice of veterinary technology, ed 3, St Louis, 2011, Mosby.)

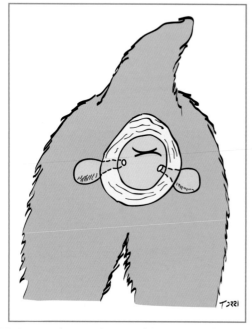

FIGURE 8-17 Schematic diagram of the anatomy of the canine anal sacs located approximately at the 4 and 8 o'clock positions. (From Mc-Curnin DM, Bassert JM: Clinical textbook for veterinary technicians, ed 6, St Louis, 2006, Saunders.)

copurulent liquid or if the discharge contains blood. Clean the perineum with a deodorizer or spot cleaner if not bathing immediately after expression.

External expression of the anal sacs is a technique that requires squeezing of the anal glands from the external anal sphincter. This technique is not recommended because of the frequent occluding of the ducts, inability to empty the sacs completely, and excessive pain that it may cause the patient.

EAR CARE

Before cleaning ears, visually examine the external ear canal and tympanic membrane for any irregularity. Cleaning the ears and instilling medication without examination may cause further damage to the tympanic membrane and result in loss of hearing, temporary loss of vestibular function, or facial nerve paralysis. The tympanic membrane must be intact before any products other than saline or water are instilled into the ear. Look for any redness, discharge, ulceration, excessive tissue formation, narrowing (stenosis) of the canal, abnormal odor, or debris in the outer ear and on the pinna. Evaluate the patient for signs of pain during the aural examination. These could indicate a bacterial or yeast infection, ear mite infestation, or tumors. Thickening of the pinna could indicate an aural hematoma. Signs of ear disease include excessive shaking of the head, scratching at the ears, head tilt, nystagmus, and ataxia.

If the animal has an ear problem, examine the less affected ear first. Most patients tolerate ear examination with minimal restraint while sitting or in sternal recumbency. Patients with painful ears or chronic ear disease typically require general anesthesia or chemical restraint for ear examination and cleaning. Use a separate, clean, otoscope cone for each ear to avoid contaminating a normal ear with organisms from an infected ear. Cytology is recommended on both ears for diagnosis.

Gently grasp the pinna and carefully insert the otoscope cone into the ear canal. Straighten the ear canal by gently pulling the pinna laterally while advancing the otoscope cone into the canal to visualize the tympanic membrane. Occasionally, the ear canal is occluded with debris and must be cleaned and flushed with saline to visualize the tympanic membrane. If cultures or cytologic samples are required, obtain the samples before cleaning the ears.

Some dog breeds, such as Poodles, have hair growth in the ear canal. This hair traps moisture and debris and increases the likelihood of infection. Hair in the ear canal should be plucked out with a hemostat or the fingertips, a few strands at a time. This procedure may be painful, so appropriate restraint of the head is necessary. Sedation or tranquilization may be necessary. Grasp a few hairs at a time with the hemostat and quickly pluck the hair out. Grasping too much hair in the hemostat is painful and may cause more inflammation.

Ensure that the tympanic membrane is intact before any cleaning. Most cleaning solutions are ototoxic if the tympanic membrane is not intact. If the membrane is not intact, use a saline solution to clean the ears. Antimicrobial agents may be used if the membrane is intact. Various ceruminolytics are available for breaking up debris and cleansing. Cleansing products with a drying agent are good for cleaning the ears of dogs with long droopy ears, such as Poodles and Cocker Spaniels (Procedure 8-1).

It is good public relations to have the patient looking better (as well as feeling better) on discharge than when it was admitted. Examine every patient before discharge to ensure that all extraneous bandages are removed. Ensure that the patient is bathed, groomed, dematted, and smelling good and that the nails are trimmed, ears cleaned, and anal sacs expressed. Brush one last time and spray with a lightly scented spray. Educating clients about proper skin care and grooming can prevent many problems and will keep the animal in better health.

ADMINISTERING MEDICATIONS

TOPICAL ADMINISTRATION

Medication applied to the skin provides a local effect and is also absorbed through the skin. Shaving and cleaning the area or parting the hair before application facilitates

absorption of the medication. Wear examination gloves and/or plastic aprons when giving a medicated bath or applying topical medication. Topical medications include medicated shampoos for skin diseases, fentanyl transdermal patches for **analgesia**, spot-on flea and tick control, topical anesthetics, nitroglycerin ointment for cardiac disease, and other various antibiotic and cortisone creams and ointments.

ORAL ADMINISTRATION

Oral administration is the route most commonly used to administer medications. Medications given orally are metabolized slowly. A different route of administration is necessary if more rapid absorption of medication is required. The patient must be able to swallow and have normal digestive function if medication is given PO.

Oral medications are available in tablet, capsule, and liquid form. If necessary, tablets can be crushed or capsule contents dissolved in water and given with a syringe or feeding tube. If multiple medications are prescribed, ensure that no contraindications exist if given simultaneously. Compounding pharmacies are now available to make medicine solutions with tasty flavorings. If the patient has a good appetite, the medication may be placed in a meatball of canned food; however, this does not work well with sick cats. If the oral cavity is damaged, the medication can be given directly into the GI tract via nasogastric or gastrostomy tube after mixing with water for easy tube passage.

A pilling device can be used to avoid being bitten. This is a plastic rod with a rubber-tipped plunger to hold the medication (Fig. 8-18). Hemostats should not be used to administer medication because they can damage the teeth or soft palate. Teach animal owners how to administer oral medication correctly and how to check the animal's mouth to ensure that all medications have been swallowed.

Place small patients at waist level and large dogs on the floor. Medicate cats by grasping the upper jaw over the top

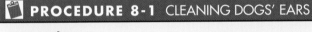

PROCEDURE 8-1 CLEANING DOGS' EARS

Materials
- Basin
- Bulb syringe
- Cotton balls or cotton swabs
- Hemostats
- Ceruminolytic agents, saline solution, cleansing solution, or dilute vinegar

Procedure
1. Obtain cytology samples (if needed) from both ears by using cotton swabs and a glass slide.
2. To clean, tip the head and ear slightly ventrally, grasp the pinna, and place the solution into the ear canal, with the bulb syringe directed ventromedially into the canal. Have the basin ready below the ear to catch the excess.
3. Massage the base of the ear to distribute the cleansing solution and loosen any debris. Flush the ear again.
4. Use cotton balls on a hemostat to clean the debris in the ear canal, or 4- × 4-inch gauze squares. Never insert cotton-tipped swabs into the canal of an inadequately restrained patient. These cotton swabs should be used for the external ear canal and interior of the pinna only.
5. Allow the patient to shake its head occasionally to loosen more debris.
6. Flush and clean the ears until debris is no longer visible. Dry the ear canal with cotton balls or 4- × 4-inch gauze squares.
7. Examine the ears with an otoscope and apply any medications necessary. Massage the ear canal to distribute the medication evenly and thoroughly.

Adapted from Sirois M: Principles and practice of veterinary technology, ed 3, St Louis, 2011, Mosby.

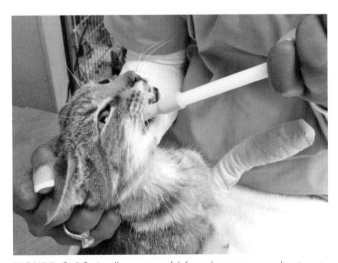

FIGURE 8-18 A pill gun is useful for administering medications to the difficult patient. (From Sirois M: Principles and practice of veterinary technology, ed 3, St Louis, 2011, Mosby.)

of the head and tipping the head back. The lower jaw will drop open, or it may need to be pried open slightly with the middle finger of the dominant hand, with the pill held between the thumb and forefinger of that hand. Place the pill in the center groove of the tongue, at the back of the throat. After swallowing, reopen the mouth to ensure pill passage. Follow this procedure with a small amount of water via a syringe for large pills. Do not scratch the soft palate with your fingers. With aggressive cats, a towel or cat bag may be necessary.

In dogs, grasp the muzzle using the fingers and thumb to press the skin against the teeth (Fig. 8-19). Slip the thumb of the left hand into the mouth and press up on the hard palate, keeping the lips against the teeth. Place the pill on the base of the tongue at the back of the throat. Keep the head slightly elevated, close the mouth, and hold it shut while rubbing the throat until the patient swallows. Swallowing can be facilitated by blowing into its nose. After administering medication, always examine the patient's mouth for complete swallowing of the medication. Follow medication with a small amount of water via syringe for large pills.

To administer liquid medication in a syringe, tilt the head back slightly and pull the lips outward slightly to form a pocket (Fig. 8-20). Place the syringe between the lips and back teeth so that the liquid flows between the molars and into the throat. Administer slowly in small boluses to allow the patient to swallow and not aspirate. Buccal or transmucosal administration of medications can also be effectively achieved in the feline patient. Specifically, use of the buccal route to deliver analgesia such as buprenorphine is more effective than the IV route because of the alkaline (pH 8 to 9) environment of the cat's mouth. Ease of administration of buccal medication is also an advantage to the owner, who can safely provide pain control to the pet.

RECTAL ADMINISTRATION

An enema introduces fluids into the rectum and colon to stimulate bowel activity, evacuate the large intestine for diagnostic procedures, and irrigate the colon (Procedure 8-2). Enemas soften feces and stimulate colonic motility. Tap water or saline adds bulk, whereas petrolatum oils soften, lubricate, and promote evacuation of hardened feces. Glycerin and water, mild soap and water, or commercial enema preparations can also be used for enema solutions. However, phosphate enemas (e.g., Fleet) should not be administered to cats or small dogs. Large volumes of warm water are administered with a bucket elevated above the patient and attached to soft red rubber tubing. Smaller volumes can be administered with a 60-mL syringe attached to the tubing. The solution should be at room temperature or tepid.

Enemas are contraindicated if the bowel is perforated or recent colon surgery has been performed. Complications

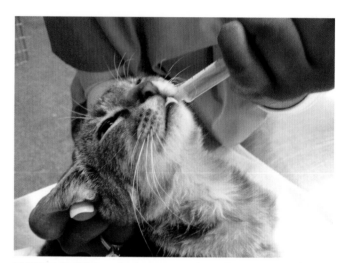

FIGURE 8-20 Liquid administration. (From Sirois M: Principles and practice of veterinary technology, ed 3, St Louis, 2011, Mosby.)

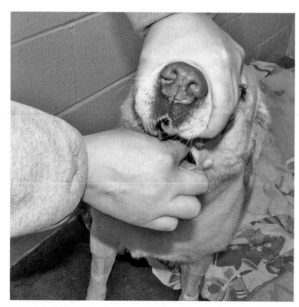

FIGURE 8-19 Oral administration of a tablet or pill. (From Sirois M: Principles and practice of veterinary technology, ed 3, St Louis, 2011, Mosby.)

PROCEDURE 8-2 GIVING AN ENEMA

1. For an evacuation enema, place the animal in a tub, run, or large cage. Lubricate the tubing with water-soluble lubricating jelly.
2. Wearing gloves and with the animal restrained in a standing position, insert the lubricated tube into the rectum, at least 5 cm cranial to the anal sphincter, and administer the solution slowly.
   - Warm water enemas to evacuate the bowel are safely given at 10 to 20 mL/kg of body weight. Rapid administration may cause the patient to vomit.
   - A small amount of liquid soap (½ tsp) and 1 to 2 tsp of sterile lubricating jelly may be safely added to the warm water solution.
3. Remove the tubing from the rectum and allow the animal to evacuate in a large area. This may take minutes to hours.

From Sirois M: Principles and practice of veterinary technology, ed 3, St Louis, 2011, Mosby.

of enema administration include perforating the colon and leakage of fluid into the peritoneal cavity, vomiting if fluid is administered too quickly, and hemorrhage if the colon is irritated. Hydration status is important to evaluate in the constipated patient. IV or subcutaneous fluids, in addition to the enema, may be indicated for colonic emptying and to prevent or correct dehydration or poor perfusion.

NASAL ADMINISTRATION

Some medications may be administered into the nasal cavity to be absorbed through the nasal mucosa. Occasionally, nasal cannulas are inserted through the nares to administer oxygen and humidified air to the lungs; nasoesophageal and nasogastric tubes are inserted to provide nutrition. Respiratory vaccines and local anesthetics also may be placed into the nasal passages. Nasal administration, via syringe or dropper, is usually not stressful, and most dogs and cats tolerate it well.

Have all medications and materials ready and within reach before starting. With the patient in sternal recumbency or sitting, tip the animal's head back so that the nose is slightly elevated and instill the medication into the nares (Fig. 8-21). It may be helpful to cover the eyes during the procedure with the hand that is holding the head back. Once the medication is administered, keep the nose elevated until the medication is absorbed through the mucosa.

OPHTHALMIC APPLICATION

Medication can be applied topically onto the eye to treat the cornea, conjunctiva, and anterior chamber. Ophthalmic medications are available in liquid and ointment forms. Most eye conditions are very painful and may require restraint for application. Before applying the medication, the eye must be cleaned of any exudates, including any excess hair that might deter application. An ophthalmic irrigating solution and cotton balls are used to clean the surrounding area. A clean comb can be invaluable when removing exudate from

hair surrounding the eye. Have all materials and medications ready and within reach before restraining the patient.

Restrain the patient in a sternal position or sitting, with the head tipped back and the nose pointed toward the ceiling. Grasp the muzzle to prevent the patient from moving its head. Gently clean the eye area with wet cotton balls. Flush the cornea and conjunctival sac by everting the eyelids and applying a gentle stream of irrigating solution from medial to lateral. If excessive ocular discharge has caused irritation of surrounding skin, apply a thin layer of petrolatum-based ointment onto the skin.

Ophthalmic solutions are easier to administer than ointments but may need to be administered more frequently. Most solutions are applied every few hours to maintain their effect. With the dropper or bottle held 1 or 2 inches above the eye and the upper eyelid pulled up, apply the solution directly onto the sclera; then release the eyelid (Fig. 8-22). To avoid contaminating the dropper bottle or tube, do not touch the eye or eyelid with it. If more than one solution is to be applied, wait a few minutes between applications. If both a solution and ointment are to be used, apply the solution several minutes before the ointment. If administration of autologous serum is prescribed by the veterinarian, place the blood into a serum-separating blood collection tube and centrifuge the sample. Using sterile technique, remove the serum and store in a sterile tube in the refrigerator until needed. An insulin or tuberculin syringe may be used to draw serum out of the tube for ocular administration. Always wipe the top of the tube with alcohol to keep its contents sterile. Because the patient may paw or scratch its eye after medications, an Elizabethan collar is generally recommended.

Ointment is slightly more difficult to apply. Ointments are usually applied every 4 to 6 hours; they do not wash out but may soil the skin around the eye. The ointment tube must be held close to but not in contact with the eye. Evert the eyelid and place a 1/8- or 1/4-inch strip of ointment medially to laterally onto the cornea or lower border of the eyelid,

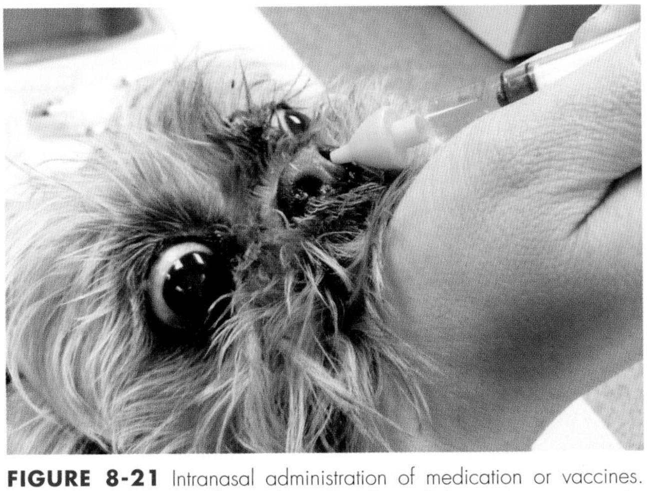

FIGURE 8-21 Intranasal administration of medication or vaccines. Note that the head is elevated to allow flow of the medication into the nasal passages. (From Sirois M: *Principles and practice of veterinary technology,* ed 3, St Louis, 2011, Mosby.)

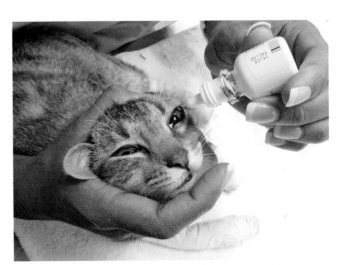

FIGURE 8-22 Instillation of ophthalmic drops to the eye. Note that the container does not touch the eye. (From Sirois M: *Principles and practice of veterinary technology,* ed 3, St Louis, 2011, Mosby.)

making sure not to touch the tube to the eye or eyelid. Gently pinch together the upper and lower eyelids to disperse the ointment.

CRITICAL CONCEPT

If multiple eye medications are prescribed, wait several seconds between administrations. Ophthalmic solutions should be applied first, followed by ointments.

OTIC APPLICATION

Liquids can be instilled into the ear canal to medicate or clean the ear. The ear should be cleaned before instilling medication to ensure that the medication is absorbed and fully dispersed. Otoscopic examination is necessary to ensure that the tympanic membrane is intact before ear cleaning or applying medication. Obtain culture or cytologic samples, if necessary, before the ears are cleaned.

The simplest technique to clean ears is to rinse with a cleanser. The ears are first filled with a cleanser followed by gentle massage of the ear cartilage. After the dog shakes the material out or after tilting the head, swab the external orifice with gauze sponges or cotton-tipped applicators. Never put cotton-tipped applicators down the vertical canal.

The ear can also be cleaned by using a bulb syringe. This is more effective than an ear rinse with the cleanser. Fill the bulb syringe with lukewarm cleanser or cerumenolytic agent; a mixture of white vinegar and water solution mixed in equal parts can also be used as a disinfectant. Place a bulb syringe loosely into the external orifice of the ear canal (Fig. 8-23). Squeeze the bulb gently to administer the cleanser, followed by gentle massage of the ear cartilage. Remove fluid and debris by gauze sponges and/or cotton-tipped applicators.

Most patients tolerate medication of the ear with minimal restraint. Start with the less affected ear first to avoid contaminating the other ear. To straighten the ear canal, apply lateral tension on the pinna (ear flap).

PARENTERAL ADMINISTRATION

Fluids and medications administered parenterally are injected via sterile syringe and needle or through a catheter.

Parenteral routes include intradermal (ID), subcutaneous (SC), intramuscular (IM), IV, **intraosseous** (IO), epidural, and intraperitoneal (IP) (Fig. 8-24). Veterinary assistants may administer SC injections and will restrain patients for the veterinary technician to administer IV, IM, and other injections. Local inflammation, pain, infection, nerve damage, anaphylactic or allergic reactions, and necrosis at the injection site are possible complications of parenteral administration.

Before aspirating medications into a syringe, swab the rubber stopper of the medication vial with alcohol. Select the appropriate syringe and needle size for the dose and route chosen (22- to 27-gauge for ID, 18- to 22-gauge for SC, 22-gauge for IM, 20- to 25-gauge for IV, 20- to 22-gauge for IP, and 22-25 gauge for epidural injections). Aspirate the medication into the syringe, hold the syringe vertically, and tap it to expel any air bubbles. Change the needle before

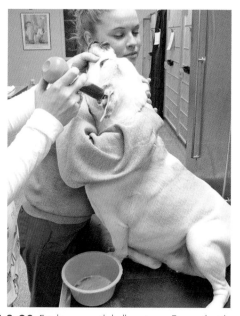

FIGURE 8-23 Ear lavage with bulb syringe. Ensure that the syringe is directed ventromedially into the canal. A basin should be ready below the ear to catch the irrigant solution. (From Sirois M: Principles and practice of veterinary technology, ed 3, St Louis, 2011, Mosby.)

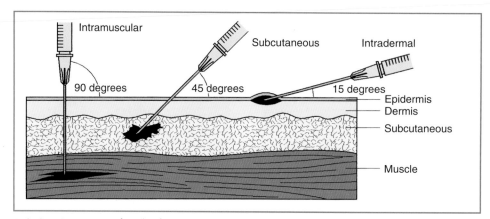

FIGURE 8-24 Comparison of angle of injection and location of medication deposit for IM, SC, and ID injections. (From Bassert JM, McCurnin DM: McCurnin's clinical textbook for veterinary technicians, ed 7, Philadelphia, 2009, WB Saunders.)

patient administration. The technician and animal handler must wear latex or chemotherapy gloves when administering chemotherapeutic agents by any route. Protective eyewear, gowns, and masks may also be indicated.

INTRADERMAL ADMINISTRATION

ID injections are used primarily for skin testing and local anesthesia. Skin testing may require sedating the patient before placing in lateral recumbency. Local anesthesia may or may not require sedation.

The veterinary technician will hold the skin taut between the thumb and forefinger of the left hand and insert the needle (bevel up) into the skin at an angle of approximately 10 degrees. The bevel of the needle is within the dermis and not visible. A small amount of allergen or local anesthetic is injected intradermally to form a bleb at the site. If no bleb forms, the injection may have been SC and not ID.

SUBCUTANEOUS ADMINISTRATION

SC injections are used for sustained absorption of fluids and medications and administration of some vaccines. Medication and fluids are absorbed slowly over 20 or 30 minutes or longer for larger volumes of fluids (6 to 8 hours). Clients can easily be taught to give SC injections of medication (e.g., insulin) and fluids to patients at home.

Fluids are not readily absorbed when injected SC in severely dehydrated or debilitated patients or in patients with poor perfusion or shock. The IV route should be used in these cases. Hypertonic, caustic, or irritating solutions administered SC can cause damage and sloughing of the skin and should not be administered by this route. Fluids given SC should not contain any additives such as those with a dextrose or potassium chloride concentration exceeding 20 mEq/liter. Read the drug's package insert before administering medications subcutaneously.

Large volumes of room-temperature fluids may be administered by gravity flow via fluid bag and administration set with a needle attached (Fig. 8-25). This allows for patient comfort during the long process of administering larger volumes of fluid. The needle should be changed with each injection site change to prevent formation of an abscess. For the average size cat or dog, 18-gauge needles are recommended and 16-gauge needles for large dogs. The patient should be restrained in a comfortable sitting, standing, or sternal position. Most cats and dogs tolerate SC administration well. Carefully part the hair, clean the skin if excessively dirty, and apply a skin antiseptic, such as 70% alcohol. Between 50 and 100 mL of fluid may be safely administered at each site without discomfort. Common sites of SC fluid administration include the dorsal scapula (between the shoulder blades) as well as the dorsal spine (thoracolumbar region). The skin is tented and the needle inserted gently. As the fluid is administered, the needle should be held in place and fluid should not leak out during initial administration. Remove the needle after administration, gently pinch the injection site, and massage the area. This prevents leakage and facilitates dispersal and absorption of fluid or medication. Large volumes of fluid may gradually migrate ventrally before being absorbed completely.

To give a single SC injection, grasp the skin between the thumb and forefinger along the dorsal aspect of the neck or back and lift gently to form a tent (Fig. 8-26). Insert the needle into the skin fold and aspirate. If blood is aspirated, withdraw the needle and use another injection site. If no blood is aspirated, inject the medication or fluid slowly. Multiple injection sites can be used along the dorsum and lateral to

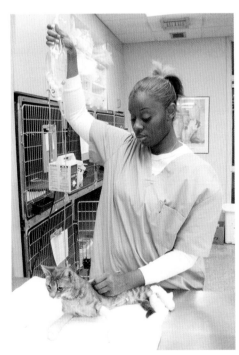

FIGURE 8-25 Administration of SC fluids. Hang the fluid bag above the patient and use a large-gauge needle for faster administration. (From Sirois M: *Principles and practice of veterinary technology,* ed 3, St Louis, 2011, Mosby.)

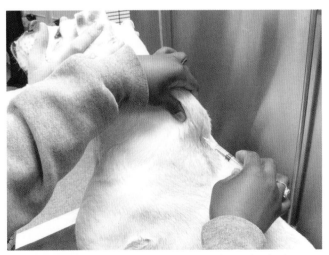

FIGURE 8-26 To give a single SC injection, grasp the skin between the thumb and forefinger along the dorsal aspect of the neck or back and lift gently to form a tent. (From Sirois M: *Principles and practice of veterinary technology,* ed 3, St Louis, 2011, Mosby.)

the spine. Patient restraint may be necessary because some substances can be painful on injection.

INTRAMUSCULAR ADMINISTRATION

Muscles are more vascular than SC tissue, and medication is more readily absorbed after IM administration than if given SC. However, muscle tissue cannot accommodate more than 2 to 5 mL of medication at any one site, and IM injections can be painful. Slow-to-moderate rates of administration with small-gauge (22- to 25-gauge) needles may be less painful than rapid injections. IM administration is never used for fluid therapy. Some medications that are poorly soluble and mildly irritating can be administered IM but not SC or IV.

Large muscle groups are used for IM injections, such as the epaxial muscles lateral to the dorsal spinous process of lumbar vertebrae 3 to 5 (L3-5), quadriceps muscles of the cranial thigh, and triceps muscles caudal to the humerus (Fig. 8-27). The epaxial muscles are the best site for IM injections in small patients. The semimembranosus and semitendinosus muscles on the caudal thigh should be avoided because of possible sciatic nerve damage from incorrect IM injection. If that muscle group must be used, the veterinary technician will insert the needle at a 45-degree angle directed caudally to avoid the sciatic nerve. Repeated IM injections should be alternated between muscle groups and given on different sides of the body.

Proper patient restraint is necessary to avoid painful injections. The veterinary assistant must restrain the patient's head and body during IM administration. After locating the muscle group by palpation, the veterinary technician swabs the injection site with a disinfectant. With the needle attached to the syringe, the needle is quickly inserted 1 to 2 cm at a 45- to 90-degree angle. The veterinary technician will aspirate the syringe to ensure that the needle is not placed in a blood vessel. If blood is aspirated, the needle is withdrawn and inserted into a different site. This step is crucial when injecting potent medications, oil-based drugs, or microcrystalline suspensions. If no blood is aspirated, the veterinary

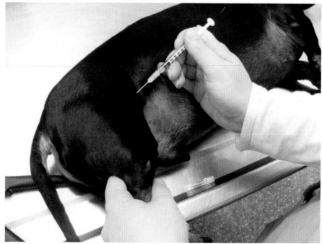

FIGURE 8-27 Large muscle groups are used for IM injections. (From Sirois M: Principles and practice of veterinary technology, ed 3, St Louis, 2011, Mosby.)

technician injects the medication at a slow to moderate rate. The needle is then removed and the muscle massaged to disperse the medication.

INTRAVENOUS ADMINISTRATION

Medications and fluids administered IV are rapidly absorbed and reach a higher blood level faster than by other routes. Large volumes of solutions may be given in a short time. Caustic, irritating, or hypertonic medications can be given IV with fewer problems than with other routes. IV injections typically do not produce a lasting effect unless a continual infusion is given. A general rule is that if the solution is opaque, it cannot be safely given IV, except for parenteral nutrient solutions and propofol. Vaccines are never administered IV. All IV injections should be performed using sterile technique. The veterinary assistant prepares supplies and restrains the patient for IV administration.

Drugs can be given IV with a syringe and needle, winged infusion set, or catheter (Procedure 8-3). The most

---

📋 PROCEDURE 8-3 INTRAVENOUS INJECTION

1. The assistant restrains the patient, immobilizes the limb, and occludes the vessel proximal to the administration site to distend the vein.
2. Shave the venipuncture site to visualize the vessel easier.
3. Prepare the site using 70% alcohol swabs to moisten the hair, clean the skin, and aid in visualization of the vein. Surgical preparation of the site is not necessary for IV administration with a syringe and needle, unlike catheter placement.
4. The veterinary assistant restrains the patient, usually in a sitting position or sternal recumbency.
5. The assistant compresses the vessel proximal to the venipuncture site.
6. The veterinary technician grasps the metacarpal-metatarsal area and straightens the leg.
7. The veterinary technician palpates by using forefinger and swabs the site with alcohol.
8. With the bevel of the needle directed up, the veterinary technician inserts the needle at a 30-degree angle through the skin and into the vessel lumen.
9. The technician aspirates blood into the syringe to ensure venipuncture.
10. Once the needle is in the vessel, the veterinary technician's assistant releases pressure on the vein while still holding the limb immobile.
11. The veterinary technician injects the medication slowly or rapidly, depending on the drug (e.g., thiopental is injected fairly rapidly; chemotherapeutic agents are given slowly and through a winged infusion set or catheter).
12. After the medication is administered, the veterinary technician withdraws the needle and the assistant applies pressure at the venipuncture site. A light compression bandage can minimize hematoma formation.

Adapted from Sirois M: Principles and practice of veterinary technology, ed 3, St Louis, 2011, Mosby.

commonly used veins for IV administration using a syringe and needle are the cephalic and saphenous veins. The patient should be restrained sitting or in sternal recumbency if the cephalic vessel is being used, and in lateral recumbency if the saphenous vessel is used. The use of rubbing alcohol on the targeted area may facilitate vessel identification and provide a cleaner surface for injection.

Patient restraint is important if using a syringe and needle for administration of medication. It is the responsibility of the veterinary assistant to ensure that the limb being used remains immobile during administration. Any movement of the patient may lacerate the vessel with the needle and/or result in extravascular administration of medication. When injecting a caustic or irritating solution, an IV catheter or winged butterfly set should be placed to prevent extravascular injection. Light pressure should be applied at all venipuncture sites to prevent hematoma formation.

INTRAOSSEOUS AND INTRAPERITONEAL ADMINISTRATION

IO administration is used to inject medication and fluids in pediatric patients into which an IV cannot be placed. Medication or fluids may be administered into the peritoneal space in neonates with vessels too small for IV catheterization or in patients needing peritoneal lavage (e.g., with pancreatitis). Debilitated or hypovolemic patients do not absorb IP fluids or medication readily. IP is the least desirable route of administration because of the serious potential complications. The only routine uses of IP procedures in small animal practice are diagnostic peritoneal lavage or IP administration of chemotherapy.

INTRAVENOUS CATHETERIZATION

IV catheters provide access to circulating blood for administration of medication, fluids, nutrients, and blood products, as well as for monitoring blood pressure and collecting blood samples. Catheters are available in a wide variety of lengths and diameters (Fig. 8-28). Types of catheters include winged

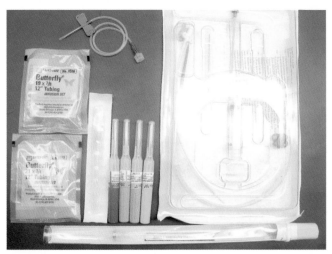

FIGURE 8-28 Catheters are available in a wide variety of lengths and diameters. (From Sirois M: Principles and practice of veterinary technology, ed 3, St Louis, 2011, Mosby.)

infusion needles (butterfly catheters), over-the-needle catheters, and through-the-needle catheters. Common insertion sites are the cephalic vein, saphenous vein, and jugular vein. The medial or lateral auricular (ear) vein can be accessed in some patients in which peripheral catheterization is difficult, such as in the Basset Hound or Dachshund breeds.

The longer the catheter, the more stable it is in the vessel and the less likely it is to cause mechanical irritation, with resulting phlebitis. A short, peripheral, over-the-needle catheter may be inserted distal to an area of flexion, such as in a cephalic vein distal to the elbow. A **central catheter** placed in a large vessel, such as the jugular vein, is less likely to cause mechanical or chemical irritation.

The diameter (gauge) of the catheter chosen depends on the diameter of the vessel. In general, although smaller-diameter catheters may be easier to place and can be less traumatic to a vessel, rapid fluid administration of fluids can become problematic. Larger, more rigid catheters are typically easier to advance through the skin but have the potential to cause more damage to vessel walls compared with the smaller-diameter catheters. The general recommendation is to place the largest-bore catheter possible without causing significant vascular trauma or stress in any patient requiring IV access. A fluid pump can facilitate delivery of fluids through a small catheter. Because small-diameter catheters are easily occluded with fibrin clots, blood sample collection through the catheter is not recommended.

WINGED INFUSION (BUTTERFLY) CATHETERS

Winged infusion (butterfly) catheters are for patients that need multiple IV medications (e.g., chemotherapeutic agents) but not long-term fluid therapy. Several medications can be given if the catheter is flushed with 0.9% saline between infusions of each medication. These catheters are simple to insert and cause the fewest local infections. However, they can cause irritation and may perforate the vessel. Winged infusion catheters require constant monitoring while in place, and stabilization of the catheter can be difficult. Once the blood starts flowing into the catheter tubing, the veterinary technician will attach the heparinized saline-filled syringe, aspirate the air out of the tubing, and flush to ensure catheter patency before administering medications. Once the medication has been administered, the veterinary technician will flush the tubing and catheter with saline before removing the catheter. If multiple drugs are to be administered, the veterinary technician will flush between medications with saline.

> ### CRITICAL CONCEPT
> The cap should be removed before insertion of the butterfly catheter or there will be no "flash" of blood flow indicating correct placement into the vessel.

OVER-THE-NEEDLE PERIPHERAL CATHETERS

Over-the-needle peripheral catheters are quick and relatively atraumatic to place, inexpensive, and easily stabilized with a light bandage. They are used for infusion of fluids, medication, anesthetics, and blood products. Proper skin preparation before catheter placement is essential to prevent phlebitis and infection. Strict aseptic technique must be followed during catheterization to avoid sepsis. Proper hand washing is done after clipping and before catheter placement. Sterile surgical gloves should be worn. All catheters must be secured with tape or sutures and covered with a light bandage to protect the insertion site and catheter from contamination. Winged infusion catheters require only taping. Daily bandage changes should be performed and the site inspected for signs of phlebitis, irritation, or infection.

The selected vessel is occluded by the veterinary assistant to raise the pressure in the vessel and allow for easier visualization and palpation. For the cephalic vein, the patient's elbow is supported with the handler's fingers, while the thumb is placed over the vessel on the medial side and slightly rotated laterally (Fig. 8-29). The lateral saphenous vein is occluded by placing one hand on top of and around the stifle, medially to laterally; the medial saphenous is occluded by applying pressure on the vessel in the inguinal (femoral) area and stabilizing the stifle.

Securing the catheter reduces movement of the catheter in the vessel and can decrease the likelihood of phlebitis. The veterinary technician will anchor a piece of ½-inch tape around the catheter hub and loosely wrap it around the limb (Fig. 8-30). Additional tape is added to secure the catheter in place, and a light bandage applied to protect the catheter from contamination.

INTRAVENOUS CATHETER CARE

Conscientious nursing care of the catheter is necessary to maintain the catheter and prevent complications from catheterization. Catheter management can prevent sepsis, the most serious complication associated with catheters. **Phlebitis**, or local venous inflammation, can be caused by contamination of the catheter during placement or chemical or mechanical

irritation. Signs of phlebitis include swelling at the catheter site, redness, pain, thickening, pitting edema, and general irritation of the vessel (Fig. 8-31). Septicemia, thrombosis, or bacterial endocarditis can be caused by indwelling catheters. Signs of septicemia and bacterial endocarditis include cardiac arrhythmias or murmurs, injected mucous membranes, fever, and leukocytosis. Signs of thrombosis include a vein that stands up without being held off and a thick, cordlike feel to the vein; the limb may feel cold and painful to the patient.

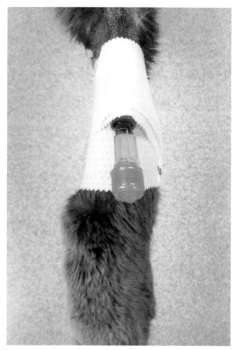

FIGURE 8-30 Securing the catheter with tape reduces movement of the catheter in the vessel and can decrease the likelihood of phlebitis. (From Sirois M: *Principles and practice of veterinary technology,* ed 3, St Louis, 2011, Mosby.)

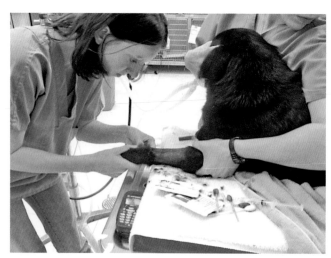

FIGURE 8-29 For easy cephalic vessel access, the patient's elbow is supported with the handler's fingers while the thumb is placed over the vessel on the medial side and slightly rotated laterally. (From Sirois M: *Principles and practice of veterinary technology,* ed 3, St Louis, 2011, Mosby.)

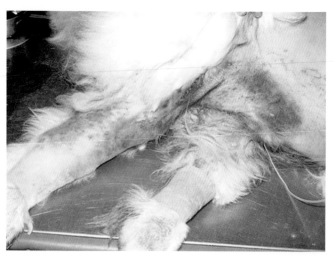

FIGURE 8-31 Signs of phlebitis include swelling at the catheter site, redness, pain, thickening, pitting edema, and general irritation of the vessel. (From Sirois M: *Principles and practice of veterinary technology,* ed 3, St Louis, 2011, Mosby.)

When signs of phlebitis or thrombosis are apparent, the catheter should be removed and a new one placed at a different site.

The catheter bandage must be kept clean and dry, the catheter and extension set clear of any blood clots, and a closed administration system established to prevent contamination. The patient's body temperature should be measured at least once daily, the site proximal to the catheter monitored for any signs of phlebitis or subcutaneous fluid accumulation, and the toes checked for swelling. The catheter should be removed at the first sign of phlebitis, thrombosis, sepsis, or catheter malfunction. Routine changing of the catheter depends on hospital policy for the type of catheter placed. Catheters not in constant use should be flushed with saline or heparinized saline several times a day.

> **CRITICAL CONCEPT**
> Any unexplained fever in the patient should warrant IV catheter replacement.

When the catheter bandage becomes wet or soiled with organic material, it must be changed and the catheter evaluated for problems. The catheter may need to be covered with plastic to keep it clean in incontinent patients. Swabbing the injection port with alcohol or a disinfectant before flushing or injecting medications can help decrease the chance of sepsis. Kinked or malfunctioning catheters and extension tubing with blood clots occluding the ports must be replaced.

URINARY TRACT CATHETERIZATION

Urinary catheters provide access to the urinary bladder via the urethra to administer radiographic contrast material directly into the bladder, collect urine for urinalysis, relieve urethral obstruction, maintain urine flow, and provide a closed urinary collection system for precise monitoring of urine output, collection of contaminated urine, and patient cleanliness. Urinary catheters are available in a variety of materials, diameters, and lengths (Fig. 8-32).

Metal urethral catheters can be used to catheterize a female dog temporarily but can cause hematuria and potentially serious injury to the urethra and bladder. Sterile polypropylene urinary catheters are ideal for temporary female catheterization in lieu of a metal urethral catheter; short, olive-tipped metal catheters can be used to relieve an obstruction at the tip of a male cat's penis. Softer, red rubber catheters should be used for male urinary catheterization or for continuous urine collection in male cats or small dogs.

> **CRITICAL CONCEPT**
> Red rubber urinary catheters can be kept in a freezer so that they remain stiff for ease of placement in a blocked cat or small dog.

Careful placement of the most flexible, smallest-diameter catheter minimizes trauma to the urethra and bladder.

However, an overly small catheter diameter may allow leakage of urine around the catheter unless a Foley catheter (containing a balloon) is used. Always examine the catheter for defects and test the bulb of a Foley catheter before use by gently inflating with sterile water or saline before placement. Overinflation of the Foley balloon may cause urethral trauma or rupture; use the smallest amount of saline required. Most Foley catheters will indicate the amount of saline needed for balloon dilation on the inflation port.

Complications of urethral catheterization include iatrogenic ascending urinary tract infections, catheter breakage, and trauma to the urethra or bladder. Urinary catheters must be placed aseptically. Indwelling urinary catheters that are left open and exposed can lead to infection. A closed urinary system can decrease infection rates. Changing the collection system—and, only if possible to replace easily, the urinary catheter—every 72 hours also helps prevent infection. Daily nursing duties include inspecting the system for kinks and blood clots, cleansing the vulva or prepuce with an antiseptic, and emptying the urine bag at scheduled times. Urinary collection bags that prevent retrograde flow are also beneficial for preventing urinary tract infections.

Most healthy cats require sedation or general anesthesia to place a urinary catheter, but very sick cats may not require chemical restraint. Most dogs do not require any chemical restraint and can be physically restrained. All patients should be placed in lateral recumbency for urinary catheterization. However, female dogs may also remain standing or be placed in sternal recumbency. Male cats may also be placed in dorsal or lateral recumbency.

> **CRITICAL CONCEPT**
> A laryngoscope blade can be used to visualize the urethral orifice or papilla. Hyperextend the vaginal fold ventrally and insert the blade slightly.

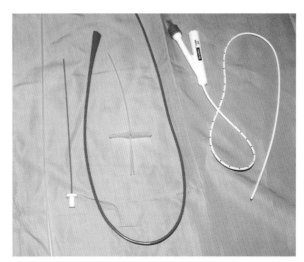

FIGURE 8-32 Urinary catheters are available in a variety of materials, diameters, and lengths. (From Sirois M: Principles and practice of veterinary technology, ed 3, St Louis, 2011, Mosby.)

GASTRIC INTUBATION

Orogastric tubes are inserted through the mouth to the stomach and used for administering liquid medication and barium, short-term feeding of gruel-type diets, and flushing the stomach (gastric lavage). The animal must have a swallowing reflex to prevent aspiration if the patient regurgitates. Another cause of aspiration is passing the orogastric tube into the trachea, instead of the esophagus, and administering the medication. Nasogastric tubes are inserted through the nares through the esophagus to the stomach.

FLUID THERAPY

Fluid therapy is one of the most commonly used supportive measures in veterinary medicine and is an important aspect of almost every critical care case. It is primarily used to correct fluid deficits, electrolyte disturbances, and acid-base imbalances. The veterinarian will determine the need for fluid administration based on assessment of the patient's state of hydration and estimation of fluid deficits through subjective patient evaluation. Formulation of a fluid therapy regimen is based on information gathered from an accurate history, thorough physical examination, and laboratory tests. There are many routes through which fluid solutions can be administered. An appropriate route is chosen after careful evaluation of the following factors:

- Volume of fluid loss
- Rate of fluid loss (acute virtually chronic)
- Fluid solution selected for administration
- Volume and rate of infusion
- Patient status

These factors will be influenced by the cause and severity of the condition. In small animal medicine, medical, practical, and economic considerations may affect the fluid solution chosen and administration route used. The IV route of fluid administration is preferable when treating animals that are critically ill, severely dehydrated, hypovolemic, or experiencing some electrolyte or metabolic disorder. Many factors influence the rate of fluid administration (e.g., disease process, rate of fluid loss, severity of clinical signs, fluid composition and delivery route, cardiac and renal function).

Regular monitoring of fluid therapy patients is needed to detect overhydration or underhydration. The patient's weight, body temperature, mucous membrane color, capillary refill time, heart and respiratory rate, respiratory rhythm, pulse rate and quality, and urine output are recorded at regular intervals for the duration of fluid therapy. The catheter and IV fluid line are also checked regularly for signs that might indicate that the catheter has become dislodged or contaminated. Edema (swelling) around the catheter site often indicates that the catheter is no longer in the vein and must be replaced. Any redness or excessive warmth around the catheter site also signifies problems that must be addressed.

WOUND CARE AND BANDAGING

A wound is a disruption of cellular and anatomic functional continuity. Wound healing is the restoration of this continuity.

Acute wounds are those induced by surgery or trauma that heal normally, with healing time determined by the depth and size of the lesion. Examples of acute wounds include surgical incisions, blunt trauma, bite wounds, burns, gunshots, and avulsion injuries. Chronic wounds have various causes and, as determined by their underlying pathology, may take months or years to heal completely. Decubital ulcers (pressure sores), diabetic ulcers, and vascular ulcers are examples of chronic wounds.

WOUND CONTAMINATION AND INFECTION

Wound contamination is not the same as wound infection. Microorganisms in the environment contaminate all wounds, even those created during surgery using strict aseptic technique. Initially, these organisms are loosely attached to tissues and do not invade adjacent tissue; there is no host immune response to these organisms. Over time, these microorganisms multiply. Infection is the process whereby organisms bind to tissue, multiply, and then invade viable tissue, eliciting an immune response. Tissue infection depends on the number and pathogenicity (or virulence) of the microorganisms. In general, a wound is infected when the number of microorganisms reaches 100,000/g of tissue or milliliter of fluid. At these numbers, the microorganisms have exceeded the host's defense mechanisms to control them. If the patient presents for treatment more than 12 hours after injury, any wounds should be considered infected. Infection is characterized by erythema, edema, pus, fever, elevated neutrophil count, pain, change in color of exudate, and/or uncharacteristic odor. Contaminated wounds may become infected under the following circumstances:

- Foreign bodies are present (e.g., organic material, bone fragments, suture material, glove powder, bone plates, screws).
- Excessive necrotic tissue is left in the wound.
- Excessive bleeding results in higher levels of ferric ion (necessary for bacterial replication).
- Local tissue defenses are impeded (e.g., excessive hemoglobin level in burn patients or patients receiving immunosuppressive drugs).
- The vascular supply is altered.
- Dirt and debris are present.

Appropriate treatment soon after injury is important to avoid infection.

WOUND CATEGORIES

Open traumatic wounds can be categorized according to the degree of contamination present (Box 8-7). Management of these wounds varies according to the severity of the injury and the patient's condition. In general, wounds that are grossly contaminated and/or dirty may not be good candidates for primary closure. Until contamination and infection can be eliminated, open wound management is necessary. Dead and dying tissues must be excised (débrided) to minimize the potential for bacterial infection and create a viable wound bed.

USE OF ANTIBACTERIALS

The decision to use antibacterials systemically or topically in a surgical wound depends on several preoperative factors, including the patient's condition and immune status, nature of the surgery (emergency versus elective), location of the wound (orthopedic versus abdominal), predicted duration of the surgical procedure, surgeon's experience, and environment in which the procedure is performed. It is generally thought that antibacterials are not needed for patients in good health with an adequate immune status that are undergoing a relatively short (<90 minutes) elective orthopedic or soft tissue surgical procedure (not abdominal), performed by an experienced surgeon using aseptic technique in a clean surgical facility.

In clean surgical wounds, preoperative antibacterials should be considered in cases of shock, severe systemic trauma, long procedures, traumatic procedures, poor blood supply, foreign bodies, dead space (seromas, hematomas), malnutrition, obesity, or in the presence of other factors altering host defense mechanisms. When systemic (injected) antibacterials are used, they are most effective if administered just before surgery is begun and continued every 90 to 120 minutes thereafter during the surgical procedure.

Traumatic wounds, as opposed to clean surgical wounds, may contain devitalized tissue and/or foreign material and are contaminated by microorganisms. Traumatized tissue provides a suitable environment for bacterial multiplication and provides a route of entry for penetration of pathogens into adjacent viable tissue. Chronic (longstanding) wounds offer an ideal environment for bacterial proliferation, with copious wound fluid, necrotic tissue, and deep cracks and crevices on the wound surface. In these cases, antibacterials with a broad spectrum of antimicrobial activity are given systemically.

It is likely that we often do more harm than good by applying topical medications to wounds. The adverse effect of these products on wound healing is independent of their antimicrobial action. Generally, water-soluble antibacterial products tend to impede wound healing more than ointments or creams. Solutions tend to evaporate, contributing to drying of the wound surface. Ointments and creams remain in contact with the wound longer than solutions, preventing drying of the wound surface but also trapping bacteria in the wound and allowing for infection. A clean wound in a healthy patient can heal optimally without application of, for example, ointments or salves. Certain topical products may be beneficial at times; however, a focus on aseptic technique and appropriate clean management of wounds is more appropriate.

FIRST AID

In the field and/or before transport to a treatment facility, the wound should be protected with a bandage. An occlusive bandage is preferred. This type of bandage controls hemorrhage, prevents additional contamination, and provides immobilization of the extremity. Open fractures should be splinted. In open or compound fractures, exposed bone should not be forced into position below the skin. This avoids additional soft tissue trauma and reduces the chance of deep tissue contamination. The wound should be evaluated for antimicrobial therapy at the treatment facility. The wound should be protected during preparation of the surrounding area (e.g., clipping, scrubbing).

> **CRITICAL CONCEPT**
> Wound management revolves around three considerations—cleansing, closing, and covering.

WOUND ASSESSMENT

Wound assessment includes evaluation of the wound's location, size, and depth, exudate (drainage), tissue in the wound bed, and any signs of infection. Wound management revolves around three considerations—cleansing, closing, and covering. Control of hemorrhage is usually the first step in wound management. After initial hemostasis, it is important to evaluate the wound for bacterial contamination and the potential for bacterial growth. To avoid introduction of microorganisms, the wound should be cleaned under aseptic or at least sanitary conditions.

CLIPPING

In initial wound treatment, the wound must be protected while areas around the wound are clipped and cleaned. Before the area around the wound is clipped and cleaned, cover the wound with a water-soluble sterile ointment (e.g., K-Y Lubricating Jelly, Johnson & Johnson, New Brunswick, NJ) or moistened sterile gauze sponges. This helps prevent loose hairs from contaminating the wound further. The wound can also be temporarily closed with towel clamps or continuous sutures, which may require analgesia. Before clipping and shaving areas around head or face wounds, an ophthalmic ointment should be instilled in the conjunctival sac to protect the cornea and conjunctiva.

If the patient is covered with dirt and debris and is not in critical condition, it should be bathed before clipping. This reduces further contamination. Clipper blades also stay sharper longer when cutting clean hair. Clipping removes sources of contamination (e.g., hair, dirt, debris) and allows better visualization of the wound. Two pairs of clipper blades are advantageous; the second set of blades is disinfected for use in areas of elective surgical sites. Hair at wound edges may be trimmed with scissors or a handheld no. 10 scalpel blade dipped in mineral oil, K-Y jelly, or water so that the hair sticks to the blade and does not enter the wound.

> **CRITICAL CONCEPT**
>
> Cover a wound with K-Y jelly or gauze sponges when clipping and cleaning around it to help reduce potential contamination.

SCRUBBING

After the area around the wound has been clipped, replace the gauze sponges or gel over the wound. Gently scrub the surrounding intact skin, not the wound itself. The most commonly used surgical scrubs for skin preparation contain an antimicrobial agent plus a detergent-surfactant, such as chlorhexidine or povidone-iodine (Betadine). Rinsing with saline or 70% isopropyl alcohol does not seem to influence the antimicrobial effect.

LAVAGE

Cleansing of the wound (lavage) and **débridement** begins after the surrounding area has been cleaned. Obvious foreign bodies and gross contamination must be removed. Usually, a noncaustic solution is used to clean the wound without creating further irritation. Lavaging with a sterile solution and gentle scrubbing are the primary methods used for cleaning the wound. Take care not to use forceful lavage or scrub too vigorously; this may force bacteria into the wound and spread contamination. Often, more than one session of lavage and additional débridement may be necessary to remove debris and necrotic tissue. Bandaging with a wet wound dressing can facilitate this process. As a general rule, wound lavage should be discontinued before the tissues take on a waterlogged appearance.

Lavage solutions are most effective when delivered to the wound with a fluid jet with a pressure of at least 7 pounds per square inch (psi). This can be achieved by forcefully expelling solution from a 35- to 60-mL syringe through an 18-gauge needle (Fig. 8-33). Lavage solutions can also be delivered using a fluid bag (with administration set, three-way stopcock, and 35- to 60-mL syringe on one side and 18-gauge needle

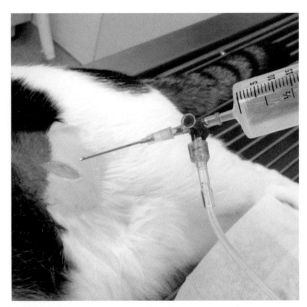

FIGURE 8-33 Demonstration of the lavage system, lavaging an open wound. (From Sirois M: Principles and practice of veterinary technology, ed 3, St Louis, 2011, Mosby.)

on the other) or Waterpik. The Waterpik should be used with care because it can deliver fluids at up to 70 psi. Adequate fluid pressure cannot be achieved with gravity flow, bulb syringe, or turkey baster.

Isotonic (normal) saline, lactated Ringer's solution, or plain Ringer's solution may be used for lavage. These physiologic solutions (isotonic, isosmotic, and sterile) do not damage tissue but have no antibacterial properties.

Povidone-iodine solution is commonly used to lavage wounds because of its broad antimicrobial spectrum. Dilutions of povidone-iodine in the range of 1% to 2% are more potent and more rapidly bactericidal than commercial 10% povidone-iodine solution, because dilution makes more free iodine available. A 1% solution can be prepared by diluting one part commercial 10% povidone-iodine with nine parts sterile water or electrolyte solution. The bactericidal effect of povidone-iodine lasts only 4 to 6 hours. It is inactivated by blood, exudate, and organic soil, reducing the period of residual action. The detergent form of povidone-iodine (scrub) is deleterious to wound tissues, causing irritation and potentiation of wound infection.

Chlorhexidine diacetate solution has a broad antimicrobial spectrum and is commonly used on small animals. In dogs it is more effective against *Staphylococcus aureus* than povidone-iodine. When chlorhexidine is applied to intact skin, the antimicrobial effect is immediate, with a lasting residual effect. Prolonged tissue contact with solutions of 0.5% or more concentrated solutions may be harmful. Currently, 0.05% chlorhexidine solutions are recommended for use in wound lavage. A 0.05% solution can be prepared by diluting 1 part 2% stock solution with 40 parts water. Chlorhexidine has sustained residual activity. Systemic absorption, toxicosis, and inactivation by organic material do not seem to be problematic.

Hydrogen peroxide is commonly used as a foaming wound irrigant. It has little antimicrobial effect, except on some anaerobes. It is more effective as a sporicide. In concentrations of 3% and higher, hydrogen peroxide is damaging to tissues. It also causes thrombosis in the microvasculature adjacent to the wound margins, impairing proliferation of blood vessels. Hydrogen peroxide should be reserved for one-time initial irrigation of dirty wounds. It should not be delivered to wounds under pressure because its foaming action forces debris between tissue planes, enlarging the wound and allowing for the accumulation of air in tissues.

CRITICAL CONCEPT

Hydrogen peroxide can be used only for initial wound cleaning.

ANESTHESIA AND ANALGESIA

After preparation of the surrounding area, the wound is prepared for analgesia and débridement. Local, regional, or general anesthesia may be used for wound management. General anesthesia is preferred if the patient can tolerate it. Tranquilizers or sedatives (e.g., xylazine, acepromazine, diazepam) are often used in conjunction with local and regional anesthesia.

Local anesthetics, such as lidocaine and bupivacaine, are used for pain control if the patient is not a candidate for general anesthesia. It may be beneficial to lavage a wound initially with 2% lidocaine for 1 or 2 minutes before irrigating to make the removal of foreign bodies less painful. Local anesthetics do not usually offer sufficient analgesia for surgical débridement.

Epinephrine is included in some local anesthetic products. It causes vasoconstriction and helps reduce hemorrhage and prolong the anesthetic effect. Epinephrine may cause tissue necrosis along the wound edge, adversely affect tissue defenses, and potentiate infection. In general, local anesthetics containing epinephrine should not be used in wound care.

DÉBRIDEMENT

Débridement is the removal of devitalized or necrotic tissue. Necrotic tissue must be removed because epithelium will not migrate over nonviable tissue, a wound will not contract without débridement, and necrotic tissue may act as a growth medium for bacteria. Débridement also removes sources of contamination, infection, and mechanical obstructions to healing.

Débridement is complete when the wound bed consists of only healthy tissue, commonly referred to as a clean wound. However, this does not mean that the wound is free of bacteria. Acute traumatic wounds are usually débrided to facilitate surgical closure, whereas chronic wounds are usually débrided to reduce the risk of infection and facilitate second-intention healing.

Wounds are generally débrided by mechanical means, such as with surgical instruments, irrigation, and dry-to-dry or wet-to-dry dressings (Procedure 8-4). Nonmechanical

débridement techniques include application of enzymatic agents or chemicals. In many cases, a combination of techniques is used.

Débridement should be performed as an aseptic procedure. To protect the wound from further contamination, sterile surgical gloves and mask should be worn and the area draped. Ideally, several sets of sterile instruments should be used to prevent reintroducing contaminated instruments into the wound (Fig. 8-34).

After a wound is cleansed and free of devitalized tissue, the surgeon explores the wound using sterile techniques. Other diagnostic procedures, such as radiographic studies using contrast materials, collection and assessment of fluid samples, and cytologic examination, may be performed to assist in the overall evaluation. Once this process is completed, a decision is made regarding how the wound will be

---

PROCEDURE 8-4 APPLYING A WET-TO-DRY DRESSING

1. This is performed using antiseptic technique and after initial cleaning and débridement of the wound has taken place.
2. Open the sterile dressings (usually gauze pads), irrigation and cleaning solution (this varies but sterile saline works well), and instrument set to provide a sterile field.
3. Gently remove and discard the old tape and soiled dressing. If the dressing sticks to the wound, moisten with sterile saline before removing.
4. Cleanse the wound. Clean from the least to the most contaminated area.
5. Apply saline to sterile gauze and place the wet material directly on the wound.
6. Apply dry gauze on top of the wet gauze.
7. Use cling gauze to hold the material in place followed by Vet Wrap.

Adapted from Sirois M: Principles and practice of veterinary technology, ed 3, St Louis, 2011, Mosby.

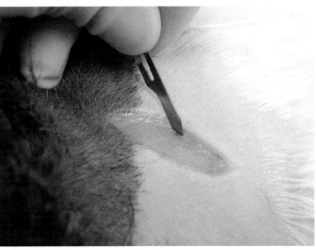

FIGURE 8-34 Débridement of a wound. (From Sirois M: Principles and practice of veterinary technology, ed 3, St Louis, 2011, Mosby.)

managed, including whether drainage is required. If primary closure is elected, decisions are made concerning anesthesia, antibacterials, nonsteroidal anti-inflammatory drugs (NSAIDs), tetanus status (if the injured animal is a horse), and bandaging, if required. The wound is then prepared for suturing.

DRAINAGE

Drains implanted in a wound provide an escape path for unwanted air and/or wound fluids, thus preventing or reducing seroma or hematoma formation in tissue pockets or dead space. The accumulation of exudate in a wound favors infection. Excessive fluid prevents phagocytic cells from reaching bacteria within a wound and provides a medium for bacterial growth. Drains are needed when wounds produce fluids and exudates for several days after initial treatment. They are indicated as follows:

- For treatment of an abscess cavity
- When foreign material and nonviable tissue are present and cannot be excised
- When contamination is inevitable (e.g., wounds near the anal area)
- To obliterate dead space
- As prophylaxis against anticipated fluid or air collection after a surgical procedure

Penrose drains are made of soft latex rubber. Their size ranges from ¼ to 1 inch in diameter and 12 to 18 inches long (Fig. 8-35). They provide a simple conduit for gravity flow. If a bandage covers the drain, there may be some capillary action. Fluid flows through the drain's lumen and around the tube and is related to the surface area of the tubing. The fenestrations (holes) in the drain decrease the surface area and reduce its effectiveness. Cutting the Penrose drain in half lengthwise increases the surface area by 100%. Penrose drains should not be left in place for more than 3 to 5 days

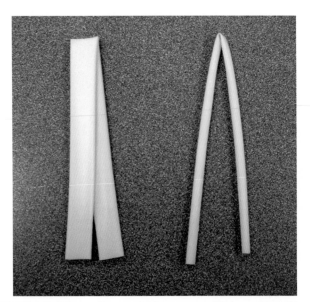

FIGURE 8-35 A collection of different sizes of Penrose drains. (From Sirois M: *Principles and practice of veterinary technology,* ed 3, St Louis, 2011, Mosby.)

because most gravitational drainage has subsided by that time.

Closed-suction drains provide drainage with a vacuum applied to the drain lumen, with no air vent. Closed-suction drains allow wounds and dressings to stay dry, prevent bacterial movement through and around the drain, afford continuous drainage, and eliminate the need for irrigation.

These drains help hold the skin grafts in contact with the granulating wound bed to enhance revascularization. Excessively high negative pressure in the drain system can injure tissue. The vacuum for these drain systems can be generated by glass vacuum bottles, compressible plastic canister (Hemovac), compressible plastic canister with two one-way valves (low-pressure suction drain), or a simple syringe (usually a modified 60-mL syringe).

Gauze or umbilical tape setons may be passed into a wound opening to keep the wound from closing before all exudates have drained. They are unsatisfactory for drainage purposes because they do not promote drainage once the gauze is saturated. They act as wicks, retaining bacterial contaminants, and can be mechanically irritating.

WOUND CLOSURE

The patient's ability to tolerate anesthesia influences initial wound management. It is usually best to close fresh wounds as quickly as possible, when the risk of infection and complication is low. Wounds with minor contamination may be cleaned, débrided, and closed. Sometimes, a drain is installed to facilitate removal of tissue fluids associated with significant soft tissue trauma. Wounds that require optimal wound drainage because of gross contamination, tissue necrosis, and/or infection are managed as open wounds until they can be closed at a later time. Table 8-3 summarizes the types of closure used with different types of wounds. A wound should be closed only when the veterinarian is certain that all devitalized and contaminated tissue has been removed and there is adequate skin to appose the wound edges. Veterinarians should consider covering the wound and allowing it to heal by second intention or delayed closure. Unfortunately, wounds are sometimes closed prematurely, resulting in dehiscence (opening) and infection a few days later. If there is any doubt about the advisability of a surgical closure, the clinician may cover the wound with a proper dressing and manage the wound with frequent dressing changes (at least daily), lavage, débridement, and reassessment, as required.

NONCLOSURE

In second-intention healing (nonclosure), the wound is not sutured but heals by contraction and epithelialization. Second-intention healing is selected for wounds involving significant tissue loss. In horses, it is especially useful for wounds of the neck, body, and proximal limbs. Although these wounds are prepared with the same care as for primary closure and delayed primary closure, wounds of the extremities in horses are often left uncovered or managed with a pressure bandage or cast. If left open to heal by second

TABLE 8-3	Types of Wound Closures	
TYPE OF CLOSURE	**TYPE OF WOUND HEALING**	**CONDITIONS OF USE**
Primary closure	First-intention healing	Wound closed with sutures or staples Full-thickness apposition of wound edges Tissues in direct apposition Minimal edema No local infection No serous discharge Minimal scar formation Rapid healing
Nonclosure	Second-intention healing	Wound left open because of infection, extensive trauma, tissue loss, or incorrect apposition of tissues Healing by contraction and epithelialization, from inner layers to outer surface Contraction starts after ≈72 hr; stops when wound edges meet or tension exceeds strength of contraction Epithelialization starts within 24 hr after injury; requires a moist, oxygen-rich environment Delayed by healing
Delayed primary closure	Form of third-intention healing	Closure 3 to 5 days after cleaning and débridement, but before granulation tissue forms Wound strength and rate of healing not affected by delaying primary closure
Secondary closure	Form of third-intention healing	Closure after >3 to 5 days after granulation tissue has formed in the wound bed
	Third-intention healing	Safe method for repair of dirty, contaminated, or infected wounds with extensive tissue damage Allows for management of infection or necrosis before closure Surgeon débrides damaged tissue; wound closed, with accurate apposition of tissues
Adnexal reepithelialization	Second-intention healing	Partial-thickness skin loss with epithelialization primarily from compound hair follicles (so-called *road burns*)

Adapted from Sirois M: Principles and practice of veterinary technology, ed 3, St Louis, 2011, Mosby.

intention, the wound should be cleaned daily at first to remove accumulated exudate. Skin distal to the wound is also cleaned and protected with petroleum jelly or a similar product to prevent skin maceration (so-called *serum burns*).

COVERING WOUNDS

Nature provides natural bandages as a part of normal healing. A partial-thickness wound that forms a blister rarely becomes infected and heals more rapidly if the blister is not broken. The scab of a full-thickness wound and the **eschar** (necrotic layer that sloughs off) of a burn also serve as natural bandages. The scab protects from external contamination, maintains internal homeostasis, and provides a surface beneath which cell migration and movement of skin edges occur. The eschar of large burn wounds serves as a biologic dressing that is protective and is considered by many surgeons to be superior to artificial bandaging materials.

PRINCIPLES OF BANDAGE APPLICATION

In veterinary application, bandages have the following functions:
- Protect wounds.
- Hold clean or sterile dressings in place.
- Absorb exudate and débride a wound.
- Serve as a vehicle for therapeutic agents.
- Serve as an indicator of wound secretions.
- Pack the wound.
- Provide support for bony anatomic structures.
- Support and stabilize soft tissue.
- Secure splints.
- Prevent weight bearing.
- Provide compression to control hemorrhage, dead space, and tissue edema.
- Discourage self-grooming.
- Restrict motion to eliminate stress of the wound edges.
- Provide patient comfort.
- Provide an aesthetic appearance.
  The basic principles of bandage application are as follows:
  - Properly prepare the area before application of a bandage. This may require clipping the hair, wound débridement, and/or cleaning of surrounding skin.
  - Use porous materials when possible. This allows circulation of air and escape of excessive moisture.
  - Use absorbent materials when exudates may be a problem. Change absorbent dressings when they become saturated and before saturation is evident externally.

- Use appropriate materials of adequate width to avoid producing a tourniquet effect.
- Apply bandage materials as smoothly as possible. Ridges and lumps lead to skin irritation and necrosis.
- Secure protective wound pads to the skin so that they do not shift from the site.
- Check bandages frequently to determine whether there is persistent swelling, skin discoloration, or coolness. A bandage applied too tightly can impair circulation, resulting in serious damage to soft tissues.
- Instruct clients on basic care of bandages and signs of bandage failure. This includes the physical appearance of the bandage, as well as behavior of the patient. Box 8-8 lists key points in discharge instructions.

Ideally, materials used for bandaging should have the following properties:

- Permeable to oxygen and other gases
- Conform to body contours
- Acceptable appearance
- Inert
- Long storage life
- Inexpensive
- Easily sterilized
- Unaffected by disinfecting and cleaning solutions
- Nonflammable
- Will not shred (so particles do not contaminate the wound)
- Compatible with topical therapeutic agents
- Will not adhere to the wound but can remove exudate and debris from the wound
- Maintains a moist wound surface that is free from exudate

BANDAGE COMPONENTS

> ### CRITICAL CONCEPT
> It is best to have all necessary materials laid out and ready for use (i.e., out of packaging) before starting a bandage.

In most situations, bandages are generally composed of three layers, each with its own properties and function. The primary layer rests on the wound and may or may not be adherent. The secondary layer provides absorbency and padding. The tertiary layer is the outer layer that holds the underlying layers in place. This is usually the only layer that the client sees. Clients often judge the quality of treatment solely on the appearance of this outer bandage layer.

PRIMARY LAYER. The primary layer is in contact with the wound itself (Fig. 8-36). When débridement is the goal, an adherent layer is used for the primary bandage. Once the wound is in the proliferation phase and granulation tissue has formed, use a nonadherent dressing to avoid disruption of the new tissue. The primary layer should be sterile and comfortable, allow fluids to pass to the secondary layer, protect the wound from exogenous contamination, and be nontoxic and nonirritating to tissue.

Adherent bandaging material, such as sterile gauze sponges with wide mesh openings and noncotton filler, can be used to provide débridement during the early stage of wound healing. This layer removes devitalized tissue and wound exudate when it is taken off during a bandage change. Adherent dressings may be wet or dry, depending on the nature of the wound. Some bandages are applied wet and then allowed to dry. Use of an adherent primary layer should be discontinued after the wound has been cleared of necrotic debris and heavy exudate.

If loose necrotic tissue or foreign material is present on the surface of the wound, a dry-to-dry dressing may be the best type to use. Dry gauze with a large mesh is placed directly on the wound. An absorbent layer is placed over this primary layer and fluid is absorbed from the wound and allowed to dry. Necrotic material adheres to the gauze and is removed with the bandage. Although this type of bandage

BOX 8-8	Key Points in Discharge Instructions for Bandages

1. Strict confinement initially and then restricted activity during healing
2. Keep the pet from licking or chewing the bandage. Many pets require an Elizabethan collar.
3. Monitor the pet for any sign of excessive discomfort. If the pet is trying to remove the bandage, it could mean that there is a problem beneath the support. Pay particular attention to the toes and area at the top of the bandage. Look for swelling of the toes or any sores and pay attention to bad odors from the bandage.
4. If the bandage appears loose, soiled, or wet, it should be checked.
5. Schedule rechecks as prescribed by the veterinarian.

Adapted from Sirois M: Principles and practice of veterinary technology, ed 3, St Louis, 2011, Mosby.

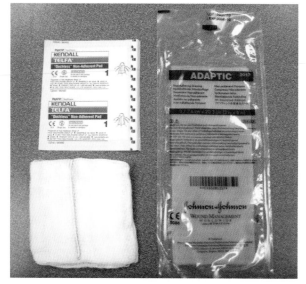

FIGURE 8-36 *Primary bandage materials. (From Sirois M: Principles and practice of veterinary technology, ed 3, St Louis, 2011, Mosby.)*

removes tissue debris, bandage removal is painful and may also remove viable tissue. Thus, dry-to-dry dressings should be used only when necessary.

If the exudate is especially viscous or dried foreign matter must be removed, a wet-to-dry dressing may be appropriate. The bandage is applied wet, which dilutes the exudate for absorption. As the bandage dries, the foreign material adheres to the bandage and is later removed with the bandage. Solutions used to wet the primary layer include physiologic (0.9%) saline or a water-soluble bacteriostatic or bactericidal compound, such as 0.05% chlorhexidine diacetate solution.

For wounds with copious exudate or transudate, a wet-to-dry dressing may be best. Wet dressings absorb fluid more rapidly than dry dressings. They may be used to transport heat to a wound and/or enhance capillary action to promote wound drainage. A water-soluble bacteriostatic or bactericidal solution can be used to wet the dressing to help control microorganisms. The primary layer is applied wet and kept wet after the secondary and tertiary layers have been applied. This bandage is also removed wet. Wet-to-wet dressings cause less pain than dry dressings when removed; by using a warm solution, patient comfort is increased. A disadvantage is that these bandages tend to cause tissue maceration and have little débriding capacity.

A nonadherent primary layer is indicated during the reparative stage of wound healing, with the formation of granulation tissue and production of a more serosanguineous exudate. In the early repair stage, petrolatum-impregnated products can be used in the presence of exudate and when little or no epithelialization has taken place. Later, when there is little fluid, and during epithelialization, nonadherent dressings are indicated. Nonadherent dressings are used to cover lacerations, skin graft donor sites, minor burns, abrasions, and surgical incisions. The main goal is to minimize tissue injury on removal. They do not absorb much fluid; draining wounds usually require a secondary dressing. Examples of nonadherent dressing materials include Adaptic and Release (Johnson & Johnson), and Telfa adhesive pads (Kendall Curity, Covidien, Mansfield, MA). These semiocclusive nonadherent materials leave the granulation bed undisturbed but still move fluid away from the wound.

SECONDARY LAYER. The secondary (intermediate) layer provides support and moves exudate or transudate away from the wound (Fig. 8-37). Materials used in this layer include gauze bandaging material (e.g., Sof-Band, Kling, Sof-Kling, Johnson & Johnson), cast padding, and bandaging cotton.

The secondary layer should be thick enough to absorb moisture, pad the wound from trauma, and inhibit wound movement. If the bandage allows evaporation of fluid from absorbed exudate, this partially dry environment retards bacterial growth. With wounds producing copious fluids, evaporation does not keep the bandage dry. If such a moist bandage is not changed frequently, the wound fluids serve as a growth medium for bacteria.

TERTIARY LAYER. The tertiary (outer) layer holds the underlying bandage layers in place (Fig. 8-38). Materials used in this layer include adhesive tapes (e.g., Zonasdont, Johnson & Johnson), elastic bandages (Elastikon, Johnson & Johnson; Vet Wrap; Kendall Conform, Covidien; Medi-Rip, Conco Medical, Rock Hill, SC), and conforming stretch gauze. This layer should be applied carefully to provide support without constricting.

CRITICAL CONCEPT

If using Vet Wrap, it is best to unroll the wrap and then loosely reroll it before placing.

Porous adhesive tape allows evaporation of fluid from the bandage. It can also allow movement of fluid (e.g., saliva, rainwater) into the wound, which may be undesirable. Waterproof adhesive tape repels water but also prevents evaporation. If the wound is producing considerable exudate, the tissues may become macerated from retained fluids. The resultant damp environment favors bacterial growth.

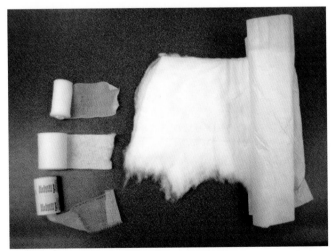

FIGURE 8-37 *Secondary layer bandage materials. (From Sirois M: Principles and practice of veterinary technology, ed 3, St Louis, 2011, Mosby.)*

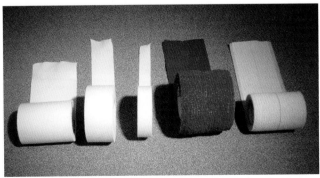

FIGURE 8-38 *Tertiary layer bandage materials. (From Sirois M: Principles and practice of veterinary technology, ed 3, St Louis, 2011, Mosby.)*

Elastic adhesive tape is compliant and applies continuous dynamic pressure to the wound as the patient moves. Elastic tape products should be wrapped over the underlying bandage materials carefully to apply even but not excessive pressure. Elastic adhesive tapes tend to adhere to themselves, so minimal external taping is needed. Self-adherent products (e.g., Vet Wrap, MediRip) have no adhesive undercoat. Although these products tend to adhere to themselves, in veterinary practice, some external tape is usually required at the ends to keep the bandage from coming apart during movement.

> **CRITICAL CONCEPT**
>
> Always make sure that the bandaging is smooth; wrinkles in the material can cause pressure points or sores to develop.

NURSING CARE FOR RECUMBENT PATIENTS

A number of conditions can cause recumbency in patients, including pelvic fractures, head trauma, and herniated intervertebral discs. A major concern in recumbent patients is the formation of **decubital ulcers** (e.g., bed sores, pressure sores). Increased skin moisture and irritation contribute to the development of decubital ulcers; therefore, patients should be kept clean and dry and should be bathed frequently. Because decubital ulcers are primarily caused by pressure, they can be avoided or minimized by using bedding such as sheepskin, foam or air mattresses, or trampolines, or with bandaging techniques. The best treatment is prevention; animals must be kept clean. Urine and feces should not be allowed to remain on the skin and hair coat. Poor sanitation promotes skin breakdown and the formation of decubital ulcers. Shaving the hair around the perineal region on animals that are incontinent or have diarrhea can save time in baths and drying. Sponge baths can be done instead.

Decubital ulcers (Fig. 8-39) develop rapidly, within 2 or 3 days, but heal slowly. The extent of tissue damage is often graded from least severe (grade I, darkened area of thickened skin, no exposure of subcutaneous tissue) to most severe (grade IV, deep tissue loss with exposure of bone). Grade II decubital ulcers involve exposure of subcutaneous fat and grade III ulcers involve tissue defects to the level of deep fascial layers. Once the underlying muscle and/or bone is exposed, it can become infected. Small superficial ulcers can be managed conservatively with doughnut bandages and topical astringents and antibiotics. Ointments with a petroleum base are not recommended because these can trap moisture and harbor bacteria. If bone is exposed, proper care should be taken to prevent the periosteum from drying. Prevention and treatment of infection are essential. Areas affected most are the sternum, shoulders, sides of the fifth digits, stifles, and hips. Surgical intervention may be required for decubital ulcers, especially if they are grade III or IV in severity. Such intervention may include débridement and primary closure, delayed wound closure, or use of cutaneous or myocutaneous flaps.

> **CRITICAL CONCEPT**
>
> Preparation H (Pfizer, New York) is believed to stimulate wound healing when applied to decubital ulcers.

TURNING

Turning the patients every 2 to 4 hours helps prevent formation of ulcers and dependent pulmonary **atelectasis**. After turning, the pressure points should be checked. Redness should be only temporary. If redness persists 30 minutes or longer, decrease the time on that side. After a position change, stimulate areas over pressure points by massage and flexion and extension exercises, which will increase circulation to the affected areas.

PADDING

Padding the recumbent patient is essential in preventing the formation of decubital ulcers and is also used when treating decubital ulcers. Paralyzed animals frequently thrash about; padding helps prevent animals from harming themselves. Any animal with paralysis or paresis, seizures, vestibular problems, encephalopathy resulting from neoplasia of the brain, orthopedic disease, or metabolic disease should have padding placed in the cage. Animals with vestibular disease, neoplasia of the brain, or frequent seizures should be placed in cages with padded doors and walls. Types of padding include fleece pads, sponge rubber egg crates, diapers, and waterbeds. Household items such as blankets, sheets, and foam rubber placed in plastic bags can be used as padding. Fleece pads are synthetic sheep skins. They are washable, absorbent, very soft, and airy. These can be combined with other forms of padding. If used alone, they are best for patients weighing under 25 pounds.

Foam rubber egg crates are especially good for larger patients. A big disadvantage, however, is that they act like a sponge, absorbing urine and water. Place them in plastic bags to keep them clean and dry. Owners can purchase these

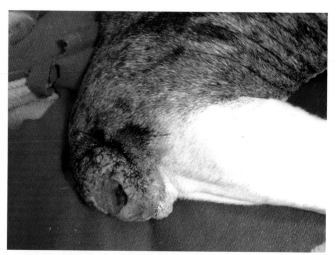

FIGURE 8-39 A major concern in recumbent patients is the formation of decubital ulcers, commonly referred to as bed sores or pressure sores. (From Sirois M: Principles and practice of veterinary technology, ed 3, St Louis, 2011, Mosby.)

crates at medical supply stores or in the bedding department of retail stores. Veterinary trampolines or cots can also facilitate patient cleanliness and may help prevent the formation of pressure sores.

Waterbeds are especially good for preventing decubital ulcers. Animal waterbeds are made in various sizes so that most standard veterinary cages will accommodate them. The bed should be placed in a cage of almost the same area so that the patient will not fall off and become stuck between the bed and cage wall. Animal waterbeds are thermostatically heated and provide warmth and comfort to animals placed on them. If they become unplugged, they require about 12 hours to heat up before they can be used. The temperature can be adjusted easily on the waterbed to prevent the animal from becoming overheated or too cold. Heat eases muscle soreness, stimulates circulation, and helps animals relax. Waterbeds should never be used without turning on the heat. A cold waterbed draws heat from the animal and results in hypothermia.

Disposable diapers or bed pads are placed on top of all padding to help keep the padding clean. Use of diapers saves valuable nursing time. Soiled diapers are simply thrown away, leaving the underlying padding reasonably clean and dry. In pet stores, these are called puppy training pads.

EUTHANASIA METHODS

The term **euthanasia** is derived from the Greek *eu-*, meaning good, and *-thanatos,* meaning death. The goal is to provide the animal with a quick and painless death while minimizing stress and anxiety. Considerations that help determine the method of euthanasia include safety of the individual performing the task and of the animal, ability of the agent to produce rapid loss of consciousness and death without pain, distress, or anxiety, reliability and availability of the agent, and age and species limitations. Depending on the technique used, death is produced by hypoxia, depression of neurons vital for life's function, or disruption of brain activity.

Animals can be euthanized by inhalation or injection methods. An enclosed chamber or induction mask is used to deliver inhalant anesthetics such as isoflurane. Inhalant anesthetics can also be used to render an animal unconscious while a second procedure is used to cause death.

IV injection of a barbiturate anesthetic is the most rapid, reliable, and desirable method for performing euthanasia. An animal that is anxious, wild, or aggressive should be sedated before IV administration of any euthanasia agent. Once the animal is sufficiently sedated, an IV or butterfly catheter will provide a controlled means for administration of the barbiturate. In small animals such as neonates (<2 kg), IP injection is acceptable, provided that the euthanasia agent is nonirritating. Intracardiac injection is acceptable for an animal that is heavily sedated, anesthetized, or comatose.

When it becomes necessary to euthanize any animal, death should be induced as quickly and painlessly as possible. It should be carried out by individuals trained and qualified to do so. When a necropsy is to be performed immediately after euthanasia, the method of euthanasia should be one that causes the least amount of artifactual changes in the tissues and leaves the animal as intact as possible.

RECOMMENDED READINGS

Lane DR: *Veterinary nursing*, Burlington, MA, 2003, Butterworth Heinemann.

Macintire DK: *Manual of small animal emergency and critical care medicine*, New York, 2005, Wiley-Blackwell.

Schaer M: *Clinical medicine of the dog and cat*, ed 2, London, 2010, Manson.

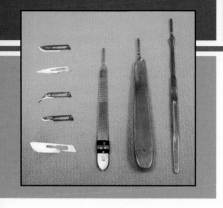

OUTLINE

Surgery Suite, *243*
Preparation Area, *243*
Scrub Area, *243*
Surgery Room, *243*
Principles of Asepsis, *244*
Contamination and Infection, *244*
Rules of Aseptic Technique, *244*
Sterilization and Disinfection, *245*
Surgical Instruments, *247*
Scalpels and Blades, *247*
Scissors, *248*
Needle Holders, *248*
Forceps, *248*
Retractors, *249*
Miscellaneous Instruments, *250*
**Sutures and Other Materials Used in Wound
   Closure,** *250*
Sutures, *250*
Other Materials, *253*
**Care and Maintenance of Surgical Instruments and
   Supplies,** *253*
Instrument Cleaning, *253*
Instrument Lubricating and Autoclaving, *254*
Wrapping Instrument Packs, *255*
Sterilization, *256*
Folding and Wrapping Gowns and Drapes, *257*
Storing Sterilized Items, *258*
Basic Surgical Terminology, *260*
Incisions, *260*
Common Surgical Procedures, *260*
Preoperative and Postoperative Considerations, *261*

Preoperative Evaluation, *261*
Patient Preparation, *261*
Preparation of the Operative Site, *262*
Hair Removal and Skin Scrubbing, *262*
Positioning, *264*
Sterile Skin Preparation, *265*
Preparation of the Surgical Team, *265*
Surgical Attire, *265*
Surgical Scrub, *266*
Gowning and Gloving, *266*
Anesthetic Equipment and Supplies, *267*
Supplies for Intravenous Fluid Administration, *267*
Endotracheal Tubes, *267*
Laryngoscope, *268*
Medical Gas Supply, *268*
Anesthesia Machines, *269*
Breathing Circuits, *272*
Anesthesia, *274*
Preanesthetic Medication, *274*
Induction, *275*
Maintenance of Anesthesia, *275*
Anesthetic Monitoring, *276*
Responding to Adverse Events, *278*
Surgical Assisting, *278*
Draping and Organizing the Instrument Table, *279*
Unwrapping or Opening Sterile Items, *280*
Recovery, *280*
Postoperative Evaluation, *280*
Pain Management, *281*
Postoperative Complications, *282*
Suture Removal, *283*

LEARNING OBJECTIVES

After reviewing this chapter, the reader will be able to:

1. Describe and explain surgical terminology.
2. Discuss principles of aseptic technique.
3. Give examples of methods used to disinfect or sterilize surgical instruments and supplies.
4. Describe procedures for preparing the surgical site and surgical team.
5. Identify surgical instruments and explain their uses and maintenance.

[1]Elsevier and the author acknowledge and appreciate the original contributions from Sirois M: Principles and practice of veterinary technology, ed 3, St Louis, 2011, Mosby, and Tear M: Small animal surgical nursing, ed 2, St Louis, 2011, Elsevier, whose work forms the heart of this chapter.

6. Compare and contrast types of suture needles and suture materials.
7. Define the role of veterinary staff members in anesthesia and perioperative pain management.
8. Describe the equipment used for anesthetizing animals.
9. Prepare and maintain anesthetic machines and the associated equipment.

10. List and describe the steps involved in anesthetizing animals for induction.
11. Explain the procedures used in medicating and monitoring animals before, during, and after anesthesia.
12. Prepare a small animal patient, anesthetic equipment, anesthetic agents, and accessories for general anesthesia.

KEY TERMS

Analgesia	General anesthesia	Ovariohysterectomy	Sedation
Anamnesis	Hypercarbia	Pain	Sterilization indicators
Anesthesia	Laparotomy	Peritonitis	Suture
Aseptic technique	Laryngoscope	Pressure manometer	Tidal volume
Autoclave	Mayo stand	Pulse deficit	Vaporizer
Breathing circuit	Narcosis	Pulse oximeter	Vasoconstriction
Electrocautery	Nociception	Pulse quality	Ventilation
Esophageal stethoscope	Non–rebreathing system	Rebreathing system	
Eviscerate	Nosocomial infection	Reservoir bag	
Flow meter	Orchiectomy	Scavenging system	

The role of the veterinary assistant in surgical procedures is diverse. During the presurgical period, the veterinary assistant may be responsible for preparation of the patient, surgical instruments and equipment, and surgical environment. During surgery, the veterinary assistant may aid the veterinary technician with monitoring the anesthetized patient. The veterinary assistant is often responsible for obtaining and opening surgical packs, suture materials, and other supplies for the surgeon. It is vital that the veterinary assistant know how to function in a sterile surgical environment without causing contamination. In the postsurgical period, the veterinary assistant is frequently responsible for postoperative patient care and monitoring, instructing clients on patient care during the recovery period, and removing sutures.

SURGERY SUITE

The American Animal Hospital Association (AAHA) recommends three distinct and separate areas for a surgical facility—the preparation area, scrub area, and surgery room. Although AAHA certification is not a legal requirement for veterinary facilities, a surgical facility should create the best environment for the patient. In addition, some state licensing boards have specific requirements regarding surgical facilities that a veterinary hospital must meet to pass inspection and to receive authorization to offer surgery.

PREPARATION AREA

Ideally, the preparation area should be adjacent to the surgery room. The prep room can be used for patient preparation and the storage of surgical supplies. AAHA also recommends placement of storage and cabinets in the prep area, not the

surgery room. The surgeon and veterinary technician can use the preparation area to scrub and gown for surgery if a separate scrub area is not available. It is ideal to have a separate **anesthesia** machine for the prep room so that cross-contamination does not occur when the machine is moved from one room to another. The prep area is used for clipping the patient. Procedures classified as dirty should be done in the prep area. Procedures such as abscessed wound care, débridement of old wounds, and treatment of impacted anal sacs are often defined as dirty.

SCRUB AREA

The scrub area may be a small area with the scrub sink, autoclave, and room to gown and glove (Fig. 9-1). This is a transitional area in which the veterinarian and staff can prepare to move into the surgery room. Adding the autoclave to the space makes it a dual-purpose area that works well for personnel because the counter area would not be in use for pack preparation while the surgeon and technician are gowning and gloving for surgery.

SURGERY ROOM

Ideally, the surgery room is a separate room that should be used only for surgery. The AAHA recommends that the surgery room be easily cleanable and be closed off as needed. Closing the door minimizes traffic, maximizes cleanliness, and helps ensure that the surgery room is used only for aseptic procedures. The room should be a dedicated room reserved for sterile surgical procedures. It should be used only for surgery, not for other types of procedures that could introduce bacteria into the room. The surgery room should be large enough that personnel can easily move around the surgery table without contaminating the surgical field or the surgeon. If present, cabinets should be off the floor and constructed of nonporous material. Keeping cabinets off the floor allows for adequate cleaning underneath and prevents dust and debris from collecting around the base of the cabinets. The cabinets that hold sterile supplies should have doors that can be closed to protect the packs and other supplies from dust, debris, and other contaminants (Fig. 9-2).

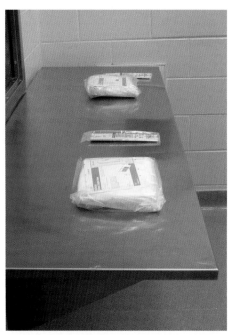

FIGURE 9-1 Gowning table. Note the absence of clutter on the table and the sufficient space to allow two people to gown and glove simultaneously. (From Tear M: Small animal surgical nursing, ed 2, St Louis, 2011, Mosby.)

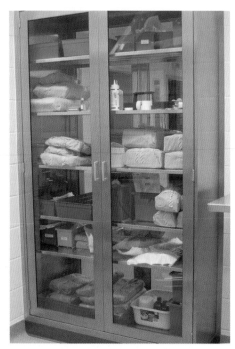

FIGURE 9-2 "Pass-through" storage cabinet. (From Tear M: Small animal surgical nursing, ed 2, St Louis, 2011, Mosby.)

The surgery room should also be free of clutter and items that may collect dust or harbor bacteria. It should have a door that can be closed; this door should be opened only when necessary to limit the amount of traffic and air flow in and out of the room. If possible, the air pressure should be greater in the surgery room to reduce the influx of bacteria from the rest of the veterinary facility.

PRINCIPLES OF ASEPSIS

Aseptic technique is the term used to describe all the precautions taken to prevent contamination, and ultimately infection, of a surgical wound. Its purpose is to minimize contamination so that postoperative healing is not delayed.

CONTAMINATION AND INFECTION

Contamination of an object or a wound implies the presence of microorganisms within or on it. Contamination of a wound can, but does not necessarily, lead to infection. With infection, microorganisms in the body or a wound multiply and cause harmful effects. Fungal, protozoal, viral, and bacterial organisms can all cause contamination of the surgical area and harmful effects to the patient. Four main factors determine whether infection occurs:

- Number of microorganisms: There must be a sufficient number of microorganisms to overcome the defenses of the animal.
- Virulence of the microorganisms: This is their ability to cause disease.
- Susceptibility of the animal: Some individuals have a greater natural resistance to infection than others.
- Route of exposure to the microorganisms: Some routes of exposure are more likely to result in infection than others.

The route of exposure to microorganisms during surgery is determined by the surgical procedure. The factor that can be most significantly influenced is the number of microorganisms that enter the surgical wound by application of strict aseptic technique before and during surgery. Improper application of methods of sanitation, sterilization, and disinfection can lead to microbial resistance and increase the risk of **nosocomial** (hospital-acquired) **infection**.

> **CRITICAL CONCEPT**
>
> Antibiotics should be used only perioperatively and postoperatively when indicated by patient status, surgery performed, or duration of surgery to reduce the risk of developing antibiotic-resistant microbes.

RULES OF ASEPTIC TECHNIQUE

During surgery, aseptic technique protects the exposed tissues of the patient from four main sources of potential contamination: the operative personnel, surgical instruments and equipment, patient itself, and surgical environment. Proper operating room conduct and adherence to a few general rules will help minimize the possibility of contamination. All personnel must be aware of which items are sterile and which are nonsterile. Sterile items should be grouped together in the operating room and kept separate from nonsterile items. Body movements should be restricted to reduce air currents. Only sterile items should touch patient tissues. When the sterility of an item is in question, always consider it contaminated.

STERILIZATION AND DISINFECTION

Sterilization refers to the destruction of all microorganisms (e.g., bacteria, viruses, spores) on a surface or object. It usually refers to objects that come into contact with sterile tissue or enter the vascular system (e.g., instruments, drapes, catheters, needles).

Disinfection is the destruction of most pathogenic microorganisms on inanimate (nonliving) objects; antisepsis is the destruction of most pathogenic microorganisms on animate (living) objects. Antiseptics are used to kill microorganisms during patient skin preparation and surgical scrubbing; however, the skin cannot be sterilized. Most disinfectants are microbicidal—that is, they kill microbes. Some disinfectants are bacteriostatic; they inhibit the growth of microbes. Common antimicrobial agents are listed in Table 9-1.

Disinfectants can be classified according to their spectrum of activity as the following:
- Bactericidal (kills bacteria)
- Bacteriostatic (inhibits growth of bacteria)
- Sporicidal (kills spores)
- Virucidal (kills viruses)
- Fungicidal (kills fungi)

MODE OF ACTION

Different physical and chemical methods destroy or inhibit microorganisms in several ways. Some act by damaging microbial cell walls or membranes. Others act by interfering with microbial cell enzyme activity or metabolism or by destroying microbial cell contents by oxidation, hydrolysis, reduction, coagulation, protein denaturation, or the formation of salt. The effectiveness of all microbial control methods depends on the following factors:

1. Time: Most methods have minimum effective exposure times.
2. Temperature: Most methods are more effective as the temperature increases.
3. Concentration and preparation: Chemical methods require appropriate concentrations of agent; disinfectants may be adversely affected by mixing with other chemicals.
4. Organisms: These are the type, number, and stage of growth of target organisms.
5. Surface: The physical and chemical properties of the surface to be treated may interfere with the method's activity; some surfaces are damaged by certain methods.
6. Organic debris or other soils: If present, these will dilute, render ineffective, or interfere with many control methods.
7. Method of application: Items may be sprayed, swabbed, or immersed in disinfectants; cotton and some synthetic materials used to apply or store chemicals may reduce their activity.

Methods used for the control of microorganisms consist of chemical and physical methods. Physical methods include

TABLE 9-1	Common Antimicrobial Chemical Agents	
AGENTS	**MAJOR MODE OF ACTION**	**APPLICATIONS**
Soaps	Disrupt cell membranes and increases permeability	Cleansing, mechanical removal of microorganisms
Detergents	Disrupt cell membranes by combining with lipids and proteins; leak N and P compounds out of cells	Cleansing, bactericidal action
Quaternary ammonium compounds	Cause changes in cell permeability; neutralize phospholipids	Disinfection of surfaces
Bisdiguanide compounds (e.g., chlorhexidine)	Alter cell wall permeability, protein precipitation; rapid action, broad spectrum	Routine skin preparation
Povidone-iodophor compounds	Damage cell wall, form reactive ions and protein complexes; rapid action	Routine skin preparation
Phenol, cresols, Lysol, hexylresorcinol	Bactericidal; denaturation and precipitation of proteins	Disinfection of laboratory equipment, instruments, bench tops, garbage pails, toilets
Bisphenols (e.g., hexachlorophene)	Bacteriostatic	Deodorants in soaps, inhibition of gram-positive bacteria; require repeated use
Cl_2 and sodium hypochlorite (bleach)	Bactericidal, oxidation of -SH and -NH_2 groups	Purification of water, kennel sanitation
Iodine	Bactericidal; oxidation of indole nucleus of enzymes or coenzymes	Skin disinfection, especially as tincture
H_2O_2 (hydrogen peroxide)	Bacteriostatic; mildly bactericidal	Antisepsis of cuts, minor wounds
$HgCl_2$ (zinc)	Highly bacteriostatic; precipitation of proteins	Antisepsis of cuts, minor wounds
$AgNO_3$ (silver nitrate)	Chemical cauterizing agent	Stops minor bleeding

Adapted from Sirois M: Principles and practice of veterinary technology, ed 3, St Louis, 2011, Mosby.

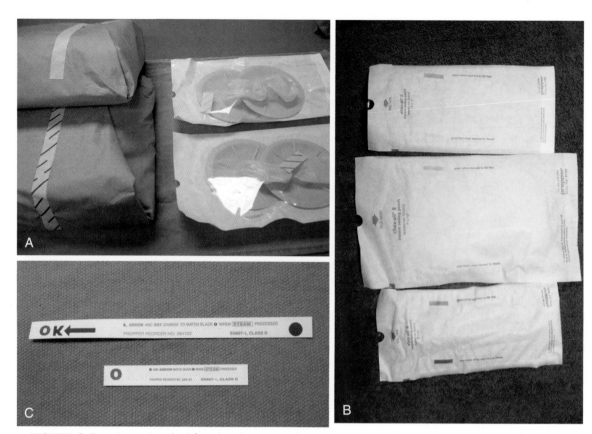

FIGURE 9-3 **A,** Surgical packs *(left)* and sterilization pouches *(right)* showing sterilization indicator tape before *(top)* and after *(bottom)* sterilization. The pack was autoclaved and the pouch was gas- sterilized. **B,** Sterilization pouches showing paper side indicators before processing *(top)*, after ethylene oxide (EO) gas sterilization *(middle)*, and after autoclave sterilization *(bottom)*. **C,** Sterilization indicators typically packed inside surgical instrument packs, after *(top)* and before *(bottom)* autoclave sterilization. (From Sirois M: Principles and practice of veterinary technology, ed 3, St Louis, 2011, Mosby.)

dry heat, moist heat, radiation, filtration, and ultrasonic vibration. Of these methods, only moist heat, in the form of steam under pressure, is routinely used for sterilization in the veterinary clinic. Chemical control methods include the application of soaps, detergents, disinfectants, and gases.

QUALITY CONTROL FOR STERILIZATION AND DISINFECTION

The effectiveness of any method of microbial control must be monitored regularly. Verification of the effectiveness of microbial control should be performed at least monthly. Simply placing an item in a sterilizer and initiating the sterilization process does not ensure sterility. Failure to achieve sterility may be caused by improper cleaning (if an item cannot be disassembled and all surfaces cleaned, it cannot be sterilized), mechanical failure of the sterilizing system, improper use of sterilizing equipment, improper wrapping, poor loading technique, and/or failure to understand the underlying concepts of sterilization processes.

INDICATORS. Chemical indicators, or **sterilization indicators**, are generally paper strips or tape impregnated with a material that changes color when a certain temperature or chemical exposure is achieved (Fig. 9-3). Most also indicate that a specific duration of exposure has been achieved, which is critical to the sterilization process. Therefore, it is important to remember that chemical indicators do not indicate sterility. Their response

indicates only that certain conditions for sterility have been met. Chemical indicators can be used with autoclaves and ethylene oxide systems and must be placed deep inside packs before sterilization. Indicator tape (Fig. 9-4) is often used to secure surgical packs and mark smaller packages of sterilized items. The tape incorporates an indicator that changes color when the sterilization temperature or duration of chemical exposure has been reached. The color change in the tape does not allow for any evaluation of duration of exposure to sterilization conditions.

BIOLOGIC TESTING. Because the purpose of the sterilization procedures is to eliminate the hardiest microorganisms, the presence or absence of bacterial spores can help verify proper sterilization conditions. To perform a biologic test of sterility conditions, commercially available bacterial spores are exposed in an autoclave or to ethylene oxide and then cultured. Bacterial spores should be killed by sterilization so that no bacterial colonies should be present after culturing. This is the recommended method for verification of proper autoclave operation in veterinary clinics.

Another test used to verify sterility is the surface sampling technique. The procedure involves swabbing the test surface (i.e., surgical equipment) with a sterile swab. The swab is then transferred to a suitable media plate for growth. This method is recommended for ensuring proper disinfection of surgical suites in veterinary clinics.

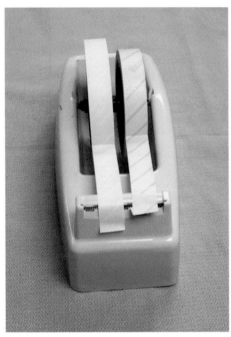

FIGURE 9-4 Sterilization indicator tape may be used on all types of pack wrapping—paper, cloth, or plastic. Shown are autoclave indicator tape *(left)* and ethylene oxide indicator tape *(right)*. (From Sirois M: Principles and practice of veterinary technology, ed 3, St Louis, 2011, Mosby.)

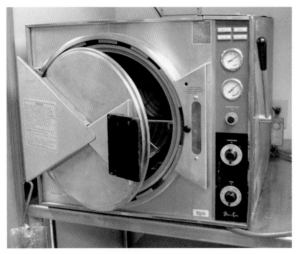

FIGURE 9-5 Large autoclave found in veterinary hospitals. This model is installed on a custom metal shelf. It will process four large surgical packs and a number of individually wrapped items in each load. (From Sirois M: Principles and practice of veterinary technology, ed 3, St Louis, 2011, Mosby.)

STEAM STERILIZATION

Pressurized steam is the most efficient and common method of sterilization used in veterinary clinics. Steam destroys microbes via cellular protein denaturation. To destroy all living microorganisms, the correct relationship among temperature, pressure, and exposure time is critical. If steam is contained in a closed compartment under increased pressure, the temperature increases as long as the volume of the compartment remains the same. If items are exposed long enough to steam at a specified temperature and pressure, they become sterile. The unit used to create this environment of high-temperature, pressurized steam is called an **autoclave**.

Several types of autoclaves are available. Gravity displacement autoclaves use water that is heated in a chamber. The continued application of heat by an electric element creates pressure within the chamber; this pressure raises the boiling point of the water and thus the ultimate temperature of the steam. These are the most common type of autoclave in veterinary clinics and are known as gravity displacement autoclaves because the steam gradually displaces the air contained within the chamber; the air is forced out through a vent (Fig. 9-5). A prevacuum autoclave is a much larger and more costly machine that is equipped with a boiler to generate steam and a vacuum system. Air is forced out of the loaded chamber by means of the vacuum pump. Steam at a temperature of 121° C (250° F) or higher is introduced into the chamber; the steam immediately fills the chamber to eliminate the vacuum.

Autoclaves consistently achieve complete sterility, are inexpensive, and are easy to operate. They are safe for most surgical instruments and equipment, drapes and gowns, suture materials, sponges, and some plastics and rubber items.

Achieving complete sterility depends on saturated steam of the appropriate temperature having contact with all objects in the autoclave for a sufficient length of time. Heat is the killing agent in the autoclave, and steam is the vector that supplies the heat and promotes penetration of the heat. Pressure is the means to create adequately heated steam. Complete sterilization of most items is achieved after 9 to 15 minutes of exposure to a temperature of 121° C (250° F). The temperature of steam at sea level is 100° C (212° F); an increase in pressure results in an increase in the temperature of the steam. The minimum effective pressure of the autoclave is 15 psi, which provides steam at 121° C (250° F).

SURGICAL INSTRUMENTS

SCALPELS AND BLADES

Scalpels are the primary cutting instrument used to incise tissue (Fig. 9-6). Reusable scalpel handles with detachable blades are most commonly used in veterinary medicine; disposable handles and blades are also available. Blades are available in various sizes and shapes, depending on the task for which they are used. Scalpels are usually used in a slide-cutting fashion, with pressure applied to the knife blade at a right angle to the direction of scalpel pressure.

LASER SCALPEL

Laser is an acronym for **l**ight **a**mplification by the **s**timulated **e**mission of **r**adiation. Laser technology has been used to treat patients safely and effectively for almost 2 decades. The most commonly used surgical laser is a carbon dioxide laser, which produces an invisible beam of light that vaporizes the water normally found in the skin and other soft tissue. Lasers have the unique ability both to coagulate and cut tissue. Although there are a variety of lasers, the most common types used in veterinary practice are carbon dioxide (CO_2) and diode.

Because the laser seals nerve endings and small blood vessels as it cuts, it results in less bleeding and less pain for the patient. Because laser scalpels do not crush, tear, or bruise tissue, as do traditional scalpels, swelling is minimized. Laser surgery is commonly used in soft tissue surgical procedures, such as cat declawing, spaying, neutering, amputations, oral and dental procedures, dermatology, and avian and exotic procedures.

ELECTROSCALPEL

The electroscalpel functions by passing an electrical current through the unit to the patient's tissues. This causes microco-

> **CRITICAL CONCEPT**
>
> Every surgical instrument is designed for a specific purpose—holding, clamping, cutting, or retracting.

agulation of tissue proteins as the unit cuts the tissue.

SCISSORS

Scissors are available in a variety of shapes, sizes, and weights, and are generally classified according to the type of points (blunt-blunt, sharp-sharp, sharp-blunt), blade shape (straight, curved), or cutting edge (plain, serrated; Fig. 9-7). Curved scissors offer greater maneuverability and visibility, whereas straight scissors provide the greatest mechanical advantage for cutting tough or thick tissue. Metzenbaum or Mayo scissors are most commonly used in surgery. Metzenbaum scissors are more delicate and should be reserved for fine, thin tissue. Mayo scissors are used for cutting heavy tissue, such as fascia. Tissue scissors should not be used to cut suture material; suture scissors should be used. Suture scissors used in the operating room are different from suture removal scissors. The latter have a concavity at the top of one blade that prevents the suture from being lifted excessively during removal. Delicate scissors, such as tenotomy scissors or iris scissors, are often used in ophthalmic procedures and other surgeries, in which fine, precise cuts are necessary. Bandage scissors have a blunt tip that when introduced under the bandage edge, reducing the risk of cutting the underlying skin.

NEEDLE HOLDERS

Needle holders are used to grasp and manipulate curved needles (Fig. 9-8). Mayo-Hegar and Olsen-Hegar needle holders have a ratchet lock just distal to the thumb. Castroviejo needle holders have a spring and latch mechanism for locking. Mathieu needle holders have a ratchet lock at the proximal end of the handles of the holder, permitting locking and unlocking simply by a progressive squeezing together of the needle holder handles.

FORCEPS

TISSUE FORCEPS

Tissue forceps are used to clamp and hold tissue and blood vessels. Thumb forceps are tweezerlike, nonlocking tissue forceps used to grasp tissue (Fig. 9-9). The proximal ends are joined to allow the grasping ends to spring open or be squeezed together. They are available in a variety of shapes and sizes; tips

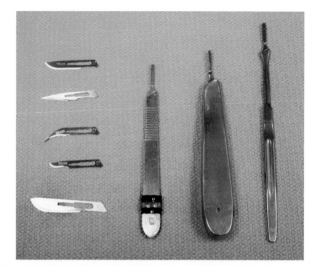

FIGURE 9-6 *Left,* Scalpel blades: *top to bottom,* nos. 10, 11, 12, 15, and 20. *Right,* Scalpel handles: *left to right,* nos. 3, 5, and 7. (From Sirois M: Principles and practice of veterinary technology, ed 3, St Louis, 2011, Mosby.)

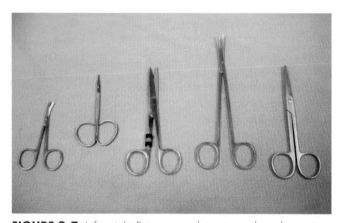

FIGURE 9-7 *Left to right,* Suture removal, tenotomy, sharp-sharp suture, Metzenbaum, and Mayo scissors. (From Sirois M: Principles and practice of veterinary technology, ed 3, St Louis, 2011, Mosby.)

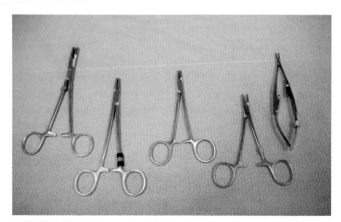

FIGURE 9-8 *Left to right,* Olsen-Hegar, Mayo-Hegar, derf, Halsey, and Castroviejo needle holders. (From Sirois M: Principles and practice of veterinary technology, ed 3, St Louis, 2011, Mosby.)

(grasping ends) may be pointed, flattened, rounded, smooth, or serrated, or have small or large teeth. The most commonly used tissue forceps, Brown-Adson, have small serrations on the tips that cause minimal trauma but hold tissue securely. Allis tissue forceps and Babcock forceps (Figs. 9-10 and 9-11) are also used for tissue grasping and retraction.

HEMOSTATIC FORCEPS

Hemostatic forceps, commonly called hemostats, are crushing instruments used to clamp blood vessels (Fig. 9-12). They are available with straight or curved tips and vary in size from smaller (3-inch) mosquito hemostats with transverse jaw serrations to larger (9-inch) angiotribes. Serrations on the jaws of larger hemostatic forceps may be transverse, longitudinal, or diagonal, or a combination of these. Longitudinal serrations are generally gentler on tissue than cross serrations. Serrations usually extend from the tips of the jaws to the box locks, but in Kelly forceps, transverse (horizontal) serrations extend over only the distal portion of the jaws. Similarly sized Crile forceps have transverse serrations that extend over the entire jaw length. Kelly and Crile forceps are used on larger

vessels. Rochester-Carmalt forceps are larger crushing forceps, often used to control large tissue bundles (e.g., during ovariohysterectomy). They have longitudinal grooves with cross grooves at the tip ends to prevent tissue slippage.

HEMOSTATIC TECHNIQUES AND MATERIALS

Hemostasis, or the arrest of bleeding, allows visualization of the surgical site and prevents life-threatening hemorrhage. During surgery, the veterinary technician will control low-pressure hemorrhage from small vessels by applying pressure to the bleeding points with a gauze sponge. Once a thrombus has formed, the sponge is gently removed to avoid disrupting clots. Large vessels must be ligated (tied off) by the veterinarian. Hemostatic agents used to control hemorrhage during surgery include bone wax and hemostatic materials made of gelatin or cellulose (e.g., Surgicel, Gelfoam).

The veterinarian may use metal clips or staples (Surgiclips, LDS staple gun, Covidien, Mansfield, MA) for vessel ligation (Fig. 9-13). They are particularly useful when the vessel is difficult to reach or multiple vessels must be ligated.

Electrocoagulation can be used to achieve hemostasis in vessels smaller than 2 mm in diameter. The term **electrocautery** is often erroneously used in place of electrocoagulation. With electrocautery, the needle tip or scalpel is heated before it is applied to the tissue; with electrocoagulation, heat is generated in the tissue as a high-frequency current is passed through it. Excessive use of electrocautery or electrocoagulation retards healing.

RETRACTORS

Retractors are used to retract tissue and improve exposure. The ends of handheld retractors may be hooked, curved, spatula-shaped, or toothed. Some handheld retractors may be bent (i.e., malleable) to conform to the structure being retracted or area of the body in which retraction is being performed. Senn (rake) retractors are double-ended retractors (Fig. 9-14). One end has three fingerlike, curved prongs; the other end is a flat, curved blade. Self-retaining retractors maintain tension on tissues and are held open with a box lock (e.g., Gelpi, Weitlaner) or other mechanism

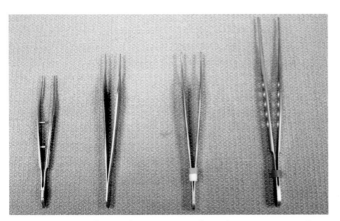

FIGURE 9-9 *Left to right,* Dressing, Adson dressing, Brown-Adson, and DeBakey tissue forceps. (From Sirois M: Principles and practice of veterinary technology, ed 3, St Louis, 2011, Mosby.)

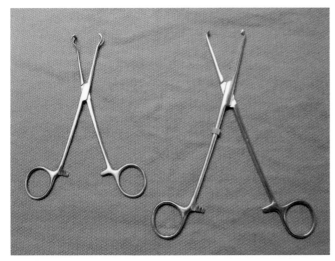

FIGURE 9-10 Tissue forceps: Babcock *(left),* Allis *(right).* (From Sirois M: Principles and practice of veterinary technology, ed 3, St Louis, 2011, Mosby.)

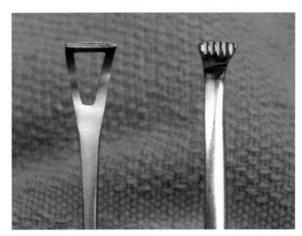

FIGURE 9-11 Tissue forceps, close-up view: Babcock *(left),* Allis *(right).* (From Sirois M: Principles and practice of veterinary technology, ed 3, St Louis, 2011, Mosby.)

(e.g., set screw). Examples of the latter are Balfour retractors and Finochietto retractors. Balfour retractors are generally used to retract the abdominal wall, whereas Finochietto retractors are commonly used during thoracotomies.

MISCELLANEOUS INSTRUMENTS

Instruments are available to suction fluid, clamp drapes or tissues, cut and remove bone pieces (rongeurs), hold bones

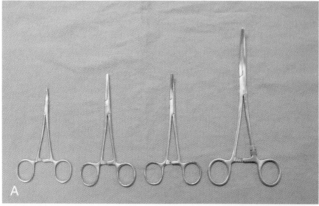

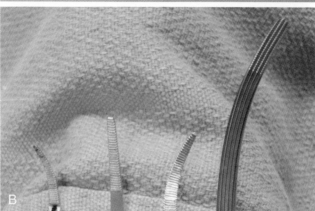

FIGURE 9-12 A, Hemostatic forceps *(left to right)*: mosquito, Kelly, Crile, and Rochester-Carmalt. **B,** Hemostatic forceps, close-up view *(left to right)*: mosquito, Kelly, Crile, and Rochester-Carmalt. (From Sirois M: Principles and practice of veterinary technology, ed 3, St Louis, 2011, Mosby.)

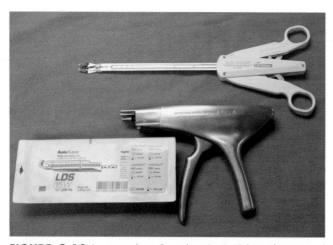

FIGURE 9-13 Ligating clips: Surgiclips *(top)*, LDS staple gun and cartridge *(bottom)*. (From Sirois M: Principles and practice of veterinary technology, ed 3, St Louis, 2011, Mosby.)

during fracture repair, scrape surfaces of dense tissue (curettes), remove periosteum (periosteal elevators), cut or shape bone and cartilage (osteotomes and chisels), and bore holes in bone (trephines).

SUTURES AND OTHER MATERIALS USED IN WOUND CLOSURE

SUTURES

SUTURE CHARACTERISTICS

The word **suture** refers to any strand of material used to approximate tissues or ligate blood vessels. The ideal suture material is easy to handle, reacts minimally in tissue, inhibits bacterial growth, holds securely when knotted, resists shrinking in tissues, is noncapillary, nonallergenic, noncarcinogenic, and nonferromagnetic, and is absorbed with minimal reaction after the tissue has healed. Such an ideal suture material does not exist; therefore, surgeons must choose one that most closely approximates the ideal for a given procedure and/or tissue to be sutured.

Monofilament sutures are made of a single strand of material. They create less tissue drag than multifilament suture material and do not have interstitial spaces that may harbor bacteria. Care should be used in handling monofilament sutures because nicking or damaging them with forceps or needle holders weakens them and predisposes to breakage.

Multifilament sutures consist of several strands that are twisted or braided together. Multifilament sutures are generally more pliable and flexible than monofilament sutures. They may be coated to decrease tissue drag and enhance handling characteristics.

The most commonly used standard for suture size is the USP (U.S. Pharmacopeia) standard, which denotes suture diameters from fine to coarse according to a numeric scale; size 10-0 material has the smallest diameter (finest) and size 7 has the largest diameter (most coarse). USP uses different

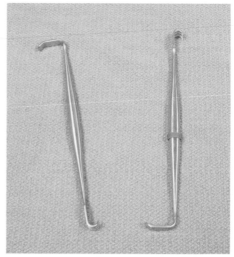

FIGURE 9-14 Senn (rake) retractor. (From Sirois M: Principles and practice of veterinary technology, ed 3, St Louis, 2011, Mosby.)

size notations for various suture materials (Table 9-2). The smaller the suture diameter is, the lower is its tensile strength. Stainless steel wire is usually sized according to the metric or USP scale or by the Brown and Sharpe wire gauge.

ABSORBABLE SUTURE MATERIALS

Absorbable suture materials lose most of their tensile strength within 60 days after placement in tissue and eventually are absorbed from the site and replaced by healthy tissue during the healing process. Absorbable sutures are used when sutures must be buried within body cavities (Fig. 9-15).

SURGICAL GUT. Surgical gut is commonly called catgut. Surgical gut is made from the submucosa of sheep intestine or the serosa of bovine intestine. It is comprised of approximately 90% collagen. Plain surgical gut is broken down by phagocytosis and elicits a marked inflammatory reaction, as compared with other materials. Tanning, by

exposure to chrome or aldehyde, slows absorption. Surgical gut so treated is called chromic surgical gut. Surgical gut is rapidly absorbed from infected sites or where it is exposed to digestive enzymes. Knots in surgical gut may loosen when wet.

SYNTHETIC ABSORBABLE MATERIALS. Synthetic absorbable materials (e.g., polyglycolic acid, polyglactin 910, polydioxanone, polyglyconate) are generally broken down by hydrolysis. There is minimal tissue reaction to synthetic absorbable suture materials. The rate of tensile strength loss and rate of absorption are fairly constant in different tissues. Infection or exposure to digestive enzymes does not significantly influence their rates of absorption.

NONABSORBABLE SUTURE MATERIALS

There are four basic groups of nonabsorbable suture materials—organic sutures, braided synthetic sutures, monofilament synthetic sutures, and metallic sutures (Fig. 9-16).

ORGANIC NONABSORBABLE MATERIALS. Silk is the most common organic nonabsorbable suture material and is used as a braided multifilament suture that is uncoated or coated. Silk has excellent handling characteristics and is often used in cardiovascular procedures; however, it does not maintain significant tensile strength after 6 months in tissues and is therefore contraindicated for use with vascular grafts. It also should be avoided in contaminated sites because it increases the likelihood of wound infection. Cotton suture has less tissue reaction than silk, but it supports bacterial growth and is not generally used for skin closure.

SYNTHETIC NONABSORBABLE MATERIALS. Synthetic nonabsorbable suture materials are available as braided multifilament (e.g., polyester, coated caprolactam) or monofilament (e.g., polypropylene, polyamide, polyolefins, polybutester) threads. They are typically strong and induce minimal tissue reaction. Nonabsorbable suture materials consisting of an inner core and outer sheath (e.g., Supramid) should not be buried in tissues because the outer sheath tends to degenerate, allowing bacteria to migrate to the inner core. This predisposes to infection and fistula formation.

TABLE 9-2	Systems Used to Indicate Suture Sizes			
DIAMETER (MM)	METRIC GAUGE	SYNTHETIC SUTURE MATERIALS (USP)	SURGICAL GUT (USP)	WIRE GAUGE (BROWN AND SHARPE)
0.02	0.2	10-0		
0.03	0.3	9-0		
0.04	0.4	8-0		
0.05	0.5	7-0	8-0	41
0.07	0.7	6-0	7-0	38-40
0.1	1	5-0	6-0	35
0.15	1.5	4-0	5-0	32-34
0.2	2	3-0	4-0	30
0.3	3	2-0	3-0	28
0.35	3.5	0	2-0	26
0.4	4	1	0	25
0.5	5	2	1	24
0.6	6	3,4	2	22
0.7	7	5	3	20
0.8	8	6	4	19
0.9	0	7		18

Adapted from Sirois M: Principles and practice of veterinary technology, ed 3, St Louis, 2011, Mosby.

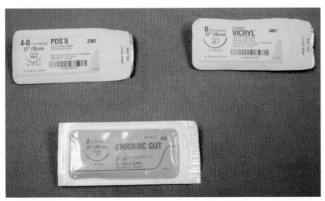

FIGURE 9-15 Absorbable suture materials. (From Sirois M: Principles and practice of veterinary technology, ed 3, St Louis, 2011, Mosby.)

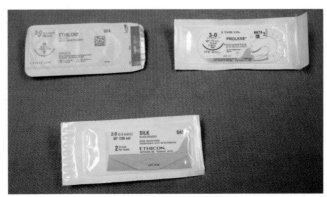

FIGURE 9-16 Nonabsorbable suture materials. (From Sirois M: Principles and practice of veterinary technology, ed 3, St Louis, 2011, Mosby.)

METALLIC SUTURES. Stainless steel is the most commonly used metallic suture. It is available as monofilament wire or twisted multifilament wire. The tissue reaction to stainless steel is generally minimal; however, the knot ends evoke an inflammatory reaction. Wire tends to cut tissue and may fragment. It is stable in contaminated wounds.

SUTURE NEEDLES

Suture needles are available in a wide variety of shapes and sizes. The type of suture needle used depends on the characteristics of the tissue to be sutured (e.g., penetrability, density, elasticity, thickness), wound topography (e.g., deep, narrow), and characteristics of the needle (e.g., type of eye, length, diameter). Most surgical needles are made from stainless steel because it is strong and corrosion-free and does not harbor bacteria.

The three basic components of a suture needle are the attachment end (swaged or eyed), body, and point (Fig. 9-17, *A*).

With swaged needles, the needle and suture are joined in a continuous unit, minimizing tissue trauma and increasing ease of use. Suture material must be threaded onto eyed needles. Because a double strand of suture is pulled through the tissue, a larger hole is created than when a swaged needle is used. Eyed needles may be closed (round, oblong, or square) or French (with a slit from the inside of the eye to the end of the needle for ease of threading; see Fig. 9-17, *B*). Eyed needles are threaded from the inside curvature.

The needle body comes in a variety of shapes (see Fig. 9-17, *C*); tissue type and depth and size of the wound determine the appropriate needle shape. Straight (Keith) needles are generally used in accessible places in which the needle can be manipulated directly with the fingers (e.g., placement of purse-string sutures in the rectum). Curved needles are manipulated with needle holders. One-fourth (¼) circle needles are primarily used in ophthalmic procedures. Three-eighths (⅜) and

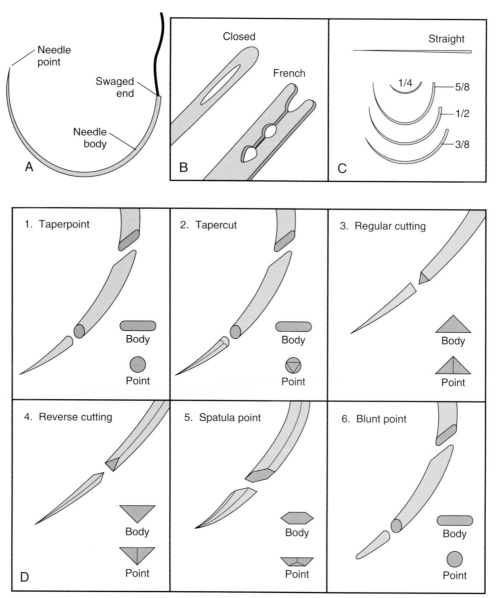

FIGURE 9-17 *A*, Basic components of a needle. *B*, Types of eyed needles. *C, D*, Needle body shapes and sizes. (From Sirois M: *Principles and practice of veterinary technology,* ed 3, St Louis, 2011, Mosby.)

one-half (½) circle needles are the most commonly used surgical needles in veterinary medicine (e.g., abdominal closure). A one-half or five-eighths (⅝) circle needle, despite requiring more wrist manipulation, is easier to use in confined locations.

The needle point (cutting, taper, reverse-cutting; see Fig. 9-17, *D*) determines the sharpness of a needle and type of tissue in which the needle is used. Cutting needles generally have two or three opposing cutting edges. They are used in tissues that are difficult to penetrate (e.g., skin). With conventional cutting needles, the third cutting edge is on the inside (concave) curvature of the needle.. Reverse-cutting needles have a third cutting edge located on the outer (convex) curvature of the needle. Side-cutting needles (spatula needles) are flat on the top and bottom. They are generally used in ophthalmic procedures.

Tapered needles (round needles) have a sharp tip that pierces and spreads tissues without cutting them. They are generally used in easily penetrated tissues (e.g., intestine, subcutaneous tissues, fascia). Tapercut needles have a reverse-cutting edge tip and a taper point body. They are generally used for suturing dense, tough fibrous tissue (e.g., tendon) and for some cardiovascular procedures (e.g., vascular grafts). Blunt point needles have a rounded blunt point that can dissect through friable tissue without cutting. They are occasionally used for suturing soft parenchymal organs (e.g., liver, kidney).

OTHER MATERIALS

TISSUE ADHESIVES

Cyanoacrylates (known as super glue) are commonly used for tissue adhesion during some procedures (e.g., declawing, tail docking, ear cropping). A variety of products are available for use in veterinary patients. These adhesives rapidly polymerize in the presence of moisture and produce a strong flexible bond. Adhesion of tissue edges generally takes less than 15 seconds, but may be delayed by excessive hemorrhage.

SKIN STAPLES

Metal staples (skin staples or Michel clips) are used to appose wound edges or attach drapes to the skin. Care must be used to ensure that the staple is appropriately bent so that when staples are used for skin closure, they cannot be easily removed by the animal. A special staple remover facilitates clip removal after healing (Fig. 9-18).

SURGICAL MESH

Surgical mesh may be used to repair hernias (e.g., perineal hernias) or reinforce traumatized or devitalized tissues (abdominal hernias). Occasionally, it is used to replace excised traumatized or neoplastic tissues. Surgical mesh is available in nonabsorbable or absorbable forms.

CARE AND MAINTENANCE OF SURGICAL INSTRUMENTS AND SUPPLIES

Good surgical instruments are a valuable investment and must be used and maintained properly to prevent corrosion, pitting, and/or discoloration. Instruments should be rinsed in cool water as soon after the surgical procedure as possible to avoid drying of blood, tissue, saline, or other foreign matter on them. Many manufacturers recommend that instruments be rinsed, cleaned, and sterilized in distilled or deionized water because tap water contains minerals that may cause discoloration and staining. If tap water is used for rinsing, instruments should be dried thoroughly to avoid staining. Instruments with multiple components should be disassembled before cleaning. Delicate instruments should be cleaned and sterilized separately. All surgical supplies and equipment that come into contact with the patient or other surgical equipment, such as Mayo instrument stands, must be cleaned and disinfected before use.

> **CRITICAL CONCEPT**
> Daily and weekly cleaning schedules should be maintained for the operating room.

INSTRUMENT CLEANING

Ultrasonic and enzymatic methods of cleaning are effective and efficient (Fig. 9-19). Before putting soiled instruments in an ultrasonic cleaner, they should be washed in cleaning solution to remove all visible debris. Dissimilar metals (e.g., chrome and stainless steel) should not be mixed in the same

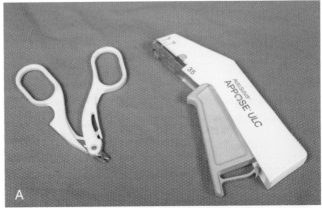

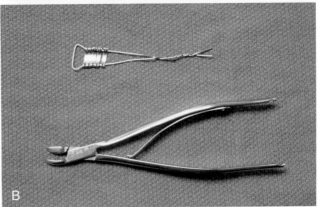

FIGURE 9-18 **A**, Skin staples (gun, *right*) and staple removal device (*left*). **B**, Michel clips (*top*) and applying and removing forceps (*bottom*). (From Sirois M: Principles and practice of veterinary technology, ed 3, St Louis, 2011, Mosby.)

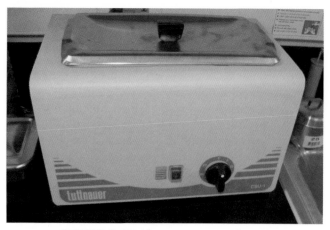

FIGURE 9-19 Ultrasonic instrument cleaner.

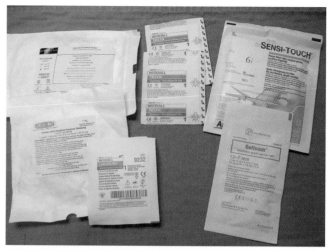

FIGURE 9-20 Presterilized items packaged in paper. Paper is generally suitable for steam or gas sterilization. (From Sirois M: Principles and practice of veterinary technology, ed 3, St Louis, 2011, Mosby.)

cycle. All instruments should be placed in the ultrasonic cleaner with their ratchets and box locks open. Instruments should not be piled on top of each other to avoid damaging delicate instruments. Instruments must not be left in the ultrasonic cleaner for longer than the cleaning cycle because this could lead to rust. They should be removed from the cleaner, rinsed, lubricated, and dried at the completion of the cycle.

If an ultrasonic cleaner is not available, instruments should be manually cleaned as thoroughly as possible, paying particular attention to box locks, serrations, and hinges. Nylon brushes and a cool cleaning solution may be used for most instruments. Rasps and serrated parts of instruments may require a wire brush. A cleaning solution with a neutral pH should be used to avoid staining. Cleaning solutions should be prepared as instructed by the manufacturer and changed frequently. Enzymatic solutions may be used to remove proteinaceous materials from general surgical instruments and endoscopic equipment. Autoclaving is not a substitute for proper instrument cleaning.

INSTRUMENT LUBRICATING AND AUTOCLAVING

Before they are autoclaved, instruments with box locks and hinges and power equipment should be lubricated with instrument milk or surgical lubricants. Do not use industrial oils to lubricate instruments because they interfere with steam sterilization. All instruments should be allowed to thoroughly air-dry before packing them into a surgical pack. The procedure for wrapping items is based on enhancing the ease of sterilization and preserving sterility of the item, not for convenience or personal preference. Before they are packed, instruments are separated and placed in order of their intended use. If steam or gas sterilization is used, the selected wrap should be penetrable by steam or gas, impermeable to microbes, durable, and flexible.

Specific guidelines should be followed when preparing packs for steam and gas sterilization to allow maximal penetration. Small items may be wrapped, sterilized, and stored in self-sealing (peel and seal) or heat-sealable paper or plastic peel pouches (Fig. 9-20), or regular cloth, muslin, or drape wrapping material.

Packed instruments can be placed in a tray or wrapped individually. The pack is wrapped using at least two layers of material. A presterilization wrap for steam sterilization consists of two thicknesses of two-layer muslin or nonwoven (paper) barrier materials. The poststerilization wrap (after sterilization and proper cool-down period) consists of a waterproof, heat-sealable plastic dust cover; this wrap is not necessary if the item is used within 24 hours of sterilization. Always take care to wrap packs tightly so that the drape material does not contact the inner wall of the autoclave. The instrument pack is sealed with autoclave tape and labeled with the date, contents, and initials of the person preparing the pack. Autoclave tape provides verification that the outside of the pack was exposed to appropriate sterilization temperatures. Surgical packs should not exceed 30 × 30 × 50 cm (12 × 12 × 20 inches) in size and 5.5 kg (12 lb) in weight.

Individual instruments can also be placed into sterilization pouches (see Fig. 9-3*B*). These pouches usually incorporate a chemical sterilization indicator. Many sterilization pouches are transparent, allowing easy visualization of contents. The pouches are often self-sealing, or you may use autoclave tape to close the pouch. Double wrapping in pouches can be used for particularly delicate or sharp instruments. Always mark items with the date that the item was autoclaved.

For steam and gas sterilization, instruments should be organized on a lint-free towel placed on the bottom of a perforated metal instrument tray. A chemical sterilization indicator is included in every pack. This provides verification that the inside of the pack was exposed to appropriate sterilization temperatures for the correct amount of time.

Instruments with box locks should be autoclaved opened. A 3- to 5-mm space between instruments is recommended for proper steam or gas circulation. Complex instruments should be disassembled when possible, and power equipment should be lubricated before sterilization. Items with a lumen should have a small amount of water flushed through them immediately before steam sterilization because water vaporizes and forces air out of the lumen.

Conversely, moisture left in tubing placed in a gas sterilizer may decrease the sterilization efficacy. Containers (e.g., saline bowl) should be placed with the open end facing up or horizontally; containers with lids should have the lid slightly ajar. Multiple basins should be stacked with a towel between each. A standard count of radiopaque surgical sponges should be included in each pack. A sterilization indicator is placed in the center of each pack before wrapping. Solutions should be steam-sterilized separately from instruments using the slow exhaust phase. Linens may be steam-sterilized.

WRAPPING INSTRUMENT PACKS

Packs may not be completely sterilized if they are wrapped too tightly or improperly loaded in the autoclave or gas sterilizer container (Procedure 9-1). Instrument packs should

---

PROCEDURE 9-1   WRAPPING A PACK

1. Place a large, unfolded wrap diagonally in front of you.
2. Place the instrument tray in the center of the wrap so that an imaginary line drawn from one corner of the wrap to the opposite corner is perpendicular to the two sides of the instrument tray (Fig. 1).

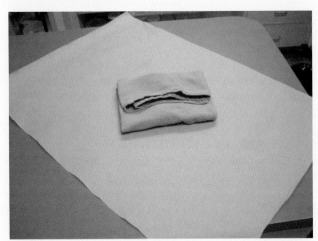

FIGURE 1

3. Fold the corner of the wrap that is closest to you over the instrument tray and to its far side, tucking it underneath the tray (Fig. 2).

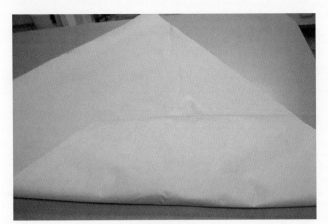

FIGURE 2

4. Fold the right corner over the pack as shown in Figure 3.

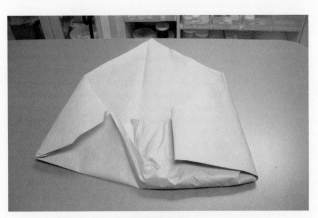

FIGURE 3

5. Fold the left corner over the pack in a similar fashion (Fig. 4).

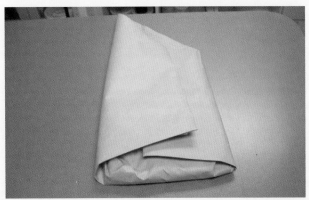

FIGURE 4

6. Fold the final corner over the wrap over the tray, tucking it in tightly under the previous two folds. Fold the tip of the final fold so that it is exposed for easy unwrapping (Fig. 5).

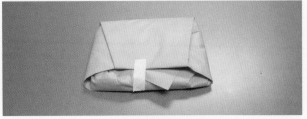

FIGURE 5

7. Wrap the pack in a second layer of cloth or paper, securing the final tab with autoclave or gas sterilization indicator tape for ease of grasping and opening.

From Sirois M: Principles and practice of veterinary technology, ed 3, St Louis, 2011, Mosby.

be positioned vertically (on edge) and longitudinally in an autoclave. Heavy packs should be placed at the periphery, where steam enters the chamber. Allow a small amount of air space between each pack to facilitate steam flow (1 to 2 inches between each pack and surrounding walls). Load linen packs so that the fabric layers are oriented vertically, on edge. Do not stack linen packs on top of one another because the increased thickness decreases steam penetration. Careful attention to exact standards for preparing, packaging, and loading of supplies is necessary for effective steam and gas sterilization.

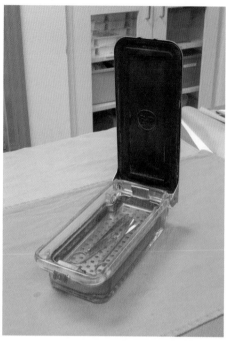

FIGURE 9-21 Cold sterilization tray. A gasket on the inner surface of the lid forms a seal when the lid is closed, preventing airborne microbes from contaminating the contents and preventing evaporation of the chemical disinfectant. (From Sirois M: Principles and practice of veterinary technology, ed 3, St Louis, 2011, Mosby.)

STERILIZATION
GAS STERILIZATION

Ethylene oxide is the most common form of gas sterilization used in the veterinary hospital. It is a flammable explosive liquid that becomes an effective sterilizing agent when mixed with carbon dioxide or Freon. Equipment that cannot withstand the extreme temperature and pressures of steam sterilization (e.g., endoscopes, cameras, plastics, power cables) can be safely sterilized with ethylene oxide. Environmental and safety hazards associated with ethylene oxide are numerous and severe. It is critical to the safety of the patient and hospital personnel that all materials sterilized with ethylene oxide be aerated according to instructions provided by the manufacturer of the ethylene oxide gas sterilization unit. Porous materials or those that will be used as implants in patients should generally be aerated for 24 hours following gas sterilization.

Items should be clean and dry before ethylene oxide sterilization; moisture and organic material bond with ethylene oxide and leave a toxic residue. If an item cannot be disassembled and all surfaces cleaned, it cannot be sterilized. Items are packed and loaded loosely to allow gas circulation. Complex items (e.g., power equipment) are disassembled before processing. Items that cannot be sterilized with ethylene oxide include acrylics, some pharmaceutical items, and solutions.

COLD CHEMICAL STERILIZATION

Liquid chemicals used for sterilization must be noncorrosive to the items being sterilized. These items are usually placed in a special tray kept in the surgery area (Fig. 9-21). Glutaraldehyde solution is noncorrosive and provides a safe means of sterilizing delicate, lensed instruments (e.g., endoscopes, cystoscopes, bronchoscopes). Most equipment that can be safely immersed in water can be safely immersed in 3% glutaraldehyde. Table 9-3 lists some commonly used cold sterilization agents. Items for sterilization should be clean and dry; organic matter (e.g., blood, pus, saliva) may prevent penetration of instrument crevices or joints. Residual water causes chemical dilution. Complex instruments should be disassembled before

TABLE 9-3	Antimicrobial Activity of Commonly Used Cold Sterilants				
	DESTRUCTIVE ACTION AGAINST				
AGENT	**BACTERIA**	**TUBERCLE BACILLI**	**SPORES**	**FUNGI**	**VIRUSES**
Alcohol, ethyl (70% to 90%)	+	+	0	+	±
Alcohol, isopropyl (70% to 90%)	++	+	0	+	±
Alcohol, iodine (2%)	++	+	±	+	+
Formalin (37%)	+	+	+	+	+
Glutaraldehyde (buffered, 2%; Cidex)	++	+	++	+	+
Iodine (2%-5% aqueous)	++	+	±	+	+
Iodophors (1%; povidone-iodine complex)	+	+	±	±	+
Mercury-containing (e.g., Merthiolate)	±	0	0	+	±
Phenolic derivatives (0.5%-3%)	+	+	0	+	±
Quaternary ammonium cation (quat; e.g., benzalkonium chloride, 1:750-1:1000)	++	0	0	+	0

++, Very good; +, good; ±, fair (greater concentration or more time needed); 0, no activity.
Adapted from Sirois M: Principles and practice of veterinary technology, ed 3, St Louis, 2011, Mosby.

immersion. Immersion times suggested by the manufacturer should be followed (e.g., for sterilization in 3% glutaraldehyde, 10 hours at 20° C [68° F] to 25° C [77° F]; for disinfection, 10 minutes at 20° to 25° C). After the appropriate immersion time, instruments should be rinsed thoroughly with sterile water and dried with sterile towels to avoid damaging the patients' tissues.

FOLDING AND WRAPPING GOWNS AND DRAPES
GOWNS

Surgical gowns must be folded so that they can be easily donned without breaking sterile technique (Fig. 9-22). Place the gown on a clean, flat surface with the front of the gown

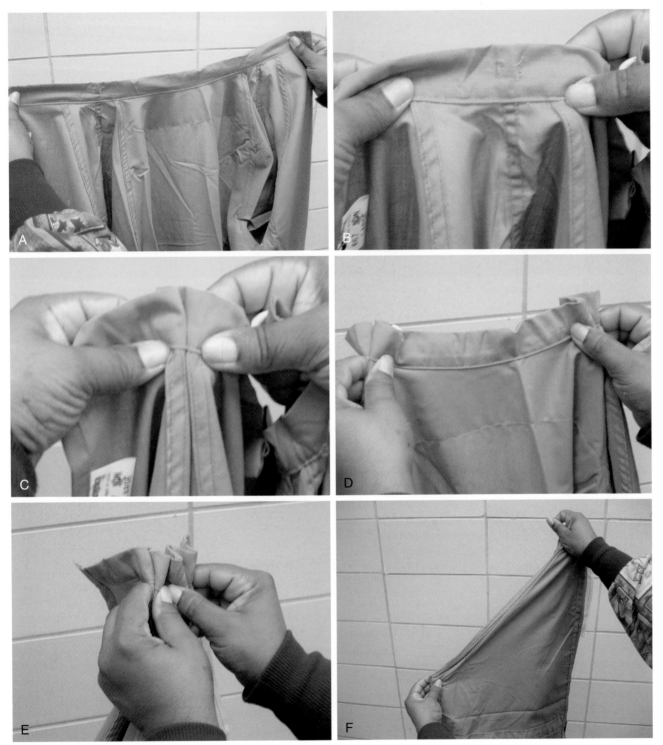

FIGURE 9-22 Method of folding a cloth surgical gown. **A,** The gown is held by the neck to see the shoulder seams on the inside of the gown. **B,** Close-up of the three seams of one shoulder. **C,** The gown is folded so that the outer two seams of one shoulder are touching. **D,** The same fold is done with the other shoulder. **E,** The gown is folded so that the seams of both shoulders are touching. **F,** The shoulders are held in one hand while the other hand aligns the armpit seams.

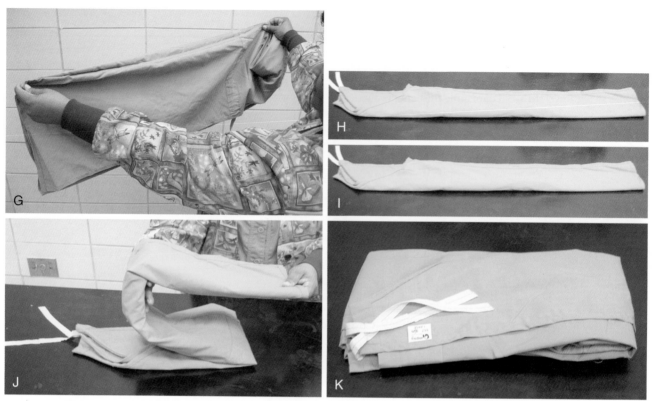

FIGURE 9-22, cont'd **G,** The shoulders and armpits are held in one hand while the other hand aligns the gown hem. **H,** The gown is laid flat on the table. (A tabletop method of folding is first to lay the gown open flat on the countertop, with the outside of the gown facing up, sleeves on top. The side edges of the gown are each folded to meet near the middle and then the gown is folded in half.) Only the inside surfaces of the gown are now exposed. **I,** The gown is folded in half lengthwise. **J,** The gown is folded in accordion fashion. **K,** The gown is laid on the table so that the neck ties are uppermost. (From Bassert JM, McCurnin DM: McCurnin's clinical textbook for veterinary technicians, ed 7, St Louis, 2010, Saunders.)

facing up. Fold the sleeves neatly toward the center of the gown with the cuffs of the sleeves facing the bottom hem. Fold the sides to the center so that the side seams are aligned with the sleeve seams. Then fold the gown in half longitudinally (sleeves inside the gown). Ties should be placed so that they can be touched without contaminating the gown. Starting with the bottom hem of the gown, fan-fold it toward the neck. Fan folding allows compact storage and simple unfolding. Fold a hand towel in half horizontally and fan-fold it into about four folds. Place it on top of the folded gown, leaving one corner turned back to allow it to be easily grasped. Wrap the gown and towel in two layers of paper or cloth wrap as described.

DRAPES

Drapes should be folded so that the fenestration (or the center of an unfenestrated drape) can be properly positioned over the surgical site without contaminating the drape (Fig. 9-23). Lay the drape out flat, with the ends of the fenestration perpendicular and the sides of the fenestration parallel to you. Grasp the end of the drape closest to you and fan-fold half of the drape toward the center. Make sure that the edge of the drape is on top to allow it to be easily grasped during unfolding. Then turn the drape around and fan-fold the other half toward the center in a similar fashion. Next, fan-fold one end of the drape to the center; repeat with the other end. Note that

when the drape is properly folded, the fenestration is on the ventral outermost aspect of the drape. Fold the drape in half and wrap it in two layers of paper or cloth wrap, as described.

> ### CRITICAL CONCEPT
> Drapes are folded accordion fashion to allow easy unfolding and placement, without the possibility of contamination.

STORING STERILIZED ITEMS

Packs are allowed to cool and dry individually on racks when removed from the autoclave; placing instrument packs on top of each other during cooling may promote condensation of moisture, resulting in contamination via strike-through (wick action). After sterile packs are completely dry, they should be stored in waterproof dust covers in closed cabinets, rather than uncovered on open shelves, to protect them from moisture or exposure to particulate matter, such as dust-borne bacteria. Sterile packs are labeled with the date on which the item was sterilized and a control lot number to trace an unsterile item. Heat-sealed waterproof dust covers are placed on items not routinely used. The shelf life of a sterilized pack varies with the type of outer wrap (Table 9-4).

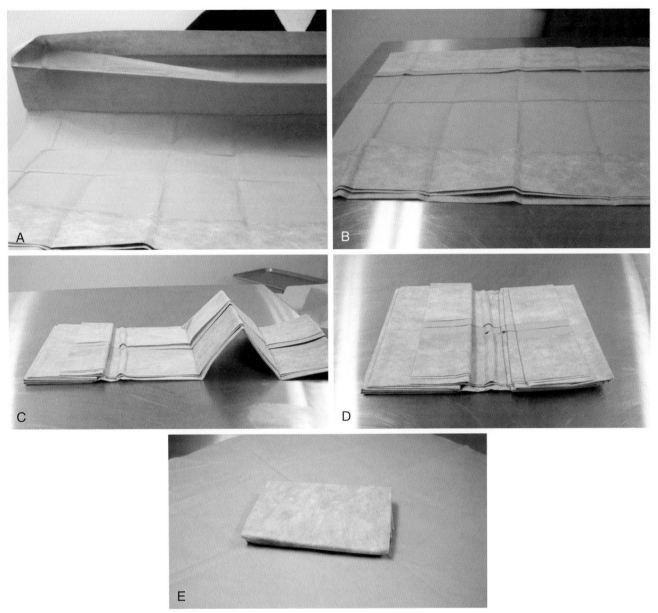

FIGURE 9-23 Accordion pleat-folding technique. **A, B,** Fold the item (drape) lengthwise, as shown. **C, D,** Fold the item accordion style again, widthwise. **E,** Position the item as shown to wrap. (From Sirois M: Principles and practice of veterinary technology, ed 3, St Louis, 2011, Mosby.)

TABLE 9-4	Recommended Storage Times for Sterilized Packs*	
WRAPPER		**SHELF LIFE**
Double-wrapped, two-layer muslin		4 wk
Double-wrapped, two-layer muslin, heat-sealed in dust covers after sterilization		6 mo
Double-wrapped, two-layer muslin, tape-sealed in dust covers after sterilization		2 mo
Double-wrapped nonwoven barrier materials (paper)		6 mo
Paper, plastic peel-back pouches, heat-sealed		1 yr
Plastic peel-back pouches, heat-sealed		1 yr

*Note that sterilized items from hospitals adopting event-related sterility assurance have an indefinite shelf-life.
Adapted from Sirois M: Principles and practice of veterinary technology, ed 3, St Louis, 2011, Mosby.

BASIC SURGICAL TERMINOLOGY

Surgical procedures are described using anatomic terms combined with word roots (suffixes; see Chapter 3). The most common suffixes used for describing surgical procedures are presented in Box 9-1.

INCISIONS
ABDOMINAL INCISIONS

Abdominal surgery is commonly performed in animal species. Entry into the abdomen is usually gained by any of four common abdominal incisions. Named according to its location, each incision offers different advantages and a different exposure of the abdomen (Fig. 9-24):

- A ventral midline incision is located on the ventral midline of the animal. It offers excellent exposure of the entire abdominal cavity.
- A paramedian incision is located lateral and parallel to the ventral midline of the animal. It is usually used when exposure of only one side of the abdomen is needed, such as for removal of a cryptorchid (retained) testis.
- A flank incision is generally performed on a standing animal or one in lateral recumbency. It is oriented perpendicular to the long axis of the body, caudal to the last rib. A flank incision provides good exposure of the organ(s) immediately deep to (beneath) the incision but does not allow exploration of much of the remainder of the abdomen. It is, therefore, useful for such procedures as nephrectomy, in which the organ in question lies directly beneath the incision.

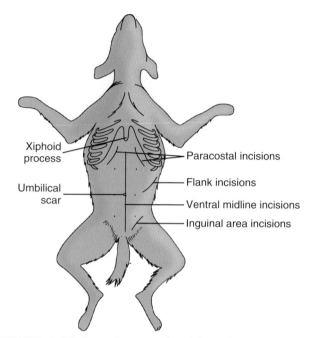

FIGURE 9-24 Surgical incisions for abdominal procedures. (From Sirois M: *Principles and practice of veterinary technology*, ed 3, St Louis, 2011, Mosby.)

- A paracostal incision is oriented parallel to the last rib and offers good exposure of the stomach and spleen in monogastric animals.

THORACIC INCISIONS

Thoracic surgery may be indicated because of pathology in the chest or traumatic injuries. Two common incisions are used in veterinary medicine:

- A median sternotomy is used for many cardiac procedures, or when all lung fields need to be visualized or approached. This incision is along the patient's midline, on the ventral thorax, moving cranially from the xiphoid process or caudally from the first sternebrae, always leaving two to three sternebrae intact.
- A lateral intercostal thoracotomy may be used if only one side of the chest needs to be approached, such as in cases of lung lobe torsion or mass. This is done on the side of the patient's thorax, perpendicular to the spine and between ribs.

COMMON SURGICAL PROCEDURES
SOFT TISSUE PROCEDURES

- An **ovariohysterectomy**, commonly referred to as a spay, involves removal of the ovaries and uterus.
- A cesarean section is a method of delivering newborn animals in cases of dystocia (difficult labor). It consists of an abdominal incision (flank or ventral midline) and then an incision into the uterus through which the newborn(s) is (are) delivered.
- An **orchiectomy** (castration) is the surgical removal of the testes.

BOX 9-1	Common Suffixes Used to Describe Surgical Procedures

- -*ectomy* = to remove (excise). For example, a splenectomy is a surgical procedure to remove the spleen.
- -*otomy* = to cut into. For example, a cystotomy (incision into the urinary bladder) is often performed to remove urinary calculi (bladder stones).
- -*ostomy* = surgical creation of an artificial opening. For example, a perineal urethrostomy is a surgical procedure often performed on male cats for relief of urethral obstruction. It involves excision of the penis (penectomy) and creation of a widened, new urethral opening.
- -*rrhaphy* = surgical repair by suturing. For example, abdominal herniorrhaphy is the surgical repair of an abdominal hernia by suturing the defect in the abdominal musculature.
- -*pexy* = surgical fixation. For example, gastropexy (suturing of the stomach to the abdominal wall to fix it in place) is often performed in cases of gastric torsion.
- -*plasty* = surgical alteration of shape or form. For example, pyloroplasty enlarges the pyloric orifice of the stomach to facilitate gastric emptying.

From Sirois M: *Principles and practice of veterinary technology*, ed 3, St Louis, 2011, Mosby.

- A lateral ear resection is often performed in animals with chronic external ear infection. It involves removal of the lateral wall of the vertical portion of the external ear canal to allow improved **ventilation** and establish drainage for exudates.
- A **laparotomy** is an incision into the abdominal cavity, often through the flank.
- A celiotomy is another term for laparotomy.
- A cystotomy is an incision into the urinary bladder, frequently for the removal of urinary calculi (bladder stones).
- A gastrotomy is an incision into the stomach.
- Gastropexy involves suturing of the stomach to the abdominal wall to fix it in place. This procedure is frequently done in cases of gastric torsion.
- A splenectomy is the removal of the spleen.
- A thoracotomy is an incision into the thoracic cavity (chest).
- A herniorrhaphy is the surgical repair of a hernia by suturing the abnormal opening(s) closed.
- An enterotomy is an incision into the intestine, often for removal of a foreign body.
- An intestinal anastomosis involves removal of a portion of the intestine (resection) and suturing the cut ends together to restore the continuity of the intestinal tube (anastomosis).
- A perineal urethrostomy involves incision into the urethra and suturing of the splayed urethral edges to the skin to create a larger urethral orifice. This procedure is frequently performed on male cats with recurrent urethral obstruction.
- A urethrotomy is an incision into the urethra, most commonly to retrieve stones that have traveled out of the bladder and become lodged in the urethra.
- A mastectomy involves removal of part or all of one or more mammary glands.

ORTHOPEDIC (BONE) PROCEDURES

- An onychectomy is the surgical removal of a claw, commonly called declawing.
- An intervertebral disc fenestration is done to remove prolapsed intervertebral disc material causing pressure on the spinal cord.
- An intramedullary bone pinning involves insertion of a metal rod (bone pin) into the medullary cavity of a long bone to fix fracture fragments in place.
- Joint stabilization via lateral suture technique or tibial tuberosity advancement is performed when the cranial cruciate ligament in the stifle joint has ruptured. Lack of an intact cranial cruciate ligament creates instability in the stifle, causing abnormal movement. This can damage the joint surfaces of the distal femur and proximal tibia.
- A femoral head ostectomy involves amputation of the head of the femur. It is usually performed in animals with severe damage to the femoral head or neck, or with a damaged acetabulum.

PREOPERATIVE AND POSTOPERATIVE CONSIDERATIONS

PREOPERATIVE EVALUATION

Anesthesia and surgery are stressful events that put an animal's life at risk. The role of a proper preoperative evaluation is to gather enough pertinent information to minimize that risk. That information can be gathered through a patient history, physical examination, and appropriate laboratory tests. The veterinary assistant will work closely with the veterinary technician who is performing the evaluation.

PATIENT EVALUATION

Patient evaluation means to judge a patient's medical history and physical condition carefully to determine health status and predict potential complications. This is the most important step because all anesthetic decisions are based on health status. The medical history and physical examination are absolutely critical before anesthesia. All abnormalities discovered should be pursued to determine their potential effect on anesthetic outcome. Patient evaluation includes consideration of patient characteristics, medical history, physical examination, and laboratory test results.

Patient characteristics include species, breed, age, and gender. Patient medical history should include signalment and **anamnesis**, including the vaccine status, medical and surgical history, injuries, diseases, past anesthetic complications, changes in the patient's condition since last observed, purpose of the appointment, including specific location, observance of fasting recommendations, and concurrent medication. The physical examination includes general body condition scoring (see Chapter 7) and evaluation of the cardiovascular, respiratory, hepatic, renal, and central nervous systems (Table 9-5). Preanesthetic laboratory tests may include hematocrit (PCV), total plasma protein, liver enzyme (e.g., alanine aminotransferase [ALT]), bile acid, blood urea nitrogen (BUN), blood glucose, and electrolyte levels, blood smear, heartworm status, fecal analysis, acid-base balance, urinalysis, blood gas values, and blood coagulation screens, depending on the condition and age of the animal. Thoracic radiography and electrocardiography also may be useful in evaluating a patient.

PATIENT PREPARATION

Patient preparation requirements vary depending on the anticipated procedure. It is also important to prepare for the possibility of unanticipated situations. Standard practice is to withhold food for 8 to 12 hours and water for 2 to 4 hours before anesthetic induction. However, special preparation may be required in complex procedures. Pediatric or smaller patients should be fasted for shorter time periods. Chronically compromised patients should have their condition stabilized, when possible, before anesthesia. For example, anemic patients (PCV < 20%) should have a transfusion

TABLE 9-5	Preanesthetic Physical Examination Checklist	
SYSTEM	**CHECK**	**NOTE SIGNS**
General body condition	Temperature, weight, body score, skin turgor, temperament	Obesity, dehydration, cachexia, hypothermia, hyperthermia, pregnancy, recent changes in weight, aggressiveness
Central nervous system	Level of consciousness	Bright, alert, responsive (BAR); quiet, alert, responsive (QAR); obtunded, depressed, lethargic, stuporous, comatose, seizures, syncope
Cardiovascular	Heart rate and rhythm, arterial blood pressure quality and regularity, concurrent pulse and auscultation, capillary refill time	Cyanosis or icterus, pale mucous membranes, prolonged CRT, heart murmurs, weak or irregular pulse, arrhythmias
Respiratory	Respiratory rate, depth and effort, character, mucous membrane color	Pallor, cyanosis, increased effort or rate, abnormal lung sounds (e.g., wheezing, crackles), dyspnea, nasal discharge
Hepatic	Color	Jaundice, failure of blood to clot, coma, seizures
Renal	Volume and discharges	Vomiting, polyuria-polydipsia, oliguria-anuria, hematuria
Gastrointestinal	Abnormalities	Diarrhea, vomiting, distention
Musculoskeletal	Stance, activity	Weakness, abnormal gait, recumbency
Exterior surfaces	Integument, coat condition, lymph nodes, mammary glands, body openings	Wounds, parasites, tumors, lesions, exudates, hair loss, roughness, redness, inflammation, enlarged lymph nodes, discharges, odors, vaginal discharge
EENT	Ears, eyes, nose, and throat	Discharges, inflammation, swelling, abnormal pupil size and response, redness, odor, stridor, dental tartar
Abdominal palpation	Abnormalities	Hardness, pain, distention

Adapted from Sirois M: Principles and practice of veterinary technology, ed 3, St Louis, 2011, Mosby.

to ensure adequate oxygen-carrying capacity. Dehydrated patients should receive sufficient intravenous fluids to restore hydration status. Patients with low total plasma protein levels (<3 g/dL) may benefit from the administration of plasma.

> **CRITICAL CONCEPT**
>
> An accurate weight should be obtained just before any anesthetic procedure. Use a pediatric scale for animals weighing less than 5 kg and a gram scale for those weighing less than 1 kg.

It is important to obtain a current and accurate weight for the patient. Clipping the surgical site and placing an IV catheter before induction minimizes anesthesia time. Maintaining patient calmness reduces stress and may lower anesthetic induction requirements. Avoid unnecessary handling and noisy personnel or equipment. Provide an environment free of excitement or anxiety. Oxygenation before and during induction may be beneficial to patients with cardiopulmonary compromise, especially during mask or chamber induction.

Preanesthetic checklists should be completed before all procedures to ensure that appropriate items are readily available, important health issues have been addressed, and all persons involved have been informed. This is especially important in high-volume clinics, when several people are involved in patient evaluation and preparation. Anesthetic induction must not be initiated until the checklist is completed (Box 9-2).

> **CRITICAL CONCEPT**
>
> If food is not withheld, pulmonary aspiration leading to pneumonia, permanent disability, or immediate respiratory arrest and death of the patient may occur. Adhere to veterinary instructions.

PREPARATION OF THE OPERATIVE SITE

Surgery puts a patient at risk for nosocomial infections (hospital-acquired infections). Because most surgical infections develop from bacteria that enter the incision during surgery, proper preparation of the surgical site is crucial to reduce the likelihood of infection. Resident skin flora (particularly *Staphylococcus aureus* and *Streptococcus* spp.) are the most common sources of surgical wound contaminants. Although it is impossible to sterilize skin without impairing its natural protective function and interfering with wound healing, proper preoperative preparation reduces the likelihood of infection.

HAIR REMOVAL AND SKIN SCRUBBING

Before preparing the patient for surgery, verify the patient's identity, surgical procedure being performed, and surgical site. It may be useful to bathe the animal the day before the surgical procedure to remove loose hair, debris, and external parasites. Preparing patients for surgery includes clipping hair and scrubbing the skin at the surgical site. These procedures should be performed outside of the surgical suite.

The extent and location of hair removal are based on the type of surgical procedure to be performed (Fig. 9-25). Hair

BOX 9-2 | Preanesthesia Checklist

Personnel
1. Select personnel and identify roles.
2. Review procedure.
3. Review emergency procedures.

Patient
1. Identify patient properly.
2. Verify patient was fasted (as appropriate).
3. Weigh patient.
4. Perform special prep (as needed; e.g., bowel prep).
5. Perform preanesthetic examination (signalment, anamnesis).

Drugs
1. Select drugs; confirm they are available.
2. Review routes of drug administration.
3. Check crash cart inventory.

Fluid Administration
1. Select IV fluids; maintain at proper temperature.
2. Confirm sufficient fluids available for adverse events.
3. Gather necessary equipment:
   - IV catheters (18- to 24-gauge, 1- to 2-inch size)
   - Injection caps

- Materials for securing IV catheter (tape, adhesive)
- Saline flush or heparinized saline (2 to 4 IU/mL), in syringe with needle
- Fluid delivery sets (60 drops/mL for <10 kg, 15 drops/mL for 11-40 kg, 10 drops/mL for >40 kg)

Endotracheal Intubation
1. Select and inspect three sizes of endotracheal tubes.
2. Gather necessary equipment:
   - Lubricating gel
   - Rolled gauze for securing
   - Laryngoscope and appropriate blades
   - Stylets
   - Lidocaine spray or swab if needed

Equipment
1. Review anesthetic machine checklist (see Box 9-3).
2. Select and inspect monitoring equipment.

Miscellaneous Supplies
- Ophthalmic ointment
- Circulating warm water blanket, table insulation, or heated table
- Face mask

Adapted from Sirois M: Principles and practice of veterinary technology, ed 3, St Louis, 2011, Mosby.

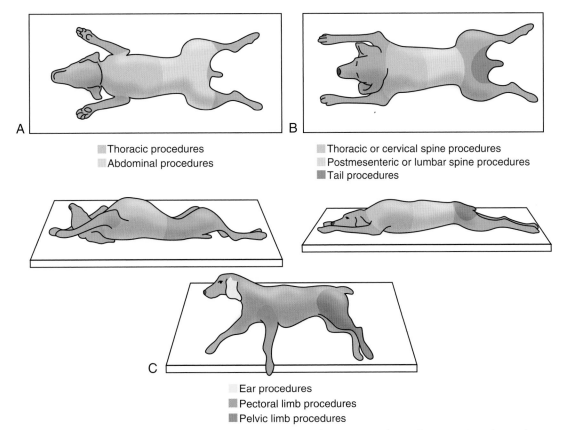

FIGURE 9-25 Hair removal patterns for selected surgical procedures. **A,** Dorsal recumbency. **B,** Sternal recumbency. **C,** Lateral recumbency. (From Sirois M: Principles and practice of veterinary technology, ed 3, St Louis, 2011, Mosby.)

should be liberally clipped around the proposed incision site so that the incision can be extended, if needed, while still remaining within a sterile field. A general guideline is to clip 20 cm on each side of the incision. The hair can be removed most effectively with an Oster-type clipper and a no. 40 clipper blade. Patients with a dense hair coat may be clipped first with a medium blade (no. 10). The higher the blade number, the shorter the remaining hair. Clippers should be held using a pencil grip and initial clipping should be done with the grain of the hair growth pattern. Subsequent clipping should be against the pattern of hair growth to obtain a closer clip. This will minimize the likelihood of irritation to the patient's skin (commonly referred to as clipper burn). Depilatory creams are less traumatic than other hair removal methods, but they induce a mild dermal lymphocytic reaction. They are most useful in irregular areas in which adequate hair clipping is difficult. Razors are occasionally used for hair removal (e.g., around the eye), but they cause microlacerations in skin that may increase irritation and promote infection. After hair has been clipped from the site, loose hair is removed with a vacuum. To enhance manipulation of limbs during surgery, a hanging leg preparation may be done. This requires that the limb be circumferentially clipped; the limb is hung from an IV pole during preparation to allow the sides of the limb to be scrubbed (Fig. 9-26).

CRITICAL CONCEPT

Sterile patient preparation generally consists of three rounds of alternating antiseptic solution with saline rinse; every pass with gauze moves in a circular motion from the anticipated incision, site radiating outward.

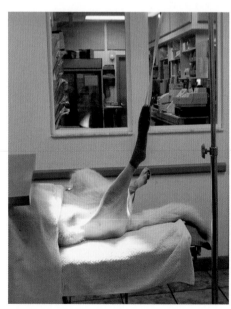

FIGURE 9-26 Manipulation of the limb during orthopedic procedures may be facilitated with a hanging leg preparation. The limb is clipped circumferentially and carefully suspended from an IV pole with tape. The patient is positioned for medial rear limb surgery. (From Sirois M: Principles and practice of veterinary technology, ed 3, St Louis, 2011, Mosby.)

Before transporting the animal to the surgical site, the incision is given a general cleansing scrub and ophthalmic antibiotic ointment or lubricant may be placed on the cornea and conjunctiva. In male dogs undergoing abdominal procedures, the prepuce may be flushed with an antiseptic solution. The skin is scrubbed with germicidal soap to remove debris and reduce bacterial populations in preparation for surgery. The area is lathered well until all dirt and oils are removed. This is a generous scrub that often encompasses the hair surrounding the operation site to remove unattached hair and dander that may be disturbed during draping. This so-called dirty prep (done outside the operating room [OR]) will often consist of chlorhexidine and saline, and the lather step may be left in place for 60 to 120 seconds to ensure adequate contact time. Other options for scrubbing solutions include iodophors, alcohols, hexachlorophene, and quaternary ammonium salts. Alcohol is not effective against spores, but it kills bacteria rapidly and acts as a defatting agent. However, it must not be used on critical patients when the possibility of defibrillator use exists. Using alcohol by itself is not recommended, but it is sometimes used in conjunction with povidone-iodine. Hexachlorophene and quaternary ammonium salts are less effective than other available agents.

CRITICAL CONCEPT

Chlorhexidine and povidone-iodine are the most commonly used antiseptic scrub and prep agents.

POSITIONING

Before sterile application of the epidermal germicide, the animal is moved to the OR and positioned so that the operative site is accessible to the surgeon and secured with ropes, sandbags, troughs, or tape. The animal is generally placed on a water-circulating heating pad and provided with a warm air–circulating blanket (Fig. 9-27); if electrocautery is being used, a ground plate should be positioned under the patient.

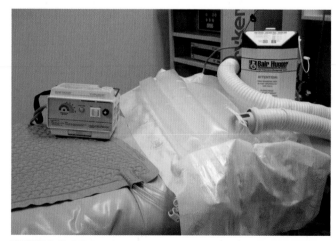

FIGURE 9-27 Patient warming systems used in the OR—warm water circulating blanket (L), warm air circulating system (R). (From Sirois M: Principles and practice of veterinary technology, ed 3, St Louis, 2011, Mosby.)

Anesthetic monitoring equipment is then attached and baseline vital signs evaluated before proceeding with the sterile prep.

STERILE SKIN PREPARATION

Sterile preparation of the surgical site begins after transporting and positioning the animal on the operating table. Scrubbing the skin for surgery is a multistep process (Procedure 9-2). An appropriate antiseptic solution should be applied using sterile gauze.

Frequently, when using povidone-iodine and alcohol, the site is scrubbed alternatively with each solution three times to allow for 5 minutes of contact time. However, using alcohol between the povidone-iodine scrubs decreases the contact time of povidone-iodine with the skin and may decrease its efficacy. Excess solution on the table or accumulated in body pockets should be blotted with a sterile towel or sponges. When the final povidone-iodine scrub is completed, a 10% povidone-iodine solution should be sprayed or painted on the site. If chlorhexidine is the preparation solution, it may be rinsed with

saline. Because chlorhexidine binds to keratin, contact time is less critical than with povidone-iodine. Two 30-second applications are considered adequate for antimicrobial activity.

PREPARATION OF THE SURGICAL TEAM

SURGICAL ATTIRE

All persons entering the operating room suite, regardless of whether a surgery is in progress or not, should be dressed in appropriate surgical attire. To minimize microbial contamination from OR personnel, wear dedicated surgical scrub clothes rather than street clothes in the operating suite. With two-piece pant suits, tuck loose-fitting tops into the trousers. Tunic tops that fit close to the body may be worn outside the trousers. The sleeves of the top should be short enough to allow the hands and arms to be scrubbed. Pants should have an elastic waist or drawstring closure. Nonscrubbed personnel should wear long-sleeved jackets over their scrub clothes.

📋 PROCEDURE 9-2 PATIENT SKIN SCRUB (STERILE PREP)

1. Gauze sponges for use in the surgical site preparation are sterilized in a pack, along with bowls into which the germicides and rinse can be poured.
2. Sponges are handled with sterile sponge forceps or the gloved hand, using aseptic technique.
3. The scrub should begin at the intended incision (Fig. 1)

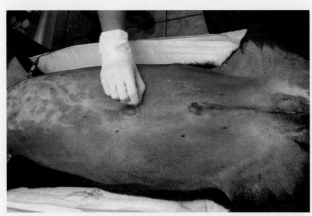

FIGURE 1

and continue out in concentric circles to an area at least 2 inches larger than the expected size of the sterile field needed (Fig. 2).

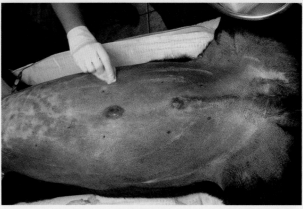

FIGURE 2

4. The scrub should be completed three times and may incorporate a rinse with saline or sterile water between each scrub.
5. Sponges are discarded after reaching the periphery (Fig. 3).

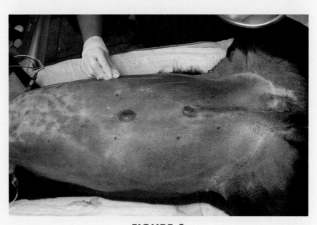

FIGURE 3

Jackets should be buttoned or snapped closed during use to minimize the risk of the edges' inadvertently contaminating sterile surfaces. Scrub clothes should be laundered between wearings and changed if they are visibly soiled or wet to prevent transfer of microorganisms to the environment. Wearing scrub clothes outside the surgical environment increases microbial contamination. If a scrub suit must be worn outside the surgery room, a laboratory coat or single-use gowns should be used to cover it.

Other surgical attire includes hair coverings, masks, shoe covers, gowns, and gloves. Hair is a significant carrier of bacteria; when left uncovered, it collects bacteria. Because bacterial shedding from hair increases surgical wound infection rates, complete hair coverage is necessary. Even when surgery is not in progress, caps and masks should be worn in the surgical suite. Caps should completely cover all scalp and facial hair, and masks should cover the mouth and nostrils (Fig. 9-28). Sideburns and/or beards require a hood for complete coverage. Skull caps that fail to cover the side hair above the ears and hair at the nape of the neck should not be worn.

Any comfortable footwear can be worn in the surgery area. Shoe covers should be donned when first entering the surgical area and should be worn when leaving it to keep shoes clean. New shoe covers are donned when returning to the surgical area. Shoe covers are generally made of reusable or disposable materials that are water-repellent and tear-resistant.

Masks, constructed from lint-free material containing a hydrophilic filter web sandwiched between two outer layers, should be worn whenever entering a sterile area. Their major function is to filter and contain droplets of microorganisms expelled from the mouth and nasopharynx during talking, sneezing, and coughing. Masks must be fitted over the mouth and nose and secured in a manner that prevents venting. The dorsal aspect of the mask is secured by shaping the reinforcing top edge tightly around the nose.

Surgical gowns may be reusable and made of woven materials (usually cotton), or disposable. Disposable (single-use) gowns are nonwoven and made directly from fibers rather than yarn. Loosely woven cotton is commonly used for reusable gowns. This fabric is instantly permeable to bacteria when it becomes wet. Fewer microorganisms contaminate the surgical environment when disposable (single-use) nonwoven materials are used.

SURGICAL SCRUB

Surgical scrubbing cleans the hands and forearms to reduce the numbers of bacteria that come into contact with the wound from scrubbed personnel during surgery. The veterinarian and veterinary technician must perform a hand and arm scrub before entering the surgical suite. Objectives of a surgical scrub include mechanical removal of dirt and oil, reduction of the transient bacterial population (bacteria deposited from the environment), and reduction of the skin's resident bacterial population.

GOWNING AND GLOVING

Gowns are another barrier between the skin of the surgical team and patient. They should be constructed of a material that prevents passage of microorganisms between sterile and nonsterile areas. Gowns should be resistant to fluid, lint accumulation, stretching, and tearing, especially at the forearm, elbow, and abdominal areas, and should be comfortable, economical, and fire- resistant. Reusable or single-use disposable gowns are available. Gowning and gloving should occur away from the surgical table and patient to avoid dripping water onto the sterile field and contaminating it.

ASSISTED GLOVING

When gloving another person, the person assisting with the gloving should have on a sterile gown and/or gloves. The assistant's hands should not touch the nonsterile surface of the person being gloved. If both gloves are being replaced, have the assistant pick up one glove and place his or her fingers and thumb under the cuff of the glove (Fig. 9-29, *A*). With the thumb of the glove facing you, have the assistant hold the glove open for you to slip your hand into (see Fig. 9-29, *B*). The assistant then brings the cuff of the glove up and over the cuff of your gown and gently lets it go. The assistant picks up the other glove. Assist him or her by holding the cuff of the glove open with the fingers of your sterile hand while putting your ungloved hand into the open glove (see Fig. 9-29, *C*). The assistant keeps her or his thumbs under the cuff while you thrust your hand into it. Ensure that the glove cuff is above your gown cuff before the assistant gently releases it (she or he should not let the cuff snap sharply).

GLOVE REMOVAL DURING SURGERY

If gloves become contaminated during surgery, they must be replaced. Both gloves may routinely be changed during

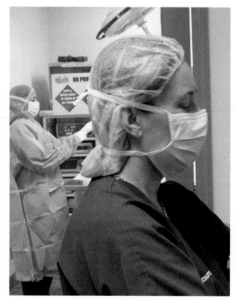

FIGURE 9-28 Hair should be covered by a bouffant-style surgical cap. This is the correct way to tie a surgical mask. (From Sirois M: *Principles and practice of veterinary technology,* ed 3, St Louis, 2011, Mosby.)

so-called dirty procedures (open gastrointestinal [GI] tract caused by perforation, or by gastrotomy or enterotomy). Most surgeons are adept at removing gloves themselves, pulling their hands back into surgical gown sleeves as they do so. New gloves may be dropped (in their inner sterile wrapper) on the instrument stand or drape. If only one glove is contaminated, or if the scrubbed personnel needs assistance for any reason, nonsterile personnel may easily assist (Fig. 9-30). The cuffs of the gown of the sterile person are grasped through the cuff of the glove. A firm grip is used, but care must be taken not to break the glove or touch the gown. The cuff of the glove is pulled toward the nonsterile assistant and, in turn, the cuff of the gown is pulled back down over the hand of the wearer. The glove is pulled free and the sterile personnel may again proceed with closed gloving.

ANESTHETIC EQUIPMENT AND SUPPLIES

More anesthetic mishaps are attributed to poor planning and preparation than to improper use of drugs. Correct selection, preparation, and use of anesthetic equipment are essential for patient safety. All equipment should be prepared and checked to be in good working order before the administration of

anesthetic compounds; intubation and oxygenation may be required unexpectedly. The use of a preanesthetic checklist ensures that all items are completed before induction (Box 9-3). The veterinary assistant will work closely with the veterinary technician who is performing these tasks.

SUPPLIES FOR INTRAVENOUS FLUID ADMINISTRATION

Placement of an IV catheter is essential for patient safety during anesthesia. IV catheters provide immediate access for IV injection and administration of fluids. Catheters should be placed before induction of anesthesia, when possible, because most anesthetic agents produce hypotension or **vasoconstriction** and may complicate catheter placement. Appropriately sized catheters, infusion sets, needles, syringes, and other supplies necessary for aseptic catheterization should be arranged for easy access.

ENDOTRACHEAL TUBES

Endotracheal intubation ensures a patent airway, facilitates patient ventilation, and provides easy delivery of volatile anesthetics. Endotracheal tube (ETT) diameter and length are important. The diameter should be the largest size that will fit into the trachea with ease. If too large, the larynx and

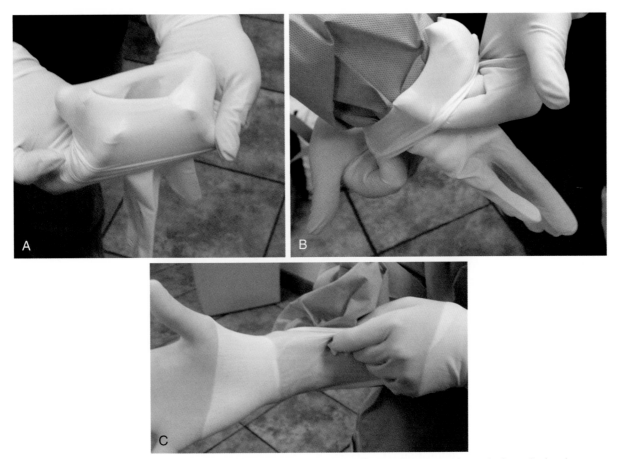

FIGURE 9-29 Assisted gloving. **A,** The assistant holds the glove open for a sterile team member to slip her or his hand in. Note that the hand remains in the gown cuff until it is within the glove cuff. **B,** The assistant then brings the cuff of the glove up and over the cuff of the gown. **C,** The sterile team member may then adjust the cuff(s). (From Sirois M: Principles and practice of veterinary technology, ed 3, St Louis, 2011, Mosby.)

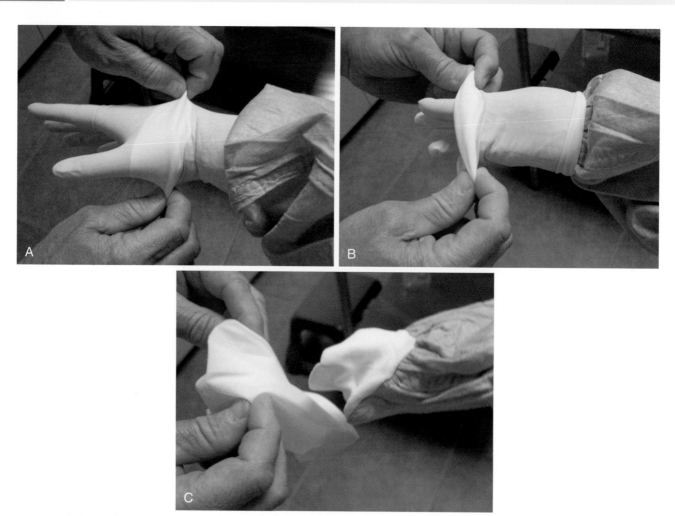

FIGURE 9-30 Assisted glove removal. **A,** Nonsterile assistant grasps the gown cuffs through the glove cuffs. **B,** Both cuffs are pulled toward the assistant together, and the sterile personnel's hand retreats into the gown. **C,** The sterile team member may then proceed again with closed gloving. (From Sirois M: Principles and practice of veterinary technology, ed 3, St Louis, 2011, Mosby.)

trachea may be traumatized. If too small, the patient will have difficulty breathing through the tube. To illustrate this for yourself, try breathing through a straw for 2 or 3 minutes. Generally, the internal diameter (ID) is used. Cats usually require 3 to 4.5 mm, whereas dogs need 6 to 14 mm (Fig. 9-31).

A fairly accurate assessment for tube size can be based on the weight of the dog, keeping in mind that body condition, confirmation, brachycephalic breed, obesity, and small size may alter the final size chosen. Use a 9- to 9.5-mm tube for a 40-pound (18.2-kg) dog. As the weight changes by 5 lb (2.3 kg), change the size of the ETT by 0.5 mm. Thus, a 50-lb dog (22.7 kg) would require approximately a 10- to 10.5-mm-ID tube. The trachea also can be palpated to feel the approximate size, or an approximation can be made by measuring the nasal septal width with the outer diameter of an endotracheal tube.

Proper length of the ETT is also important. The inserted tip of the tube should not extend beyond (caudal to) the thoracic inlet to prevent bronchial intubation. The adapter end of the tube should not extend more than 1 or 2 inches beyond (rostral to) the mouth to limit mechanical dead space and prevent the rebreathing of exhaled gas.

The ETT should be clean and free of defects or obstructions. If it has an inflatable cuff, it should be checked for leaks. The connector must be securely attached. Stylets may be used to facilitate intubation with small-diameter or very flexible tubes.

LARYNGOSCOPE

The **laryngoscope** facilitates visualization of the glottis as the endotracheal tube passes through into the trachea. Laryngoscopes consist of a handle and detachable blade in a variety of sizes and shapes (Fig. 9-32). The blade is curved to match the curvature of the tongue and allow even pressure along its length.

MEDICAL GAS SUPPLY

Medical gases may be delivered from compressed gas cylinders by a central pipeline or direct attachment to the anesthetic machine. Medical grade oxygen and nitrous oxide are the gases commonly used in veterinary medicine, although the benefits of nitrous oxide in veterinary practice are limited. The nitrous oxide source must be independent of the oxygen source; nitrous oxide is mixed with oxygen just before passing through the vaporizer.

| **BOX 9-3** | Checklist for Daily Inspection of Anesthetic Equipment |

- Sufficient oxygen available—check cylinder pressure.
- Flow meter bobbin or float moves freely through length of tube.
- Unidirectional valves properly functioning
- Vaporizer filled and filler caps tightened
- All gas lines correctly connected
- Sufficient and fresh CO_2 absorbent time available
- Scavenger system properly connected and operational
- Cuff syringe available
- Attach breathing circuit, tubes, and reservoir bag.
- Check for leaks:
  1. Close pop-off valve.
  2. Occlude patient end of breathing circuit (where endotracheal tube attaches).
  3. Fill circuit with oxygen to a pressure of 20 cm H_2O.
  4. Turn on oxygen flow to 100 mL/min (0.1 liter/min).
  5. If pressure increases, leaks are within acceptable limits.
  6. If pressure drops, increase the flow rate until pressure remains stable.
  7. Leaks exceeding 200 mL/min (0.2 liter/min) must be corrected via machine maintenance.
  8. Open the pop-off valve while occluding the Y piece; pressure should drop to 0 cm H_2O.

Adapted from Sirois M: *Principles and practice of veterinary technology,* ed 3, St Louis, 2011, Mosby.

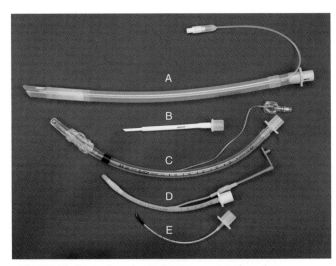

FIGURE 9-31 Endotracheal tube type, material, and size comparison. **A,** Cuffed 11-mm silicone rubber tube. **B,** 2.5-mm Cole tube. **C,** Cuffed 8-mm polyvinyl chloride (PVC) tube. **D,** Cuffed 4-mm red rubber tube. **E,** Uncuffed 2-mm PVC Murphy tube. (From Sirois M: *Principles and practice of veterinary technology,* ed 3, St Louis, 2011, Mosby.)

The most commonly used sizes of compressed medical gas cylinders are the E cylinder (4.25 × 26 inches) and the H cylinder (9.25 × 51 inches). All medical gas cylinders are color coded; oxygen cylinders are green (white in Canada), and nitrous oxide cylinders are blue. E cylinders attached directly to the anesthetic machine for backup should be kept in the off position until in use to ensure that they remain full until needed.

Pressure regulators attached to the cylinder valve on H cylinders and near the hanger yokes for E cylinders (Fig. 9-33) passively reduce oxygen pressure to the normal working pressure of the anesthetic machine to a gauge of 50 pounds per square inch (psi). If there is a line pressure gauge, it should be checked before every procedure to verify correct pressure in the intermediate pressure gas lines (40 to 50 psi; Fig. 9-34). Pressure reduction is necessary to prevent damage to the anesthetic machine and allow a constant rate of oxygen delivery to the **flow meter**. Cylinder pressure gauges are associated with the pressure regulator and may be used to estimate the relative volume of gas remaining in a cylinder. Oxygen cylinders contain only compressed oxygen vapors, and the pressure is proportional to the content. The pressure in a fully charged oxygen cylinder, regardless of size, is almost 2200 psi.

CRITICAL CONCEPT

Handle compressed gas cylinders with care. Turn a tank on only when it is attached to a yoke or pressure regulator. Avoid contact with flames, store tanks properly, and make sure that the tanks fit properly to the yoke.

Mark tanks as full, in use, or empty to indicate their status, and be sure that a full backup tank is always kept on the machine as a spare in case the primary tank runs out. Change the tanks at no less than 100 psi of oxygen for an E tank and 680 psi for an H tank.

ANESTHESIA MACHINES

Several companies manufacture anesthesia machines for veterinary use. Anesthetia machines deliver a mixture of oxygen and inhalation anesthetic to the **breathing circuit**. The components of an anesthetia machine include the oxygen source, pressure regulator, oxygen pressure valve, flow meter, vaporizer, breathing circuit, reservoir bag, circuit manometer, positive pressure relief valve, carbon dioxide absorbent, and unidirectional dome valves (Fig. 9-35).

FLOW METERS

Flow meters receive medical gases from the pressure regulator. Their purpose is to measure and deliver a constant gas flow to the vaporizer, common gas outlet, and breathing circuit. The flow meter also further reduces the pressure of the gas in the intermediate-pressure line from approximately 50 to 15 psi. This pressure is only slightly above atmospheric pressure (≈14.7 psi), making it ideal for the breathing circuit and the patient's lungs.

Oxygen enters the flow meter near the bottom and travels upward through a tapered, transparent flow tube. A floating indicator inside the flow tube, a ball or plumb bob, indicates the amount of gas passing through the control valve. The flow rate is indicated on a scale associated with the flow tube. When the control valve is open, oxygen enters the tube, pushing the floating indicator upward. Where the indicator hovers in equilibrium, the rate of flow is determined by reading the calibrated scale from the center of the ball or the top of the plumb bob (Fig. 9-36).

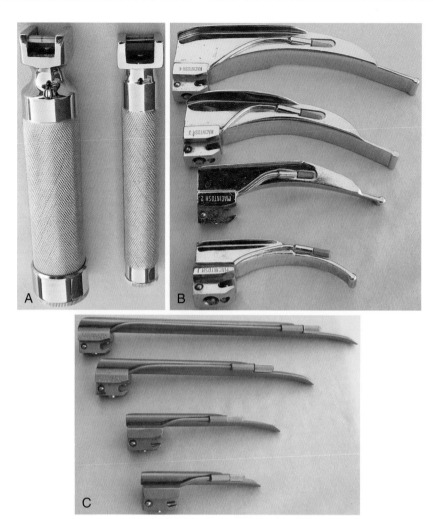

FIGURE 9-32 Laryngoscopes. **A,** Laryngoscope handle. **B,** MacIntosh laryngeal speculum. **C,** Miller laryngeal speculum. (From Sirois M: Principles and practice of veterinary technology, ed 3, St Louis, 2011, Mosby.)

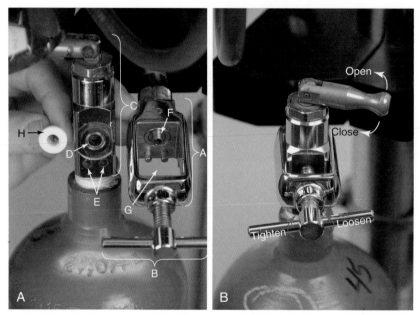

FIGURE 9-33 A, Parts of compressed gas cylinder and yoke. *A,* Yoke. *B,* Wing nut. *C,* Outlet valve. *D,* Valve port. *E,* Pin holes. *F,* Nipple of yoke. *G,* Index pins. *H,* Nylon washer. **B,** Opening and closing the outlet valve; loosening and tightening the wing nut. (From Thomas JA, Lerche P: Anesthesia and analgesia for veterinary technicians, ed 4, St Louis, 2011, Mosby.)

Flow meters are gas-specific and must not be interchanged; an oxygen flow meter cannot safely be replaced with a nitrous oxide flow meter. Control knobs to regulate the flow of medical gases must be distinguishable from each other.

CRITICAL CONCEPT

The oxygen control knob must be green, permanently marked with the word or symbol for oxygen, and the valve should be fluted, project beyond other knobs, and be larger in diameter than other knobs.

Flow meters are common sources of leaks and should be checked at regular intervals for cracks in the flow tube. Dirt or static electricity may cause a float to stick, which makes the flow appear to be higher or lower than indicated. Excessive tightening easily damages control knobs, leading to expensive repair. Overtightening may prevent the flow meter from closing completely, causing significant leaking in the off position. Leaking may lead to an unexpected shortage of medical gases and exhaustion (saturation) of carbon dioxide absorbent from the constant flow of gas through the absorbent.

VAPORIZERS

Inhalation anesthetic agents are volatile liquids that vaporize at room temperature. The primary function of a **vaporizer** is controlled enhancement of anesthetic vaporization. Each vaporizer is designed to be used with a specific inhalant anesthetic and is color coded—isoflurane is purple, sevoflurane is yellow, halothane is red, and desflurane is blue.

Precision vaporizers, designed for a specific anesthetic agent, deliver a constant concentration (as a percentage) that is automatically maintained with changing oxygen flow rates and

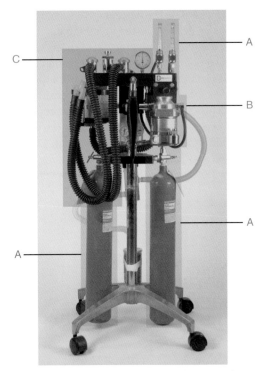

FIGURE 9-35 Small animal anesthesia machine; anesthetic machine systems. **A,** Carrier gas supply. Note the two size E compressed gas oxygen cylinders next to the As at the bottom of this image. **B,** Anesthetic vaporizer. **C,** Breathing circuit. Note that the scavenging system is not visible in this view. (From Thomas JA, Lerche P: Anesthesia and analgesia for veterinary technicians, ed 4, St Louis, 2011, Mosby.)

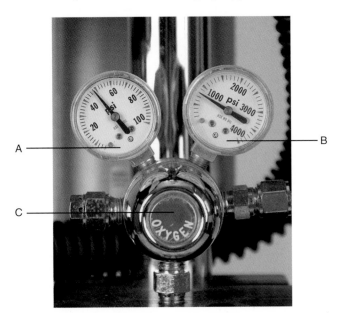

FIGURE 9-34 A, Line pressure gauge (registering 48 psi). **B,** Tank pressure gauge (registering 800 psi). **C,** Pressure-reducing valve. (From Thomas JA, Lerche P: Anesthesia and analgesia for veterinary technicians, ed 4, St Louis, 2011, Mosby.)

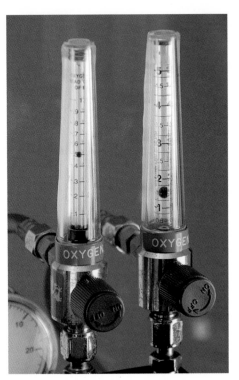

FIGURE 9-36 Oxygen flow meters with ball indicators. The flow meter on the *left* is adjusted to 0.5 L/min, and the flow meter on the *right* is adjusted to 1.5 L/min, for a total oxygen flow of 2 L/min. (From Thomas JA, Lerche P: Anesthesia and analgesia for veterinary technicians, ed 4, St Louis, 2011, Mosby.)

temperature (Fig. 9-37). The percentage setting on the control dial approximates delivery to the breathing circuit. Precision vaporizers are designed to function out of the breathing circuit (VOC, vaporizer out of circuit)—that is, between the flow meter and breathing circuit—so that oxygen from the flow meter flows into the vaporizer before entering the breathing circuit.

Several hazards are associated with vaporizers. Filling with the incorrect agent can lead to delivery of an excessively high or low concentration of vapor to the patient. Delivering an unknown agent may lead to varied cardiovascular effects. Tipping the vaporizer may allow liquid agent to enter the fresh gas line, increasing the anesthetic concentration. Overfilling the chamber decreases the volume of vapor available to mix with fresh gas and may allow liquid anesthetic to reach the common gas outlet line. Leaks are also common at the inlet fitting, outlet fitting, filling port, and drain port. Vaporizers located incorrectly in the common gas outlet can deliver excessive anesthetic concentrations when the oxygen flush is activated. The additional flow through the vaporizer (35 to 75 L/min) increases the volume of vapor delivered to the breathing circuit.

BREATHING CIRCUITS

Medical gases pass from the anesthetic machine to the patient through tubing known as a breathing circuit. Breathing circuits deliver fresh gases (oxygen and anesthetic vapor) to the patient and transport exhaled gases from the patient. The breathing circuit is classified as a **rebreathing system** (circuit), where it is incorporated into the machine and carbon dioxide is eliminated from the circuit by soda lime absorption, or a **non–rebreathing system**, in which the carbon dioxide is eliminated using high gas flow rates and not a carbon dioxide absorber.

REBREATHING CIRCUITS

The term rebreathing means "to breathe again" and refers to exhaled gases (carbon dioxide, oxygen, anesthetic). Rebreathing circuits (circle system) are most commonly used in veterinary practice. The amount of carbon dioxide rebreathed depends on the degree of carbon dioxide absorption and fresh gas flow rate. The components of the circle system include a reservoir bag, manometer, positive-pressure relief valve (pop-off valve), carbon dioxide absorbent, unidirectional valves, fresh gas inlet, and removable set of breathing tubes (Fig. 9-38). Some circuits also have a negative-pressure relief valve.

Advantages of the rebreathing circuit include conservation of body heat and fluids, reuse of exhaled oxygen and anesthetic gases, and cost-efficient, lower flow rates. Disadvantages of the rebreathing circuit include the danger of

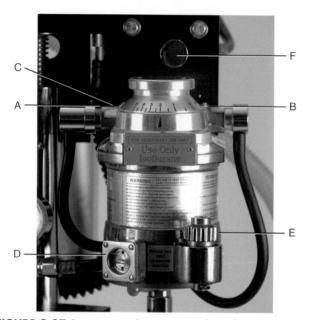

FIGURE 9-37 Precision anesthetic vaporizer for isoflurane set on 2%. **A,** Inlet port with keyed fitting leading from the flow meters. **B,** Outlet port with keyed fitting leading to the fresh gas inlet. **C,** Safety lock. **D,** Indicator window. **E,** Fill port. **F,** Oxygen flush valve (part of the compressed gas supply). (From Thomas JA, Lerche P: Anesthesia and analgesia for veterinary technicians, ed 4, St Louis, 2011, Mosby.)

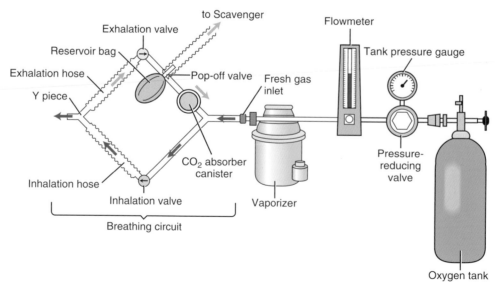

FIGURE 9-38 Diagram of an anesthetic machine with a rebreathing circuit and vaporizer outside the breathing circuit. (From Bassert JM, McCurnin DM: McCurnin's clinical textbook for veterinary technicians, ed 7, St Louis, 2010, Saunders.)

hypercarbia resulting from malfunction of the carbon dioxide absorbent or unidirectional valves, particularly at flow rates low enough to produce a closed system.

The **reservoir bag** (rebreathing bag) provides a gas volume sufficient for the patient to inhale maximally without creating negative pressure in the circuit. It is also used for positive-pressure ventilation or to inflate the lungs when needed. Reservoir bag sizes of 0.5 to 5 liters are used for small animals. The ideal reservoir bag is five to six times the patient's normal **tidal volume** of 10 mL/kg.

> ### CRITICAL CONCEPT
> At peak expiration, the reservoir bag should be approximately 75% full.

The circuit manometer is useful to monitor circuit pressure. Excessive circuit pressure (>4 cm H_2O) may prevent normal respiration and increase intrathoracic pressure, resulting in decreased venous return and a subsequent drop in cardiac output. During positive-pressure ventilation (bagging), the manometer allows delivery of the correct circuit pressure. Typically, healthy dogs and cats are ventilated to pressures of 15 to 20 cm H_2O to ensure adequate tidal volume. When breathing spontaneously, the manometer should not read more than 0 to 2 cm H_2O.

The positive-pressure relief (pop-off) valve prevents excessive pressure in the rebreathing circuit and allows for the removal of excess waste gases. A common cause of anesthetic mishap is leaving the pop-off valve closed after performing positive-pressure ventilation. The pop-off valve is equipped with a scavenger interface, permitting connection to a waste gas removal system to prevent waste gas discharge into the room air.

The carbon dioxide–absorbent canister removes carbon dioxide from the exhaled gases before the gases are returned to the patient. The gases are directed to the canister by the expiratory unidirectional valve of the breathing circuit. The canister contains absorbent granules such as calcium hydroxide, which removes CO_2 from the expired air. Exhaustion of the granules depends on gas flow rates and patient size. The absorbent should be changed monthly or after 6 to 8 hours of use, whichever is first. Look for signs to determine whether the granules need to be changed earlier (Table 9-6). Precautionary measures to ensure that the absorbent is reasonably fresh include logging of date changed and amount of time used for anesthesia.

The unidirectional valves maintain one-way flow of gases within the breathing circuit. The inhalation or inspiratory unidirectional valve opens so that fresh gas and anesthetic can flow to the patient; the exhalation or expiratory valve passes through the carbon dioxide absorbent before reaching the patient again.

> ### CRITICAL CONCEPT
> When the velocity of the gas is very slow, the unidirectional valves appear to flutter in response—thus, the alternative name, flutter valves.

Corrugated inspiratory and expiratory breathing tubes carry the anesthetic gases to and from the patient. Each tube is connected to a unidirectional valve at one end, and the Y piece at the other end. Standard breathing tubes are 22 mm in diameter and 1-m long for small animal patients weighing 7 to 135 kg. Shorter 15-mm–diameter tubes are preferred for patients weighing less than 7 kg. Large animal tubes are 500 mm in diameter and 1.7-m long. The classic setup uses separate inhalation and exhalation tubes connected via a Y piece to the endotracheal tube adapter. The Universal F-circuit was developed to place the inhalation tube inside the exhalation tube. The advantages of this arrangement include warming of inhaled gases by exhaled gases.

The air intake valve admits room air to the circuit in the event that negative pressure (a partial vacuum) is detected in the breathing circuit, a situation indicated by a collapsed reservoir bag. An air intake valve can be present on some machines either separately or integrated into the inspiratory unidirectional valve or pop-off valve.

NONREBREATHING CIRCUITS

Nonrebreathing circuits do not have a carbon dioxide absorber. The exhaled gases are immediately vented from the system through another hose, usually into a reservoir bag, where the gases are released into the **scavenging system** through an overflow valve. If properly used, nonrebreathing circuits allow no significant rebreathing of exhaled gases. Because nonrebreathing systems do not resist air, they are recommended for patients less than 7 kg in body weight so that work required to breathe is minimized. As with the rebreathing system, the oxygen or nitrous oxide enters the circuit from the tank, through the flow meter and into the vaporizer, but instead of the fresh gas passing into the circle, as with a rebreathing system, the fresh gas goes directly to the patient. Thus, the carbon dioxide absorber

TABLE 9-6	Comparison of Fresh and Exhausted CO_2 Granules	
FEATURE	**FRESH CO_2 GRANULES**	**EXHAUSTED CO_2 GRANULES**
Consistency	$Ca(OH)_2$—chip or crumble with finger pressure	$CaCO_3$—hard and brittle
Color	White	Slightly off white
pH indicator	Pink or white depending on brand	When one third to half of granules change color to white instead of original pink; violet instead of original white*
Capnographic monitor	[CO_2]—peak inspiration, near 0 mm Hg	[CO_2] → 0 mm Hg (could also result from other causes; e.g., dysfunctional expiratory unidirectional valve)

*May not occur in small patients and returns to original color in a few hours.
Adapted from Sirois M: Principles and practice of veterinary technology, ed 3, St Louis, 2011, Mosby.

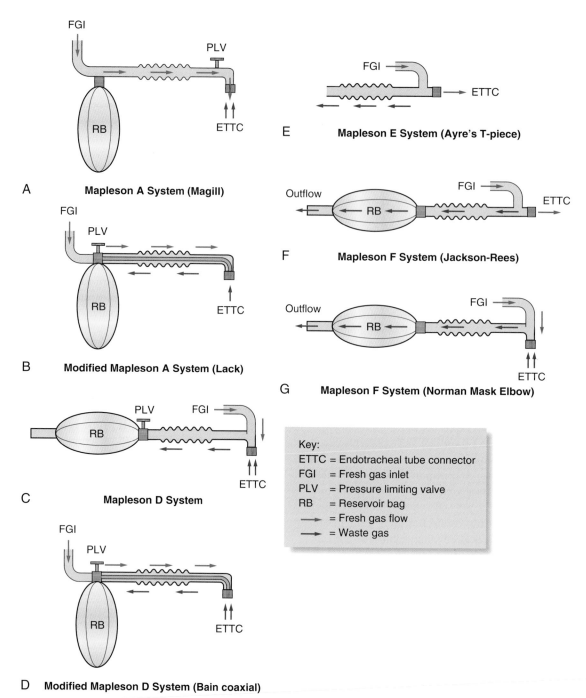

FGI

PLV

RB

ETTC

A   **Mapleson A System (Magill)**

FGI

PLV

RB

ETTC

B   **Modified Mapleson A System (Lack)**

PLV   FGI

RB

ETTC

C   **Mapleson D System**

FGI

PLV

RB

ETTC

D   **Modified Mapleson D System (Bain coaxial)**

FGI

ETTC

E   **Mapleson E System (Ayre's T-piece)**

Outflow   FGI

RB   ETTC

F   **Mapleson F System (Jackson-Rees)**

Outflow   FGI

RB

ETTC

G   **Mapleson F System (Norman Mask Elbow)**

Key:
ETTC = Endotracheal tube connector
FGI = Fresh gas inlet
PLV = Pressure limiting valve
RB   = Reservoir bag
———→ = Fresh gas flow
———→ = Waste gas

FIGURE 9-39 Nonrebreathing circuits. (From Sirois M: Principles and practice of veterinary technology, ed 3, St Louis, 2011, Mosby.

canister, **pressure manometer**, and unidirectional valves are not present in a nonbreathing circuit.

Nonrebreathing circuits used in veterinary medicine include the Mapleson A (Magill and Lack circuits), modified Mapleson D (Bain coaxial circuit), Mapleson E (Ayre's T piece and Bain circuits), and Mapleson F circuits (Jackson-Rees' modification of Ayre's T-piece circuit and Norman mask elbow), and the Humphrey ADE circuit, which can switch among Mapleson A, D, and E circuits (Fig. 9-39).

ANESTHESIA

PREANESTHETIC MEDICATION

Preanesthetic medication is usually beneficial to the patient and should be considered for all patients. Selection of preanesthetics is based on the patient's health status, not on the surgical procedure. Various drugs are used for premedication, including calming agents, analgesics, and anticholinergics.

INDUCTION

A primary goal of proper anesthetic technique is to provide maximum safety for the patient and personnel (Box 9-4). Recognize that induction is short-term **general anesthesia** and induction agents are frequently used alone to perform short surgical or diagnostic procedures. When gas anesthesia is to be used, anesthetic induction is the transition from the conscious preanesthetic state to the level of anesthesia at which the patient may be intubated.

It is important to minimize or avoid personnel exposure to anesthetic waste gases (Box 9-5). Anesthetic techniques have evolved to avoid specific problems that were previously encountered. Although the consequences of error or mishap in any one step of a procedure may seem negligible, the cumulative effects of marginal technique may produce serious consequences.

BOX 9-4	Patient Positioning, Comfort, and Safety

Keep the following in mind throughout anesthetic induction and maintenance:

- Support patient's body as it is losing consciousness.
- If using an IV agent for induction and if not using an indwelling catheter, remove the needle and syringe once the animal is induced.
- Lay the animal in lateral recumbency after intubation.
- Secure the endotracheal tube before inflating the cuff.
- Constantly check for endotracheal tube patency.
- When turning the patient, temporarily disconnect the endotracheal tube to prevent trauma to the trachea.
- Ensure that the anesthetic tubing does not apply force on the endotracheal tube.
- Minimize hyperflexion and hyperextension of the neck or limbs during the procedure.
- Keep the patient warm by placing it on a heat-retaining surface.
- Do not apply pressure to the chest with instruments or restraint devices.
- Ensure that the leg restraint devices are not overly tightened.
- Put sterile lubricant in the eye initially and then every 90 minutes.
- To prevent pressure on the diaphragm, do not elevate the caudal aspect of the body more than 15 degrees.
- Record vital signs every 5 minutes throughout anesthesia as well as postoperatively.
- Constantly note reflexes and other indicators of anesthetic depth.
- Periodically, manually ventilate the lungs to help expand collapsed alveoli, keeping the reading on the pressure manometer below 20 cm H_2O.
- Know normal values and when to inform the veterinarian.
- If properly monitoring, you are noting circulation, oxygenation, and ventilation.
- Keep administering O_2 for 5 minutes after anesthetic is turned off; use mask if too light.
- Postoperatively, keep the patient warm and turn every 10 to 15 minutes.

Adapted from Sirois M: Principles and practice of veterinary technology, ed 3, St Louis, 2011, Mosby.

DRUGS FOR ANESTHETIC INDUCTION

Several methods are used for induction before inhalation anesthesia; each has its advantages and disadvantages. IV administration of the induction agent is preferred in most cases. Anesthetic induction may proceed after a vein is catheterized, the equipment is readied, and the surgeon is available. Administration of the induction or maintenance agent should provide a smooth and safe transition to unconsciousness. When jaw muscle tone and orolaryngeal reflexes are lost, intubate the patient.

ENDOTRACHEAL INTUBATION IN DOGS AND CATS

Dogs and cats are placed in a sternal position, with the head and neck extended in a straight line to aid visualization of the larynx. The veterinary assistant will position the head by grasping the maxilla behind the canine teeth while the anesthetist places the endotracheal tube. Lubrication of the cuff with sterile, water-soluble lubricant facilitates intubation and protects the tracheal mucosa from drying where the inflated cuff contacts the mucosa. Pulling the tongue forward also helps improve visualization of the glottis.

Once the tube is placed, the veterinary technician will attach the breathing circuit to the endotracheal tube adapter before inflating the cuff.

MAINTENANCE OF ANESTHESIA

Once the patient is fully anesthetized by the inhalation anesthetic, the induction period is over and the stage of maintenance anesthesia begins. The amount of anesthetic needed to maintain an appropriate level of anesthesia is not a constant. Anesthetic depth is a product of the amount of drug reaching the brain, degree of painful stimulus applied, and patient's health status . In a typical abdominal surgical procedure, minimal anesthesia is needed during the surgical preparation, moderate anesthesia during the skin incision, maximal anesthesia during the intra-abdominal phase, and

BOX 9-5	Techniques for Minimizing Exposure to Waste Anesthetic Gases

1. Check for and correct leaks in anesthesia machine and breathing circuit.
2. Use a cuffed endotracheal tube of the proper size; inflate the cuff if needed.
3. Do not disconnect the patient from the breathing circuit immediately after anesthesia; if possible, wait several minutes for gases to dissipate.
4. Connect pop-off valve to a scavenger system, preferably one that discharges outdoors.
5. Connect a nonrebreathing system to a scavenger system.
6. Avoid use of chamber or mask induction techniques.
7. Avoid spilling liquid anesthetic while filling the vaporizer; recap bottle and vaporizer immediately.
8. Maintain adequate ventilation of the area.

Adapted from Sirois M: Principles and practice of veterinary technology, ed 3, St Louis, 2011, Mosby.

moderate anesthesia during skin suturing. Hypothermia and hypotension reduce anesthetic requirements.

Once anesthesia with the inhalant agent is accomplished, the vaporizer setting and oxygen flow are reduced to maintenance levels. The anesthetist's attention now focuses on monitoring and support of vital organ function. Connect all monitoring instruments and begin recording all pertinent information on the patient's anesthetic record. Monitoring should be continuous and data should be recorded every 5 to 10 minutes, or when significant changes occur. An anesthetic record provides important documentation of your vigilance and notes adverse trends and important events occurring in the perioperative period (Fig. 9-40). A well-organized anesthetic record serves as legal documentation of anesthetic events, drug dosages used, and patient values during anesthesia and guides the actions of the anesthetist by tracking trends in cardiopulmonary function.

> **CRITICAL CONCEPT**
>
> The vaporizer setting controls where anesthetic concentration in the circuit is going; the oxygen flow rate controls how fast it will get there.

ANESTHETIC MONITORING

Comprehensive monitoring of the anesthetized patient involves observing anesthetic equipment and evaluating the central nervous system (CNS), pulmonary function, and

MONITORING	"EARLY WARNING"				RECOVERY PERIOD
Time:	10 20 30 40 50	10 20 30 40 50	10 20 30 40 50	10 20 30 40 50	
AGENTS:	ml/hr	ml/hr	ml/hr	ml/hr	TOTALS
Fluids:					Fluids:
Blood:					Blood:
Plasma:					Plasma:
Meds:					Meds:
Oxygen Flow:					Vaporizer Off:
Vaporizer Setting:					ETT Removed:
End Tidal Conc:					Sternal:
PLANE: Light … Deep					Standing

			SUPPORT
Anesthesia	A	250	1. None
		240	2. Heating
Operation	⊙	230	3. Fluids
		220	4. Oxygen
End ⊙⊗		210	5. ICU
		200	6. Other
End A	A	190	**COMPLICATIONS**
		180	1. None
Systolic P	V	170	2. Arrhythmias
		160	3. Aspiration
Diastolic P	Λ	150	4. Cardiac Arrest
		140	5. Convulsions
Mean P	X	130	6. Cyanosis
		120	7. Death
Heart Rate	•	110	8. Excitement
		100	9. Hypothermia
Resp. Rate	O	90	10. Injury
		80	11. Laryngospasm
Spont.	S	70	12. Panting
		60	13. Regurgitation
Assist.	A	50	14. Resp. Arrest
		40	15. Resp. Depression
Ventil.	V	30	16. Resp. Obstruction
		20	17. Salivation
		10	18. Other
		0	

Temperature (°F)	
E.C.G.	
pH	
Pco_2	
Po_2	
HCO_3	
Base Balance	
Event	

Complications:

1. None	5. Cardiac Arrest	9. Hyperthermia	13. Panting	17. Resp. Obstruct.
2. Apnea	6. Cyanosis	10. Hypotension	14. Regurgitation	18. Salivation
3. Arrythmias	7. Death	11. Hypothermia	15. Resp. Arrest	19. Tympany
4. Aspiration	8. Hemorrhage	12. Inadequate Relaxation	16. Resp. Depression	20. Variable Depth

Assigned to Student Clinician at:__________

Student Anesthetist:

Student Clinician:

FIGURE 9-40 This is a typical anesthetic record for recording information related to an anesthetic procedure. (From Sirois M: Principles and practice of veterinary technology, ed 3, St Louis, 2011, Mosby.)

cardiovascular function. Early detection of equipment failure and/or depression of vital organ function allow for the execution of corrective measures, which are more effective than treating complications (Box 9-6). Corrective actions to maintain or restore tissue perfusion are determined by integrating information from all body systems. Monitoring anesthesia covers a wide range of parameters and situations. It is important to "expect the unexpected."

BOX 9-6 | Monitoring of Anesthetic Equipment

1. All anesthetic equipment should be clean, calibrated, maintained in good working order, and functionally checked before and continuously throughout the procedure. Observe the oxygen source, anesthetic machine, and breathing circuit for leaks, and check that carbon dioxide absorbent is not exhausted.
2. During anesthesia, frequently check connections to the patient and anesthetic circuit. Power sources to monitoring equipment and heat sources should be verified throughout the procedure.
3. Verify monitoring device readings with quick, simple observations, such as mucous membrane color, capillary refill time, pulse rate, and pulse quality. If the blood pressure reads zero but the mucous membranes are pink and well perfused, common sense dictates that the blood pressure reading is probably incorrect.

Adapted from Sirois M: Principles and practice of veterinary technology, ed 3, St Louis, 2011, Mosby.

CRITICAL CONCEPT
The most essential monitor is a well-prepared, highly skilled individual performing continuous monitoring.

MONITORING PHYSIOLOGIC CONDITIONS
The patient's physiologic conditions are monitored to ensure that excessive derangement of vital functions is not developing. A variety of equipment is available for this purpose (Table 9-7). This process is focused on the respiratory and cardiovascular systems, and the goal is to maintain adequate delivery of oxygenated blood to the tissues or tissue perfusion.

MONITORING RESPIRATORY FUNCTION
Equipment useful for monitoring respiratory function includes a blood gas machine, **pulse oximeter** (Fig. 9-41), end-tidal carbon dioxide analyzer (capnometer), and rate monitor. Hearing, vision, and touch can be used to monitor the respiratory system and airway. Good indicators that air is moving in and out of the lungs are auscultation of

---

TABLE 9-7 | Monitoring Equipment Used in Veterinary Medicine

MONITORING DEVICE	OVERVIEW	CONCERNS
Stethoscope	Always accessible; evaluates heart rate (HR), rhythm, and sounds	More difficult to hear beat in anesthetized patient
Esophageal stethoscope	Amplifies heart beat audible from a distance, can alert to possible arrhythmia, inexpensive	Does not give quantitative information; if sounds are muffled, difficult to hear; complicated if mouth or throat surgery
Electrocardiograph	Monitors HR and rhythm	Heart can stop beating even though electrical activity continues
Pulse oximeter	Detects changes in oxygen saturation of hemoglobin by calculating the difference between levels of oxygenated and deoxygenated blood; also determines HR; during oxygenation saturation, level should be >95%; probe transmissive—place over nonpigmented skin that allows light transmission (e.g., tongue, lip) or reflective (in hollow organ; rectum or esophagus)	To help minimize signal loss, light source must be oriented toward the tissue; decreased signal strength in hypotension, hypothermia, and altered vascular resistance; inaccurate if carboxyhemoglobin or methemoglobin is present
Apnea monitor	Sensor placed between ETT connector and breathing circuit; audible beep is heard when the patient breathes and the difference in temperature between warm expired and cold inspired air is monitored; will hear an alarm if no breath for a preset time period	Increased mechanical dead space can be a problem in smaller animals if not using a special ETT connector; does not warn of inadequate respiratory depth; alarm may sound with decreased tidal volume (V_T) or hypothermic patient
Ultrasonic Doppler	Monitors HR and rhythm by detecting flow of blood through small arteries; converts into an audible beep; when combined with cuff and sphygmomanometer, can indirectly determine systolic BP; fairly accurate in dogs	Must clip hair, cover skin with ultrasonic gel, be parallel to and directly over artery, and use firm contact; if using cuff, must be 30%-50% of circumference of the extremity; manually performed so is labor-intensive; probe is expensive and easily damaged; underestimates systolic BP in cats by 15 mm Hg; prone to artifacts and technical problems such as movement, shivering, contact pressure

TABLE 9-7	Monitoring Equipment Used in Veterinary Medicine—cont'd	
MONITORING DEVICE	**OVERVIEW**	**CONCERNS**
Oscillometric BP monitor	Monitors HR and indirect BP; cuff with an internal pressure-sensing bladder is placed around tail or leg, then connected to computerized base that automatically inflates and deflates the cuff and interprets the signals sent by machine; more expensive but measures BP automatically and, in addition to systolic pressure, notes diastolic and MAP	Expensive and not as accurate in animals <7 kg; also prone to artifacts and technical problems as well as hypotension, tachycardia, and arrhythmias; best to keep the cuff at the same horizontal plane as the heart; inaccurate at low BPs
Capnometer	Determines respiratory rate and end-tidal CO_2 by estimating partial CO_2 in bloodstream at the end of expiration, when CO_2 levels of the expired gas are approximately equal to alveolar and arterial CO_2 ($Paco_2$); the fitting is placed between ETT and breathing circuit; monitor measures CO_2 in inspired and expired air; one of the best indicators of adequate respiration; levels for anesthetized patients should be 40-45 mm Hg	Abnormal readings if lung, cardiovascular, or tissue disease; hypoventilation; abnormal breathing problems; or malfunctioning equipment; interpretation of capnogram is complex; levels higher than normal indicate hypoventilation; lower levels indication of hyperventilation
Central venous pressure	Monitors hydration and efficacy of fluid therapy by inserting catheter into anterior vena cava; catheter is connected to water manometer for measurement of mean right arterial pressure	Invasive; best used in conjunction with other parameters and to monitor trends; zero mark of manometer must be at level of distal catheter tip

NOTE: If alarm signals occur when using monitoring equipment, it is important to confirm by physically examining the patient.
MAP, Mean arterial pressure.
Adapted from Sirois M: Principles and practice of veterinary technology, ed 3, St Louis, 2011, Mosby.

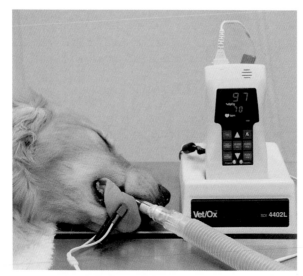

FIGURE 9-41 Pulse oximeter with transmission lingual probe. The upper number (97) represents the percentage of oxygen saturation (% SpO₂). The lower number (70) represents the heart rate (in beats/min). (From Thomas JA, Lerche P: Anesthesia and analgesia for veterinary technicians, ed 4, St Louis, 2011, Mosby.)

breathing and lung sounds using a standard or **esophageal stethoscope** (Fig. 9-42), observation of the chest wall and the reservoir bag for movement, and feeling the reservoir bag for resistance.

MONITORING CARDIOVASCULAR FUNCTION

Cardiovascular function is monitored to ensure that cardiac output and forward movement of blood are contributing to tissue perfusion. Cardiovascular function is evaluated by the heart rate, heart sounds, **pulse quality** and rate, mucous membrane color, and capillary refill time. Electrocardiography is recommended for the evaluation of rhythm and conduction disturbances. Ordinarily, smaller patients have faster heart rates than larger patients of the same species. Blood pressure, urine output, and body temperature are also indicators of cardiovascular function.

Auscultation of the heart while simultaneously palpating the peripheral pulse is an excellent method of recognizing **pulse deficits** that may result from cardiac arrhythmias. Abnormal heart rates, irregular rhythm, and weak or muffled heart sounds may indicate diminished cardiac function.

RESPONDING TO ADVERSE EVENTS

All adverse events should be brought to the veterinarian's attention immediately. Be prepared to execute the veterinarian's directives quickly and accurately. The administration of drugs to counteract specific conditions should be under the veterinarian's direction.

SURGICAL ASSISTING

The veterinary technician serves as the sterile surgical assistant and must don a sterile gown and gloves when entering the surgical suite. Care must be taken not to contaminate the gown by brushing against tables or other individuals when entering the surgical suite.

The veterinary assistant serves as the circulating assistant (nonsterile) and should be available to place needed supplies

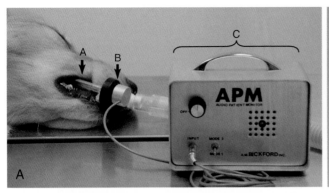
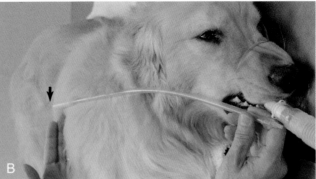

FIGURE 9-42 *A,* Esophageal stethoscope. *A,* Catheter. *B,* Sensor. *C,* Base unit. **B,** *Measurement of the catheter to the level of the fifth rib or caudal border of the scapula (arrow).* (From Thomas JA, Lerche P: Anesthesia and analgesia for veterinary technicians, ed 4, St Louis, 2011, Mosby.)

and equipment on the **Mayo stand**. This is the primary role of the veterinary assistant in surgery. All personnel should have their cap and mask on before placing sterile items on the Mayo stand. Materials should be opened facing away from the body and allowed to fall on the stand so that the assistant's arms are not directly over the top of the Mayo stand. The surgical assistant should arrange the instruments and supplies on the Mayo stand before the start of surgery. The assistant may also be responsible for operating the surgical suction and passing and holding instruments for the surgeon. A circulating (nonsterile) assistant should be present to provide any additional items that may be needed by the surgeon.

The assistant must be familiar with the procedure to be performed and be able to anticipate the instruments and supplies that the surgeon may need. Instruments should be passed to the surgeon by pressing the instrument firmly into the surgeon's hand. Instruments are usually passed so that they will be placed in the surgeon's hand in a ready-to-use position. Curved instruments are passed with their concave side up.

The veterinary assistant may also responsible for ensuring that the surgical lighting is focused on the surgical site and the site remains dry. Blotting the site gently with gauze sponges or removing excess blood and tissue fluid can be used to accomplish this task. When a body cavity is opened, sponges should be counted at the beginning of the procedure (before the first incision) and before closure to ensure that none have been inadvertently left in the body cavity. Contaminated instruments or soiled sponges should not be placed back on the instrument table. Surgical assistants may also be required to hold clamps on tissues or vessels. Always handle tissues gently and keep tissues moistened with sterile saline when they are removed from body cavities.

DRAPING AND ORGANIZING THE INSTRUMENT TABLE
ORGANIZING THE INSTRUMENT TABLE
Instrument tables should be height-adjustable to allow them to be positioned within reach of surgical personnel. The instrument packs should not be opened until the animal has been positioned on the surgical table and draped.

Large, water-impermeable table drapes should be used to cover the entire instrument table. To open these drapes, the drape and outer wrap are positioned on the instrument table, the exposed undersurface of the drape is gently grasped, and the ends and then the sides are unfolded. Once the drape has been opened, nonsterile personnel should not reach over it. Mayo stands are often used in procedures that require additional instruments (e.g., bone plating); specially designed Mayo stand covers are available to cover these tables. When the instrument pack has been opened, instruments should be positioned so that they can be readily retrieved. The instrument layout is generally determined by the surgeon's preference, but grouping similar instruments (e.g., scissors, retractors) facilitates their use.

DRAPING
Once the animal has been positioned and the skin prepared, the animal is ready to be draped. The drapes maintain a sterile field around the operative site. If electrocautery is being used, sufficient time should elapse between skin preparation and application of the drapes to permit complete evaporation of flammable substances (e.g., alcohol) from the skin. If an abdominal incision extends to the pubis in males, the prepuce should be clamped to one side with a sterile towel clamp.

Draping is performed by a gowned and gloved surgical team member (veterinarian and/or veterinary technician) and begins with placement of field drapes (quarter drapes) to isolate the unprepared portion of the animal. These towels should be placed one at a time at the periphery of the prepared area. Field (quarter) drapes may be lint-free towels or disposable nonabsorbent towels. Drapes should not be flipped, fanned, or shaken, because rapid movement of drapes creates air currents onto which dust, lint, and droplet nuclei can migrate. Drapes, supplies, and equipment extending over or dropping below the table level should be considered nonsterile because they are not within the surgeon's visual field and their sterility cannot be verified. Towels are secured at the corners with Backhaus towel clamps (Fig. 9-43). When the animal and incision site are protected by field drapes, final draping can be performed. A large drape is placed over

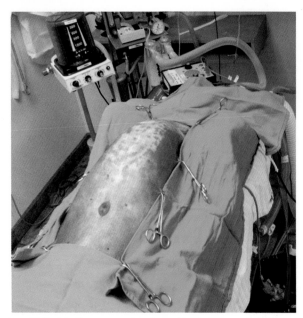

FIGURE 9-43 The patient is positioned for thoracic and abdominal incisions. Field drapes are secured at the corners and midpoints with towel clamps. (From Sirois M: Principles and practice of veterinary technology, ed 3, St Louis, 2011, Mosby.)

the animal by the veterinarian or veterinary technician and entire surgical table to provide a continuous sterile field. Cloth drapes should have an appropriately sized and positioned opening that can be placed over the incision site while the drape covers the remaining surfaces.

UNWRAPPING OR OPENING STERILE ITEMS
UNWRAPPING STERILE LINEN OR PAPER PACKS

If you are right-handed, hold the pack in your left hand (and vice versa). Using the right hand, unfold one corner of the outside wrap at a time, being careful to secure each corner in the palm of the left hand to keep it from recoiling and contaminating the contents. Hold the final corner with your right hand. When the pack is fully exposed and all corners of the wrap secured, gently pass the pack to sterile personnel or set the pack on the table cover, being careful not to allow your hand and arm to reach across or over the sterile field.

UNWRAPPING STERILE ITEMS IN PAPER OR PLASTIC OR PLASTIC PEEL-BACK POUCHES

Identify the edges of the peel-back wrapper and carefully separate them. Peel the edges of the wrapper back slowly and symmetrically to ensure that the sterile item does not contact the torn edge of the wrapper, which is nonsterile. If the item is small, place it on the sterile area as described, being careful not to lean across the sterile table. If the item is long or cumbersome, have a sterile team member grasp it and gently pull it from the peel-back wrapper, taking care not to brush the item against the peeled edge of the wrapper. Packages containing scalpel blades and suture material are opened similarly.

RECOVERY

Recovery means to restore to a normal state; it begins when the administration of anesthetic is discontinued. Pain relief and maintenance of a patent airway are important during recovery. The critical period has passed when the body temperature is normal, sternal recumbency is achieved, and oropharyngeal reflexes are restored. However, observation should continue until the patient can stand and is free of all drug effects.

When recovering, the patient should be maintained on 100% oxygen to ensure oxygenation and allow exhaled anesthetic gases to enter the scavenger system rather than the room air. As the patient begins to awaken, the endotracheal tube cuff should be deflated and the tie undone. When the patient exhibits swallowing reflexes, the tube should be gently removed. Close observation is essential immediately after extubation because the patient may regurgitate or have difficulty breathing. Brachycephalic dogs are especially notorious for developing breathing difficulties after extubation.

Fluid administration should continue until recovery is adequate. Premature removal of the IV catheter may result in the inability to administer IV medications quickly in the event of an emergency. Recovery is considered adequate, but not complete, when the body temperature is normal, the patient's vital signs are stable, and sternal recumbency is maintained. Observation should continue until the patient can stand and walk without assistance.

POSTOPERATIVE EVALUATION

The postoperative period should be considered critical for all patients. Because of the possibility of unforeseen complications, it is essential that patients be continually monitored after any type of surgery.

BODY TEMPERATURE

After surgery, every patient should have its rectal temperature measured hourly until it reaches 100° F (37.8° C) and then every 4 to 12 hours based on orders prepared by the doctor. A 1° or 2° F increase in rectal temperature for the first few postoperative days is a normal physiologic response to the trauma of major surgery. A higher or more prolonged temperature increase may indicate infection.

BODY WEIGHT

Daily monitoring of a surgical patient's body weight provides a measure of the animal's nutritional status and general body condition. One of the most frequently neglected aspects of postoperative patient care is provision of adequate nutrition. The healing process after surgery increases an animal's nutritional needs, particularly for protein. Those needs must be met so that healing can proceed without delay.

ATTITUDE

An animal's behavior during the immediate postoperative period can yield important information about the amount of pain it is enduring and possible complications that might be developing. If a patient is depressed, the reasons for that state must be determined and appropriate treatment quickly instituted.

APPETITE AND THIRST

Surgical patients must receive adequate nutrition and fluid intake. Animals should begin eating and drinking as soon as possible after surgery. Opioid medications used for pain control may reduce appetite, so encouragement or temptation to eat is sometimes needed by postoperative patients. A genuine lack of interest in food or obvious nausea may indicate problems that should be investigated without delay.

URINATION AND DEFECATION

Elimination patterns provide important information about kidney and GI tract function in patients recovering from surgery. GI motility and defecation may be reduced if opioids are used for pain management, but this should resolve within 1 or 2 days of discontinuing the medications. Assuming adequate fluid intake, urination should proceed normally.

APPEARANCE OF THE SURGICAL WOUND

The surgical incision should be examined at least daily during the immediate postoperative period. It should be evaluated by visual inspection as well as gentle palpation. Abnormalities such as excessive or prolonged bleeding, fluid accumulation, dramatic inflammation, and impending dehiscence (opening) of the surgical wound can be detected and corrected early if the incision is carefully evaluated.

PAIN MANAGEMENT

Pain is defined as an unpleasant sensory or emotional experience associated with actual or potential tissue damage. Physiologic pain results from the stimulation of nerve endings called nociceptors, which are found throughout the tissues (Fig. 9-44). Pain may be classified as peripheral, neuropathic, clinical, or idiopathic. Pain causes many deleterious effects on the body, possibly affecting each of the systems (Box 9-7).

Nociception is different from pain. General anesthesia controls the perception of intraoperative pain. Unconsciousness or unresponsiveness is not lack of pain; nociception still occurs. Anesthetics vary in analgesic efficiency and may not completely disrupt the nociceptive mechanisms of the nervous system. This is why it is important to check the depth of anesthesia and monitor the patient closely, using the response to painful stimuli.

Pain recognition is difficult because responses to pain vary among species and individuals. Some individuals tolerate considerable discomfort without any reaction. Other individuals vocalize loudly when given a minor injection. Anticipation of possible pain enters into the animal's response as well. It is helpful to know the normal behavior of the individual when assessing for pain (Box 9-8). Obvious inflammation (e.g., redness, swelling, heat) is generally accompanied by pain. Animals recovering from anesthesia are not able to exhibit a normal range of behavioral signs and may be experiencing pain long before it becomes apparent to the observer. Research guidelines indicate that any condition that would cause pain in humans should be assumed to cause pain in animals. Accordingly, we assume

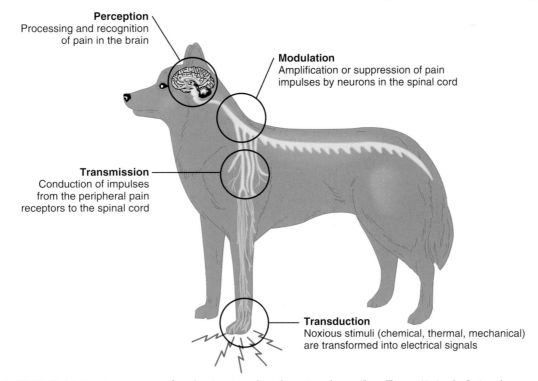

Perception
Processing and recognition of pain in the brain

Modulation
Amplification or suppression of pain impulses by neurons in the spinal cord

Transmission
Conduction of impulses from the peripheral pain receptors to the spinal cord

Transduction
Noxious stimuli (chemical, thermal, mechanical) are transformed into electrical signals

FIGURE 9-44 Nociception—site of analgesic action along the pain pathway. (From Thomas JA, Lerche P: Anesthesia and analgesia for veterinary technicians, ed 4, St Louis, 2011, Mosby.)

BOX 9-7	Effects of Clinical Pain

1. Immunosuppression
2. Increased tissue catabolism
3. Reduced healing
4. Increased autonomic activity, primarily sympathetic
5. Emotional stress, distress

From Sirois M: Principles and practice of veterinary technology, ed 3, St Louis, 2011, Mosby.

BOX 9-8	Signs of Pain

1. Changes in behavior and temperament (e.g., shunning or seeking attention, postural changes, inappetence, changes in voiding behavior, reluctance to move, unusual gait)
2. Protection of the affected area (avoids touching; threatens if approached)
3. Vocalization (especially on movement or palpation of affected area)
4. Licking or biting affected area
5. Scratching or shaking affected area
6. Restlessness, pacing
7. Sweating
8. Tachycardia, hyperpnea, peripheral vasoconstriction, muscle tension, hypertension

From Sirois M: Principles and practice of veterinary technology, ed 3, St Louis, 2011, Mosby.

that a dog undergoing abdominal surgery would experience as much pain as a person would experience from a comparable procedure, even if the dog does not exhibit signs of pain. It has been demonstrated that pain is more easily managed if analgesics are given preemptively, before a patient experiences pain. To assess the patient properly, it is essential that a comprehensive and thorough history and physical assessment be completed.

PAIN RELIEF MODALITIES

Pain relief modalities take advantage of one or more means of preventing or interfering with the development or perception of pain. Refinement of surgical technique to produce less tissue damage will prevent a great deal of postoperative pain. For example, proponents of laser surgery have reported that postoperative pain is greatly reduced. To the extent that some tissue trauma is inevitable in any surgical procedure, a variety of pain management modalities may be used before, during, and after the procedure to manage the type and level of pain experienced at that time.

ANALGESIA. Most of the drugs used for **analgesia** cause various other dose-dependent effects. The opioid analgesic agents produce a dose-dependent **sedation** (called **narcosis**) that may be profound. The nonsteroidal anti-inflammatory drugs (NSAIDs), especially the older ones, have a tendency to cause GI irritation, ulceration, and bleeding. Newer analgesic agents are designed to have fewer adverse side effects.

Analgesic agents are needed to suppress the physiologic pain mechanisms that remain active during anesthesia. These will also allow a reduction in the dosage of general anesthetic needed to maintain anesthesia. In human anesthesiology, there have been recent reports of awareness of sound and pain by apparently anesthetized patients. Postoperatively, they are able to repeat conversations overheard during their procedure and describe the experience of searing pain. It is not fully understood whether this situation occurs in anesthetized animals or how to recognize it if it does.

CRITICAL CONCEPT

Using several analgesic drugs, each with a different mechanism of action, is called multimodal therapy. This results in lower dosages, which increases safety.

POSTOPERATIVE COMPLICATIONS

HEMORRHAGE

If not quickly corrected, postoperative hemorrhage can lead to serious consequences for an animal, even death from shock. External hemorrhage is usually relatively easy to evaluate and control because it is easily visible. Internal hemorrhage is not readily apparent and, therefore, often more serious. An animal can bleed to death through hemorrhage into the abdominal or thoracic cavity. The status of an animal's cardiovascular system should be frequently monitored during the immediate postoperative period for signs that might indicate hemorrhage. Pulse rate, capillary refill time, temperature of the extremities, and color of the mucous membranes can provide valuable information about cardiovascular function.

SEROMA AND HEMATOMA

Seromas (accumulations of serum) and hematomas (accumulations of blood) beneath the surgical incision are usually caused by dead space left in the incision that the body naturally fills with fluid. Small seromas and hematomas are usually of cosmetic importance only, unless the skin sutures tear out. Treatment may not be indicated in cases of small seroma or hematoma; observation only may be used to gauge resolution. Larger seromas or hematomas may be treated with warm compresses, drainage of the fluid via needle and syringe, and possibly application of a pressure bandage.

INFECTION

A persistently or drastically elevated rectal temperature, depressed attitude, poor appetite, or swollen, inflamed incision are all signs of possible postoperative infection.

Postoperative infections can be superficial, subcutaneous, within a body cavity, or spread throughout the body. Superficial infection often results in a draining wound that does not heal well. Subcutaneous infections frequently progress to abscess formation. Infection in the abdominal cavity (**peritonitis**) or thoracic cavity (pleuritis) often results from a penetrating injury or damage to organs in that body cavity. Septicemia is a generalized infection that spreads via the bloodstream. Fortunately, septicemia is not common after surgery. When the danger of postoperative infection is high, as with long or potentially contaminated procedures, the patient may be given an antibiotic during and/or following surgery.

WOUND DEHISCENCE

Wound dehiscence (disruption of the surgical wound) is one of the most common and serious postoperative complications that can occur. Possible causes of wound dehiscence include the following:

- Suture failure (loosening, untying, breakage)
- Infection
- Tissue weakness (e.g., old or debilitated animals, hyperadrenocorticism, prolonged corticosteroid use)
- Mechanical stress (e.g., stormy anesthetic recovery, chronic vomiting, chronic cough, excessive activity)
- Poor nutrition

Early signs of surgical wound dehiscence are frequently seen within the first 3 or 4 days after surgery. They may include a serosanguineous discharge from the incision, firm or fluctuant swelling deep to (under) the suture line, and palpation of a hernial ring or loop of bowel beneath the skin.

If only the muscle layer of an abdominal incision breaks down and the skin sutures remain intact, a doughy swelling can be palpated under the skin. This is a serious situation but not an acute emergency. A bandage should be applied for support and the suture line should be repaired as soon as possible.

If both the muscle layer and skin sutures of an abdominal incision break down, the animal can **eviscerate** (abdominal organs protrude through suture line). If evisceration occurs, the involved organs can become bruised and grossly contaminated, and may even be mutilated by the animal itself. This is an acute emergency that must be attended to immediately. Carefully gather the exteriorized viscera in a towel moistened with physiologic saline and hold them in place near the incision while others prepare the animal and OR for the repair.

SUTURE REMOVAL

Skin incisions are often closed with nonabsorbable suture material. These sutures are removed once healing is sufficient to prevent wound dehiscence, usually after 10 to 14 days. However, delayed healing, as in debilitated animals, may require that sutures be left in place for longer periods. Additionally, if fibrosis is desired (e.g., aural hematoma), delayed suture removal may be considered.

Skin suture removal is begun by grasping one or both of the suture ends, which were deliberately left long for that purpose, and pulling the knot away from the skin (Fig. 9-45). Using suture removal scissors, cut one of the two strands of suture beneath the knot at the skin surface and pull the suture out. It is important that only one of the strands be cut to avoid leaving some of the suture material buried beneath the skin, where it could act as an irritant. Skin staples are removed with specially designed staple removers (Fig. 9-46).

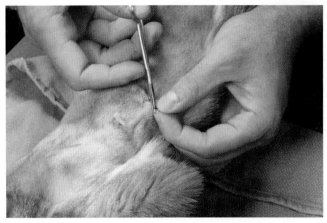

FIGURE 9-45 Suture removal. (From Sirois M: Principles and practice of veterinary technology, ed 3, St Louis, 2011, Mosby.)

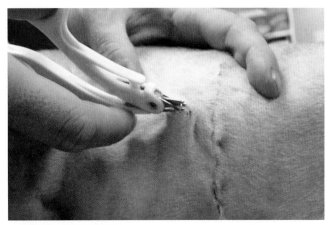

FIGURE 9-46 Skin staple removal. (From Sirois M: Principles and practice of veterinary technology, ed 3, St Louis, 2011, Mosby.)

RECOMMENDED READINGS

American College of Veterinary Anesthesiologists: Commentary and recommendations on control of waste anesthetic gases in the workplace, *J Am Vet Med Assoc* 209:75–77, 1996.

Bassert JM, McCurnin DM: *McCurnin's clinical textbook for veterinary technicians,* ed 7, St Louis, 2010, Saunders.

Doherty T, Valverde A, editors: *Manual of equine anaesthesia and analgesia,* Blackwell, 2006, Oxford, England.

Mathews KA: Pain assessment and general approach to management, *Vet Clin North Am Small Animal Pract* 30:729–755, 2000.

Muir WW, Hubbell JAE: *Equine anesthesia,* ed 2, St Louis, 2009, Mosby.

Muir WW, Hubbell JAE, Skarda R, et al.: *Handbook of veterinary anesthesia,* ed 4, St Louis, 2007, Mosby.

Riebold TW: *Large animal anesthesia: principles and techniques,* ed 2, Ames, IA 1995, Iowa State University Press.

Shaffran N: Defining pain in dogs and cats, *Vet Tech J,* August 2002.

Short CE: *Principles and practice of veterinary anesthesia,* Baltimore, 1987, Williams & Wilkins.

Sonsthagen TF: *Veterinary instruments and equipment: a pocket guide,* St Louis, 2011, Mosby.

Tear M: *Small animal surgical nursing: skills and concepts,* ed 2, St Louis, 2012, Mosby.

Thomas JA, Lerche P: *Anesthesia and analgesia for veterinary technicians,* ed 4, St Louis, 2011, Mosby.

Thurmon JC, Tranquilli WJ: *Lumb and Jones' veterinary anesthesia,* ed 3, Baltimore, 1996, Williams & Wilkins.

Thurmon JC, Tranquilli WJ, Benson GJ: *Essentials of small animal anesthesia and analgesia,* Philadelphia, 1999, Lippincott.

Tranquilli WJ, Thurmon JC, Grimm KA: *Teton NewMedia. Pain management for the small animal practitioner,* WI, 2000, Jackson.

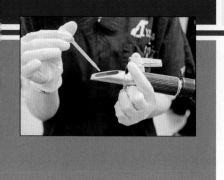

10 Laboratory Procedures[1]

OUTLINE

Laboratory Design, *285*
General Considerations, *285*
Safety Concerns and Supplies, *286*
Laboratory Measurements and Mathematics, *286*
Dilutions, *287*
Equipment and Instrumentation, *287*
Microscope, *287*
Centrifuge, *289*
Refractometer, *290*
Chemistry Analyzers, *291*
Hematology Analyzers, *293*
Incubators, *295*
Pipettes, *295*
Miscellaneous Equipment and Supplies, *296*
Quality Assurance, *296*
Laboratory Records, *297*
Internal Records, *297*
External Records, *297*
Hematology Examination Procedures, *297*
Sample Collection, *297*
Sample Type, *298*
Complete Blood Count, *299*
Coagulation Testing, *303*
Clinical Chemistry, *305*
Hepatobiliary Function Testing, *305*
Enzyme Analyses, *306*
Kidney Function Testing, *306*
Pancreatic Function Testing, *306*
Other Serum Assays, *307*

Basic Principles of Immunology, *308*
Immunologic Tests, *308*
Common Errors and Artifacts, *310*
Microbiology, *310*
Characteristics of Bacteria, *311*
Mycology, *311*
Sample Collection, *311*
Sample Processing Materials, *313*
Culture Media, *313*
Stains, *314*
Procedures, *314*
Biochemical Test Materials, *315*
Quality Control Concerns, *315*
Cytology, *315*
Collection and Preparation of Samples from Tissues and Masses, *316*
Collection and Preparation of Fluid Samples, *317*
Examination of Cytology Specimens, *317*
Histology, *317*
Urinalysis, *317*
Sample Collection, *318*
Complete Urinalysis, *318*
Parasitology, *319*
Classification of Parasites, *320*
Diagnostic Techniques, *328*
Sample Collection and Handling, *330*
Evaluation of Fecal Specimens, *330*
Evaluation of Blood Samples, *334*

LEARNING OBJECTIVES

After reviewing this chapter, the reader will be able to:

1. Describe methods used to collect samples for laboratory examination.
2. Describe the preparation of diagnostic samples for laboratory examination.
3. List and describe common procedures used for hematologic examinations.
4. List and describe methods for evaluation of hemostasis in dogs and cats.
5. List and describe equipment needed for clinical chemistry and serology testing.

[1]Elsevier and the author acknowledge and appreciate the original contributions from Sirois M: Principles and practice of veterinary technology, ed 3, St Louis, 2011, Mosby, and Hendrix CM, Sirois M: Laboratory procedures for veterinary technicians, ed 5, St Louis, 2007, Mosby, whose work forms the heart of this chapter.

LEARNING OBJECTIVES—cont'd

6. List and describe the types of tests used in clinical chemistry testing.
7. List the biochemical assays commonly performed to asses liver, kidney, and pancreatic function.
8. List the types of immunologic tests and describe the test principles used in those tests.
9. Discuss methods used to verify the accuracy of laboratory test results.
10. List and describe methods used to collect samples of body tissues and fluids for laboratory examination.

11. List and describe microbiologic tests commonly performed to identify bacterial and fungal pathogens.
12. List tests commonly performed for analyzing urine specimens.
13. List common internal parasites of dogs and cats.
14. List common external parasites of dogs and cats.
15. Describe procedures used to diagnose parasites.

KEY TERMS

Acariasis	Dermatophyte	Icterus	Polychromasia
Arthropod	Differential white blood cell	Intermediate host	Precision
Azotemia	count	Lipemia	Preprandial samples
Bacilli	Ectoparasite	Microfilaria	Refractometer
Centesis	Electrolyte	Mycology	Specific gravity
Cestode	ELISA	Myiasis	Thrombocyte
Cocci	Endoparasite	Oocyst	Trematode
Control serum	Granulocyte	Packed cell volume	Urolithiasis
Definitive host	Hemolysis	Pediculosis	Warble

Veterinarians depend on laboratory results to help establish diagnoses, track the course of diseases, and offer prognoses to clients. Veterinary assistants are often involved in aiding the veterinary technician with the collection and preparation of samples. The veterinary assistant must have a thorough knowledge of procedures and equipment used, as well as general knowledge about the tests performed.

The veterinary practice laboratory can be a significant source of income for the practice. Rapid availability of test results improves patient care and client service. Although some veterinary clinics use outside reference laboratories for test results, this may delay the implementation of appropriate treatment for patients. Most diagnostic tests can be performed in-house by the well-educated veterinary support staff. Veterinary practice laboratories have become increasingly sophisticated. Analytic instruments are affordable and readily available for inclusion in even the smallest veterinary clinic.

LABORATORY DESIGN

GENERAL CONSIDERATIONS

The veterinary clinical laboratory should be located in an area that is separate from other hospital operations (Fig. 10-1). The area must be well lit and large enough to accommodate laboratory equipment, as well as provide a comfortable work area. Countertop space must be sufficient so that sensitive equipment such as chemistry analyzers and cell counters can be physically separated from centrifuges and water baths.

Room temperature controls should provide a consistent environment, which in turn provides for optimal quality control. A draft-free area is preferable to one with open windows or with air conditioning or heating ducts blowing air onto the area. Drafts can carry dust, which may contaminate specimens and interfere with test results. Although each veterinary practice is unique, every practice laboratory has certain components, including a sink, storage space, electrical supply, and Internet access.

SINK

The laboratory area needs a sink and a source of running water to provide a place to rinse, drain, and/or stain specimens and reagents and to discard fluids. In every veterinary practice, caution should be paramount; handling and

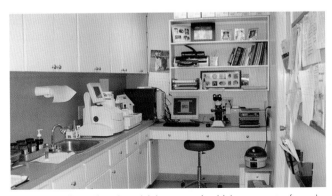

FIGURE 10-1 The clinical laboratory should be separate from the main traffic flow in the clinic. (From Hendrix CM, Sirois M: Laboratory procedures for veterinary technicians, ed 5, St Louis, 2007, Mosby.)

disposing of hazardous laboratory materials entail legal and ethical responsibilities that have increased substantially in recent decades. Certain basic laboratory practices are essential for the protection of workers and environment. Some of these practices are simply good laboratory hygiene, whereas federal, state, and local regulations have mandated others. A thorough understanding of these laws is at the foundation of proper laboratory practices regarding hazardous chemicals and specimens. When in doubt, never dispose of unknown reagents or chemicals down any sink drain.

STORAGE SPACE

Adequate storage space must be available for reagents and supplies to avoid clutter on the laboratory counter space. Drawers and cabinets should be available so that needed supplies and equipment are conveniently located near the site at which they will be used. Some reagents and specimens must be kept refrigerated or frozen. A refrigerator and freezer should be readily available. A compact counter-top refrigerator is sufficient for most practice laboratories. Frost-free freezers remove fluid from frozen samples, making them more concentrated if they are left in the freezer too long. For long-term storage of fluid samples (e.g., serum, plasma), a chest freezer or freezer that is not self-defrosting should be used.

ELECTRICAL SUPPLY

Placement of electrical equipment requires careful consideration. Sufficient electrical outlets and circuit breakers must be available. Circuits must not be overloaded with ungrounded three-prong adapters or extension cords. Avoid working with fluids around electrical wires or instruments. An uninterruptible power supply may be necessary if sensitive equipment will be used or if the practice is located in an area subject to frequent power outages.

INTERNET ACCESS

The diagnostic laboratory of the 21st-century veterinary clinic should have Internet access in the laboratory or at another location in the veterinary clinic. Many reference laboratories use e mail or fax to report the critical results of submitted diagnostic tests. Photographic images such as scanned microscopic images of blood smears and urine sediments may be sent as e mail attachments to an outside reference laboratory for diagnostic assistance.

The Internet also may be a valuable resource for veterinary medical information. However, information on the Internet may be oversimplified, incomplete, or even inaccurate. Two basic determinants are used to assess website quality. First, high-quality Internet sites are unbiased—the group providing the information should not have a vested interest (e.g., selling a product) in slanting the information a certain way. Second, sources should be staffed by recognized experts in the field, such as those from a government agency, college, or university diagnostic laboratory, or the American Veterinary Medical Association.

Other signs of the quality of a website include the following:
- Funding and sponsorship are clearly shown.
- Timeliness (date of posting, revising, and updating) is clear and easy to locate.
- Information about the source (e.g., the organization's mission statement) is clear and easy to find.
- Authors or contributors to references on the site are clearly identified.
- References and sources for information are listed.
- Experts have reviewed the site's content for accuracy and completeness.

Box 10-1 summarizes some important criteria for the evaluation of Internet resources.

SAFETY CONCERNS AND SUPPLIES

A comprehensive laboratory safety program is essential for ensuring the safety of employees in the clinical laboratory area. The Occupational Safety and Health Administration (OSHA) mandates specific laboratory practices that must be incorporated into the laboratory safety policy. The safety policy should include procedures and precautions for the use and maintenance of equipment. Safety equipment and supplies, such as eyewash stations, fire extinguishers, spill clean-up kits, hazardous and biohazard waste disposal containers, and protective gloves, must be available. All employees working in the clinical laboratory must be aware of the location of these items and thoroughly trained in their use. Laboratory safety policies must be in writing and placed in an accessible location in the clinical laboratory area. Signs should be posted to notify employees that eating, drinking, applying cosmetics, and adjusting contact lenses in the laboratory are prohibited. Chapter 1 contains more information regarding safety procedures.

LABORATORY MEASUREMENTS AND MATHEMATICS

Veterinary staff members must have knowledge and skill to perform a variety of calculations in the clinical laboratory. Reagent solutions might need to be prepared or diluted, samples must be measured and sometimes diluted, and results

---

BOX 10-1	Evaluation Criteria for Internet Sources

- Authority: Who is the author? Does the author list his or her occupation and credentials?
- Affiliation: What company or organization sponsors the site?
- Currency: When was the information created or updated?
- Purpose: What is the purpose of the site (inform, persuade, explain)?
- Audience: Who is the intended audience?
- Comparison: How does the information compare with other similar works?
- Conclusion: Is this site appropriate for research?

From Sirois M: Principles and practice of veterinary technology, ed 3, St Louis, 2011, Mosby.

must be calculated. All these mathematical operations require a thorough understanding of the metric system, as well as a strong background in basic algebra. Chapter 5 contains more information on metric system units.

DILUTIONS

It may be necessary to prepare dilutions of reagents or patient samples in the clinical laboratory. Concentrations of dilutions are usually expressed as ratios of the original volume to the new volume. A ratio is the amount of one number relative to another or the number of parts relative to a whole. Ratios may be written in a number of ways—for example, $\frac{1}{2} = 1:2 = 0.5$. These terms express the ratio that is one in two, or one to two, or one half. All three ratios are equal. The terms of a ratio are abstract numbers (no units) or of the same unit. The only ratio usually expressed as a decimal in veterinary technology is specific gravity. Specific gravity is a ratio expressed in decimal form that represents the weight of a substance relative to the weight of the same volume of water.

To prepare a 1:10 dilution of a patient sample, combine 10 microliters (μL) of sample with 90 μL of distilled water. This represents a dilution that is 10:100, which reduces mathematically to 1:10. Results from any tests on this 1:10 dilution must then be multiplied by 10 to yield the correct result for the undiluted sample.

Serial dilutions are sometimes needed when performing certain immunologic tests or when preparing manual calibration curves for some equipment. The dilutions are prepared as described, and the concentration of substance in each dilution is calculated. For example, if a standard solution of bilirubin contains 20 mg/dL and is diluted 1:5, 1:10, and 1:20, the concentration of each dilution would then be 4 mg/dL, 2 mg/dL, and 1 mg/dL, respectively.

EQUIPMENT AND INSTRUMENTATION

The size of the veterinary practice and the tests routinely performed in the laboratory determine the equipment and instrumentation needed. Minimal equipment includes a microscope, **refractometer**, microhematocrit centrifuge, and clinical centrifuge. Additional instrumentation needed, including blood chemistry analyzers, cell counters, and incubators, depends on the type and size of the practice, geographic location of the practice, and special interests of practice personnel.

> ### CRITICAL CONCEPT
> With proper care, a high-quality microscope will last a lifetime.

MICROSCOPE

A high-quality binocular, compound, light microscope is essential, even in the smallest laboratory (Fig. 10-2). It may be used to evaluate blood, urine, semen, exudates, and transudates, other body fluids, feces, and other miscellaneous specimens. It also may be used to detect internal and external parasites and initially characterize bacteria. Ideally, the practice should maintain two microscopes. One should be used for performing routine parasite studies and procedures that use corrosive or damaging materials. The second microscope should be reserved for use with cytology and hematology evaluations.

A compound light microscope is so named because it generates an image by using a combination of lenses. Compound light microscopes have many components and a light path. The mechanical stage holds a glass slide to be evaluated. The microscope should have a smoothly operating mechanical stage to allow easier manipulation of the sample. Left- or right-handed stages are generally available. Coarse- and fine-focus knobs are used to focus the image of the object being viewed.

The compound light microscope consists of two separate lens systems, the ocular system and the objective system. The ocular lenses are located in the eyepieces and most often have a magnification of 10×. This means that the ocular lens magnifies an object 10 times. A monocular microscope has one eyepiece, whereas a binocular microscope, the most commonly used type, has two eyepieces. A binocular head is needed for almost all routine laboratory evaluations. Most compound light microscopes have three or four objective lenses, each with a different magnification power. The most common objective lenses are 4× (scanning), 10× (low power), 40× (high dry), and 100× (oil immersion). The scanning lens is not found on all microscopes.

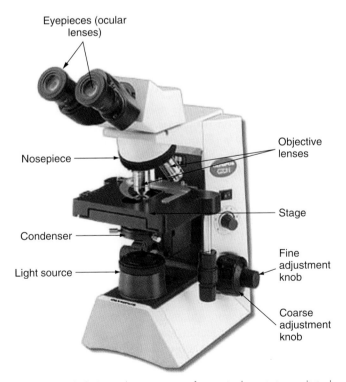

FIGURE 10-2 Binocular microscope for use in the veterinary clinical laboratory. (From Sirois M: Principles and practice of veterinary technology, ed 3, St Louis, 2011, Mosby.)

An optional fifth lens, a 50× (low oil immersion), is found on some microscopes.

Total magnification of the object being viewed is calculated by multiplying the ocular magnification power by the objective magnification power. For example, an object viewed under the 40× objective through a 10× ocular lens is 400 times larger in diameter than the unmagnified object:

$$10 \times \text{(ocular lens)} \times 40 \times \text{(objective lens)} = 400 \times \text{(total magnification)}$$

The microscope head supports the ocular lenses and may be straight or inclined. A microscope with an inclined head has ocular lenses that point back toward the user. This minimizes the need to bend over the microscope to look through the lenses. The nosepiece holds the objective lenses and should always rotate easily and provide ready access to the objective lenses for cleaning.

CRITICAL CONCEPT

Total magnification of the object being viewed is calculated by multiplying the ocular magnification power and the objective magnification power.

When viewed through a compound light microscope, an object appears upside down and reversed. The actual right side of an image is seen as its left side, and the actual left side is seen as its right side. Movement of the slide by the mechanical stage also is reversed. Travel knobs are used to move the glass slide and thus the object (or portion of the object) to be moved. When the stage is moved to the left, the object appears to move to the right.

The substage condenser consists of two lenses that focus light from the light source onto the object being viewed. Light is focused by raising or lowering the condenser. Without a substage condenser, haloes and fuzzy rings appear around the object. The aperture diaphragm is usually an iris type, consisting of a number of leaves that are opened or closed to control the amount of light illuminating the object.

In modern microscopes, the light source is contained within the microscope. The most common light sources found on compound light microscopes are low-voltage tungsten lamps or higher-quality quartz halogen lamps. The light source can be in the base or separate and should have a rheostat to adjust intensity.

USE, CARE, AND MAINTENANCE

Regardless of the features of the individual microscope, care must be taken to follow manufacturer's recommendations for use and routine maintenance (Procedure 10-1). Only high-quality lens tissue should be used to clean the lenses. If cleaning solvent is needed, methanol can be used or a specially formulated lens cleaning solution can be purchased. Excess oil may require the use of xylene for cleaning. However, xylene may also dissolve some of the adhesive used to

---

PROCEDURE 10-1 OPERATING THE MICROSCOPE

1. Lower the stage to its lowest point.
2. Turn on the light.
3. Inspect the eyepieces, objectives, and condenser lens and clean as necessary. (Consult the manufacturer's operating manual for any special cleaning instructions.)
4. Place the slide or counting chamber on the stage, appropriate side up.
5. Move the 10× objective into position by turning the turret, not the objective lens.
6. While looking through the eyepieces, adjust the distance between them so that each field appears almost identical and the two fields can be viewed as one.
7. Use the coarse and fine focus knobs to bring the image into focus.
8. Adjust the condenser and diaphragms according to the manufacturer's instructions. This allows full advantage of the microscope's resolving power.
9. When using the 40× (high-dry) objective:
   - Look for a suitable examination area using the 10× (low-power) objective.
   - Swing the high-dry objective into place.
   - Do not use oil on the slide when using the high-dry objective.
10. When using the 100× (oil immersion) objective:
    - Locate a suitable examination area using the 10× (low-power) objective.
    - Place a drop of oil on the slide.
    - Swing the oil immersion objective into place.
11. When finished:
    - Turn the light off.
    - Lower the stage completely.
    - Swing the 43× or 103× objective into place.
    - Remove the slide or counting chamber.
    - Clean the oil immersion lens if necessary.

Adapted from Hendrix CM, Sirois M: Laboratory procedures for veterinary technicians, ed 5, St Louis, 2007, Mosby.

---

secure the objective lenses and must therefore be used sparingly. Note that methanol and xylene are flammable and toxic. The microscope should be wiped clean after each use and kept covered when not in use. A dirty field of study may be caused by debris on the eyepiece. The eyepieces should be rotated one at a time while looking through them. If the debris also rotates, it is located on the eyepiece. The eyepiece is cleaned with lens paper. Cleaning and adjustment by a microscope professional should be performed at least annually.

Extra light bulbs should be available. Changing a light bulb requires turning off the power and unplugging the microscope. When the defective bulb has cooled, it should be removed and replaced with a new bulb according to the manufacturer's instructions. Replacement bulbs should be identical to those that they are replacing. Avoid touching the replacement bulb directly because oils from the skin can shorten the life of the bulbs.

Locate the microscope in an area in which it is protected from excessive heat and humidity. With proper care, a high-quality microscope can last a lifetime. The microscope should be placed in an area where it cannot be moved frequently, jarred by vibrations from centrifuges or slamming doors, or splashed with liquids. It must be kept away from sunlight and drafts. The microscope is carried with both hands, one hand securely under the base and the other holding the supporting arm.

CENTRIFUGE

Another vital instrument in the veterinary practice laboratory is the centrifuge. The centrifuge is used to separate substances of different densities that are in a solution. When solid and liquid components are present in the sample, the liquid portion is referred to as the supernatant and the solid component is referred to as the sediment. The supernatant, such as plasma or serum from a blood sample, can be removed from the sediment and stored, shipped, or analyzed. Veterinary practice laboratories often have more than one type of centrifuge. The microhematocrit centrifuge is designed to hold capillary tubes, whereas a clinical centrifuge accommodates test tubes of varying sizes.

Clinical centrifuges used in veterinary laboratories are one of two types, depending on the style of the centrifuge head. A horizontal centrifuge head, also known as the swinging arm type, has specimen cups that hang vertically when the centrifuge is at rest. During centrifugation, the cups swing out to the horizontal position. As the specimen is centrifuged, centrifugal force drives the particles through the liquid to the bottom of the tube. When the centrifuge stops, the specimen cups fall back to the vertical position.

The second type of centrifuge head available is the angled centrifuge head (Fig. 10-3). The specimen tubes are inserted through drilled holes that hold the tubes at a fixed angle, usually approximately 52 degrees. This type of centrifuge rotates at higher speeds than the horizontal head centrifuge, without excessive heat buildup. The angled centrifuge head is usually configured to accommodate just one tube size. Smaller-sized tubes require the use of an adaptor unless a small-capacity centrifuge is available (Fig. 10-4). Microhematocrit centrifuges are a type of angled centrifuge. The microhematocrit centrifuge is configured to accommodate capillary tubes.

In addition to a standard on-off switch, most centrifuges have a timer that automatically turns the centrifuge off after a preset time. A tachometer or dial to set the speed of the centrifuge is also usually present. Some centrifuges do not have a tachometer and always run at maximal speed. Most centrifuges have speed dials calibrated in revolutions per minute (rpm) times 1000. Thus, a dial setting of 5 represents 5000 rpm.

CRITICAL CONCEPT

The centrifuge brake should only be used in cases of equipment malfunction when the centrifuge must be stopped quickly.

A centrifuge also may have a braking device to stop it rapidly. The brake should only be used in cases of equipment

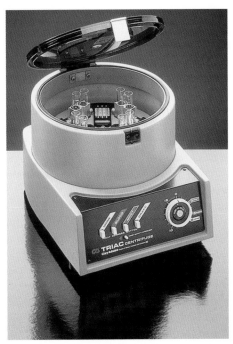

FIGURE 10-3 This centrifuge is capable of accommodating centrifuge tubes and hematocrit tubes. (From Hendrix CM, Sirois M: Laboratory procedures for veterinary technicians, ed 5, St Louis, 2007, Mosby.)

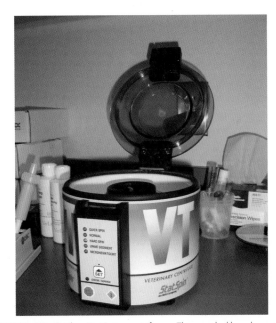

FIGURE 10-4 The StatSpin centrifuge. This angled-head centrifuge is specifically designed for small sample volumes. (From Hendrix CM, Sirois M: Laboratory procedures for veterinary technicians, ed 5, St Louis, 2007, Mosby.)

malfunction when the centrifuge must be stopped quickly. The centrifuge should never be operated with the lid unlatched. Always load the centrifuge with the open ends of tubes toward the center of the centrifuge head. Tubes must be counterbalanced with tubes of equal size and weight. Water-filled tubes may be used to balance the centrifuge. This ensures that the centrifuge will operate correctly without wobbling and that no liquid is forced from the tubes during operation. Incorrect loading of the centrifuge can cause damage to the instrument and injury to the operator. The centrifuge should be cleaned immediately if anything is spilled inside it. Tubes sometimes crack or break during centrifugation. Pieces of broken tubes must be removed when the centrifuge stops. If these are not removed, they could permanently damage the centrifuge. The operator's manual should list maintenance schedules of the different components of the centrifuge. Some centrifuges require periodic lubrication of the bearings. Most need the brushes to be checked or replaced regularly. A regular maintenance schedule prevents costly breakdowns and keeps the centrifuge running at maximum efficiency.

Specimens must be centrifuged for a specific time at a specific speed for maximum accuracy. A centrifuge that is run too fast or for too long may rupture cells and destroy the morphologic features of cells in the sediment. A centrifuge that is run too slowly or for less than the proper time may not completely separate the specimen or concentrate the sediment. Information regarding speed and time of centrifugation should be developed for all laboratory procedures and followed for maximum accuracy.

REFRACTOMETER

A refractometer, or total solids meter, is used to measure the refractive index of a solution. Refraction is the bending of light rays as they pass from one medium (e.g., air) into another medium (e.g., urine) with a different optical density. The degree of refraction is a function of the concentration of solid material in the medium. Refractometers are calibrated to a zero reading (zero refractive index) with distilled water at a temperature between 60° and 100° F (15.6° and 37.8° C). The most common uses of the refractometer are determination of the specific gravity of urine or other fluids and the protein concentration of plasma or other fluids.

The refractometer has a built-in prism and calibration scale (Fig. 10-5). Although refractometers can measure the refractive index of any solution, the scale readings in the instrument have been calibrated in terms of specific gravity and protein concentrations (in g/dL). The specific gravity or protein concentration of a solution is directly proportional to its concentration of dissolved substances.

Because no solution can be more dilute or have a lower concentration of dissolved substances than distilled water, the scale calibration and readings (specific gravity or protein concentration) are always greater than zero. The refractometer is read on the scale at the distinct light-dark interface (Fig. 10-6).

Various refractometer models are available. Most are temperature-compensated between 60° F and 100° F (15.6° and 37.8° C). As long as the temperature remains between these two extremes, even as the refractometer is held in a person's hands, the temperature fluctuation will not affect the accuracy of the reading.

CRITICAL CONCEPT

The refractometer is a delicate optical instrument that must be properly cared for to ensure accurate results.

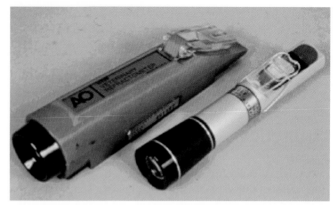

FIGURE 10-5 Refractometer used for measurement of urine specific gravity and total solids in plasma. (From Bassert JM, McCurnin DM: McCurnin's clinical textbook for veterinary technicians, ed 7, St Louis, 2010, Saunders.)

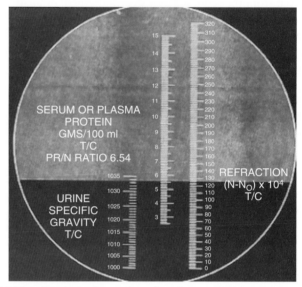

FIGURE 10-6 Reading scale in the refractometer. (From Bassert JM, McCurnin DM: McCurnin's clinical textbook for veterinary technicians, ed 7, St Louis, 2010, Saunders.)

USE, CARE, AND MAINTENANCE

Procedures for use of the refractometer are given in Procedure 10-2. The refractometer should be cleaned after each use. The prism cover glass and cover plate are wiped dry. Lens tissue should be used to protect the optical surfaces from scratches. Some manufacturers suggest cleaning the cover glass and plate with alcohol. The manufacturer's cleaning instructions should be consulted.

The refractometer should be calibrated regularly, weekly or daily, depending on use. Distilled water at room temperature placed on the refractometer should have a zero refractive index and therefore read zero on all scales. If the light-dark boundary deviates from the zero mark by more than half a division, the refractometer should be adjusted by turning the adjusting screw as directed by the manufacturer. The refractometer should not be used if it has not been calibrated to zero with distilled water. Newer refractometers are digital and contain a microprocessor that provides automatic calibration and temperature monitoring.

📋 **PROCEDURE 10-2** USE AND CARE OF THE REFRACTOMETER

1. Inspect and clean the prism cover glass and cover plate.
2. Place a drop of sample fluid on the prism cover glass, and close the cover (Fig. 1).

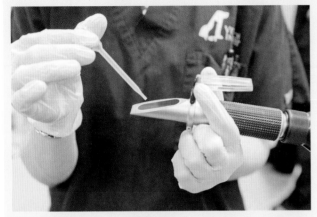

FIGURE 1

3. Point the refractometer toward bright artificial light or sunlight (Fig. 2).

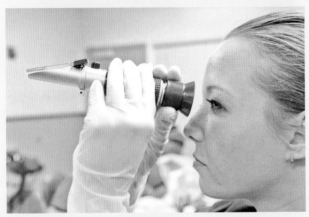

FIGURE 2

4. Bring the light-dark interface line into focus by turning the eyepiece.
5. Read and record the result with the appropriate scale (e.g., specific gravity, protein).
6. Clean the refractometer according to the manufacturer's recommendations.

Illustrations from Sirois M: Laboratory procedures for veterinary technicians, ed 6, St Louis, 2015, Mosby.

CHEMISTRY ANALYZERS

Veterinarians are better able to diagnose disease and monitor patient therapy when results are available immediately. Various chemistry analyzers are available for use in the veterinary practice laboratory. Most chemistry analyzers used in the veterinary practice use the principles of photometry to quantify constituents found in the blood. Analyzers using electrochemical methods are also available for in-house use.

PHOTOMETRY

Several types of photometers are used for in-house diagnostic equipment. Spectrophotometers are designed to measure the amount of light transmitted through a solution. The basic components of spectrophotometers are the same, regardless of the specific manufacturer of the equipment. All spectrophotometers contain a light source, prism, wavelength selector, photodetector, and readout device (Fig. 10-7). The light source is typically a tungsten or halogen lamp. The prism functions to fragment the light into its component wavelength segments. The photodetector receives whatever light is not absorbed by the sample. The photodetector signal is then transmitted to the readout device. Depending on the model of the instrument, the readout units may be in percentage transmittance, percentage absorbance, optical density, or concentration units. Some automated analyzers use variations of the basic photometric procedure. A type of photometer that uses a filter to select the wavelength is referred to as a colorimeter. Another type detects light reflected off a test substance rather than transmitted light. This type is referred to as a reflectometer.

ELECTROCHEMICAL METHODS

Some analyzers use principles of electrochemistry to determine analyte concentrations. A few analyzers combine electrochemical and photometric methods within self-contained cartridges. Electrochemical methods are used for the evaluation of electrolytes and other ionic components. These types of tests vary considerably in configuration but function in a similar manner (Fig. 10-8). Analyzers are designed with specific electrodes that are configured to allow interaction with just one ion. The most common of these systems is known as a potentiometer. These systems are designed so that ions diffuse across an area separated by a membrane; the difference in voltage, or electric potential, between the two sides of the membrane can be measured. This electrical variation corresponds to the number of active ions present in the sample.

FEATURES AND BENEFITS OF COMMON TYPES OF CHEMISTRY ANALYZERS

Most automated analyzers use liquid reagents, dry reagents, or slides that contain dry reagents. Liquid reagents may be purchased in bulk or in unitized disposable cuvettes. Dry reagents are available in unitized form. Bulk liquid reagents are the least expensive but require additional handling and storage space. Some reagents are flammable and toxic. The purchase of unitized reagents eliminates the hazards associated with handling these reagents. Dry slide reagents pose little or no handling or storage concerns but tend to be more expensive.

Analyzers that use dry systems include those with reagent-impregnated slides, pads, or cartridges. Most of these use reflectance assays. They do not require reagent handling, and the performance of single tests is relatively simple. Running profiles on these types of systems tends to be some-

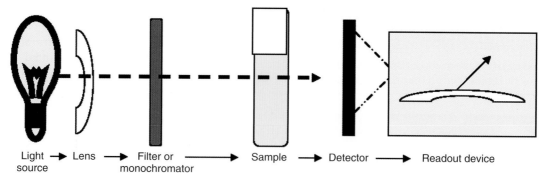

Light → Lens → Filter or → Sample → Detector → Readout device
source   monochromator

FIGURE 10-7 Principles of spectrophotometry. (From Hendrix CM, Sirois M: Laboratory procedures for veterinary technicians, ed 5, St Louis, 2007, Mosby.)

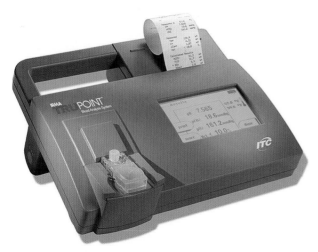

FIGURE 10-8 The IRMA analyzer (infrared motion analyzer; International Technidyne, Edison, NJ) uses electrochemical methods to measure blood gas and electrolyte levels. (Courtesy Dr. B. Mitzner.)

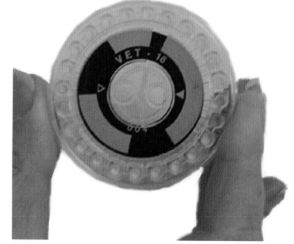

FIGURE 10-9 Reagent rotor for use in the Analyst blood chemistry analyzer. (Courtesy Dr. B. Mitzner.)

what more time consuming than it is for most other analyzer types. Some dry systems use reagent strips similar to those used for urine chemical testing.

Liquid systems include those that use a lyophilized (freeze-dried) reagent or an already prepared liquid reagent. The most common type of lyophilized reagent system for veterinary clinical practice uses rotor technology. The rotors consist of individual cuvettes to which diluted samples are added (Fig. 10-9). Cuvettes are optical quality reservoirs used in the photometer and may be plastic or glass. Rotor-based systems tend to be accurate and are usually cost-effective for profiles but are not capable of running single tests. Other liquid systems in common use include those with unitized reagent cuvettes or a bulk reagent. Unitized systems have the advantage of not requiring reagent handling but tend to be the most expensive of all the liquid reagent systems. In addition, running profiles with these systems is somewhat time consuming, but single testing is simple. Bulk reagent systems may supply reagent in concentrated form that must be diluted or is of working strength. Working-strength reagent systems do not usually require any special reagent handling. These analyzers are the most versatile in that they can perform profiling or single testing with relative ease. Most require

little preparation time. However, some have extensive maintenance time, particularly with the calibration of test parameters. Some systems that use bulk reagent may have a flow cell instead of a cuvette. Sample and reagent can be aspirated directly through the analyzer without the need for transfer of the reactants into cuvettes.

Dedicated use analyzers are available for certain tests. These analyzers sample for only one substance, such as blood glucose (Fig. 10-10). Dedicated analyzers can be used if only a single test is requested or in an emergency situation.

INSTRUMENT CARE AND MAINTENANCE

Chemistry analyzers are sensitive instruments that must be carefully maintained. Always follow the manufacturer's operating instructions. Instruments generally have a warm-up period to allow the light source, photodetector, and incubator, if present, to reach equilibrium before they are used. Ideally, laboratory personnel should turn on the instrument in the morning and leave it on all day. The instrument is therefore ready to use at any time during the day, especially in an emergency situation.

Following the manufacturer's maintenance schedule prolongs the life of the chemistry analyzer. A schedule sheet should be established for each instrument in the laboratory

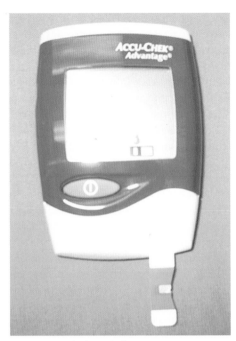

FIGURE 10-10 This dedicated glucose measuring instrument is available over the counter in many pharmacies. (From Tear M: Small animal surgical nursing, ed 2, St Louis, 2012, Mosby.)

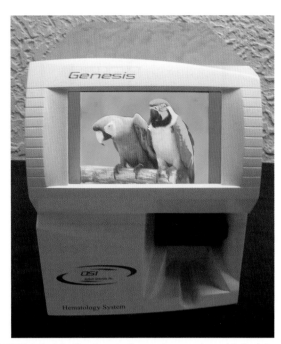

FIGURE 10-11 The Genesis hematology analyzer (Oxford Science, Oxford, CT) combines impedance and laser-based methods.

to allow quick and easy review of the maintenance history of any instrument. Most manufacturers have a toll-free number to call if problems arise.

HEMATOLOGY ANALYZERS

Instrumentation designed for veterinary hospital use is available to facilitate the generation of hematologic data for the complete blood count (CBC). Options are cost-effective and convenient in situations in which at least several CBCs are performed daily. Benefits of instrumentation include reduced labor investment, more complete information, and improvement of data reliability. Individual users are responsible for becoming familiar with the detailed documentation that accompanies specific instruments.

Instrumentation for the veterinary hospital falls into three general categories—impedance analyzers, laser-based analyzers, and the quantitative buffy coat analysis system. Some manufacturers now provide analyzers that combine several methods for performing a CBC. One commonly available system uses impedance methods for the enumeration of cells and laser-based methods for performing the differential white blood cell count (Fig. 10-11). Some hematology analyzers also have photometric capabilities to determine the hemoglobin level.

TYPES OF ANALYZERS

IMPEDANCE ANALYZERS. A number of electronic cell counters used in human medical laboratories have been adapted for veterinary use (Fig. 10-12). This adaptation was necessary because of the variation in blood cell size among different animal species. Some companies have developed dedicated veterinary multispecies hematology systems that count cells and determine the hematocrit, hemoglobin concentration, and mean corpuscular hemoglobin

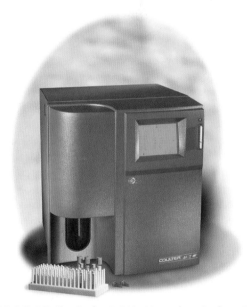

FIGURE 10-12 The Coulter AcT Vet Hematology Analyzer (Beckman Coulter, Danvers, MA), designed specifically for animal species, uses impedance technology. (From Hendrix CM, Sirois M: Laboratory procedures for veterinary technicians, ed 5, St Louis, 2007, Mosby.)

concentration (MCHC). Some also provide a partial white blood cell (WBC) differential count.

Electronic cell counters that use the impedance method are based on the passage of electric current across two electrodes separated by a glass tube with a small opening or aperture (Fig. 10-13). Electrolyte fluid on either side of the aperture conducts the current. Counting occurs by moving cells through the aperture using a vacuum or positive pressure. Because cells are relatively poor conductors of electricity compared with the electrolyte fluid, they impede the flow of current while passing through the aperture. These

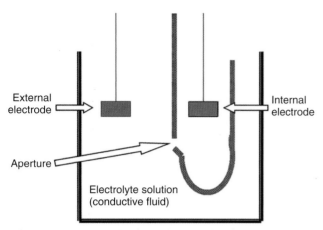

FIGURE 10-13 Principle of impedance analysis for cell counts. (From Hendrix CM, Sirois M: *Laboratory procedures for veterinary technicians*, ed 5, St Louis, 2007, Mosby.)

transient changes in current may be counted to determine the blood cell concentration. In addition, the volume or size of the cell is proportional to the change in current, allowing the system to catalog cell sizes. Size information may be displayed in a distribution histogram of the cell population. Leukocytes, erythrocytes, and platelets may be enumerated with these systems.

These instruments are calibrated to count cells in specified size ranges, defined by threshold settings, which prevents erroneous interpretation of small debris and electronic noise as cells, and to separate cell populations properly in the same dilution, such as platelets and erythrocytes. Because cell populations vary in size among species, some of the threshold settings are species specific. These settings should be established by the manufacturer and are usually set automatically by system software when the user selects the species for analysis in a software menu. Comprehensive hematology systems designed specifically for veterinary applications are now commonly used in veterinary facilities. These systems incorporate the advantages of individual cell analysis, which provides sophisticated information about blood cell populations.

The blood sample must be diluted to count cells. For WBCs, also known as leukocytes, a dilution is treated with a lytic agent that destroys cell membranes, leaving only nuclei for counting. Erythrocytes, also known as red blood cells (RBCs), may be analyzed with systems that count the RBCs and provide cell size information by using a much greater blood dilution to which no lytic agent is added. Erythrocyte analysis on automated systems provides diagnostic information about cell volume and an alternative method for determining the hematocrit (Hct). The mean corpuscular volume (MCV) may be directly measured from analysis of the erythrocyte volume distribution. The hematocrit is then calculated by multiplying the MCV by the erythrocyte concentration.

Many automated hematology systems provide a complete analysis of platelet, erythrocyte, and WBC populations, including WBC differential count information. Most provide graphic displays of cell population size analysis. Differential information is calculated from the WBC population size distribution. Normally, these systems provide an estimate of the relative percentage of granulated and nongranulated WBCs. This value has limited application for the evaluation of patients with a pathologic condition. Variations in the size of the cells introduce error into this measurement. In addition, numerous morphologic abnormalities can be present and may not be identified with this partial differential count. A thorough examination of the differential blood film must also be included when evaluating patients.

Impedance analyzers are composed of numerous pumps, tubing, and valves that must be maintained. Diluting fluid and dusty glassware may be contaminated with particles large enough to be erroneously counted as cells. The aperture may become partially or totally obstructed. The threshold setting may be improperly set on a counter with a variable threshold control. Cold agglutinins may cause a decreased RBC count because of RBC clumping. Before processing, refrigerated blood samples must be warmed to room temperature. Fragile lymphocytes, as seen with some forms of lymphocytic leukemia, may rupture in the lysing solution used to lyse RBCs. This rupturing can result in a decreased WBC count. The presence of spherocytes (abnormally small, round RBCs) may alter the mean corpuscular volume, thus reducing the calculated hematocrit. Elevated serum viscosity may interfere with cell counts. Platelet counts obtained from impedance counters are affected by platelet clumping and are often inaccurate.

QUANTITATIVE BUFFY COAT SYSTEM. The quantitative buffy coat system (QBC; Becton, Dickinson, Franklin Lakes, NJ) uses differential centrifugation and estimation of cellular elements by measurements on an expanded buffy coat layer in a specialized microhematocrit tube. It provides a hematocrit value and estimates of leukocyte concentration and platelet concentration. It extrapolates tube volumes to an estimate of concentration based on fixed cell volumes. Partial differential count information is provided in the form of total **granulocyte** and lymphocyte and monocyte categories. One limitation of these leukocyte groupings is that abnormalities such as left shift and lymphopenia may be undetected unless the blood film is examined as defined for the minimum CBC. These systems are best used as screening tools because they provide an estimation of cell numbers rather than an actual cell count.

LASER-BASED ANALYZERS. These types of analyzers use laser beams to determine the size and density of solid components. Cells scatter light differently, depending on the presence or absence of granules and nuclei. The degree and direction of light scatter allows the enumeration of monocytes, lymphocytes, granulocytes, and erythrocytes. When certain dyes are added to the sample, variations in laser light scatter can also allow the enumeration of mature and immature erythrocytes (Fig. 10-14).

INSTRUMENT CARE AND MAINTENANCE
Electronic cell counters, similar to chemistry analyzers, are sophisticated instruments that require careful maintenance. The manufacturer's recommendations for routine

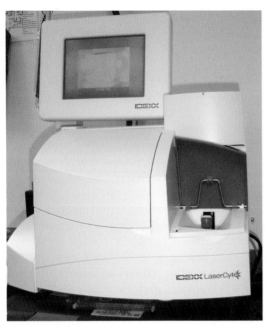

FIGURE 10-14 Laser-based analyzer for use in the veterinary practice laboratory. (From Hendrix CM, Sirois M: Laboratory procedures for veterinary technicians, ed 5, St Louis, 2007, Mosby.)

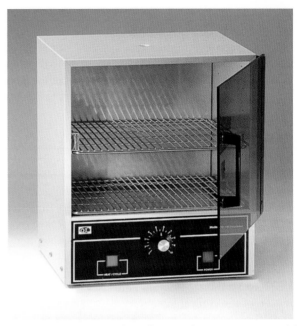

FIGURE 10-15 Small incubator for use in the veterinary practice laboratory. (Courtesy Dr. B. Mitzner.)

maintenance should be followed. Daily maintenance for many electronic cell counters requires flushing the entire system with bleach and fresh diluting solution to keep the aperture open. Background counts are periodically performed to make sure that the diluting solution is not contaminated and/or the glassware and tubing are not dirty. The vacuum pump must be checked at regular intervals to ensure that the proper amount of blood and diluting fluid is being drawn into the counter.

INCUBATORS

A variety of microbiology tests require the use of an incubator. Incubators for the in-house veterinary practice laboratory are available in a variety of sizes and configurations. The incubator must be capable of sustaining a constant temperature of 37° C (98.6° F). The incubator should be fitted with a thermometer or should have one placed inside the chamber to monitor temperature (Fig. 10-15). Heat should be provided by a thermostatically controlled element. A small dish of water should also be placed inside to maintain proper humidity. Some incubators have built-in humidity controls, but this type of equipment tends to be expensive. Larger laboratories may have incubators that automatically monitor temperature and humidity, as well as carbon dioxide and oxygen levels.

PIPETTES

Although most test kits and analyzers contain their own specific pipettes and pipetting devices, some others may be needed in the veterinary practice laboratory. The primary types of pipettes used in the practice laboratory are transfer pipettes and graduated pipettes. Transfer pipettes are used when critical volume measurements are not needed. These pipettes may be plastic or glass, and some can deliver volumes by drops. Graduated pipettes may contain a single volume designation or have multiple gradations. Pipettes with single gradations are referred to as volumetric pipettes and are the most accurate of the measuring pipettes. Larger volumetric pipettes are usually designated as TD pipettes, which means that the pipette is designed *to d*eliver the specific volume. A small amount of liquid should remain in the tip of the pipette after the volume has been delivered. Volumetric pipettes designed to deliver microliter volumes are designated TC, meaning that the pipette is designed *to c*ontain the specified volume. These pipettes must only be used to add specified volumes to other liquids. The pipette then must be rinsed with the other liquid to deliver the specified volume accurately. The small volume of fluid left in the tip of the pipette is then blown out of the pipette. Pipettes that contain multiple gradations are marked as either TD or TD with blow out, depending on whether the fluid remaining in the tip of the pipette should remain or be blown out. TD with blow-out pipettes usually contain a double-etched or frosted band at the top.

The pipette chosen for a specific application should always be the one that is the most accurate and that measures volumes closest to the volume needed. For example, a 1-mL pipette, rather than a 5-mL pipette, should be chosen if the volume needed is 0.8 mL. Pipettes are also designed for measuring liquids at a specified temperature, normally room temperature. Liquids that are significantly colder or warmer will not measure accurately. Pipetting devices must also be used correctly, and fluid must not be allowed to enter the pipetting device. Never pipette any fluid by placing your mouth directly on the pipette.

MISCELLANEOUS EQUIPMENT AND SUPPLIES

Some clinical chemistry and coagulation tests may require the use of a water bath or heat block capable of maintaining a constant temperature of 37° C (98.6° F). Slide dryers can be a useful addition to the busy veterinary practice laboratory. Aliquot mixers can also be helpful by keeping items well mixed and ready for use.

QUALITY ASSURANCE

Quality assurance refers to the procedures established to ensure that clinical testing is performed in compliance with accepted standards and that the process and results are properly documented. Unlike human medical laboratories, veterinary facilities are not subject to regulations that require quality assurance programs. However, without a comprehensive quality assurance program, the accuracy and **precision** of laboratory test results cannot be verified. A comprehensive quality assurance program addresses all aspects of the operation of the clinical laboratory. This includes qualifications of laboratory personnel, standard operating procedures for care and use of all supplies and equipment, sample collection and handling procedures, methods and frequency of performance of quality control assays, and record-keeping procedures.

ACCURACY, PRECISION, AND RELIABILITY

Accuracy, precision, and reliability are terms frequently used to describe quality control and are the standards for any quality control program. Accuracy reflects how closely results agree with the true quantitative value of the constituent. Precision is the magnitude of random errors and the reproducibility of measurements. Reliability is the ability of a method to be accurate and precise. Factors that affect accuracy and precision are test selection, test conditions, sample quality, operator skill, electrical surges, and equipment maintenance.

ANALYSIS OF CONTROL MATERIALS

Control serum is used for assessment of the instrument and operator. Producing valid results with control materials provides assurance that the procedure was performed correctly and that all components (e.g., reagents, equipment) are functioning correctly. Controls are handled in exactly the same way as patient test samples and should be regularly assayed with each test batch, daily or weekly, at the same time that patient serum samples are assayed. The frequency of control testing depends on the laboratory's goals. To ensure reliability, control samples must be tested when a new assay is set up, a new staff member runs the test, a new lot number of reagents is used, or an instrument is known to perform erratically. Ideally, a control sample is tested with each batch of patient samples. A problem with a particular assay may require an increase in the frequency of control testing.

After the assay is completed, the control value should fall within the manufacturer's reported range. If it does not, the assays of the patient and control samples must be repeated. The results of the analysis of control serum are recorded on a chart or log for each assay (Fig. 10-16). The values for tests performed on control serum should not vary significantly each time that the tests are performed. Data may be analyzed in two ways, by detecting shifts or trends and by determining whether results for control samples are within the range established by the manufacturer. If a control serum result does not fall within this range, it should be retested. If it still fails to fall in this range, the reagents, instrument, and technique

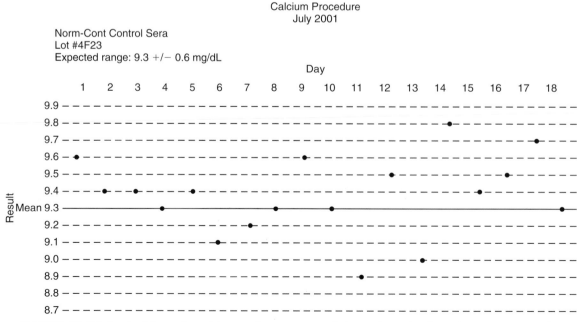

FIGURE 10-16 Results of the analysis of the control serum are recorded on a chart or log for each assay. (From Hendrix CM, Sirois M: Laboratory procedures for veterinary technicians, ed 5, St Louis, 2007, Mosby.)

must be checked. When control values are successively distributed on one or the other side of the mean, the mean has shifted and a systematic error is involved.

APPLIED QUALITY CONTROL

Instrument maintenance is required to prolong the life of the instrument and prevent expensive down-time. All instruments are accompanied by an owner's manual. If the manual has been misplaced, the manufacturer should be contacted for a replacement. The manual lists the instrument components that must be inspected and attended to regularly. A notebook listing a schedule with the types of maintenance required for each instrument facilitates instrument maintenance. A page is dedicated to each instrument and includes the following:

- Instrument name
- Serial number
- Model number
- Purchase date
- Points to be checked
- Frequency of checks
- Record of test readings
- Changes made to restore accuracy and precision of readings
- Cost and time associated with necessary repairs and restoration
- Name or initials of the person performing the maintenance

Results obtained with the control serum are recorded and kept in a permanent record. The results are graphed so that changes or trends can be detected visually.

If attention is paid to detail and as many sources of all three types of error as possible can be eliminated, the laboratory can provide reliable results. Sloppy, inattentive work habits can lead to diagnostic and therapeutic disasters that could result in the death of an animal. Careful attention to detail ensures that the veterinarian has all the correct information needed to make a proper diagnosis, prescribe appropriate treatment, and offer an educated prognosis.

LABORATORY RECORDS

Laboratory records are divided into internal and external record systems. Complete, up-to-date records are necessary for both systems. A number of computer systems are now available for almost all the records generated in the veterinary clinic or hospital. Patient information, inventory, ordering information, sales records, and laboratory data can be stored on a computer. Clinics using a computer system should be sure to keep backup records in case of computer failure or damage by computer viruses.

INTERNAL RECORDS

By using internal records, the laboratory tracks assay results and obtains methods. The records consist of a standard operating procedure (SOP) and quality control data and graphs. The SOP contains the instructions for all analyses run in the laboratory. Each procedure is described on a separate page. The easiest way to maintain the book is to insert the instruction sheets accompanying each commercial test kit in a three-ring binder, along with pages for any other procedures performed in the laboratory. Each procedure not performed with a commercial kit is described on a separate page, including the name of the test, synonyms (if any) for the test, the rationale for use of the procedure, reagent list, and stepwise instructions for a single analysis. Individual pages can be inserted into plastic overlays for protection. The SOP book is reviewed periodically and updated as needed. Those who keep an SOP book on a computer should make sure that an up-to-date hard copy backup is available.

EXTERNAL RECORDS

Laboratory personnel communicate with people throughout the veterinary clinic or hospital and in other laboratories with the use of external records. These consist of request forms that accompany the sample to the laboratory, report forms for assay results, laboratory log books with individual test results, and a book containing pertinent information on samples sent to reference laboratories. In a clinic or hospital with an internal computer network, all personnel can access much of this information as needed.

Information provided on a request form includes the patient's full identification (including identification number, if available) and presenting signs, date and method used to obtain the sample, pertinent history, tests desired, any special notes regarding sample handling, and to whom and by which method results are to be reported (telephone, fax, e mail, or written report).

The report form should include complete patient identification and presenting signs, test results (including appropriate units), and notation of any extraordinary observations or explanatory comments, if applicable. For additional backup, the laboratory staff should keep a log book to record test results. If the original laboratory report form is lost in transit, the results are retrievable.

HEMATOLOGY EXAMINATION PROCEDURES

Hematologic examination, or the analysis of blood, is a powerful diagnostic tool. Hematologic procedures include collecting and handling blood samples, performing a CBC, assisting with bone marrow examination, and performing routine blood coagulation tests.

SAMPLE COLLECTION

Sample quality has a significant impact on test accuracy. Careful attention to collection procedures will minimize these problems. When preparing to collect blood, the technician first determines which specific test procedures will be needed. This will determine, in part, the equipment and supplies needed and the choice of a particular blood vessel from which to collect the sample. Unless the purpose of the test is to monitor therapy, the blood sample is always collected before any treatment is given. It is important to remember that treatment, such as fluid therapy, may affect results. Certain test methods cannot be accurately performed once the patient has received certain pharmaceutical therapies. **Preprandial samples**, or samples from an animal that has not eaten for some time, are ideal. Postprandial samples, or samples collected after the animal has eaten, may produce many erroneous results. Increased amounts of lipid (**lipemia**) may also be present in postprandial blood samples. Lipemia also increases the likelihood of hemolysis in the sample, and further complicates analyses.

Improper handling of blood may render a blood sample unusable for analysis or result in inaccurate results. The methods and sites of blood collection depend on the species, amount of blood needed, and personal preference. Venous blood is preferred for use in hematologic testing and is easily accessible in most species. The cephalic vein is the preferred site in dogs and cats when relatively small volumes of blood are needed. The saphenous vein (lateral in the dog, medial in the cat) is a reasonable substitute, especially in fractious cats. Jugular venipuncture is an efficient way to collect a large volume of blood.

The veterinary assistant should clip the collection site to remove hair. Clean the site with alcohol or another suitable antiseptic and allow it to dry before proceeding with the venipuncture. Take care not to stress the animal during blood collection. Use only the amount of restraint necessary to immobilize the animal. Excitement and stress can cause splenic contraction, which can alter the results of tests performed on RBCs. Results of several WBC tests are also affected.

COLLECTION EQUIPMENT

A variety of collection equipment is available for use with veterinary patients. Blood may be collected in a syringe or specialized vacuum device, such as the Vacutainer system (Becton, Dickinson). When the needle-syringe method is used, the needle chosen should always be the largest one that the animal can comfortably accommodate. For most small animals, 20- to 25-gauge needles work well. The syringe chosen should be one that is closest to the required sample volume. Use of a larger syringe could collapse the patient's vein. Using a large syringe with a small-bore needle can result in **hemolysis** (rupture of red blood cells) when the syringe plunger is pulled back with great speed and force. Remove the needle before expelling the blood into the collection tube. Erythrocytes (RBCs) may hemolyze (rupture) if forced back through the needle.

Vacutainers are useful for multiple samples and when blood can be collected from a larger vessel, such as the cephalic or jugular vein. The Vacutainer system consists of a special needle, a needle holder, and vacuum-filled tubes that may be empty (clot tubes) or may contain a premeasured amount of anticoagulant (Fig. 10-17). A fixed amount of blood is drawn into the tube, based on tube size and amount of vacuum in the tube. Collapse of veins, especially in smaller animals, may occur because of excessive negative pressure exerted by the vacuum. Using small vacuum tubes may remedy this problem.

Fill collection tubes with the proper amount of blood, regardless of the method used to collect the sample. Unless otherwise directed, fill the tube approximately two-thirds to three-quarters full. This ensures a proper blood-to-anticoagulant ratio. Mix the blood adequately by inverting the tube gently for 10 to 20 seconds after transferring the blood. A precise venipuncture prevents the formation of blood clots in the sample resulting from platelet activation after multiple attempts at venipuncture. Note that serious errors may result if a sample is not labeled immediately after it has been collected. Label the tube with the date and time of collection, owner's name, patient's name, and patient's clinic identification number. If submitted to a laboratory, include with the sample a request form that includes all necessary sample identification and a clear indication of which tests are requested.

SAMPLE TYPE
WHOLE BLOOD

Whole blood is composed of cellular elements (erythrocytes, leukocytes, and platelets) and a fluid called plasma. To collect a whole blood sample, place the appropriate amount of blood into a container with the proper anticoagulant and gently mix the sample by inverting the tube multiple times. Whole blood may be refrigerated if analysis is to be delayed, but it should never be frozen unless the plasma has been separated from the cellular elements. If the blood has been refrigerated, warm the sample to room temperature and mix gently before analysis.

PLASMA

To obtain a plasma sample, collect the appropriate amount of blood in a container with the proper anticoagulant and mix well by gentle inversion. Centrifuge the closed container for 10 minutes at 2000 to 3000 rpm to separate the fluid from

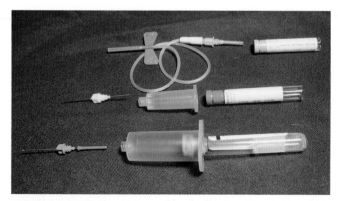

FIGURE 10-17 The Vacutainer blood collection system (Becton, Dickinson, Franklin Lakes, NJ) consists of a needle, holder, and collection tube. Several types of systems are available. (From Sirois M: Principles and practice of veterinary technology, ed 3, St Louis 2011, Mosby.)

the cells. After the sample is centrifuged, remove the plasma from the cells, being careful not to contaminate the plasma with any pelleted cells, and transfer the plasma into another appropriately labeled container. Separate plasma from the cellular elements as soon as possible after collection to minimize any artifactual changes. Plasma can be refrigerated or frozen until analysis is performed, depending on the specific requirements of the desired test(s).

ANTICOAGULANTS

Anticoagulants are used when whole blood or plasma samples are required. The choice of a particular anticoagulant should be based on the tests needed. Some anticoagulants can interfere with certain test methods. The most commonly used anticoagulant is ethylenediaminetetraaectic acid (EDTA). Tubes that contain EDTA have a lavender or purple rubber stopper (Fig. 10-18).

EDTA functions as an anticoagulant by binding calcium, which is necessary for clotting to occur. It is preferred for routine hematologic studies because it preserves cell morphology better than other anticoagulants. Even if collected in an EDTA tube, blood should be analyzed as quickly as possible, preferably within 2 hours after collection. Blood preserved in EDTA remains fresh for several hours or even overnight if stored in a refrigerator at 4° C (39.2° F). However, morphologic changes in the cells, such as cytoplasmic vacuolation, irregular cell membranes, and crenation (shrinkage of RBCs), may occur in stored samples, especially when the ratio of blood to anticoagulant is incorrect. This can make interpretation of observations difficult and result in inaccuracies. It is for this reason that blood smears are best

made immediately with fresh blood or within 1 hour after collection in an EDTA tube.

> ### CRITICAL CONCEPT
> EDTA is the preferred anticoagulant for hematology testing.

Heparin is not a permanent anticoagulant; it inhibits coagulation for only 8 to 12 hours. Tubes containing heparin (green-topped tubes) may be used if tests run on whole blood are done promptly. Heparin may cause cells to clump and stain poorly. Heparin tubes may be a good choice for storing small blood samples from birds because you can use the whole blood for hematologic tests and then collect plasma after spinning the sample.

Sodium citrate (blue-topped tubes) anticoagulant is used for coagulation tests. However, it is generally not suitable for routine hematologic studies because it can cause distortion in cell morphology.

COMPLETE BLOOD COUNT

The CBC is a cost-effective way to obtain valuable hematologic information about a patient. CBCs are indicated for the diagnostic evaluation of disease states, well-animal screening (e.g., geriatric animals), and as a screening tool before surgery. A CBC includes total erythrocyte and leukocyte counts, **packed cell volume**, hemoglobin concentration, differential white blood cell count, and RBC indices. Additional tests that should be included at the time of the CBC are the following:

- Measurement of total solids
- Evaluation of serum color and clarity
- Buffy coat evaluation
- Platelet estimate
- Platelet assessment

Most components of the CBC are performed with automated analyzers. Manual methods are rarely performed in clinical practice. Automated analyzers can provide accurate and cost-effective results. Hematology analyzers for the veterinary practice use impedance methods, buffy coat analysis, or laser methods when evaluating a sample. Some analyzers may incorporate a combination of methods. Each method has specific advantages and disadvantages. Regardless of which analyzer you use, an understanding of the test principles used with your analyzer is essential. Knowing the limitations of the analytic system enhances the validity of your test results. Regular quality control is also essential for ensuring the accuracy of your test results.

> ### CRITICAL CONCEPT
> Hemoglobin and PCV testing and RBC indices help determine the cause of anemia.

The packed cell volume (PCV) is another vital part of the CBC. The PCV, also known as the microhematocrit (Hct), is an expression of the percentage of whole blood occupied by RBCs. The PCV assay is usually performed with the microhematocrit technique (Procedure 10-3). A blood-filled

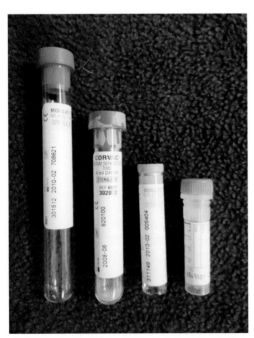

FIGURE 10-18 From left to right: red-top plain blood collection tube; tiger-top tube; ethylenediaminetetraacetic acid tube; and heparin tube. (From Sirois, M: *Laboratory procedures for veterinary technicians, ed 6,* St Louis, 2015, Mosby.

📋 PROCEDURE 10-3 MICROHEMATOCRIT PROCEDURE

1. Fill two microhematocrit tubes ≈ ¾ full with whole blood. Wipe the excess blood from the outside of the tube. Use plain (anticoagulant-free) microhematocrit tubes with anticoagulated blood. Use heparinized tubes when collecting blood from a venipuncture site (Fig. 1).

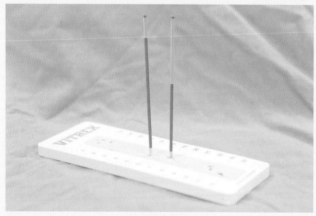

FIGURE 1

2. Push sealing clay into one end of each microhematocrit tube. Rotate each tube as it is pressed into the clay to ensure a tight seal (Fig. 2).

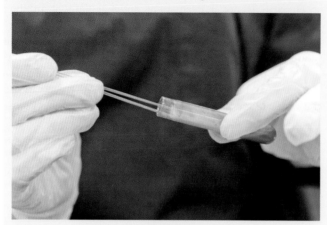

FIGURE 2

3. Put the tubes in a microhematocrit centrifuge, with the clay seal to the outside. Centrifuge for 2 to 5 minutes, depending on the model of the centrifuge used (Fig. 3).

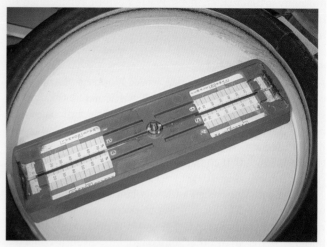

FIGURE 3

4. Determine the PCV for each tube by measuring the length of the RBC column using a microhematocrit tube reader. Average the two readings (Fig. 4).

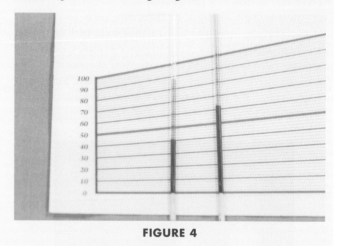

FIGURE 4

Adapted from Sirois M: Laboratory procedures for veterinary technicians, ed 6, St Louis, 2015, Mosby.

capillary tube is centrifuged for 2 to 5 minutes, depending on the type of centrifuge. The blood separates into a plasma layer, a white buffy coat composed of WBCs and platelets, and a layer of packed red cells (Fig. 10-19). Measuring the RBC layer in the capillary tube determines the PCV. The precision of a PCV is approximately 1%, making it a very accurate test.

> **CRITICAL CONCEPT**
>
> The PCV is a measure of the percentage of the blood that is occupied by red blood cells.

A low PCV may indicate anemia. There are many causes of anemia, including blood loss, neoplasia, parasitism, and chronic infection. An increased PCV also has several possible causes, including dehydration and splenic contraction in an excited animal. PCV values may be erroneously high because of clots in the sample, failure to mix the EDTA and blood adequately, and insufficient centrifugation time. PCV values may be erroneously low if the microhematocrit tube contains excessive plasma because of inadequate mixing of the sample. Sample dilution because of a low blood-to-anticoagulant ratio may also cause a spurious decrease in the PCV.

After determining the PCV, evaluate the plasma for turbidity and color (Box 10-2). An icteric, or yellow, plasma layer

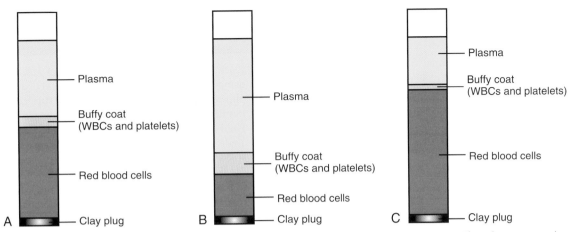

FIGURE 10-19 Separated layers in a centrifuged hematocrit tube. (From Colville T, Bassert JM: Clinical anatomy and physiology for veterinary technicians, ed 2, St Louis, 2008, Mosby.)

BOX 10-2	Visual Assessment of Plasma Turbidity and Color

- Normal: Clear and colorless to light straw-yellow
- Icterus: Clear and yellow
- Hemolysis: Clear and red
- Lipemia: Turbid and white

From Sirois M: Principles and practice of veterinary technology, ed 3, St Louis, 2011, Mosby.

may occur with liver disease or hemolytic anemia. A hemolytic, or red, sample can occur from improper sample collection and handling or with hemolytic anemia (Fig. 10-20). Sometimes the buffy coat is red tinged, especially in very sick animals or if there is an increased number of immature RBCs in the circulation. Lipemic plasma appears cloudy (turbid) and white, indicating excessive lipids in the blood. This can occur if blood was collected from an animal that was not fasted, or it may be pathologic. **Icterus**, hemolysis, and lipemia may be quantified as slight, moderate, or marked. The width of the buffy coat should be assessed.

TOTAL PLASMA PROTEIN DETERMINATION

The serum or plasma total protein level can be rapidly and reliably measured using a handheld refractometer (see Procedure 10-2). Accurate plasma protein determination is difficult in lipemic samples because the turbidity produces an indistinct line of demarcation on the scale. Hemoglobinemia caused by hemolysis can falsely increase plasma protein levels because of the presence of the heme portion of hemoglobin. The yellow color of an icteric sample does not interfere with refractometry.

ERYTHROCYTE INDICES

Erythrocyte indices are calculated values that use the RBC count, hemoglobin measurement, and PCV. Erythrocyte indices include the MCV, mean corpuscular hemoglobin (MCH), and MCHC. The term *corpuscular* is an old term used to describe red blood cells. These measurements provide data

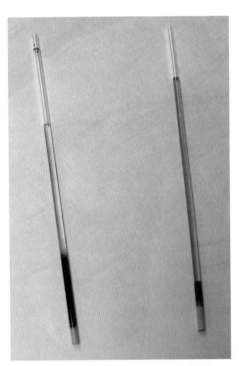

FIGURE 10-20 Icteric *(left)* and hemolyzed *(right)* plasma in a PCV tube. (From Sirois M: Principles and practice of veterinary technology, ed 3, St Louis 2011, Mosby.)

on the overall size of the RBCs as well as the relative amount of hemoglobin within the individual RBCs. The equations used to calculate the RBC indices are given in Table 10-1.

DIFFERENTIAL BLOOD FILM

Although most veterinary hematology analyzers provide at least a partial differential white blood cell count, a blood film must still be prepared and evaluated. There are a large number of abnormalities that are not routinely reported by automated analyzers. These include nucleated red blood cells, Heinz bodies, cellular inclusions (e.g., parasites, viral materials), toxic granulation, platelet clumps, **polychromasia**, target cells, and hypersegmentation.

TABLE 10-1	Equations Used to Calculate Red Blood Cell Indices	
PARAMETER	EQUATION	UNIT
MCV	(PCV × 10)/RBC count	fl (femtoliter; 10^{-15} liter)
MCH	(Hb × 10)/RBC count	pg (picogram; 10^{-12}g)
MCHC	(Hb × 100)/PCV	%

Adapted from Sirois M: Principles and practice of veterinary technology, ed 3, St Louis, 2011, Mosby.

EVALUATING THE BLOOD FILM. The CBC must include a differential blood film that enumerates various types of white blood cells present and also describes the morphology of red and white blood cells and platelets. A platelet estimate is also performed on the differential blood film. In addition to reporting the morphologic changes, a rating system is used to characterize the relative numbers of abnormal cells seen on the differential blood film.

Only one drop of blood is needed to make a smear (Procedure 10-4). It is best to use blood from the tip of the needle immediately after the blood is collected. This prevents the development of artifacts related to the presence of anticoagulant. If you cannot make a smear immediately, make the smear as soon as possible after collection.

CRITICAL CONCEPT

The preferred sample for preparation of the differential blood cell film is the blood drop on the tip of the needle immediately after the blood is collected.

The two methods of preparing blood smears are the wedge (glass slide) method and the coverslip method. Always use precleaned, glass microscope slides and coverslips and always hold slides by their edges to avoid smudging with grease or fingerprints. Even precleaned slides need to be cleaned because they have a thin film that aids in preventing them from sticking to one another but that also inhibits the blood cells from adhering to the glass slide or coverslip. Clean the slides with alcohol and allow them to dry before making the blood film. The wedge method is the most common type of smear used for routine hematology. The coverslip method is often preferred for avian blood smears because it renders a thinner film, which facilitates cell identification. It is also less traumatic on fragile avian blood cells. Coverslip smears are made by putting one small drop of blood in the center of a clean, square coverslip (Fig. 10-21). Place a second clean coverslip diagonally on top of the first so that the blood spreads evenly between the two surfaces. Then, pull the coverslips apart horizontally in a single smooth motion just as the blood has spread completely.

Improper technique and inappropriate staining can result in inferior or useless blood smears. Jerky movements and dirty slides may cause streaks on the film. Using too little or too much blood results in improper smear length. Clots or fat in the blood can cause small holes in the smear and an uneven, feathered edge. If the blood is from an anemic patient (decreased PCV),

PROCEDURE 10-4 MAKING A WEDGE SMEAR

1. Place a small drop of blood at the end of a clean glass slide using a microhematocrit tube or the end of a wooden applicator stick. Place this slide on a flat surface or suspend in midair between the thumb and forefinger.
2. Hold a second slide (the spreader slide) at a 30-degree angle and pull back into contact with the drop of blood, spreading blood along the edge of the spreader slide. Push the spreader slide forward in a rapid, steady, even motion to produce a blood film that is thick at one end and tapers to a thin feathered edge at the other (Fig. 1). The blood film should cover ≈ ¾ of the length of the slide.

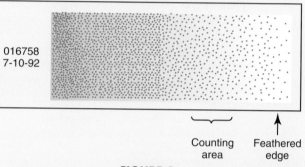

016758
7-10-92

Counting area   Feathered edge

FIGURE 1

3. Air-dry the smear by waving the slide in the air. This fixes the cells to the slide so that they are not dislodged during staining.
4. Label the slide at the thick end of the smear. If the slide has a frosted edge, this may be written on.
5. After drying, stain the smear with Wright stain or a Romanowsky-type stain, available in commercial kits (e.g., Wright Dip Stat3; Medi-Chem, Santa Monica, CA). These kits contain an alcohol fixative, methylene blue mixture to stain cell nuclei and certain organelles bluish-purple, and eosin to stain hemoglobin and some WBC granules reddish-orange. Follow the directions packaged with the staining kit. Smears usually must be immersed in each solution for 5 to 10 seconds.
6. After staining, rinse the slide with distilled water. Allow the slide to dry upright with the feathered edge pointed upward. This allows the water to drip off the slide away from the smear.

Adapted from Sirois M: Principles and practice of veterinary technology, ed 3, St Louis, 2011, Mosby.

increase the spreader slide angle to approximately 45 degrees. Conversely, the angle should be decreased to approximately 20 degrees if the blood is concentrated (increased PCV). Increasing the spreader slide angle makes a thicker smear, whereas decreasing it makes a thinner smear (Fig. 10-22).

PERFORMING THE DIFFERENTIAL. The evaluation of the differential blood film is the responsibility of the veterinary technician, although the veterinary assistant may aid in preparing the materials for the evaluation. The technician

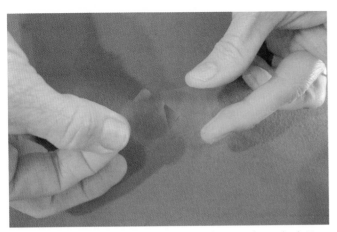

FIGURE 10-21 Preparing a blood film by the coverslip method. (From Sirois M: Principles and practice of veterinary technology, ed 3, St Louis 2011, Mosby.)

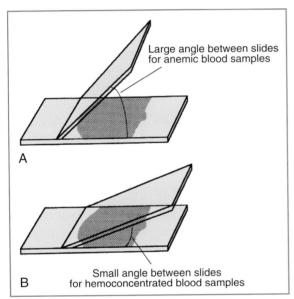

FIGURE 10-22 Difference in slide angle necessary for making blood films from anemic or hemoconcentrated blood. **A,** Large angle for anemic blood. **B,** Small angle for hemoconcentrated blood. (From Sirois M: Principles and practice of veterinary technology, ed 3, St Louis 2011, Mosby.)

will examine the blood smear in a systematic manner. The smear is scanned at low power (100× magnification) to assess overall cell numbers and distribution. Platelet clumps (aggregates) and blood parasites (e.g., **microfilariae**) are sometimes found at the feathered edge and must be noted on the hematology report.

A monolayer (single layer of blood cells) is located adjacent to the feathered edge. The cells should have even distribution and not be overlapping. Using the oil immersion objective (1000× magnification), it is here that the differential WBC count takes place. The procedure requires that 100 WBCs be counted, identified, and recorded. Because 100 WBCs are counted, the number of each WBC type observed is recorded as a percentage. This is called the relative WBC count. Various counting devices are available to aid the differential WBC count. Once the relative percentages of each cell type have been determined, the absolute value of each

cell type must be calculated. This is accomplished by multiplying the total white blood cell count by the percentage of each cell type.

The morphology of RBCs and WBCs is then assessed and recorded. The presence of any abnormal cells or toxic changes is reported and semiquantified. A platelet estimate and evaluation is also performed. Normal erythrocyte morphology varies greatly among different species. Veterinary technicians are responsible for identifying normal and abnormal RBC morphology. Morphology is evaluated using the oil immersion objective (1000× magnification) in the monolayer portion of the smear.

Changes in the appearance of erythrocytes occur in a variety of conditions. In general, these changes fall into one or more of the following categories: (1) changes in size; (2) changes in shape; (3) changes in color; (4) changes in cell behavior; and (5) appearance of inclusions. A variety of blood parasites can also be seen on a peripheral blood film. Most of these are found on or within erythrocytes. Parasites may also be found free of cells and within leukocytes and platelets.

Leukocytes seen on blood smears from mammals include neutrophils, basophils, eosinophils, lymphocytes, and monocytes. Segmented neutrophils, also known as segs or polymorphonuclear (PMN) cells, are mature WBCs that function mainly as phagocytes and are involved in inflammation. Lymphocytes have functions within the immune system. Monocytes are very large WBCs that are phagocytic and have immune system functions. Eosinophils are associated with allergic responses and are more numerous in patients with parasitic infections. Basophils are involved in the mediation of the immune system, and increased numbers are seen with a variety of inflammatory and infectious conditions.

Changes in the appearance of leukocytes generally occur as a result of disease processes that affect the appearance and/or function of the cell. These changes can also occur as normal reactions to a disease process and may be nonpathologic. Leukocyte changes may affect the cell nucleus, cytoplasm, or both.

Platelets are sometimes referred to as **thrombocytes**. In mammals, they are derived from the bone marrow cell called a megakaryocyte. Mammalian platelets are fragments of the cytoplasm of this bone marrow cell. Platelets function to provide an initiating coagulation factor. They are also capable of plugging small ruptures in small blood vessels.

COAGULATION TESTING

Hemostasis refers to the ability of the body systems to maintain the integrity of the blood and blood vessels and is a complex interaction among blood vessel walls, platelets, and coagulation factors.

HEMOSTATIC DEFECTS

Coagulation disorders are rare in cats. Most bleeding disorders found in veterinary species are in canine species and are secondary to some other disease process. The most common inherited coagulation disorder of domestic animals is von

Willebrand disease. This disease results when the production of von Willebrand factor is decreased or deficient. The disease occurs with relative frequency in Doberman dogs and has been reported in other canine breeds, as well as in rabbits and swine.

> **CRITICAL CONCEPT**
>
> The most common inherited coagulation disorder of domestic animals is von Willebrand disease.

Other coagulation disorders result from the decreased production or increased destruction of platelets as well as nutritional deficiencies, liver disease, and ingestion of certain medications or toxic substances. Thrombocytopenia refers to a decreased number of platelets and is the most common bleeding disorder of hemostasis in veterinary patients. This can occur as a result of bone marrow depression that reduces the production of platelets or autoimmune disease that increases the rate of platelet destruction. A large number of infectious agents, such as *Ehrlichia, Dirofilaria,* and parvovirus, can also affect thrombocyte production and destruction. Because the liver is the site of production of most coagulation factors, any condition that affects liver function can result in a coagulation disorder. Ingestion of toxic substances such as warfarin can also create bleeding disorders. Warfarin is a common component of rodenticides and acts to inhibit vitamin K function. Because vitamin K is required for the synthesis of coagulation factors II, VII, IX, and X, this can create a deficiency in several necessary components of the coagulation cascade. Ingestion of medications such as aspirin can also cause bleeding disorders.

DISSEMINATED INTRAVASCULAR COAGULATION. Although not a disease entity on its own, disseminated intravascular coagulation (DIC) is associated with many pathologic conditions. DIC is often seen in trauma cases and a large number of infectious diseases. Many types of events can trigger DIC. The resulting hemostatic disorder may manifest as systemic hemorrhage or microvascular thrombosis. Because the triggering event and the resulting disorder are diverse, the laboratory findings are highly variable. Schistocytes may be seen on the blood film on DIC patients because of the intravascular destruction of erythrocytes.

The clinical presentation of patients with bleeding disorders include petechia (pinpoint hemorrhage), ecchymoses (superficial hemorrhage ≈1 cm in diameter), purpura (bruising), epistaxis (bleeding from the nares), and prolonged bleeding following trauma or surgery. Patients may exhibit hematuria as a result of bleeding into the urinary bladder, melena as a result of bleeding into the digestive tract, or bleeding into joint cavities.

ASSESSMENT OF COAGULATION AND HEMOSTASIS

Coagulation tests may be appropriate if a bleeding disorder is suspected or as part of a presurgical screening protocol. Coagulation tests are designed to evaluate specific portions of the hemostatic mechanisms. All patients should be evaluated for coagulation defects before undergoing surgery. Most coagulation tests can be completed with minimal time and equipment and are relatively inexpensive. Plasma samples for coagulation testing are collected into an appropriate anticoagulant. Tests to determine the concentration and/or function of specific coagulation factors are not routinely performed in veterinary practice.

PLATELET COUNTS AND ESTIMATES

Platelet counts are part of all coagulation profiles as well as evaluation of the blood film for platelet morphology and clumping. A platelet estimate is performed when the veterinary technician completes the differential blood film evaluation. Most automated analyzers provide a platelet count.

BUCCAL MUCOSAL BLEEDING TIME

This test detects abnormalities in platelet function. The test requires a standard spring-loaded bleeding time device, blotting paper or no. 1 Whatman filter paper, stopwatch, and tourniquet. The test is performed with the patient anesthetized and placed in lateral recumbency (Fig. 10-23).

OTHER COAGULATION TESTS

The activated clotting time (ACT) test uses a preincubated tube that contains a diatomaceous earth material. A clean venipuncture is performed, and 2 mL of blood is collected in the tube. A timer is started as soon as the blood enters the tube. The tube is gently mixed three times and placed in a 37 °C (98.6 ° F) incubator or water bath. The tube is observed at 60 seconds and then at 5-second intervals for presence of a clot.

The prothrombin time (PT) and activated partial thromboplastin time (aPTT) tests are usually determined with automated analyzers (Fig. 10-24). These analyzers use whole

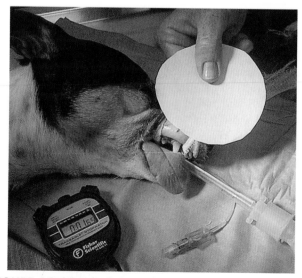

FIGURE 10-23 Buccal mucosa bleeding time test. (From Sirois M: Principles and practice of veterinary technology, ed 3, St Louis, 2011, Mosby; courtesy Dr. B. Mitzner.)

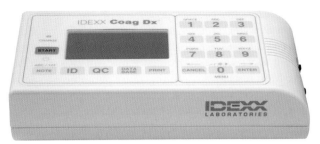

FIGURE 10-24 The Coag Dx Analyzer (IDEXX Laboratories, Westbrook, ME) provides measurements of prothrombin time and activated partial thromboplastin time. (From Sirois M: Principles and practice of veterinary technology, ed 3, St Louis, 2011, Mosby.)

blood or plasma samples collected in citrate anticoagulant tubes. The tests are simple and rapid and provide an accurate evaluation of the PT and aPTT.

CLINICAL CHEMISTRY

Laboratory analysis of blood biochemical constituents is performed for a variety of reasons. A blood sample may be collected from a patient as part of a general wellness screening process, to confirm or rule out a specific disease, as part of management of a clinical case to evaluate the status of a previously diagnosed condition, or as part of emergency medical therapy. Biochemistry profiles, or groups of tests, are routinely performed using serum as the preferred sample type, although heparinized plasma may also be used with some analyzers. Determinations of levels of the various chemical constituents in blood can provide valuable diagnostic information. The chemicals being assayed are usually enzymes associated with particular organ functions or metabolites and metabolic by-products that are processed by certain organs.

> ### CRITICAL CONCEPT
> Clinical chemistry testing usually requires either a serum or plasma sample.

HEPATOBILIARY FUNCTION TESTING

Hepatic (liver) cells exhibit extreme diversity of function and are capable of regeneration if damaged. As a result, there are over 100 types of tests to evaluate liver and gallbladder function. In most cases, evaluation of several liver function test results is required to assess the overall status of the liver. Liver cells also compartmentalize the work, so damage to one zone of the liver may not affect all liver functions. Liver function tests are often done with serial determinations. Usually, liver disease has greatly progressed before clinical signs appear. Liver function tests are designed to measure substances that are produced by the liver (primarily proteins), modified by the liver (e.g., bilirubin), or released when hepatocytes are damaged (primarily liver enzymes).

> ### CRITICAL CONCEPT
> The most commonly performed hepatobiliary tests in small animal practice are ALT, ALP, Bilirubin, and Total Protein.

PROTEIN

In the small veterinary practice, total protein is usually measured with a refractometer (see Procedure 10-2). Total serum protein concentrations include all plasma proteins except fibrinogen and other coagulation proteins that have been removed during the coagulation process. Most serum proteins are produced by hepatocytes. Chemical analyzers also measure total protein concentration.

Serum protein levels are affected by the rate of protein synthesis in the liver, the rate of protein catabolism in the animal, hydration status, and alterations in the distribution of proteins in the body. Dehydrated animals usually have elevated total protein values; overhydrated animals usually have decreased total protein values. Marked hemolysis falsely increases total protein levels. Do not use lipemic samples, especially if the refractometric method is used. Moderate icterus has no effect on the refractometric method. Heat, ultraviolet light, surfactant detergents, and chemicals can break down proteins, leading to artificially low results.

ALBUMIN. Albumin is one of the most important proteins in plasma or serum. It makes up approximately 35% to 50% of the total serum protein concentration. Albumin is synthesized by the liver. Albumin levels are also influenced by dietary intake, renal disease, and intestinal protein absorption. Albumin functions as a transport and binding protein of the blood and is responsible for maintaining osmotic pressure of plasma.

GLOBULIN. Globulins are a complex group of proteins that include all the proteins (plasma or serum) other than albumin and coagulation proteins. The globulins are separated into three major classes by electrophoresis—alpha, beta, and gamma globulins. Most alpha and beta globulins are synthesized by the liver. The gamma globulins (immunoglobulins) are synthesized by plasma cells and are responsible for the body's immunity provided by antibodies. Immunoglobulins identified in animals include immunoglobulin G (IgG), IgD, IgE, IgA, and IgM.

Direct measurement of globulin is not usually performed. Globulin concentration is calculated by subtracting the albumin concentration from the total serum protein.

BILIRUBIN

Bilirubin is assayed to determine the cause of jaundice (icterus), evaluate liver function, and check the patency of bile ducts. Bilirubin is an insoluble molecule derived from the breakdown of hemoglobin in the spleen. Two types of bilirubin, conjugated and unconjugated, are present in the plasma. Alterations in the ratios of the various bilirubin compounds help determine whether liver damage is present or if other conditions (e.g., bile duct obstruction) are contributing to disease.

BILE ACIDS

Bile acids are produced from cholesterol in the liver and serve many functions, including aiding in fat absorption and modulating cholesterol levels. The gallbladder stores bile acids, which are then released into the intestinal tract. Most bile acids are actively resorbed in the ileum and carried to the liver, where they are reconjugated and excreted as part of the enterohepatic circulation of bile acids. Blood levels of bile acids in normal animals are very low, especially in fasted animals.

ENZYME ANALYSES

Enzymes are specialized proteins that catalyze various chemical reactions. Most enzymes work intracellularly at a specific pH. Enzymes are usually not present in high concentrations in serum. Increased concentrations of enzymes in serum often indicate cellular damage. Enzyme assays usually involve measurement of the outcome of enzyme activity rather than specific measurement of the enzyme itself. Enzymes related to liver function in most mammals include the phosphatases and transaminases.

PHOSPHATASES

The primary phosphatases are the alkaline phosphatases (ALPs) and acid phosphatases (ACPs). Determinations of ACP levels are not usually carried out but may help in the diagnosis of certain types of hemolytic anemia. ALPs have multiple organ sources, including the liver, kidney, bone, and intestine. The extent of the increase aids in determining whether the patient has intrahepatic or extrahepatic damage. The ALP assay is most often used to detect cholestasis in dogs and cats. ALP levels can be increased in young, growing animals because of bone remodeling and increases in the bone isoenzyme level.

TRANSFERASES

This group of enzymes is found primarily in tissues that have high rates of protein metabolism, especially the kidney, liver, and muscle. In small animal veterinary medicine, the transferases of clinical significance are alanine aminotransferase (ALT) and aspartate aminotransferase (AST).

In dogs and cats, damage to hepatocytes results in the release of large amounts of ALT. In other species, ALT levels have little clinical significance. ALT is a liver-specific enzyme and a good indicator of hepatocellular damage in dogs, cats, and primates because the primary or major source of serum ALT is the hepatocyte. AST assays are used primarily to evaluate the extent of skeletal muscle damage in the equine and may also be used to evaluate cardiac muscle damage in some species.

KIDNEY FUNCTION TESTING

The primary chemical tests of kidney function are determination of urea nitrogen and creatinine levels. Blood urea nitrogen (BUN) is the principal product of protein catabolism. Normally, all urea passes through the glomerulus, and approximately 50% is resorbed by passive diffusion. **Azotemia**, an increase in BUN levels, can occur when blood flow through the kidneys alters the glomerular filtration rate or when the urinary tract is obstructed. Dehydration will also

result in azotemia because urea must be excreted in a large amount of water. Differences in rates of protein catabolism between male and female animals, young and adult animals, different species, and nutritional status will also affect BUN levels. Most tests for urea nitrogen use photometric analysis.

Serum creatinine is produced from the metabolic breakdown of phosphocreatine in muscle tissue. The daily rate of creatinine production is relatively constant in any animal and is dependent on muscle mass. Creatinine is also primarily cleared by the kidney. Glomerular filtration is the primary mode of elimination. Creatinine is used to evaluate renal function based on the ability of the glomeruli to filter creatinine from the blood and eliminate it in urine. Similar to BUN, if serum creatinine values are increased because of decreased renal function, this indicates that approximately 75% of the nephrons are nonfunctional.

> **CRITICAL CONCEPT**
> The primary chemical tests of kidney function are urea nitrogen and creatinine.

URIC ACID

Uric acid is an end product of the catabolism of nucleic acids. It is the primary end product of nitrogen metabolism in avian species and is actively secreted by the renal tubules. Measurement of the plasma or serum uric acid level is therefore preferred over the urea level as an indicator of kidney function in birds. In most animals, uric acid is bound to albumin, passes through the glomerulus, and then is resorbed. It is usually converted to allantoin and excreted in the urine. In Dalmatian dogs, the liver is unable to convert uric acid, so these animals excrete uric acid rather than allantoin. This also predisposes the breed to urate **urolithiasis**. Photometric analysis of uric acid is a complex procedure not commonly performed in veterinary clinical practice. However, newer methods of chemical analysis using liquid-stable reagents can enable uric acid testing in the veterinary practice laboratory.

PANCREATIC FUNCTION TESTING

The pancreas functions as an endocrine and exocrine organ. The endocrine part of the pancreas contains small nodules of endocrine cells, the islets of Langerhans. Two hormones are produced within the islets, insulin and glucagon. Insulin is necessary for the body's cells to use glucose for fuel. It prevents abnormally high blood glucose levels and allows glucose to enter the cells for use. A defect in insulin secretion or action leads to diabetes mellitus, characterized by abnormally high blood glucose levels and many metabolic difficulties. The other pancreatic hormone, glucagon, has the opposite effect, and tends to increase the blood glucose level.

AMYLASE

Amylase is produced in a variety of tissues, including the salivary glands, small intestine, and pancreas, and functions in the breakdown of starch to glucose. Serial determinations of amylase in conjunction with lipase provide the best indication of pancreatic function. Increased levels of amylase can occur with acute pancreatitis, flare-ups of chronic pancreatitis, and obstruction of the pancreatic ducts.

> **CRITICAL CONCEPT**
>
> Serial determination of both amylase and lipase are commonly performed to diagnose and manage pancreatitis in small animals.

LIPASE

Lipase functions to break down the fatty acids of lipids. Not all animals with pancreatitis have elevated lipase levels. Lipase activity may also be elevated by nonpancreatic factors such as chronic renal failure, exploratory surgery, and corticosteroid use. Almost all serum lipase is derived from the pancreas. Excess lipase is easily filtered through the kidneys, so lipase levels tend to remain normal in the early stages of pancreatic disease. Gradual increases are seen as disease progresses.

GLUCOSE

A small portion of the pancreas is involved in the production of insulin. Insulin is required to facilitate the uptake of glucose by body cells. Blood glucose measurements provide an indicator of the status of pancreatic endocrine activity. However, these can be affected by a variety of factors, including diet and stress. The blood glucose level reflects the net balance between glucose production (dietary intake, conversion from other carbohydrates) and glucose use (energy expended, conversion to other products). It also reflects the balance between blood insulin and glucagon levels.

Glucose use depends on the amount of insulin and glucagon being produced by the pancreas. As the blood insulin level increases, so does the rate of glucose use, resulting in decreased blood glucose levels. Glucagon acts as a stabilizer to prevent blood glucose levels from becoming too low. As the insulin level decreases, so does glucose use, resulting in increased blood glucose concentration. Although excess serum glucose can result from a variety of disease conditions, the highest blood glucose values are seen in diabetes mellitus. This condition results from decreased or defective production of insulin. Without sufficient insulin, the body cells are unable to take up glucose. Although the nephron normally resorbs blood glucose from the filtrate, excess glucose cannot be effectively resorbed by the nephron. This results in glycosuria—glucose in the urine. Glycosuria alters the solute concentration of the filtrate and causes an increased loss of electrolytes and nitrogen into the urine.

A variety of methods are available to evaluate blood glucose levels. Dedicated instruments for blood glucose testing are also readily available. Most of these were initially designed for use in human medicine to allow diabetic patients to monitor their own blood glucose levels. It is vital that the blood serum or plasma be removed from contact with the erythrocytes immediately after blood collection. If the sample is left in contact with the erythrocytes, the blood glucose levels can drop up to 10%/hour at room temperature. Erythrocytes use glucose for energy. In a blood sample, erythrocytes may decrease the glucose level enough to give false-normal results if the original sample had an elevated glucose level. If the sample originally had a normal glucose level, a falsely low level may result. If the blood sample cannot be centrifuged and the serum or plasma is not separated from the erythrocytes, collect the sample in a sodium fluoride tube. Sodium fluoride inhibits the use of glucose by erythrocytes and therefore stabilizes glucose levels for up to 12 hours at room temperature, and for 48 hours if the sample is refrigerated. Refrigeration slows glucose use by erythrocytes. Because eating raises the blood glucose level and fasting decreases it, a 12-hour fast is recommended when possible for all animals, except for mature ruminants, before the blood sample is collected.

FRUCTOSAMINE

Fructosamine is a more specific indicator of pancreatic endocrine activity than glucose. Fructosamine results from a reaction between glucose and serum protein. Fructosamine levels provide an indication of the average glucose levels over the life span of the protein ($\approx$1 to 3 weeks).

OTHER SERUM ASSAYS
ENZYMES AND LACTATE

Creatine kinase (CK), also referred to as creatine phosphokinase (CPK), is a cytoplasmic enzyme that appears in the serum in increased concentrations after cellular injury. Lactate dehydrogenase (LD) is a serum enzyme present in almost all tissues, although liver, muscle, and erythrocytes are the major sources of increased blood LD levels.

Lactate, also referred to as lactic acid, is an indication of tissue hypoxia. Lactate values are frequently used to monitor and develop prognostic indicators for critically ill patients. Handheld meters for in-house use are available for lactate testing. However, few of these have been validated for veterinary species (Fig. 10-25).

ELECTROLYTES

Electrolytes are minerals that exist as positively charged or negatively charged particles in an aqueous solution. Positively charged particles are called cations and negatively charged particles are called anions. These particles function primarily in the regulation of acid-base and osmotic balance of the body. The primary method for electrolyte evaluation involves the use of ion-specific electrodes. Automated ion-specific instruments are readily available and reasonably priced, so many veterinary practices can now perform electrolyte testing (Fig. 10-26).

> **CRITICAL CONCEPT**
>
> Electrolyte analyzers used in veterinary practice employ ion-specific electrode methodology.

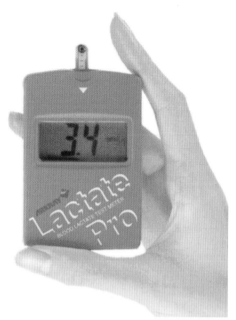

FIGURE 10-25 Handheld lactate meter. (From Sirois M: Principles and practice of veterinary technology, ed 3, St Louis, 2011, Mosby.)

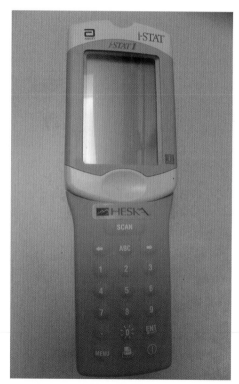

FIGURE 10-26 Electrolyte analyzer for veterinary practice use. (From Sirois M: Principles and practice of veterinary technology, ed 3, St Louis, 2011, Mosby.)

The electrolytes that are most commonly measured are sodium (Na^+), potassium (K^+), chloride (Cl^-), calcium (Ca^{2+}), inorganic phosphorus (P), and magnesium (Mg^{2+}). Electrolytes can be measured using serum or heparinized plasma. It is important to remember that different salts of heparin are available—sodium heparin, potassium heparin, ammonium heparin, and lithium heparin. When selecting an anticoagulant, do not choose a form of heparin that contains the substance that is being measured.

BASIC PRINCIPLES OF IMMUNOLOGY

The term *immune system* refers to a variety of cells, tissues, organs, and organ systems that are involved in the body's defense mechanisms. Some components are present and active in the body at all times. Others are created or activated in response to a foreign substance.

Immunity can generally be divided into two types, passive and active. Passive immunity includes maternal antibodies from colostrum and physicochemical barriers, such as the skin and mucous membranes. Active immunity is developed or acquired and is classified as humoral or cell-mediated immunity. Humoral immunity is mediated by the production of unique proteins (antibodies), which are responsible for the specific recognition and elimination of antigens. Foreign substances that are capable of generating a response from the immune system are referred to as antigens. Antigens include bacteria, viruses, parasites, or even the body's own tissues (autoimmunity). Specific substances on the surface of the antigen are responsible for the recognition of an antigen by the body's immune system. These substances are usually proteins and act as markers for the immune system. Recognition of these markers often results in the formation of antibody by the immune system. When antibodies are produced, the immune system retains a memory of the antigen and can respond more quickly to future attacks by the same antigen. Cell-mediated immunity is dependent on cells, in particular lymphocytes. Similar to antibodies, these lymphocytes recognize specific antigens, such as those of fungi, parasites, intracellular bacteria, or tumor cells, and help remove them from the animal by lysing the infected or cancerous cell or organism.

IMMUNOLOGIC TESTS

Dysfunction of the immune system can lead to an overactive immune system that produces immune-mediated disease or an underactive immune system that produces immunodeficiency disorders. These disorders can involve any component of the immune system (e.g., passive, humoral, cell mediated). Serologic testing is based on the ability to detect antibody-antigen interactions. Immunoassays usually contain monoclonal antibodies to an antigen or part of an antigen, such as a viral capsule or surface protein of a parasite. The tests, therefore, detect that portion of the antigen for which the test kit manufacturer has created a specific antibody. A few tests detect circulating antibody, rather than antigen, but these are used only when the antigen is not readily available for testing. Serologic tests formerly required a reference laboratory; however, many kits are now available for in-house testing for various infectious agents.

> **CRITICAL CONCEPT**
>
> ELISA tests are the most common immunoassays performed in clinical practice.

ENZYME-LINKED IMMUNOSORBENT ASSAY

Enzyme-linked immunosorbent assay (**ELISA**) tests are the most common types of immunologic tests performed in veterinary clinics. Every ELISA test has the same basic components:

- Solid phase
- Conjugate
- Chromogen

The solid phase may be a microwell, wand, flow-through membrane, or chromatographic strip. Conjugate reagents are embedded on the solid phase and usually consist of monoclonal antibodies bound to an enzyme. The chromogen is a photosensitive reagent that produces a color change in the test system. Adding patient sample to the solid phase is the first step in the test. The sample is then allowed to incubate. If specific antigen is present in the sample, it will bind to the antibody on the test surface. After the appropriate incubation time, the patient sample is washed away. If antigen has bound to the solid phase, it will not be washed away. Chromogen is then added that can react with the bound enzyme-antigen-antibody complex, if present, and produce a color change in the test system (Fig. 10-27). The SNAP test is a type of filter format ELISA (Fig. 10-28).

RAPID IMMUNOMIGRATION ASSAY

The rapid immunomigration (RIM) assay, also known as immunochromatography, is similar to the ELISA method except that gold staining is used to replace the chromogen. This format has become more common in veterinary practice in recent years. In these test formats, also known as lateral flow assays, the conjugate is an antibody bound to colloidal gold or latex, instead of an enzyme. The solid phase of a RIM test is a chromatographic strip. Most RIM tests require a flow solution, usually a buffered saline, to aid in the movement of the sample across the chromatographic strip. Some RIM tests do not require flow solution because the sample volume is large enough to flow onto the solid phase without additional steps. The RIM method does not use temperature-sensitive enzymes, so the test kit can be kept at room temperature.

The RIM test is performed by adding the patient sample to the absorptive pad on the solid phase. The absorptive pad functions to absorb the sample and filter out solid substances, such as blood cells. The conjugate is released as the sample flows onto the solid phase. The sample and conjugate then pass across two test areas. The first test area, known as the patient line, contains antibodies to the antigen that the test is designed to detect. If the antigen is present in the sample, it will bind to the antibodies on the patient line. When that occurs, the conjugate also reacts and produces a color change on the patient line. The sample and conjugate continue to flow to the second test area. The second area is a control line that contains antibodies to the conjugate. A color change is produced on this line and indicates that the test is functioning correctly.

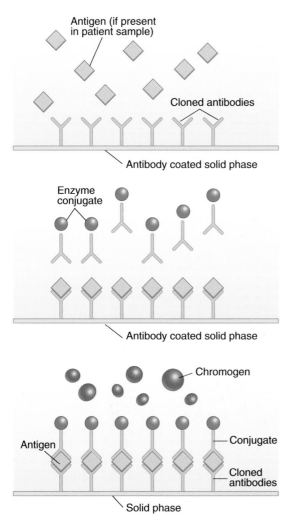

FIGURE 10-27 Principle of ELISA reaction. (From Sirois M: Principles and practice of veterinary technology, ed 3, St Louis, 2011, Mosby.)

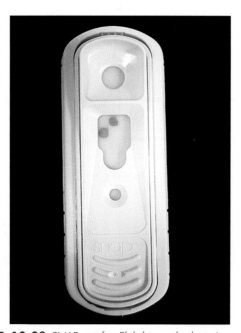

FIGURE 10-28 SNAP test for *Ehrlichia* antibodies. A positive test result is indicated on the ELISA membrane format. A positive control spot is also seen. (Courtesy IDEXX Laboratories, Westbrook, ME.) (From Sirois M: Principles and practice of veterinary technology, ed 3, St Louis, 2011, Mosby.)

AGGLUTINATION TEST

Agglutination tests are used for the detection of antibodies to large particulate antigens. The test requires adding a specific antigen to the test sample. If the sample contains the antibody for that antigen, agglutination (clumping) occurs.

In some agglutination tests, the antigen may be coated with latex beads to induce agglutination reactions. Agglutination tests are usually performed on a slide. Latex agglutination is commonly used to diagnose brucellosis in dogs and determine blood types (Fig. 10-29).

OTHER TESTS

There are three major types of precipitation tests—immunodiffusion, radioimmunodiffusion, and immunoelectrophoresis. Several types of electrophoresis procedures are performed. These are primarily performed in reference or referral laboratories, rather than in clinical practice.

The Coombs test is used to detect autoantibodies (antibodies to one's own tissues). Although the Coombs test is fairly simple to perform, the expense of stocking the species-specific Coombs reagent for only occasional tests makes it impractical to run in house. The tests are usually sent to an outside reference laboratory.

Although not commonly performed in veterinary practices, fluorescent testing is available at most veterinary reference laboratories. These test procedures are frequently used to verify a tentative diagnosis made by the veterinarian.

INTRADERMAL SKIN TESTING

Patients with allergic skin diseases may be diagnosed with a combination of clinical signs and exclusion of suspected allergens or may require immunologic intradermal testing. Common causes of allergic skin disease include food allergy, contact dermatitis, insect bites and stings, inhalant allergy (e.g., pollen, mold), and atopy. Allergies are mediated by IgE antibody molecules and can be detected by using allergenic extracts of grasses, trees, weed pollens, molds, dust, insects, and other possibly offending antigens. The extracts are injected intradermally, and the injection sites are monitored for allergic reactions. A positive reaction appears as a raised welt, meaning that the animal is allergic to that antigen.

ANTIBODY TITERS

Results of some antibody tests may be reported as positive or negative. In other words, the test indicates the presence or absence of antibody to the particular infectious agent in the patient's serum. Results of other antibody tests may be reported as antibody titers, or levels. The patient's serum is serially diluted to different concentrations, such as $1:10$, $1:40$, and $1:160$, meaning 1 part serum in 9 parts saline, 1 part serum in 39 parts saline, and 1 part serum in 159 parts saline, respectively. A test to detect antibodies is done on each of these dilutions, and the greatest dilution that tests positive is reported. For example, if $1:10$ and $1:40$ are positive and $1:160$ is negative, the titer is reported as $1:40$. If none of the dilutions is positive, the titer may be reported as negative or the test may be repeated at lesser dilutions, such as $1:2$, $1:4$, or $1:8$. A higher titer (positive at greater dilutions) indicates that more antibody is present. More antibody is present in a sample with a titer of $1:160$ than in a sample with a titer of $1:40$.

An antibody titer in a single sample may indicate only that the animal has been previously exposed to an infectious agent; the animal may not currently have an active infection. A rising titer in two or more samples indicates an active infection.

COMMON ERRORS AND ARTIFACTS

In spite of what may seem like simplistic technology, the proper performance of these tests is vital to ensure accurate results. Each test method mentioned has specific advantages and limitations. However, if the test is not performed correctly, a number of other factors can produce false-positive or false-negative results. A false-positive result is a positive test result on a sample from a patient that is, in fact, negative for the antigen. A false-negative result is a negative test result on a sample from a patient that is, in fact, positive for the antigen. Many immunoassays incorporate controls that help determine the accuracy of the test results. A visible positive control indicates that the test kit is functional. The most common causes of false results are poor sample quality, inadequate washing (ELISA tests), improper incubation, cross-reacting proteins, or expired or improperly stored kits.

MICROBIOLOGY

The term *microbiology* refers to the study of microbes, specifically bacteria. Bacteria are small prokaryotic cells that have no nucleus and have few cellular organelles. Microbiologic evaluations of tissues and body fluids can be used to determine the presence of specific disease-causing organisms and to aid in managing patient therapy. Samples for microbiologic evaluation can be collected quickly by various

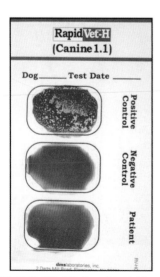
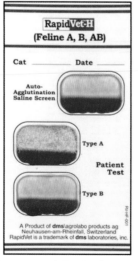

FIGURE 10-29 RapidVet-H blood typing card (DMS Laboratories, Flemington, NJ). (From Sirois M: Principles and practice of veterinary technology, ed 3, St Louis, 2011, Mosby.)

methods, including swabbing, scraping, and aspiration. The specific techniques used depend on the type of lesion and its location on the animal's body. Careful attention to aseptic technique is critical to achieving diagnostic quality results.

CHARACTERISTICS OF BACTERIA

Bacteria are variable in size, ranging from 0.2 to 2.0 μm. They can be classified into one of four general categories (cocci, bacilli, spirals, palisades) and can have a variety of arrangements (Fig. 10-30). Although most cellular organelles are absent, bacteria contain cell walls, plasma membranes, and ribosomes. Some contain capsules and flagella and can develop endospores. These characteristics are often used in the differentiation of specific bacterial pathogens.

> **CRITICAL CONCEPT**
> Bacteria can be cocci, bacilli, spirals, and palisades shapes and can occur singly or in pairs, tetrads, chains, or clusters.

Most bacteria are chemoheterotrophic. That is, they obtain nutrients from nonliving components of their environment. Growth factors such as vitamins, amino acids, and nucleotides are also essential. Oxygen and temperature requirements vary among different species. Most species require a pH in the range of 6.5 to 7.5. Bacteria reproduce primarily by binary fission and their numbers grow exponentially until essential nutrients are depleted, toxic waste products accumulate, and/or space becomes limiting.

MYCOLOGY

The study of fungi is referred to as **mycology**. Fungi are groups of organisms that are characterized by vegetative structures known as hyphae. Hyphae can grow into matted structures known as mycelia. Fungi contain eukaryotic cells with cell walls composed of chitin. The organisms are heterotrophic and may be parasitic or saprophytic. Fungi can be differentiated based on the structure of the hyphae and on the presence of spores. Different groups of fungi produce different types of spores. Various fungal organisms can affect veterinary species and cause superficial mycosis or deep my-

cosis. Table 10-2 summarizes fungal pathogens of veterinary importance, species affected, resultant diseases or lesions, and specimens required for diagnosis.

SAMPLE COLLECTION

The specific choice of collection method depends on the location of the lesion on the animal's body, as well as the specific type of testing desired. Samples that are to be processed immediately can usually be collected using sterile cotton swabs. However, this is the least suitable method of collection because contamination risk is high and cotton can inhibit microbial growth. Oxygen can also be trapped in the fibers, making recovery of anaerobic bacteria less likely. Should delays in processing the sample be expected, a rayon swab in a transport medium must be used to preserve the quality of the sample (Fig. 10-31). Aspirated samples and tissue samples can be collected in a fashion similar to that described later in this chapter for cytology samples.

The following guidelines should be kept in mind for proper specimen collection and handling:

- Collect the specimen aseptically. Specimen contamination is the most common cause of diagnostic failure. The importance of aseptic collection of microbiologic specimens cannot be overemphasized. Collect samples as soon as possible following the onset of clinical signs and before the initiation of any treatment.
- Keep multiple specimens separate from each other to avoid cross-contamination. This is essential for intestinal specimens because of the normal flora found there. In addition, samples that contain formalin should be stored and/or shipped to outside laboratories in containers that are separate from prepared slides and nonformalinized specimens. Formalin fumes can render samples unsatisfactory for further analysis.
- Label the specimen container, especially if a zoonotic condition is suspected, such as anthrax, rabies, leptospirosis, or brucellosis. Tissues from animals with suspected zoonoses should be submitted in a sealed, leakproof, unbreakable container.
- Keep the specimen cool during transport. Any sample that can be frozen should be frozen, especially in summer. Swabs must be sent in transport medium. Bacteriologic, virologic, and *Mycoplasma* tests require separate swabs for each. Samples for anaerobic culture must be submitted cool or frozen.
- If shipping involves dry ice, seal the container or swab to prevent entry of CO_2 into the container. Carbon dioxide released by dry ice may kill bacteria and viruses.
- Swabs placed in a viral transport medium cannot be used for bacterial culture. Use duplicate bacterial transport media.
- If using an outside referral laboratory, send the specimen to the diagnostic laboratory by the fastest possible means. If the sample will be arriving during a weekend, inform the laboratory ahead of time so that arrangements can be made for pickup.

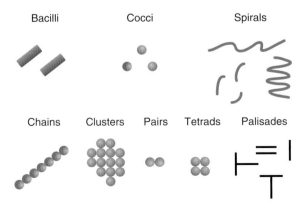

Bacilli   Cocci   Spirals

Chains   Clusters   Pairs   Tetrads   Palisades

FIGURE 10-30 Bacterial cell shapes and arrangements. (From Hendrix CM, Sirois M: Laboratory procedures for veterinary technicians, ed 5, St Louis, 2007, Mosby.)

TABLE 10-2	Summary of Pathogenic Fungi, Species Affected, Disease or Lesions Caused, and Specimens for Diagnosis		
ORGANISM	**SPECIES AFFECTED**	**DISEASE OR LESION**	**SPECIMENS**
Microsporum			
M. canis	Dogs, cats	Ringworm	Fresh plucked hair and skin scrapings from edges of lesions
M. distortum	Dogs, cats, horses, pigs	Ringworm	
M. gypseum	Horses, cats, dogs, other species	Ringworm	
M. persicolor	Voles, bats, dogs	Ringworm	
Trichophyton			
T. erinacei	Hedgehogs, dogs, people	Ringworm	
T. mentagrophytes	Most animal species	Ringworm	
T. rubrum	Primarily humans, but also dogs, cats	Ringworm	
Candida			
Candida spp. (e.g., C. tropicalis) can cause lesions	Dogs Cats	Mycotic stomatitis Enteritis of kittens	Fixed affected tissue or scrapings from affected tissue
Malassezia pachydermatis	Dogs	Chronic otitis externa	Fresh ear swabs
Cryptococcus neoformans	Humans, dogs, cats (infection frequently affects nervous systems)	Subacute or chronic affected tissue	Fresh nasal discharge, milk
Coccidioides immitis (southwest United States and South America; occurs in soil)	Humans, horses, cattle, sheep, dogs, cats, captive feral animals	Disease characterized by granulomas, often in bronchial and mediastinal lymph nodes and lungs; can cause lesions in brain, liver, spleen, kidneys	Fresh and fixed lesions and affected tissue
Histoplasma capsulatum (northeast, central, and south central United States; occurs in soil)	Humans, dogs, cats, sheep, pigs, horses	Disease that generally affects reticuloendothelial system; dogs, cats—ulcerations of intestinal canal; enlargement of liver, spleen, lymph nodes; tuberculosis-like lesions	Fresh and fixed lesions or affected tissue
Blastomyces dermatitidis (United States, Canada, and Africa; occurs in soil)	Humans, dogs, cats, sea lions	Granulomatous lesions in lungs and/or skin and subcutis	Fresh and fixed lesions and affected tissue
Sporothrix schenckii	Humans, horses, dogs, pigs, cattle, fowl, rodents	Subcutaneous nodules or granulomas that eventually discharge pus; can include involvement of bones and visceral organs	Fresh and fixed pus, granulomas
Rhinosporidium seeberi (not yet cultured in vitro)	Horses, dogs, cattle, humans	Characterized by polyps on the nasal and ocular mucous membranes	Fresh nasal discharge and polyps; fixed polyps
Aspergillus			
A. fumigatus main pathogen; potentially pathogenic A. nidulans A. niger	Many animal species and birds	Dogs—infection of nasal chambers	Fresh deep scrapings or affected tissue Abortions
A. flavus	Ducklings, domestic birds, pigs, dogs	Aflatoxicosis; affects liver and sometimes kidneys	Suspect food product

Adapted from Sirois M: Principles and practice of veterinary technology, ed 3, St Louis, 2011, Mosby.

SAMPLE PROCESSING MATERIALS

Preparation of samples for microbiology requires some unique supplies. Glass slides and coverslips are needed when performing Gram staining procedures; these can be of average quality. Inoculating loops or wires for transfer of specimens to culture media are also needed. A propane (Bunsen) burner or alcohol lamp is required to sterilize the inoculating loops and to flame the mouth of culture tubes before inoculation. When anaerobic or microaerophilic microbes are suspected pathogens, a candle jar or anaerobe jar (GasPak, Becton, Dickinson) will be required to provide the appropriate environment for microbial growth.

CULTURE MEDIA

Culture media are available in dozens of formulations. General purpose nutrient media provide basic requirements for bacterial growth. Selective media contain additives that allow certain microorganisms to grow while inhibiting the growth of others. Enriched media also promote the growth of certain microbes by providing specific growth factors for bacteria with strict nutrient requirements. These types of bacteria are referred to as fastidious. Differential media contain additives that detect certain biochemical reactions of the bacteria. Media are also available that incorporate the features of more than one type. Most small animal practice microbiology laboratories will require just a few of these. Media are also supplied as a solid form on culture plates or in tubes, liquid form in tubes, or dehydrated form. Dehydrated media are the least expensive. However, they require additional preparation time and must be autoclaved before use. This may not be financially justifiable unless the practice is performing very large numbers of microbiology tests.

CRITICAL CONCEPT

Culture media formulations include selective, enriched, and differential media.

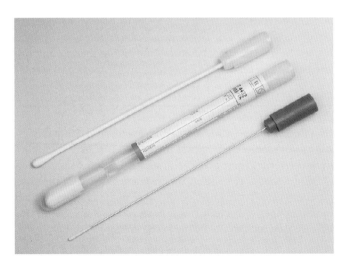

FIGURE 10-31 The Culturette consists of a rayon swab in a transport medium. (From Hendrix CM, Sirois M: Laboratory procedures for veterinary technicians, ed 5, St Louis, 2007, Mosby; courtesy Dr. B. Mitzner.)

In veterinary practice, the most commonly used solid media in culture plates are Mueller-Hinton, trypticase soy agar with 5% sheep blood (commonly called blood agar), and MacConkey or eosin–methylene blue (EMB). Mueller-Hinton is the recommended medium for culture and sensitivity testing. MacConkey and EMB are both selective media that support the growth of gram-negative bacteria and incorporate an additional indicator to allow differentiation among gram-negative enteric bacteria based on their ability to ferment lactose. Blood agar is an enriched medium that allows differentiation among specific hemolytic organisms.

CRITICAL CONCEPT

Pathogenic bacteria exhibit beta hemolysis on blood agar.

Solid media in culture tubes are used primarily for the growth of fungi and yeasts. Additional media available in this form include those used for biochemical testing of microbes. The most common types of slant media tubes are Sabouraud dextrose or bismuth-glucose-glycine yeast (commonly referred to as "biggy"). The medium is usually solidified into a slant-topped configuration. Either type is suitable for the growth of **dermatophytes** and is usually described as dermatophyte test medium (DTM), regardless of which specific medium is present. Fungal cultures of solid tissue samples may require the use of a 20% potassium hydroxide reagent for preparation of the sample.

A variety of companies produce culture plates that incorporate several different media within individual compartments on a culture plate. Items such as the Bullseye Veterinary Plate (Vetlab Supply, Palmetto Bay, FL; Fig. 10-32) and Bacti-Vet culture system (Invistra, Troy Biologicals, Troy, MI) provide five different types of media that can simultaneously

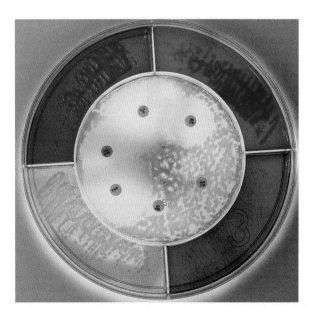

FIGURE 10-32 Bull's Eye culture medium (HealthLink, Jacksonville, FL). (From Hendrix CM, Sirois M: Laboratory procedures for veterinary technicians, ed 5, St Louis, 2007, Mosby.)

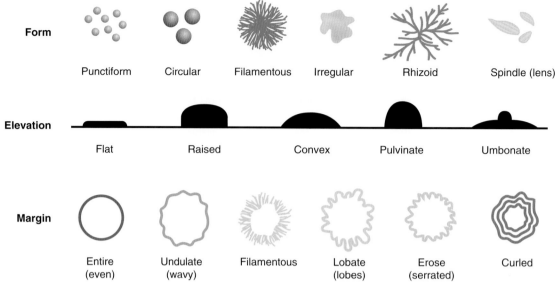

FIGURE 10-33 Bacterial colonies may be described on the basis of their form, elevation, and margins. (From Hendrix CM, Sirois M: Laboratory procedures for veterinary technicians, ed 5, St Louis, 2007, Mosby.)

select and differentiate microbes as well as provide antibiotic sensitivity data.

Broth media in tubes is necessary for blood cultures and is also available in forms to provide differentiation of gram-negative enteric bacteria. Thioglycollate broth is a general purpose medium that can be used for urine cultures. Specific blood culture tubes are available as evacuated tubes used for blood collection. These contain both anticoagulant and culture media.

Bacteria may often be partially differentiated based on their growth patterns on agar plates. Evaluation of colony characteristics should include form, elevation, margin, texture, and pigmentation (Fig. 10-33). The specific configuration made by a bacterial colony depends on the type of culture medium used as well as environmental conditions.

STAINS

Gram stain is an essential component of the microbiology laboratory. It is available in kit form or can be purchased as an individual solution (Fig. 10-34). For differentiation of certain types of bacteria, other stains are also available. Acid-fast stains are useful in the identification of *Mycobacterium*. These involve the addition of an agent such as dimethyl sulfoxide (DMSO) before addition of the primary stain. The agent allows the stain to penetrate the stain-resistant cells of *Mycobacterium*. The subsequent addition of acidic alcohol or dilute alcohol removes the stain. If the stain is not removed, the organism is said to be acid-fast. Flagella stains, capsule stains, endospore stains, and fluorescent stains are also available but have limited application in the average veterinary microbiology laboratory.

> ### CRITICAL CONCEPT
> Gram stain is the primary differential stain used in microbiology testing.

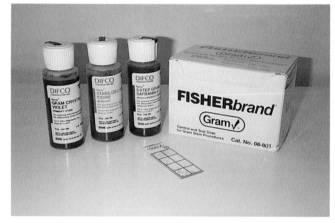

FIGURE 10-34 Gram stain kit. (From Hendrix CM, Sirois M: Laboratory procedures for veterinary technicians, ed 5, St Louis, 2007, Mosby; courtesy Dr. B. Mitzner.)

Simple stains, such as crystal violet or methylene blue, are usually used for yeasts. Lactophenol cotton blue stain is often needed to prepare fungal culture samples for analysis and can also be used for cellophane tape preparations of external lesions.

PROCEDURES

INOCULATING CULTURE MEDIA

Aseptic technique is crucial to achieving diagnostic-quality results in microbiology. Culture media and processing supplies must be sterile. There are several methods for the inoculation of culture media, depending on the characteristics of the sample and type of testing needed. Because many samples contain multiple types of bacteria, most bacterial tests involve an initial step designed to isolate the bacterium of interest.

INOCULATING DERMATOPHYTE TEST MEDIA

The procedures used for dermatophyte testing are slightly different than those used for general bacteriology testing. Either a DTM or plain Sabouraud dextrose agar can be used. DTM usually incorporates an additional reagent that causes a color change in the medium when *Microsporum canis* is present. However, it is important to note that some common contaminants can also induce this color change and some cultures of *M. canis* do not produce color change on the medium.

Suspect lesions may be gently cleaned with soap and water, and clean thumb forceps can be used to remove a few hairs and a small amount of epidermal scales from the periphery of the lesion. The hair and scale samples are then placed onto the surface of the culture medium. A portion of the sample is pressed down into the medium. The culture is loosely covered and placed in a cabinet or drawer at room temperature. Starting at 48 hours after incubation, the inoculated medium must be inspected each day for evidence of color change. A flocculent growth accompanied by color change suggests *M. canis* infection. If no growth occurs after 7 days, the specimen should be redistributed over the medium and the culture procedure repeated. If growth is evident, the material should be stained and examined microscopically. A drop of lactophenol cotton blue stain is placed in the center of a microscope slide. A 2-inch piece of clear (not frosted) cellophane tape or FungiTape (Scientific Device Laboratory, Des Plaines, IL) is pressed against the flocculent material observed growing on the plate. The tape is lifted and then pressed down into the drop of stain previously placed on the slide. The sample is evaluated microscopically for the characteristics of the organisms used to verify the species present.

BIOCHEMICAL TEST MATERIALS

Biochemical tests are often necessary to differentiate specific types of microbes. Biochemical testing may involve the use of specific liquid reagents or use media that contain the necessary reagents. The most commonly performed tests in the small veterinary practice laboratory are the oxidase and catalase tests. Reagents to perform these tests are inexpensive and readily available. Table 10-3 summarizes bacterial pathogens of veterinary importance.

QUALITY CONTROL CONCERNS

An effective quality control program is vital to achieving accurate and reliable results in any laboratory. Samples for microbiologic analysis are greatly affected by inappropriate or improperly performed collection methods. Careful attention to aseptic technique is critical. The timing of sample collection and processing must also be considered. Samples collected after medical treatment has begun or that are held for long periods of time before processing will yield unreliable results. Staining supplies and reagents must be stored and used correctly for maintenance of the integrity of these items. In addition to maintaining the sterility of collection and processing supplies, equipment used in the microbiology laboratory requires regular verification of performance. This includes verification of temperatures in autoclaves and incubators. Such routine quality control must be performed on a regular schedule and the results recorded so that equipment malfunctions can be detected early.

TABLE 10-3	Bacterial Pathogens of Veterinary Importance
GROUP	**GENERA**
Spirochetes	*Leptospira* *Borrelia* *Treponema* *Brachyspira*
Spiral and curved bacteria	*Campylobacter* *Helicobacter*
Gram-negative aerobic bacilli	*Pseudomonas* *Francisella* *Brucella* *Neisseria* *Bordatella*
Gram-negative facultative bacilli	*Escherichia* *Proteus* *Shigella* *Yersinia* *Salmonella* *Citrobacter* *Klebsiella* *Aeromonas* *Enterobacter* *Actinobacillus* *Serratia* *Haemophilus* *Pasteurella*
Gram-negative anaerobic bacilli	*Bacteroides* *Fusobacterium*
Gram-positive bacilli	*Bacillus* *Listeria* *Clostridium* *Erysipelothrix* *Lactobacillus*
Gram-negative pleomorphic	*Rickettsia* *Haemobartonella* *Ehrlichia* *Eperythrozoon* *Anaplasma* *Chlamydia* *Mycoplasma*
Gram-positive cocci	*Staphylococcus* *Streptococcus* *Enterococcus*

From Sirois M: Principles and practice of veterinary technology, ed 3, St Louis, 2011, Mosby.

CYTOLOGY

The primary goal of the cytology evaluation is the differentiation of inflammation and neoplasia. The types and numbers of cells present in a properly collected and prepared cytology specimen can provide rapid diagnostic information to the clinician. Samples for cytology evaluation can be collected quickly and do not generally require specialized materials or equipment for proper evaluation. With careful attention to appropriate collection, preparation, and staining technique, a high-quality cytology sample can be obtained. These samples yield valuable results for the clinician and often preclude the need for more invasive procedures to determine diagnosis, treatment, and prognosis for a patient.

Several different preparations are often made from each sample. This allows for additional diagnostic testing without additional collection. Samples may be processed as compression or modified compression preparations, impression smears, line smears, starfish smears, or simple smears. The exact type of preparation depends on the characteristics of the sample. Some samples may also require concentration by centrifugation. Fluid samples often require the addition of an anticoagulant and/or preservatives. A variety of staining techniques are also available for cytology specimens. Some samples will require processing with more than one staining procedure.

Collected and processed correctly, a cytology specimen is characterized as inflammatory, neoplastic, or mixed. The specimen is then described according to the presence of specific cell types. Neoplastic cells are further evaluated for malignant changes. Inflammatory processes are characterized as suppurative, pyogranulomatous, or eosinophilic when specific cell types and numbers of cells are evident on the cytology preparation. In general, samples that are inflammatory are characterized by a predominance of neutrophils and macrophages (tissue monocytes). Neoplastic samples are characterized by large numbers of tissue cells. There may be a combination of cell types present, which may indicate a neoplastic disease with secondary inflammation.

COLLECTION AND PREPARATION OF SAMPLES FROM TISSUES AND MASSES
IMPRESSION SMEARS

Impression smears are prepared from active lesions on an animal's body or from tissues removed during surgical procedures. For impression smears from active lesions, an initial impression is made before cleaning the lesion or initiating treatment. Additional smears are prepared after cleaning the lesion. To prepare the smear, gently touch a clean glass slide to several areas of the lesion. Although this type of sample can be prepared quickly and easily, it tends to yield the fewest number of cells and can also be contaminated by bacteria that may be present because of secondary bacterial infection. Impression smears of tissue samples are made in a similar manner except that a fresh section of the tissue is made; the tissue is then blotted to remove excess blood and tissue fluid. These excess fluids may prevent tissue cells from adhering to the slide (Procedure 10-5).

SCRAPINGS

Scrapings can be prepared from external lesions or from tissues removed during surgical procedures. This type of sample yields a greater number of cells than impression smears. To prepare a scraping, the lesion or tissue must be cleaned and blotted dry. If using tissue samples, a fresh section is cut before obtaining the sample. A dull scalpel blade is held at a 90-degree angle to the lesion or tissue and is gently pulled across the surface. A compression smear is then prepared

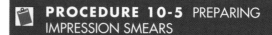

PROCEDURE 10-5 PREPARING IMPRESSION SMEARS

Materials
- Scalpel
- Forceps
- Paper towels and/or gauze sponges
- Glass slides

Procedure
1. Section the tissue to expose a fresh surface.
2. Hold the tissue fragment with forceps.
3. Blot excess fluid on a paper towel or gauze sponge until the tissue is almost dry.
4. Gently touch the tissue to the surface of a slide repeatedly down the length of the slide. Reblot as needed.
5. Allow the slide to air-dry.

Adapted from Sirois M: Principles and practice of veterinary technology, ed 3, St Louis, 2011, Mosby.

from the material on the edge of the scalpel blade. The sample can also be smeared across a slide directly from the scalpel blade.

CRITICAL CONCEPT
Cytology samples from solid masses are collected using impression smears, swabbing, scraping, or fine-needle biopsy.

SWABBINGS

Swab smears can provide valuable diagnostic information for certain types of specimens. This type of sample preparation is most useful for fistulated lesions or collections from the vaginal canal. A sterile cotton swab is moistened with 0.9% saline and lightly swabbed along the surface of the tissue. The swab is then gently rolled across the surface of a clean glass slide.

FINE-NEEDLE BIOPSY

A fine-needle biopsy sample can often provide much information to the clinician and may preclude the need for biopsy of lesions of internal organs. This type of sample preparation may also be preferred for the collection of samples from superficial lesions because bacterial contamination can be kept to a minimum. If microbiologic tests are to be performed on a portion of the sample collected or a body cavity (e.g., peritoneal and thoracic cavities, joints) is to be penetrated, the area of aspiration is surgically prepared. Otherwise, preparation is essentially the same as that which would be required for venipuncture. An alcohol swab may be used to clean the area.

The procedure may be performed using an aspirate or nonaspirate technique. For the aspiration biopsy, equipment needed includes a 3- to 20-mL syringe and a 21- to 25-gauge needle. Samples collected from softer tissue require smaller syringes and needles. Firmer tissues require larger syringes and large-bore needles. The nonaspirate procedure can be used to collect samples from solid masses.

PREPARATION TECHNIQUES FOR CYTOLOGY SAMPLES

Samples collected from organs and masses can be prepared in several ways. The veterinary assistant is responsible for preparing the supplies needed. Regardless of the preparation method chosen, the smear must be made quickly to avoid deterioration of the sample. Several smears should be made and rapidly air-dried.

COLLECTION AND PREPARATION OF FLUID SAMPLES

Fluid removed from the abdominal, thoracic, and pericardial cavities should be well mixed with an appropriate anticoagulant (e.g., EDTA) and the specimen prepared as quickly as possible to prevent cellular deterioration. Slides can be prepared directly from the nonconcentrated fluid or from concentrated sediment following centrifugation of the sample.

> **CRITICAL CONCEPT**
> Centesis refers to fluid samples collected from body cavities.

CONCENTRATION TECHNIQUES

Fluid samples may be centrifuged to concentrate the solid material before preparing smears. The technique is similar to that used for the preparation of urine sediment for microscopic analysis. The anticoagulated fluid is placed in a standard clinical centrifuge and spun for 5 minutes at 1000 to 2000 rpm (165 to 400 g). The supernatant is poured off, leaving a few drops in the tube. The sediment is gently resuspended in the remaining supernatant.

EXAMINATION OF CYTOLOGY SPECIMENS

The primary goal of the initial cytology evaluation is the differentiation of inflammation and neoplasia. In general, samples that are inflammatory are characterized by a predominance of neutrophils and macrophages or eosinophils. Neoplastic processes are characterized by large numbers of tissue cells. There may be a combination of cell types present. This mixed cell population often indicates neoplastic disease with secondary inflammation. The veterinary technician will evaluate the cell types present and record the information in the medical record.

> **CRITICAL CONCEPT**
> Fluid samples are classified as transudates, modified transudates, or exudates based on their gross appearance, total protein, and total nucleated cell count.

The gross appearance, total protein, and total nucleated cell count (TNCC) are also recorded for all fluid samples. The TNCC and total protein values for the sample will allow it to be classified as transudate, modified transudate, or exudate.

VAGINAL CYTOLOGY

Cytologic evaluation of vaginal tissues is used to determine the stage of estrus in the dog and cat and as an aid in timing of mating or artificial insemination. Samples are collected with the animal in a standing position, with the tail elevated. The external genitalia should be cleaned and rinsed. The veterinary assistant should prepare the necessary supplies, which include lubricant, vaginal speculum, and sterile moistened swabs. The veterinary technician will insert the lubricated vaginal speculum into the vagina, followed by a sterile moistened swab.

> **CRITICAL CONCEPT**
> The presence of specific types of epithelial cells, blood cells, and bacteria in a vaginal cytology sample is combined with behavioral history and clinical signs to determine estrous stage.

HISTOLOGY

Many samples collected for cytology analysis will also require histologic evaluation. Histology samples are usually collected by biopsy and require special preparation to preserve the cells for detailed evaluation. Fixation of tissues is a critical first step. The fixative must rapidly denature cellular proteins to avoid autolysis of the sample. Fixatives are chosen based on their speed and penetrating ability. They must not excessively harden or soften tissues and, ideally, be nontoxic to the user and inexpensive. Common fixatives include acetic acid, isopropyl or isobutyl alcohol, chromic acid, and formalin. The size of the tissue sample also affects the rate of fixation. Samples must be sectioned so that the fixative can penetrate the entire tissue within 24 to 48 hours. For large tissue samples, several cuts should be made into the tissue to allow the fixative to penetrate rapidly. Most fixatives are capable of penetrating approximately 2 to 4 mm/24 hours. The amount of solution needed is generally 10 to 20 times the volume of the sample. Once adequately fixed, the sample can be transferred into a smaller container.

> **CRITICAL CONCEPT**
> Samples to be used for histopathology must be sectioned so that the fixative can penetrate the entire tissue within 24 to 48 hours.

URINALYSIS

Complete examination of urine is a relatively simple, rapid, and inexpensive diagnostic procedure that can provide crucial information to the veterinarian. Urinalysis is a valuable diagnostic procedure for evaluating patients. Abnormalities in the urine may reflect a variety of disease processes involving several different organs. The basic equipment needed to perform a urinalysis is minimal and readily available in most veterinary clinics.

SAMPLE COLLECTION

Collect urine samples in clean glass or plastic containers. Sterile containers are not necessary unless you are performing a urine culture. Urine samples are collected using one of the following methods.

- Free-flow or clean catch: Collecting a specimen as the animal urinates
- Expressing the bladder: Manual compression of the bladder using gentle, steady pressure applied through the abdominal wall
- Catheterization: Placing a urinary catheter through the urethra into the bladder
- Cystocentesis: Inserting a needle into the bladder through the ventral abdominal wall

Bladder expression and cystocentesis require the bladder to be full enough to palpate and hold in position. Cystocentesis requires sterile collection equipment and aseptic technique. Only specimens collected by cystocentesis are suitable for urine culture. Cystocentesis and catheterization are also performed to relieve bladder distention in animals unable to urinate. Manual compression cannot be performed on an obstructed animal because this could rupture the bladder. Bladder expression, catheterization, and cystocentesis all cause some degree of trauma. A first-morning urine sample is the preferred specimen because this sample is the most concentrated. The first few drops should be discarded because there is a high incidence of contamination by the debris normally present at the urethral opening in the first few drops. In females, the first drops of urine may also be contaminated with material from the genital tract, such as blood from an intact bitch in proestrus.

Because physical, chemical, and microscopic characteristics of a urine specimen begin to change as soon as urine is voided, urine specimens should be analyzed immediately after collection. Samples left at room temperature for 1 hour or longer will have increases in pH, turbidity, and bacteria and decreases in glucose, bilirubin, and ketone levels. If specimens are left at room temperature for longer than 1 hour, cells and casts may also disintegrate, especially in dilute alkaline urine, or urine color may change because of oxidation or reduction of metabolites. If analysis cannot be done immediately, refrigeration will minimize deterioration of the specimen. The specimen should be brought to room temperature before testing. Chemical preservatives can also be added to urine. However, preservatives usually act as antimicrobial agents, so chemically preserved urine cannot be used for culture and may interfere with biochemical testing.

COMPLETE URINALYSIS

A complete urinalysis has the following four parts:
1. Gross examination
2. Specific gravity measurement
3. Biochemical analysis
4. Sediment examination

A systematic approach is vital to achieving high-quality, reproducible results. The gross examination includes an evaluation of color, clarity, odor, and volume. Normal canine and feline urine is light amber–colored, clear, and has a characteristic odor. Normal urine output for canine and feline patients is 10 to 20 mL/pound in a 24-hour period.

SPECIFIC GRAVITY

Specific gravity (SG) is a measure of the ratio of a volume of urine to the weight of the same volume of distilled water at a constant temperature. SG is an indicator of the concentration of dissolved materials in the urine and provides an indication of kidney function. Alteration in the concentrating ability of the kidneys is an early indicator of renal tubular damage. The preferred method for determining SG is with the use of a refractometer. SG indicator pads on urinalysis dipstick tests may be unreliable in veterinary species. SG can be measured before or after centrifugation, as long as the procedure is always performed consistently in the clinic. All individuals performing the test should perform it in the same manner on the same type of sample.

BIOCHEMICAL TESTING

The chemical evaluation of urine is used to detect substances that may have passed into the urine as a result of damage to the nephron or overproduction of specific analytes. Most in-house urinalysis chemical tests use the dipstick format (Fig. 10-35). Dipsticks can be used to perform an individual test or multiple tests. Each reagent pad on the dipstick contains reagent for one specific chemical test. The reagent pad changes color during the reaction, and the color is visually compared with a color chart. Before using the dipstick, always note the expiration date and general condition of the strips. Containers of dipsticks should be stored at room temperature with the lid tightly capped. Avoid placing containers or color charts in direct sunlight. Always use well-mixed,

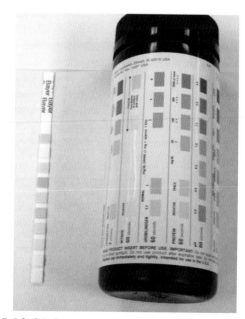

FIGURE 10-35 Reagent strip test container and combination dipstick strip. (From Hendrix CM, Sirois M: Laboratory procedures for veterinary technicians, ed 5, St Louis, 2007, Mosby.)

room-temperature urine samples and perform chemical testing before adding any chemical preservatives. Read the instructions carefully, and evaluate color changes at the correct time interval. Because dipsticks are not configured for veterinary species, some tests (e.g., SG, nitrite, leukocyte) may be unreliable with some species. Most urinalysis dipstick tests provide indicator pads for protein, glucose, ketones, pH, bilirubin, and blood.

MICROSCOPIC EXAMINATION OF URINE SEDIMENT

The primary purpose of microscopic examination of urine is to determine the presence of abnormal formed elements (e.g., cells, casts, crystals) in the sample (Fig. 10-36). The presence of specific formed elements usually provides detailed diagnostic information to the clinician. The examination requires 5 to 10 mL of fresh urine. The sample should be centrifuged at low speed for approximately 5 minutes and then the supernatant poured off, leaving approximately 1 mL of supernatant with the sediment. The remaining sediment is resuspended in the supernatant and mixed

gently. A drop of this suspension is then placed on a microscope slide, a coverslip is added, and the specimen is examined microscopically. Although stain may be added to the sample, this often creates artifacts and can add bacteria to the sample. When a stain is needed to classify cell types, it should be added after the initial evaluation of the specimen. The veterinary technician is responsible for evaluating the urine sediment.

PARASITOLOGY

Parasitology is the study of organisms that live in (internal parasites, **endoparasites**) or on (external parasites, **ectoparasites**) another organism, the host, from which they derive their nourishment. The host may be a **definitive host**, sheltering the sexual, adult stages of the parasite, or an **intermediate host**, harboring asexual (immature) or larval stages of the parasite. There are also paratenic or transport hosts for some parasites, in which the parasite survives without multiplying or developing. Parasite life cycles can be simple, with direct transmission, or complex and involve

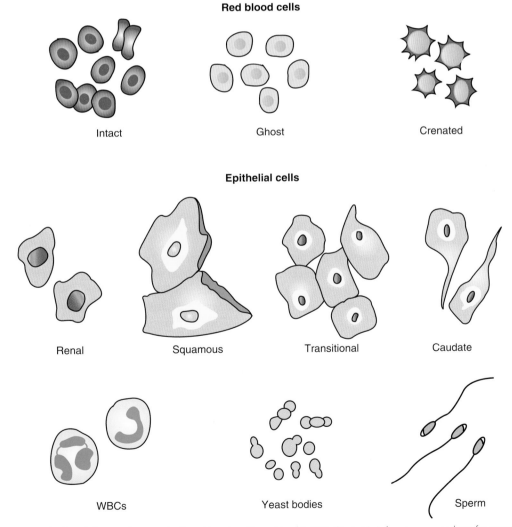

FIGURE 10-36 Cell types that may be found in urine. (From Hendrix CM, Sirois M: Laboratory procedures for veterinary technicians, ed 5, St Louis, 2007, Mosby.)

one or more vectors. A vector can be mechanical or biologic. Mechanical vectors transmit the parasite, but the parasite does not develop in the vector. Biologic vectors serve as intermediate hosts for the parasite. The term life cycle refers to the maturation of a parasite through various developmental stages in one or more hosts. For a parasite to survive, it must have a dependable means of transfer from one host to another and the ability to develop and reproduce in the host, ideally without producing serious harm to the host. This requires the following:

• Mode of entry into a host (infective stage)
• Availability of a susceptible host (definitive host)
• Accommodating location and environment in the host for maturation and reproduction (e.g., gastrointestinal, respiratory, circulatory, urinary, or reproductive system)
• Mode of exit from the host (e.g., feces, sputum, blood, urine, smegma), with dispersal into an ecologically suitable environment for development and survival

For parasites that have one or more intermediate hosts, the definitive host is the one in which sexual maturity takes place.

Parasites have a wide distribution within host animals. They can have a negative impact in a number of ways, including the following:

• Injury on entry (e.g., creeping eruption)
• Injury by migration (e.g., sarcoptic mange)
• Injury by residence (e.g., heartworms)
• Chemical and/or physiologic injury (e.g., digestive disturbances)
• Injury caused by host reaction (e.g., hypersensitivity, scar tissue)

CLASSIFICATION OF PARASITES

Parasites of domestic animals are found in the Protista and Animalia kingdoms and in a large number of phyla in those kingdoms. There is some variation in classification schemes in different references, and organisms are often reclassified when new information on their biochemistry is obtained. Box 10-3 contains a summary of the taxonomic classifications of common parasites of domestic animals.

KINGDOM PROTISTA, SUBKINGDOM PROTOZOA

There are approximately 65,000 known protozoans in a wide variety of habitats. Only a small percentage of protozoans is parasitic. Protozoa are single-celled organisms with one or more membrane-bound nuclei containing DNA and specialized cytoplasmic organelles. The life cycles of protozoa can be simple or complex. Reproduction may be asexual (binary fission, schizogony, budding) or sexual (syngamy, conjugation). With certain groups of protozoa, reproductive stages are useful in identification. The trophozoite (also known as the vegetative form) is the stage of the protozoal life cycle that is capable of feeding, movement, and reproduction. The trophozoite is often too fragile to survive transfer to a new host and generally

---

| **BOX 10-3** | Taxonomic Classifications of Parasites of Animals |

Kingdom: Animalia (animals)
Phylum: Platyhelminthes (flatworms)
   Class: Trematoda (flukes)
      Subclass: Monogenea (monogenetic flukes)
      Subclass: Digenea (digenetic flukes)
   Class: Cotyloda (pseudotapeworms)
Phylum: Nematoda (roundworms)
Phylum: Acanthocephala (thorny-headed worms)
Phylum: Arthropoda (animals with jointed legs)
   Subphylum: Mandibulata (possess mandibulate mouthparts)
   Class: Crustacea (aquatic crustaceans)
   Class: Insecta
      Order: Dictyoptera (cockroaches)
      Order: Coleoptera (beetles)
      Order: Lepidoptera (butterflies and moths)
      Order: Hymenoptera (ants, bees, and wasps)
      Order: Hemiptera (true bugs)
      Order: Mallophaga (chewing or biting lice)
      Order: Anoplura (sucking lice)
      Order: Diptera (two-winged flies)
      Order: Siphonaptera (fleas)
Phylum: Sarcomastigophora
   Subphylum: Mastigophora (flagellates)
Phylum: Sarcomastigophora
   Superclass: Sarcodina (amoebae)
Phylum: Ciliophora (ciliates)
Phylum: Apicomplexa (apicomplexans)
Phylum: Proteobacteria
   Class: Alpha Proteobacteria
      Order: Rickettsiales
         Family: Rickettsiaceae
         Family: Anaplasmataceae

From Sirois M: Principles and practice of veterinary technology, ed 3, St Louis, 2011, Mosby.

---

is not infective. Transmission to a host often occurs when the protozoan is in the cyst stage. Most metabolic functions are suspended when the parasite is encysted. The cyst wall prevents desiccation.

The phylum Sarcomastigophora (Sarcodina) includes the amoebas and flagellates. The most common parasitic organism of dogs and cats in this phylum is *Giardia* (Fig. 10-37). The phylum Apicomplexa contains the sporozoans. Sporozoal parasites are found within the host cells and commonly occur in the intestinal tract cells and blood cells. **Oocyst** is the name given to the cyst stage of this group of intestinal protozoa. The most common genera of veterinary importance include *Cystoisospora* (formerly *Isospora*) and *Toxoplasma*.

KINGDOM ANIMALIA

Three of the phyla in this kingdom contain hundreds of species that are of veterinary significance. These include (1) Platyhelminthes, the flatworms, (2) Nematoda, the

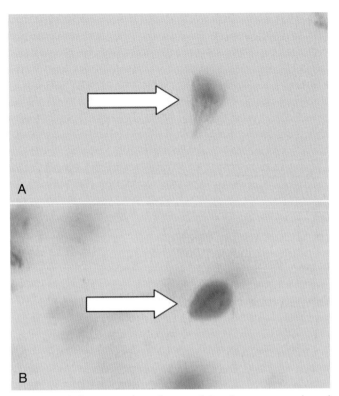

FIGURE 10-37 **A**, Motile trophozoite of *Giardia* spp. is pear shaped and dorsoventrally flattened and possesses four pairs of flagella. **B**, Mature cysts of *Giardia* spp. are oval and possess a refractile wall and four nuclei. (From Hendrix CM, Robinson E: Diagnostic parasitology for veterinary technicians, ed 4, St Louis, 2012, Mosby.)

roundworms, and (3) Arthropoda, ticks, mice, and lice. The phylum Acanthocephala contains just a few species of veterinary significance.

PHYLUM PLATYHELMINTHES. Organisms in the phylum Platyhelminthes are commonly called flatworms because of the dorsoventral flattening of their body tissues. The two groups of veterinary importance are the **cestodes** (tapeworms) and **trematodes** (flukes).

CESTODES. Two major groups of tapeworms are important in veterinary medicine. The first group is composed of the cyclophyllidean tapeworms, which typically have one intermediate host (Fig. 10-38). Organisms in this group include *Dipylidium caninum*, *Taenia* spp., and *Echinococcus* spp. The second group is composed of the pseudophyllidean tapeworms, which have two intermediate hosts (e.g., *Diphyllobothrium latum*). Typically, the larval stages of cestodes in domestic animals are more harmful (pathogenic) than the adult stages in the intestinal tract. However, the adult stages are the source of eggs, especially for cestodes, which can use humans as an intermediate host and pose a risk to human health (zoonotic).

Cestodes are multicellular organisms that lack a body cavity. The body of tapeworms is long and dorsoventrally flattened, and consists of three regions. The head (scolex) is modified into an attachment organ and bears two

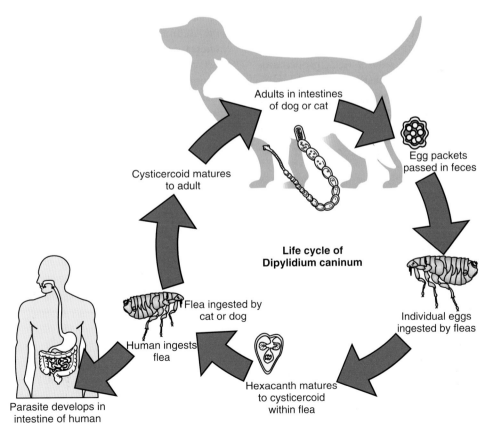

Adults in intestines of dog or cat

Egg packets passed in feces

Cysticercoid matures to adult

Life cycle of Dipylidium caninum

Individual eggs ingested by fleas

Flea ingested by cat or dog

Human ingests flea

Hexacanth matures to cysticercoid within flea

Parasite develops in intestine of human

FIGURE 10-38 Life cycle of *Dipylidium caninum*. (From Hendrix CM, Robinson E: Diagnostic parasitology for veterinary technicians, ed 4, St Louis, 2012, Mosby.)

to four muscular suckers, or bothria. The suckers may be armed with hooks. There may also be a snout (rostellum) on the head, which can be fixed or retractable. The rostellum can also be armed with hooks. Caudal to the head is a short neck of undifferentiated tissue, followed by the body (strobila). The body is composed of segments (proglottids) in different stages of maturity. Those near the neck are immature, followed by sexually mature proglottids, terminating with gravid segments containing eggs. Gravid proglottids break off and pass out of the body of the definitive host in the feces. New proglottids are continually formed from the undifferentiated tissue of the neck. Cestodes lack a digestive tract, and nutrients are absorbed directly through the body wall. The most prominent organs in cestodes are the organs of the reproductive system. Both male and female reproductive organs occur in an individual tapeworm. Cestodes also have a nervous system and an excretory system.

The cestode egg contains a fully developed embryo, which has six hooks in three pairs (hexacanth embryo, or oncosphere; Fig. 10-39), or a zygote that develops into a ciliated embryo (coracidium). The life cycle of tapeworms is always indirect and involves one or two intermediate hosts. The intermediate hosts may be **arthropods**, fish, or mammals. Domestic animals can be definitive and/or intermediate hosts for tapeworms. The larval stages of some tapeworms found in domestic animals are called bladder worms because they resemble fluid-filled sacks, with one or multiple scoleces. When ingested by a definitive host, the bladder worms are released from the tissue of the intermediate host and develop into adult tapeworms within the digestive tract of the definitive host. Some cestodes have larval forms that are solid bodies (e.g., procercoid, plerocercoid, tetrathyridium). Domestic animals become infected with the larval stages of tapeworms by ingestion of the cestode egg or procercoid. Table 10-4 summarizes the cestode parasites of veterinary species.

TREMATODES. The trematodes (flukes) are flatworms that, like cestodes, lack a body cavity. They are unsegmented and leaflike. The organs are embedded in loose tissue (parenchyma) and also possess two muscular attachment organs, or suckers. One sucker, the anterior sucker, is located at the mouth. The other sucker, the ventral sucker or acetabulum, is located on the ventral surface of the worm near the middle of the body or at the caudal end. There are three main groups of trematodes, but only the digenetic trematodes are parasites of domestic animals.

The life cycle of digenetic trematodes is complicated. They pass through several different larval stages (e.g., miracidium, sporocyst, redia, cercaria, metacercaria) and typically require one or more intermediate hosts, one of which is almost always a mollusk (e.g., snail, slug). The primary digenetic trematodes of concern is dogs is *Nanophyetus salmincola.*

PHYLUM NEMATODA. Organisms in the phylum Nematoda are commonly called roundworms because of their cylindrical body shape. The life cycle of nematodes follows a standard pattern consisting of several developmental stages—the egg, four larval stages that are also wormlike in appearance, and sexually mature adults. The infective stage may be an egg containing a larva, free-living larva, or larva within an intermediate or transport host. A life cycle is considered direct if no intermediate host is necessary for development to the infective stage. If an intermediate host is required for development to the infective stage, the life cycle is considered indirect. Transmission to a new definitive host can occur through ingestion, skin penetration of infective larvae, ingestion of an intermediate host, or deposition of infective larvae into or on the skin by an intermediate host.

Once a nematode gains entry into a new host, development to the adult stages may occur in the area of their final

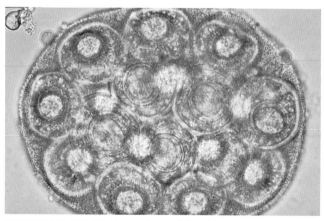

FIGURE 10-39 If fresh proglottids of *Dipylidium caninum* are teased or broken open, they may reveal thousands of egg packets, each containing 20 to 30 hexacanth embryos. (From Hendrix CM, Robinson E: *Diagnostic parasitology for veterinary technicians,* ed 4, St Louis, 2012, Mosby.)

TABLE 10-4	Selected Cestode (Tapeworm) Parasites of Dogs and Cats	
SCIENTIFIC NAME	**COMMON NAME**
Dogs	
Diphyllobothrium spp.	Broad fish tapeworm
Dipylidium caninum	Cucumber seed tapeworm
Spirometra spp.	Zipper tapeworm
Echinococcus granulosus	Hydatid disease tapeworm
Cats	
Echinococcus multilocularis	Hydatid disease tapeworm
Taenia taeniaeformis or *Hydatigera taeniaeformis*	Feline tapeworm
Diphyllobothrium spp.	Broad fish tapeworm
Dipylidium caninum	Cucumber seed tapeworm
Spirometra spp.	Zipper tapeworm

Adapted from Sirois M: *Principles and practice of veterinary technology,* ed 3, St Louis, 2011, Mosby.

location or may occur after extensive migration through the body of the definitive host. The diagnostic stages of parasitic nematodes are typically found in feces, blood, sputum, or urine. Most parasitic nematodes are found in the intestinal tracts of their respective definitive hosts, but some are found in the lungs, kidney, urinary bladder, or heart.

Table 10-5 summarizes the nematode parasites of dogs and cats. Nematodes of dogs and cats include *Toxocara* spp., *Toxascaris* spp., and *Ancylostoma* spp. *Trichuris vulpis*, the canine whipworm, derives its common name from the fact that adults possess a thin, filamentous anterior end (lash of the whip) and thick posterior end (handle of the whip).

TABLE 10-5 Selected Nematodes (Roundworms) of Veterinary Species

SCIENTIFIC NAME	COMMON NAME
Dogs	
Acanthocheilonema reconditum (formerly Dipetalonema reconditum)	Skin filariid
Ancylostoma braziliense	Hookworm
Ancylostoma caninum	Hookworm
Capillaria plica	Bladder worm
Dioctophyma renale	Giant kidney worm
Dirofilaria immitis	Canine heartworm
Dracunculus insignis	Guinea worm
Eucoleus aerophilus (formerly Capillaria aerophila)	Lungworm
Filaroides spp.	Canine lungworm
Physaloptera spp.	Stomach worm
Spirocerca lupi	Esophageal worm
Strongyloides spp.	Threadworms
Thelazia californiensis	Eyeworm
Toxocara canis	Roundworm, ascarid
Trichuris vulpis	Whipworm
Uncinaria stenocephala	Northern canine hookworm
Cats	
Aelurostrongylus abstrusus	Lungworm
Ancylostoma braziliense	Hookworm
Ancylostoma tubaeforme	Hookworm
Aonchotheca putorii (formerly Capillaria putorii)	Gastrid capillarid of cats
Capillaria feliscati	Bladder worm
Eucoleus aerophilus (formerly Capillaria aerophila)	Lungworm
Physaloptera spp.	Stomach worm
Spirocerca lupi	Esophageal worm
Thelazia californiensis	Eyeworm
Toxascaris leonina	Roundworm, ascarid
Toxocara cati	Roundworm, ascarid
Trichuris campanula	Whipworm
Trichuris serrata	Whipworm

From Sirois M: Principles and practice of veterinary technology, ed 3, St Louis, 2011, Mosby.

The egg of the whipworm is described as trichuroid or trichinelloid; it has a thick, yellow-brown, symmetrical shell with polar plugs at both ends.

D. immitis (Fig. 10-40) is the heartworm of dogs. The life cycle of *D. immitis* requires an intermediate host to be transmitted from animal to animal. The adults live in the right ventricle and pulmonary artery. The male and female adults mate, and the female produces microfilariae. The microfilariae are released into the host's bloodstream, where they are ingested by feeding female mosquitoes. The microfilariae grow and molt in the mosquito until they reach the infective stage. Once they become infective, they enter a new host the next time the mosquito feeds (Fig. 10-41). Once in the new host, the larvae migrate and molt through various body tissues on their way to the heart. It is at this time that the larvae may grow and molt to become adults in sites other than the heart.

PHYLUM ACANTHOCEPHELA. Acanthocephalans are commonly referred to as thorny-headed worms. This group of intestinal parasites is rarely encountered but occasionally is found in pigs and dogs. The life cycle of an acanthocephalan is complex and involves an intermediate host, usually a crustacean or an insect. The main acanthocephalan of concern is *Oncicola canis*, an acanthocephalan found in dogs.

RICKETTSIAL PARASITES
The rickettsia are a group of obligate, intracellular, gram-negative bacteria. The major taxonomic families are the Rickettsiaceae (Table 10-6), which include the genera *Rickettsia*, *Orientia*, and *Coxiella*, and the Anaplasmataceae, which include the genera *Anaplasma* and *Ehrlichia*. The organisms are transmitted by arthropod or helminth vectors.

PHYLUM ARTHROPODA. Organisms in the phylum Arthropoda are characterized by the presence of jointed legs. They have a chitinous exoskeleton composed of segments. Only certain groups of arthropods are parasitic. Members of other groups may act as intermediate hosts for the other parasites discussed earlier. When a parasite resides

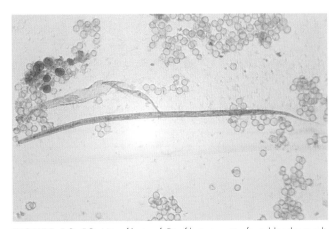

FIGURE 10-40 Microfilaria of *Dirofilaria immitis*, found by the modified Knott's technique. (From Hendrix CM, Robinson E: Diagnostic parasitology for veterinary technicians, ed 4, St Louis, 2012, Mosby.)

on the surface of its host, it is called an ectoparasite. Most ectoparasites are insects (e.g., fleas, lice, flies) or arachnids (e.g., ticks, mites).

The following general characteristics differentiate the two major classes of arthropods of veterinary importance. Insects have three pairs of legs, three distinct body regions (head, thorax, and abdomen), and a single pair of antennae. Arachnids (adults) have four pairs of legs, a body divided into two regions (cephalothorax, abdomen), and no antennae. The mouth parts of insects vary in structure, depending on feeding habits, with adaptations for chewing and biting, sponging, or piercing and sucking. The sexes are separate,

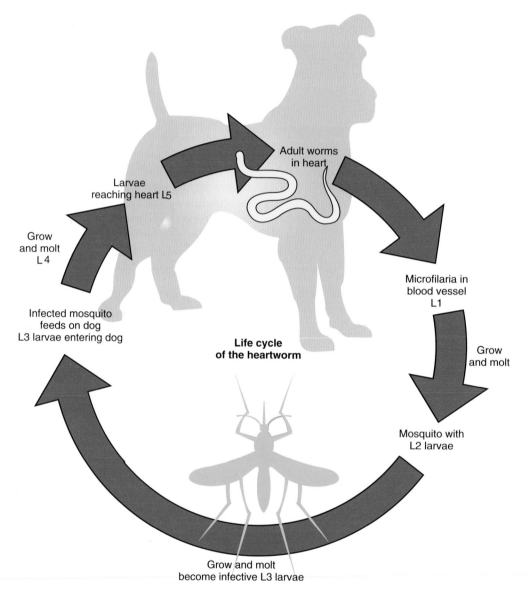

FIGURE 10-41 Life cycle of the canine *Dirofilaria immitis*. (From Hendrix CM, Robinson E: Diagnostic parasitology for veterinary technicians, ed 4, St Louis, 2012, Mosby.)

TABLE 10-6	Pathogenic Rickettsiaceae That Affect Animals		
AGENT	**DISEASE**	**VECTOR**	**GEOGRAPHIC DISTRIBUTION**
Rickettsia rickettsii	Rocky Mountain spotted fever	*Dermacentor* spp., ticks, *Amblyomma cajennense–Rhipicephalus sanguineus*	Western Hemisphere
R. felis	Cat flea typhus	*Ctenocephalides felis* (cat flea)	Western Hemisphere, Europe
R. typhi	Murine typhus	*Xenopsylla cheopis* (rat flea)	Worldwide
R. prowazekii	Epidemic typhus	Human body louse, flying squirrel louse, squirrel flea	Worldwide

Adapted from Songer JG, Post KW: Veterinary microbiology: Bacterial and fungal agents of animal disease, St Louis, 2005, Saunders.

and reproduction results in the production of eggs or larvae. Development often involves three or more larvae followed by the formation of a pupa and a change in form or transformation (complete metamorphosis) to the adult stage. In other insects, development occurs from the egg through several immature stages (nymphs), which resemble the adult in form but are smaller (incomplete metamorphosis). Fleas and flies demonstrate complete metamorphosis, and lice demonstrate incomplete metamorphosis. Insects may produce harm to their definitive host as adults and/or larvae.

Ticks and mites are the more important groups of arachnids in veterinary medicine, although some spiders and scorpions can harm domestic animals via toxic venoms. Arachnids are generally small, often microscopic. Life cycle stages consist of the egg, larva, nymph, and adult.

FLEAS. Fleas are blood-sucking parasites of dogs, cats, rodents, birds, and people. They are vectors of several diseases, such as bubonic plague and tularemia. Cat and dog fleas, *Ctenocephalides felis* and *C. canis*, respectively, can act as intermediate hosts for the common tapeworm, *Dipylidium caninum.* Heavy infestations with fleas, especially in young animals, produce anemia. Flea saliva is antigenic and irritating, causing intense pruritus (itching) and hypersensitivity, known as flea bite dermatitis or miliary dermatitis.

Fleas are laterally compressed, wingless insects with legs adapted for jumping. They move rapidly on the host and from host to host. Flea infestations are encountered most frequently on dogs and cats. They can be detected around the tail head, on the ventral abdomen, and under the chin.

Fleas demonstrate complete metamorphosis (Fig. 10-42). Eggs deposited on the host fall off and develop to larvae in the environment. The larvae can occasionally be found in the animal's bedding, on furniture, or in cracks and crevices of the animal's environment. The larvae are maggot-like, with a head capsule and bristles. Flea larvae feed on organic debris, including the excrement of adult fleas. Flea droppings

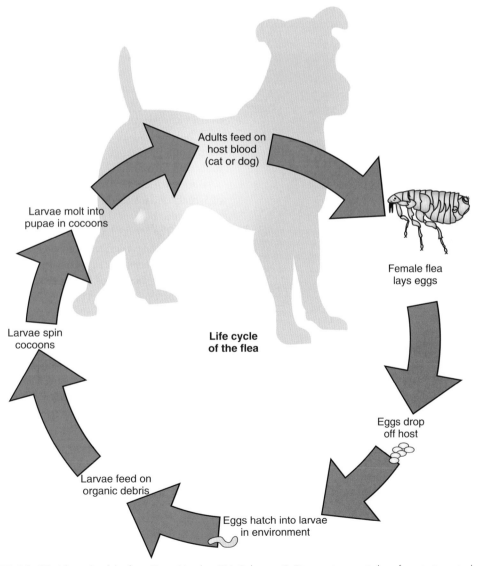

FIGURE 10-42 Life cycle of the flea. (From Hendrix CM, Robinson E: Diagnostic parasitology for veterinary technicians, ed 4, St Louis, 2012, Mosby.)

are reddish brown, comma-shaped casts of dehydrated blood (Fig. 10-43). Flea droppings in the animal's hair coat indicate flea infestation. Fleas have preferred hosts, but they attack any source of blood if the preferred host is not available. Adult fleas can also survive for extended periods off the host and can heavily infest premises.

LICE. Lice are dorsoventrally flattened, wingless insects with clawed appendages for clasping to the host's hairs. Lice are separated into two orders, based on whether their mouth parts are modified for chewing (Mallophaga) or sucking (Anoplura). Sucking lice feed on blood and move slowly on the host. They have a long, narrow head. Biting lice feed on epithelial debris and can move rapidly over the host. They have a broad, rounded head. Lice are host-specific, remain in close association with the host, and have preferred locations on the host. Lice glue their eggs or nits (Fig. 10-44) to the hairs or feathers of the host. Transmission is usually by direct contact but can occur through equipment contaminated with eggs, nymphs, or adults.

Louse infestations (**pediculosis**) tend to be more severe in young, old, or poorly nourished animals, especially in

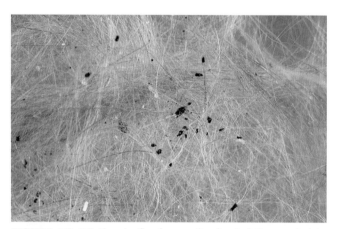

FIGURE 10-43 Flea dirt (flea feces or flea frass) of *Ctenocephalides felis,* the cat flea. (From Hendrix CM, Robinson E: Diagnostic parasitology for veterinary technicians, ed 4, St Louis, 2012, Mosby.)

overcrowded conditions and during the colder months. Sucking lice produce anemia, whereas biting lice are irritating and disturbing to the animal. Common biting lice of domestic animals include *Trichodectes canis* and *Felicola subrostratus* (cat). *Linognathus setosus* is a common sucking louse of the dog.

FLIES. Flies are a diverse group of insects that undergo complete metamorphosis. They have one pair of wings, which may be scaled or membranous, and a pair of balancing structures, called halters. The mouth parts may be adapted for sponging or piercing and sucking. Flies produce harm by inflicting painful bites, sucking blood, producing hypersensitive reactions, depositing eggs in sores, migration of larval stages through tissues of the host with escape through holes in the skin (**warbles**), causing annoyance, and acting as vectors and intermediate hosts to other pathogenic agents.

Biting midges (known as no-see-ums), *Culicoides* spp., are small flies. The females are blood suckers that inflict a painful bite. Black flies (buffalo gnats) are small flies with a characteristic humped back. They produce harm similar to that of no-see-ums and, in great numbers, can exsanguinate a host. Sand flies (*Phlebotomus* spp.) are mothlike flies, known primarily for their role in the transmission of leishmaniasis and viral diseases. The females suck blood. Mosquitoes are a large and important group of flies known for the annoying bites of the females, which suck blood, and also for their role in the transmission of numerous protozoal, viral, and nematode diseases to animals and humans.

Botflies include *Cuterebra* spp., beelike flies, the adults of which do not feed. The adult flies glue their eggs to the hairs of the host or deposit them at the entrance of animal burrows. The larvae hatch and penetrate the skin of the host (**myiasis**). Some migrate extensively through the host's body, and others develop locally. They produce large pockets in the subcutaneous tissues of the host with air holes in the skin, and are known as warbles (Fig. 10-45).

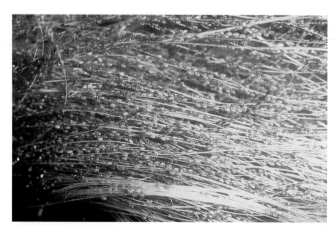

FIGURE 10-44 Thousands of nits cemented by female lice to the hair coat. (From Hendrix CM, Robinson E: Diagnostic parasitology for veterinary technicians, ed 4, St Louis, 2012, Mosby.)

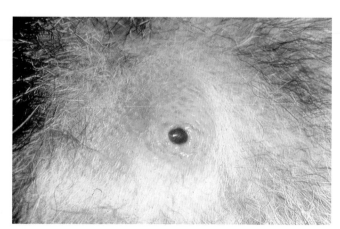

FIGURE 10-45 Larval *Cuterebra* spp. in a subcutaneous fistula. (From Hendrix CM, Robinson E: Diagnostic parasitology for veterinary technicians, ed 4, St Louis, 2012, Mosby.)

TICKS. Ticks are blood-sucking arachnids. They are dorsoventrally flattened in the unengorged state. There are two types of ticks, hard ticks (Ixodidae) and soft ticks (Argasidae).

Hard ticks are important vectors of protozoal, bacterial, viral, and rickettsial diseases. The saliva of female ticks of some species is toxic and produces flaccid ascending paralysis in animals and humans (tick paralysis). The adults, larvae, and nymphs attach to the host and feed on blood. Eggs are deposited in the environment (Fig. 10-46). Hard ticks are dorsoventrally flattened, with well-defined lateral margins in the unengorged state. They have a hard, chitinous covering (scutum) on the dorsal surface of the body. Hard ticks may have grooves, margins, and notches (festoons), which are useful for identification purposes. They may attach to and feed on one to three different hosts during a life cycle and are referred to as one-host, two-host, or three-host ticks.

Important hard ticks in North America include *Rhipicephalus sanguineus* (Fig. 10-47), *Dermacentor* spp., *Ixodes* spp., and *Amblyomma* spp. *R. sanguineus* is unusual in that it can become established in indoor dwellings and kennels.

Soft ticks lack a scutum, and their mouth parts are not visible from the dorsal surface. The females feed often, and eggs are laid off the host. There are three genera of veterinary importance—*Argas* spp., *Otobius megnini,* and *Ornithodoros* spp.

MITES. Mites are arachnids that occur as parasitic and free-living forms, some of which act as intermediate hosts for cestodes. Most parasitic mites are obligate parasites, which spend their entire life cycle on the host and produce the dermatologic condition referred to as mange. Most mite infestations (**acariasis**) are transmitted through direct contact with an infested animal. Burrowing mite infestations are diagnosed with deep skin scrapings at the periphery of lesions.

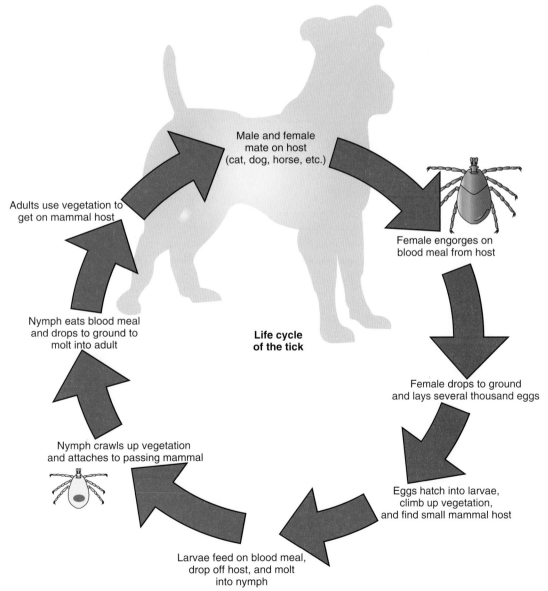

FIGURE 10-46 Life cycle of the tick. (From Hendrix CM, Robinson E: *Diagnostic parasitology for veterinary technicians,* ed 4, St Louis, 2012, Mosby.)

Mites can be divided into two main groups, burrowing mites and nonburrowing mites. Another group of mites is parasitic only as larvae, the trombiculid mites, or chiggers. The burrowing mites include *Sarcoptes scabiei* (Fig. 10-48) and *Notoedres cati*. These mites tunnel into the superficial layers of the epidermis and feed on tissue fluids. Sarcoptic mange caused by *S. scabiei* can affect most animal species, including humans, but is most commonly seen on dogs and pigs. *Demodex* spp. are also burrowing mites that live in the hair follicles and sebaceous glands of the skin. They are considered part of the normal skin fauna of most mammals. Demodectic mange is most common in dogs and can be localized or generalized. Immunodeficiency, both genetic and induced by the mites, is necessary for an infestation to become clinically apparent.

Deep skin scrapings are used to recover the cigar-shaped mites for diagnosis (Fig. 10-49).

Nonburrowing mites live on the surface of the skin and feed on keratinized scale, hair, and tissue fluids. *O. cynotis* and *Cheyletiella* spp. are examples of nonburrowing mites that are parasites of dogs and cats.

DIAGNOSTIC TECHNIQUES

Parasites may be located in the oral cavity, esophagus, stomach, small and large intestines, internal organs, and skin of animals. Diagnostic stages can be found in sputum, feces, blood, urine, secretions of the reproductive organs, and epidermal layers of the skin. Samples collected for examination should be as fresh as possible and examined as soon as possible, preferably within the first 24 hours after collection. Clients can collect fecal

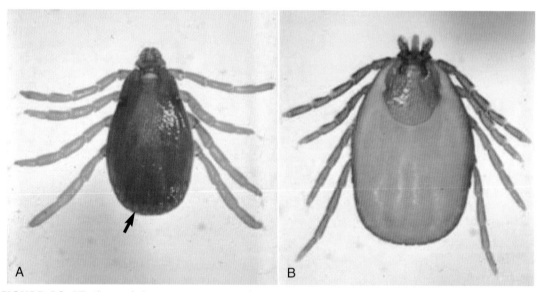

FIGURE 10-47 *Rhipicephalus sanguineus.* **A,** Male. **B,** Female. (From Bowman DD: Georgis' parasitology for veterinarians, ed 9, St Louis, 2009, Saunders.)

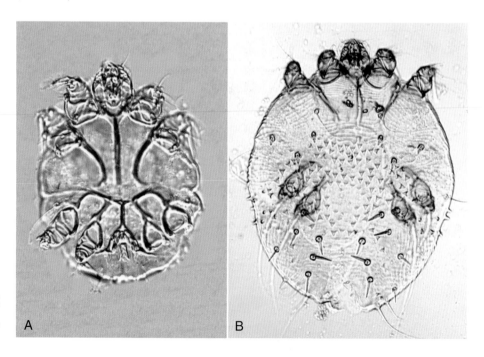

FIGURE 10-48 *Sarcoptes scabiei.* **A,** Male. **B,** Female. (From Bowman DD: Georgis' parasitology for veterinarians, ed 9, St Louis, 2009, Saunders.)

samples and store them in any clean, sealable container, or collection can occur at the clinic. Refrigeration or fixation may be necessary if prompt examination is not possible. A sample of 5 to 50 g (the size of a pecan or walnut) may be needed, depending on which procedures are necessary. Pooled samples from a herd or kennel can be used, but generally it is better to examine several samples from individual animals.

It is vital to take proper precautions when working with samples to prevent contamination of the work environment and to ensure personal health when handling agents transmissible to humans. Table 10-7 lists some zoonotic internal parasites.

Wear gloves and/or wash your hands frequently with warm water and soap. Clean and disinfect work areas after examinations. Also, clean equipment frequently.

Maintenance of good records is important. Label samples with the client's name, date of collection, species of host, and identification of the animal. Records should include identification information, procedures performed, and results. An adequate history, including clinical signs,

duration of signs, medications given, environment, vaccinations, stocking density, and number of animals affected, should accompany the sample.

Parasitologic examination of feces begins with gross examination of the sample, noting consistency, color, and the presence of blood, mucus, odor, adult parasites, or foreign bodies, such as string. Normal feces should be formed, yet soft. Diarrhea or constipation can occur with parasitic infections. Most secretions are clear and moderately cellular. A yellowish discoloration with excessive mucus could signal infection. Blood in a sample can be fresh and bright red or partially digested (hemolyzed), appearing dark reddish brown to black and tarry. Excessive mucus in a sample generally indicates irritation to a mucosal membrane, with a proliferation of mucus-producing cells. This is common in parasitic infections of the respiratory system and lower digestive tract. Adult parasites, such as roundworms and tapeworm proglottids, can be found in vomitus or feces, and can be identified.

Microscopic examination of samples is the most reliable method for detection of parasitic infections. A binocular microscope with 10×, 40×, and 100× objectives is needed. A stereo microscope is also helpful for identifying gross parasites. A calibrated ocular micrometer may be necessary to determine sizes and specific differentiation of some parasitic stages, such as microfilariae. Samples are generally mounted on a glass slide in a fluid medium, with a coverslip on top. The sample should be thoroughly and systematically viewed, beginning at one corner of the coverslip and ending at the opposite end using the 10× objective. Parasite stages usually are in the same plane of focus as air bubbles or the edge of the coverslip. Any materials or objects observed can be viewed and verified with more powerful objectives. A good working knowledge of the parts of the binocular microscope is essential to obtain proper illumination for parasitology examinations.

Parasitology testing is one of the most common activities of practicing veterinary technicians and assistants.

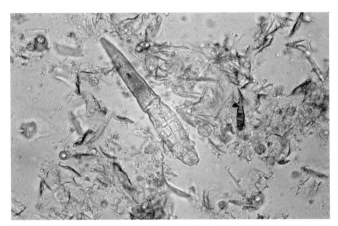

FIGURE 10-49 Adult *Demodex canis*. (From Hendrix CM, Robinson E: Diagnostic parasitology for veterinary technicians, ed 4, St Louis, 2012, Mosby.)

TABLE 10-7	Zoonotic Internal Parasites		
PARASITE	**HOST**	**RESERVOIR**	**DISEASE**
Toxocara spp.	Dogs, cats	Dogs, cats	Visceral larva migrans
Ancylostoma spp.	Dogs, cats	Dogs, cats	Cutaneous larva migrans
Uncinaria stenocephala	Dogs, cats	Dogs, cats	Cutaneous larva migrans
Toxoplasma gondii	Cats	Cats, raw meat	Toxoplasmosis
Strongyloides stercoralis	Dogs, cats, humans	Humans, dogs, cats	Strongyloidiasis
Dipylidium caninum	Dogs, cats, humans	Flea	Cestodiasis
Echinococcus granulosus	Dogs	Dogs	Hydatidosis
Echinococcus multilocularis	Dogs, cats	Dogs, cats	Hydatidosis
Spirometra mansonoides	Dogs, cats	Unknown	Sparganosis
Sarcocystis spp.	Dogs, cats	Dogs, cats	Sarcosporidiosis
Cryptosporidium	Mammals	Mammals	Cryptosporidiosis
Trichinella spiralis	Mammals	Porcine and bear muscle	Trichinellosis
Thelazia spp.	Mammals	Flies	Verminous conjunctivitis
Giardia spp.	Mammals	Mammals	Giardiasis
Babesia spp.	Rodents, humans	Hard ticks	Babesiosis
Trypanosoma	Mammals	Reduviids	Chagas' disease

Adapted from Sirois M: Principles and practice of veterinary technology, ed 3, St Louis, 2011, Mosby.

The following section provides an overview of sample collection and handling, as well as principles and general procedures for the most common parasitology tests performed.

SAMPLE COLLECTION AND HANDLING
FECAL SAMPLES

For tests to be valid, the fecal sample must be fresh and stored properly if testing is to be delayed. With small animals, it is common to provide the client with a collection container. Instruct the client to witness the animal defecating and collect the sample immediately. Samples can also be collected directly from the rectum using a fecal loop. A sample collected with a fecal loop is the least desirable because only a small quantity of sample is obtained and the quantity may not be sufficient to find evidence of parasites. The sample should be refrigerated until it is to be examined. Large animal specimens are often collected directly from the rectum. Herd animal samples are normally collected as pooled samples. Several samples are taken from the area in which the animals are confined.

BLOOD SAMPLES

The specific collection procedure varies somewhat, depending on the tests to be performed. Whole blood in EDTA or serum may be required. Standard collection methods for these sample types will yield appropriate samples for parasitologic testing.

MISCELLANEOUS SAMPLES

Skin scrapings, cellophane tape collections, transtracheal washes, urine sample collections, and swabbings are all performed in parasitology. Standard protocols for these collections will yield appropriate samples.

EVALUATION OF FECAL SPECIMENS

Depending on clinical signs and patient history, it is likely that specific parasite infestations may be suspected. This information helps guide the choice of test to be performed. All parasitology samples should undergo gross evaluation for the presence of abnormalities such as blood, mucus, and parasites that are large enough to see with the unaided eye (e.g., tapeworm segments). Additional tests can then be performed.

DIRECT SMEAR

Fecal direct smears are the simplest of the evaluation procedures. Feces, sputum, urine, smegma, and blood can be observed with the technique described in Procedure 10-6. This requires a minimum amount of equipment and materials and is a rapid scan for parasite stages. The procedure involves placing a small amount of feces on a clean glass slide and examining it microscopically for the presence of eggs and larvae. This method will also allow visualization of the trophozoite stages of protozoal parasites such as *Giardia* spp.

Unfortunately, a direct smear alone is not an adequate examination for parasites because only a small quantity of sample is examined and parasitic infections can be missed. However, it should be incorporated as a routine part of any parasitology examination.

FECAL FLOTATION

Flotation methods are based on differences in the specific gravity of the life cycle stages of parasites found in feces and fecal debris. Simple fecal flotation is an example of a flotation method (Procedure 10-7). Specific gravity refers to the weight of an object compared with the weight of an equal volume of distilled water and is a function of the total amount of dissolved material in the solution. Most parasite eggs have a specific gravity between 1.10 and 1.20 g/mL. Flotation solutions are formulated with a specific gravity higher than that of common parasite ova. Therefore, the ova float to the surface of the solution. Saturated solutions of sugar and various salts are used as flotation solutions and have a specific gravity ranging from 1.18 to 1.40 g/mL. Fecal debris and eggs with a specific gravity greater than that of the flotation solution do not float. Fluke eggs are generally heavier than the specific gravity of most routinely used flotation solutions and are not usually recovered using this technique. Nematode larvae can be recovered but frequently are distorted from crenation, making identification difficult. If the specific gravity of the flotation solution is too high, a plug of fecal debris floats and traps parasite stages in it, obscuring them from view.

Commonly used flotation solutions are sugar, sodium chloride, sodium nitrate, magnesium sulfate, and zinc sulfate. Each solution has its advantages and disadvantages, including cost, availability, efficiency, shelf life, crystallization, corrosion of equipment, and ease of use. Selection is often determined by the type of practice and common parasites encountered in the area. Some companies have packaged flotation kits using prepared solutions of sodium nitrate or zinc sulfate, disposable plastic vials, and strainers (Fig. 10-50). They are convenient but more expensive. Materials for conducting simple flotation procedures can be acquired from suppliers of scientific equipment and chemicals.

The specific gravity of flotation solutions can be checked using a hydrometer and adjusted by adding more salt or more water to the solution. Leaving extra crystals of salt on the bottom of the solution ensures that the solution is saturated.

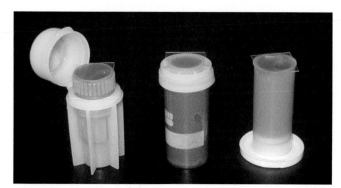

FIGURE 10-50 Three commercially available fecal flotation kits—Fecalyzer (EVSCO Pharmaceuticals, Buena, NJ; *left*), Ovassay (Pfizer, New York; *center*), and Ovatector (BGS Medical Products, Venice, FL; *right*). These kits are based on the principles of the simple flotation procedure. (From Hendrix CM, Robinson E: Diagnostic parasitology for veterinary technicians, ed 4, St Louis, 2012, Mosby.)

PROCEDURE 10-6 DIRECT SMEAR OF FECES

Materials
- Glass microscope slides (25 mm)
- Glass coverslips (22 mm², no. 1)
- Wooden applicator sticks
- Water or saline

Procedure
1. Place a drop of saline on a slide (Fig. 1).

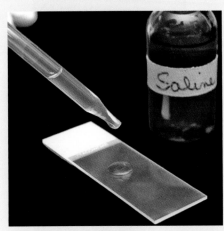

FIGURE 1

2. Dip the applicator stick into the feces; only a small amount should adhere to the stick (Fig. 2).

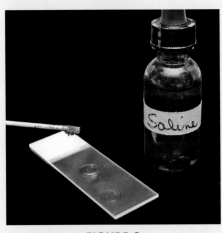

FIGURE 2

3. Mix the feces with the saline to produce a homogeneous emulsion that is clear enough to read newsprint through it. A common mistake is to make the smear too thick (Fig. 3).

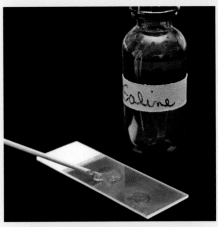

FIGURE 3

4. Place the cover slip over the emulsion.
5. Examine the slide at 100× and 400× magnification for eggs, cysts, trophozoites, and larvae.

Optional: To demonstrate diagnostic features of protozoa, add one drop of Lugol's iodine:
1. To make a 5% Lugol's stock solution, add 5 g iodine crystals to 10 g potassium iodide/100 mL distilled water.
2. Store solution in an amber bottle away from light.
3. Dilute one part 5% Lugol's stock solution with five parts distilled water to make a staining solution.

Adapted from Sirois M: Principles and practice of veterinary technology, ed 3, St Louis, 2011, Mosby.
Illustrations from Greene CE: Infectious diseases of the dog and cat, ed 4, St Louis, 2012, Saunders.

CENTRIFUGAL FLOTATION

This procedure is similar in principle to the flotation procedure except that once the sample and solution are mixed, the specimen is strained (to remove excess debris). Add a coverslip and centrifuge the specimen at 400 to 650 g for 5 minutes. Centrifugal force holds the coverslips in place during spinning, provided that the tubes are balanced. A bacteriology loop is then used to remove a drop of liquid from the surface of the tube, and the drop is examined microscopically. Centrifugal flotation is more sensitive than simple flotation. It recovers more eggs and cysts in a sample in less time (Procedure 10-8). However, it requires access to a tabletop centrifuge with a head for rotation buckets. Fixed-angle heads do not work as well for this procedure as described. They can be adapted for this procedure by not filling the tubes and omitting the coverslip during centrifugation.

PROCEDURE 10-7 SIMPLE FECAL FLOTATION

Materials

- 75 glass microscope slides (25 mm)
- Glass coverslips (22 mm², no.1)
- Wooden tongue depressors
- Waxed paper cups (90-150 mL)
- Cheesecloth, 10-cm gauze squares, or metal screen tea strainer
- Shell vial (1.25-2.0 cm or 5.0-7.5 cm) or 15-mL conical centrifuge tube
- Saturated salt or sugar flotation solution

Procedure

1. Place approximately 2-5 g of feces in the paper cup.
2. Add 30 mL of flotation solution.
3. Using the tongue depressor, mix the feces to produce an evenly suspended emulsion (Fig. 1).

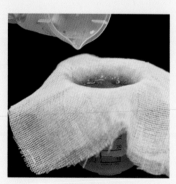

FIGURE 1

4. If using cheesecloth, bend the sides of the cup to form a spout and cover the top with the cheesecloth squares while pouring the suspension into the shell vial. If using a metal strainer, pour the suspension through the metal strainer into another cup and fill the shell vial with the filtered solution (Fig. 2).

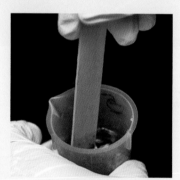

FIGURE 2

5. Fill the shell vial to form a convex dome (meniscus) at the rim. **NOTE:** Do not overfill the vial. Fresh solution can be used to form this dome (Fig. 3).

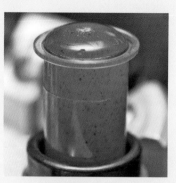

FIGURE 3

6. Place a coverslip on top of the filled shell vial (Fig. 4).

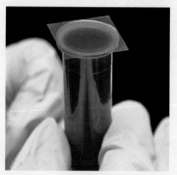

FIGURE 4

7. Allow the coverslip to remain undisturbed for 10 to 20 minutes.
8. Pick the coverslip straight up and place it on a glass slide, fluid side down (Fig. 5).

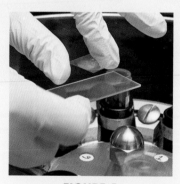

FIGURE 5

The veterinary technician will then systematically examine the surface under the coverslip at 100× magnification.

Adapted from Sirois M: Principles and practice of veterinary technology, ed 3, St Louis, 2011, Mosby.
Illustrations from Greene CE: Infectious diseases of the dog and cat, ed 4, St Louis, 2012, Saunders.

PROCEDURE 10-8 CENTRIFUGAL FLOTATION

Materials

- Glass microscope slides (25 mm)
- Glass coverslips (22 mm², no. 1)
- Waxed paper cups
- Cheesecloth, 10-cm gauze squares, or metal screen tea strainer
- Funnel
- Conical centrifuge tubes (15 mL)
- Test tube rack
- Flotation solution
- Centrifuge with rotating buckets
- Wooden tongue depressors
- Balance scale

Procedure

1. Prepare a fecal emulsion using 2-5 g of feces and 30 mL of flotation solution.
2. Strain the emulsion through the cheesecloth or tea strainer into the centrifuge tube. (Suspending a funnel over the tube facilitates filling the tube.)
3. Fill the tube to create a positive meniscus with flotation solution.
4. Place a coverslip on top of the tube.
5. Create a balance tube of equal weight, containing another sample or water.
6. Place the tubes in the centrifuge buckets and weigh them on a balance. You may add water to the buckets to make them equal weights.
7. Centrifuge the tubes for 5 minutes at 400-650 g ($\approx$1500 rpm).
8. Remove the coverslips from the tubes by lifting straight up and place them on a slide.
9. Systematically examine the slides at 100× magnification.

Adapted from Sirois M: Principles and practice of veterinary technology, ed 3, St Louis, 2011, Mosby.

PROCEDURE 10-9 FECAL SEDIMENTATION

Materials

- Waxed paper cups (90-150 mL)
- Wooden tongue depressors
- Cheesecloth, 10-cm gauze squares, or metal screen tea strainer
- Funnel
- Conical centrifuge tubes (50 mL)
- Disposable pipettes (2 mL)
- Glass microscope slides (25 mm)
- Glass coverslips (22 mm², no. 1)

Procedure

1. Mix 2-5 g of feces in a cup with 30 mL of water.
2. Strain the fecal suspension through the cheesecloth or tea strainer into a 50-mL conical centrifuge tube. (Suspending a funnel over the tube facilitates filling the tube.)
3. Wash the sample with water until the tube is filled.
4. Allow the tube to sit undisturbed for 15 to 30 minutes.
5. Decant the supernatant off, and resuspend the sediment in water.
6. Repeat steps 4 and 5 two more times.
7. Decant the supernatant without disturbing the sediment.
8. Using a pipette, mix the sediment and transfer an aliquot to a slide.
9. Place a coverslip over the sediment and systematically examine the slide with 100× magnification.
10. Repeat steps 8 and 9 until all sediment has been examined.

Adapted from Sirois M: Principles and practice of veterinary technology, ed 3, St Louis, 2011, Mosby.

FECAL SEDIMENTATION

The sedimentation procedure is used when suspected parasites produce ova too large to be recovered with standard flotation (e.g., fluke ova). The fecal sample is mixed in a small volume of water and strained into a centrifuge tube. The sample can be centrifuged at 400 g for 5 minutes or allowed to remain undisturbed for 20 to 30 minutes. The supernatant is poured off and a pipette is used to remove a drop of the sediment. A drop from the upper, middle, and lower portions of the sediment is removed. These drops are then examined microscopically. Sedimentation concentrates parasite stages as well as fecal debris (Procedure 10-9). Because of the debris, parasite stages may be obscured from view. Also, this technique is more laborious. Sedimentation is used primarily when fluke infections are suspected. Most fluke eggs do not float or are distorted by flotation solutions with a higher specific gravity, making it difficult to recognize them. A few drops of liquid detergent can be added to the water as a surfactant to help remove excess fats and debris from the sample.

CELLOPHANE TAPE PREPARATION

This method is often used to aid in identification of tapeworms. A piece of cellophane tape is wrapped around a tongue depressor, with the adhesive side out. The animal's tail is raised and the tongue depressor firmly pressed against the anus. The tape is then removed, applied to a glass slide that has a small amount of water on it, and examined microscopically (Procedure 10-10).

MISCELLANEOUS FECAL EXAMINATIONS

The Baermann technique is sometimes used to recover nematode larvae from feces, fecal culture, soil, herbage, and animal tissues but is rarely performed in small animal practice. In dogs and cats, a Baermann technique should be used when *Strongyloides* spp. infections are suspected. The procedure requires construction of a Baermann apparatus, which consists of a large funnel supported in a ring stand. A piece of rubber tubing is attached to the end of the funnel

PROCEDURE 10-10 CELLOPHANE TAPE PREPARATION

Materials
- Transparent adhesive tape
- Wooden tongue depressors
- Glass microscope slides (25 mm)

Procedure
1. Place adhesive tape in a loop around one end of the tongue depressor, with the adhesive side facing out.
2. Press the tape firmly against the skin around the anus.
3. Place a drop of water on the slide. Undo the loop of tape and stick the tape to the slide, allowing the water to spread out under the tape.
4. Examine the taped area of the slide microscopically for the presence of tapeworm eggs.

From Sirois M: Principles and practice of veterinary technology, ed 3, St Louis, 2011, Mosby.

and placed in a collection tube. The fecal sample is placed in the funnel on top of a piece of metal screen. Warm water or warmed physiologic saline is passed through the sample. The larvae are stimulated to move by the warm water and then sink to the bottom of the apparatus. A drop of the material in the collection container is examined microscopically for the presence of larvae.

Some parasites produce intestinal bleeding. This bleeding may be evident as frank blood in the fecal sample or as darkened feces. Some intestinal bleeding can only be identified with chemical testing, referred to as fecal occult blood testing. Several types of kits are available for this procedure. They primarily act to identify the presence of hemoglobin in the sample. Examination of vomitus may also aid in the diagnosis of parasitism. Some parasites (e.g., *Toxocara canis*) are often present in the vomitus of infected patients.

Fecal culture is used to differentiate parasites whose eggs or larvae are not easily distinguished by examination of a fresh fecal sample. First-stage hookworm larvae in a dog or cat sample and some free-living nematode larvae in soil or on grass cannot be easily distinguished from first-stage *Strongyloides* larvae. After fecal culture, the third-stage larvae of many of these parasites can be identified to genus level. Identification may require the help of an experienced helminthologist.

EVALUATION OF BLOOD SAMPLES

Examination of blood samples may reveal adult parasites and/or their various life cycle stages free in the blood or intracellularly. A variety of methods can be used for this determination. Thin or thick blood smears are prepared in the same way as smears for a WBC differential count (see earlier discussion). Most parasites are carried with the laminar flow to the feathered edge of the slide. Parasites may be located between cells, on the surface of cells, or in the cytoplasm of cells. Thin blood films are most effectively used to study the morphology of protozoan and rickettsial parasites. If parasitemia is low, infections

can be missed. A thick blood film or a buffy coat smear is more effective because it concentrates a larger volume of cells.

The buffy coat smear is a concentration technique for the detection of protozoa and rickettsiae in WBCs. A microhematocrit tube is centrifuged as for a PCV determination. Microfilariae and some protozoa may also be found at the top of the plasma column. The technique is quick but cannot be used to differentiate *D. immitis* from *Acanthocheilonema reconditum*.

DIRECT DROP TEST

This is the simplest of the blood evaluations, although it is the least accurate because of the small sample size. A drop of anticoagulated whole blood is examined microscopically. The movement of parasites that are extracellular can be detected with this method.

FILTER TEST

The filter technique is a method designed to concentrate microfilariae in blood. The blood is passed through a filter, which collects the microfilariae. Commercial kits use a detergent lysing solution and a differential stain. This procedure is quicker and easier than some of the other tests, but the differential characteristics of the microfilariae are not as obvious. It is primarily used in locations in which animals are expected to have circulating microfilariae (e.g., stray, shelter animal).

MODIFIED KNOTT'S TEST

This method is used to concentrate microfilaria and can help in the differentiation of *Dirofilaria* from *Acanthocheilonema*. The procedure requires a mixture of blood and formalin or acitic acid solution in a centrifuge tube. The mixture is incubated at room temperature for 1 to 2 minutes and then centrifuged for 5 minutes. The supernatant is poured off, and a drop of methylene blue is added to the sediment in the tube. A drop of this mixture is transferred to a glass slide for microscopic evaluation. The modified Knott's technique is a rapid method for the detection of microfilariae (heartworm larvae) in the blood (Procedure 10-11). It is used primarily for differentiating *D. immitis* and *A. reconditum* infections in dogs. When preparing the 2% formalin solution, it is important to remember that 37% formaldehyde is equivalent to 100% formalin. It is also important to use water, not physiologic saline, to prepare this solution because physiologic saline does not lyse red blood cells. The modified Knott's technique cannot detect occult heartworm infections.

IMMUNOLOGIC TESTS

A variety of tests are available to identify antigen and/or antibody to specific parasites. Most tests are based on the ELISA principle (see earlier). The tests are highly accurate and precise and can detect occult infections. Canine heartworm infections and *Toxoplasma* infections are routinely diagnosed with these methods. The American Heartworm Society currently recommends using antigen detection methods for routine screening. Antigen detection methods are preferred to microfilariae concentration methods in cats because these

PROCEDURE 10-11 MODIFIED KNOTT'S TECHNIQUE

Materials

- Blood collection materials
- 15-mL conical centrifuge tubes
- 2% formalin (2 mL 37% formaldehyde/98 mL water)
- 2.5% methylene blue (2.5 g methylene blue/100 mL water)
- Tabletop centrifuge
- Glass microscope slides (25-mm)
- Glass coverslips (22-mm^2, no. 1)
- Pipettes

Procedure

1. Mix 1 mL of blood with 9 mL of 2% formalin in a centrifuge tube. Agitate the tube and mix well.
2. Centrifuge the tube at 1500 rpm for 5 minutes.
3. Pour off the supernatant, and add one or two drops of methylene blue stain to the pellet at the bottom of the tube.
4. Using a pipette, mix the stain and sediment and transfer the mixture to a glass slide.
5. Apply a coverslip and examine the sediment microscopically for microfilariae at 100× and 400× magnification.

Adapted from Sirois M: Principles and practice of veterinary technology, ed 3, St Louis, 2011, Mosby.

aberrant hosts circulate microfilariae only for a short time. However, antigen levels in the blood of infected cats may also be too low to detect. Other methods, such as radiography, may be used to make a diagnosis in cats.

Approximately 25% of heartworm-infected dogs have occult infections. Occult infections are characterized by a lack of circulating microfilaria and occur if the infection is not yet patent, if the population of adult heartworms consists of only one sex, or if immune reactions of the host to microfilariae eliminate this stage from the bloodstream. Occult infections can also occur if animals infected with adult heartworms are given heartworm prevention medications of the ivermectin group. These interfere with oogenesis and sterilize the worms.

RECOMMENDED READINGS

Abbas AK: Cellular and molecular immunology, ed 6, Philadelphia, 2009, Saunders.

Baker R, Lumsden J: Color atlas of cytology of the dog and cat, St Louis, 2000, Mosby.

Bowman DD: Georgis' parasitology for veterinarians, ed 9, St Louis, 2009, Saunders.

Cowell R, Tyler R, Meinkoth J: Diagnostic cytology and hematology of the dog and cat, ed 3, St Louis, 2008, Mosby.

Dow SW, Jones RL, Rosychuk RA: Bacteriologic specimens: Selection, collection, and transport for optimum results, Trenton, NJ, 1997, Veterinary Learning Systems.

Graff L: A handbook of routine urinalysis, Philadelphia, 1992, Lippincott Williams & Wilkins.

Hendrix CM, Robinson E: Diagnostic parasitology for veterinarians, ed 4, St Louis, 2012, Mosby.

Male D: Immunology, ed 7, St Louis, 2006, Mosby.

Meyer D: Veterinary laboratory medicine: Interpretation and diagnosis, ed 3, St Louis, 2004, Saunders.

Meyer DJ: The management of cytology specimens, Trenton, NJ, 1997, Veterinary Learning Systems.

Raskin R, Meyer DJ: Canine and feline cytology: A color atlas and interpretation guide, ed 2, St Louis, 2009, Saunders.

Sirois M: Laboratory procedures for veterinary technicians, ed 6, St Louis, 2014, Mosby.

Sloss MW, Kemp RL, Zajac AM: Veterinary clinical parasitology, ed 6, Ames, IA, 1994, Iowa State University Press.

Sodikoff CH: Laboratory profiles of small animal disease, ed 3, St Louis, 2001, Mosby.

Tizard IR: Veterinary immunology: An introduction, ed 9, St Louis, 2013, Saunders.

Willard MD: Small animal clinical diagnosis by laboratory methods, ed 4, St Louis, 2004, Saunders.

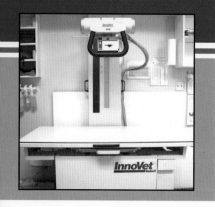

 Diagnostic Imaging[1]

OUTLINE

X-ray Generation, 337
X-ray Tube Anatomy, 337
Radiographic Image Quality, 337
Radiographic Contrast, 338
Radiographic Detail, 338
Exposure Variables, 341
Radiographic Film, 342
Intensifying Screens, 343
X-ray Equipment, 343
Digital X-ray Imaging, 344
Computed Radiography, 345
Digital Radiography, 345
Radiation Safety, 345
Terminology, 346
Darkroom Techniques, 347
Darkroom Setup, 347
Film Identification, 348
Safelights, 348
Film Processing, 349
Radiographic Artifacts, 350

Radiographic Positioning and Terminology, 352
Oblique Projections, 353
Contrast Studies, 354
Positive Contrast Media, 354
Negative Contrast Media, 355
Double-Contrast Procedure, 355
Diagnostic Ultrasound, 355
Transducers, 355
Terminology Describing Echotexture, 355
Instrument Controls, 356
Artifacts, 356
Endoscopy, 356
Types of Endoscopes, 356
Endoscopy Room, 357
Accessory Instruments, 357
Care of Endoscopes, 357
Gastrointestinal Endoscopy, 358
Computed Tomography, 358
Magnetic Resonance Imaging, 358
Nuclear Medicine, 359

LEARNING OBJECTIVES

After reviewing this chapter, the reader will be able to:

1. Describe the components of the x-ray machine and the function of each part.
2. Explain how x-rays are produced.
3. Discuss the factors that affect radiographic quality.
4. Describe techniques and devices used to optimize radiographic quality.
5. Discuss the dangers of radiation and methods to avoid radiation injury.
6. Describe the procedures used to develop radiographs.
7. Explain proper positioning of animals for various radiographic studies.
8. Describe the basic physics of ultrasound.
9. List the components of ultrasound machines and the function of each part.
10. List the non–x-ray imaging modalities and provide an overview of each.

KEY TERMS

ALARA
Anechoic
Annular array
Anode
Bucky

Cathode
Collimators
Contrast
Direct exposure film
Distance enhancement

Echoic
Film latitude
Film–focal distance (FFD)
Fluoroscopy

Focused grids
Heel effect
Hyperechoic
Hypoechoic
Intensifying screens

[1]Elsevier and the author acknowledge and appreciate the original contributions from Sirois M: Principles and practice of veterinary technology, ed 3, St Louis, 2011, Mosby, whose work forms the heart of this chapter.

KEY TERMS

Isoechoic

Kilovoltage peak (kVp)

Latent image

Maximum permissible dose
  (MPD)

Milliamperage (mA)

Mirror image

Object-film distance
  (OFD)

Penumbra effect

Radiographic density

Radiolucent

Radiopaque

Rem

Sievert (SV)

Slice thickness

Sonolucent

Source-image distance
  (SID)

Ultrasonography

Diagnostic imaging is an integral part of the diagnosis and treatment of patients. Radiography and ultrasonography are the two most common modalities available in the clinical setting, with some referral hospitals having state of the art imaging modalities such as computed tomography (CT), magnetic resonance imaging (MRI), and nuclear medicine (NM). The veterinary support staff is responsible for the operation of imaging equipment. A thorough understanding of the physics behind the various imaging modalities is needed to produce quality diagnostic studies.

X-RAY GENERATION

X-rays are a form of electromagnetic radiation. X-rays are similar to visible light but have a shorter wavelength, higher frequency, and higher energy; it is the higher energy that makes x-rays dangerous. The x-rays are generated when fast-moving electrons (from the cathode) collide with the anode (positive end of the x-ray tube). Within the x-ray tube, at the time of exposure, a stream of electrons is accelerated toward a tungsten anode target. The energy of the electrons interacting with the atoms of the target is converted to heat (99%) and x-rays (1%). Heat generation in the x-ray tube is a limiting factor in the production of x-rays.

X-RAY TUBE ANATOMY

The x-ray tube consists of a **cathode** (−) that contains a tungsten filament at which the electrons are generated when heated. This tungsten filament is housed within a focusing cup to focus the beam of electrons on the focal spot of the anode. The **anode** (+) contains a rotating tungsten target wherein x-rays are generated at the focal spot. Both the anode and cathode are enclosed in a vacuum glass or metal envelope. A beryllium window in the glass envelope allows x-rays to pass with minimal filtration. An aluminum filter is placed outside the window in the collimator housing, usually on top of the mirror, to absorb the low-energy (soft) x-rays while allowing the more energetic and useful x-rays to form the primary x-ray beam. By law, any x-ray tube that generates over 70 **kilovoltage peak (kVp)** must have a collimator because there has to be a total filtration of 2.5- mm Al equivalent. Thus, the lower-energy x-rays do not enter the patient. The entire x-ray tube is surrounded by oil that acts as an electrical barrier while absorbing heat generated by the tube. The tube and oil are encased in a lead housing to prevent damage to the glass envelope from the outside and to absorb stray radiation (Fig. 11-1).

The **heel effect** is the result of unequal distribution of the x-ray beam intensity emitted from the x-ray tube along the cathode-anode axis. Some x-ray tubes have a distribution of the x-ray beam intensity that decreases rapidly on the anode side of the tube as a result of primary x-ray beam absorption by the anode material (Fig. 11-2). This can be used as an advantage when taking x-rays of areas of unequal thickness, such as the thorax or abdomen. By placing the patient's head toward the anode side, the part of the x-ray beam with the higher intensity (cathode side) is directed to the thickest area of the patient, as in this example of radiographing a thorax. This produces a more even film density. The heel effect is most noticeable when using large film sizes, low kVp, and long focal–film distance.

> ### CRITICAL CONCEPT
> The anode heel effect refers to the unequal distribution of x-ray beam intensity along the cathode-anode axis.

RADIOGRAPHIC IMAGE QUALITY

Radiographic density is the degree of blackness on a radiograph. The dark areas are made up of black metallic silver deposits on the finished radiograph. These deposits occur in areas in which x-rays have penetrated the patient and exposed the emulsion of the film. Radiographic density can be intensified by increasing the mAs (a product of the milliamperage and time), which is a result of increasing the **milliamperage**

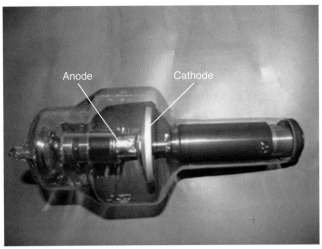

FIGURE 11-1 Anatomy of an x-ray tube. (From Sirois M: Principles and practice of veterinary technology, ed 3, St Louis, 2011, Mosby.)

(mA) or the exposure time in seconds (s). This increases the mAs by increasing the number (quantity) of x-rays produced as a result of increasing the number of electrons in the electron cloud, or the time that the electrons are allowed to travel from the cathode to the anode. A higher kVp yields more radiographic density by increasing the penetrating power (quality) of the x-ray beam.

> **CRITICAL CONCEPT**
>
> Radiographic density refers to the degree of blackness of the film, whereas radiographic contrast refers to the varying shades of gray on the film.

RADIOGRAPHIC CONTRAST

Radiographic **contrast** is defined as the differences in radiographic density between adjacent areas on a radiographic image. Radiographs that show a long scale of contrast have a few black and white shades, with many shades of gray. A short scale of contrast has black and white shades, with only a few shades of gray in between. For most studies, a long scale of contrast is desirable. Obtaining a long scale of radiographic contrast depends on four factors—subject density, kVp level, film contrast, and film fogging.

Subject density is the ability of the different tissue densities to absorb x-rays. The extent to which x-rays penetrate

the various tissues depends on the differences in atomic number and thickness.

On radiographs, air or lung tissue will appear **radiolucent**, or black, because it allows more of the radiation to pass through. With increasing density, the tissue will appear whiter, or more **radiopaque**, as it absorbs more of the radiation (Fig. 11-3). Bone absorbs more x-rays than muscle and appears whiter (radiopaque) on the finished radiograph, whereas air in the thorax will appear more radiolucent in comparison. The thickness of the area also affects the number of x-rays absorbed. If you radiograph an area that ranges from 5 to 20 cm in thickness, the 20-cm-thick area absorbs more x-rays than the 5-cm-thick area. The scale of radiographic contrast can be lengthened or shortened by increasing or decreasing the kVp.

> **CRITICAL CONCEPT**
>
> Denser tissues, such as bone, absorb greater amounts of x-rays and appear white on a radiograph, whereas less dense tissues, such as lung tissue, absorb fewer x-rays and appear black on the finished radiograph.

Film contrast also affects radiographic contrast. Some types of film can produce a long scale of contrast or long latitude. Long-latitude film allows for more variation in technique while still producing a diagnostic radiograph. The scale of contrast can be shortened by changing the exposure technique when using long-latitude film. However, the scale of contrast cannot be lengthened when using contrast film, film that produces a short scale of contrast.

Film fogging can greatly decrease radiographic contrast by decreasing the differences in densities between two adjacent shadows. Care must be taken in the storage and handling of x-ray film to prevent fogging. Film can become fogged from low-grade light leaks in the darkroom, scatter radiation, heat, and improper processing.

RADIOGRAPHIC DETAIL

A diagnostic radiograph is one with diagnostic radiographic detail. Radiographic detail is considered to be of diagnostic quality

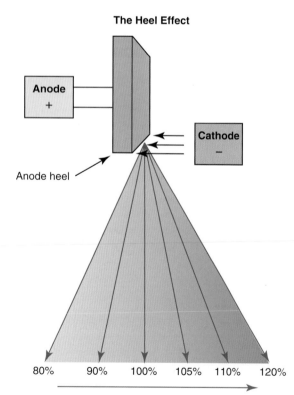

The Heel Effect

FIGURE 11-2 Anode heel effect. The x-ray beam intensity decreases toward the anode side because of absorption by the target and anode material. (Courtesy J. Johnson.) (From Sirois M: Principles and practice of veterinary technology, ed 3, St Louis, 2011, Mosby.)

Air	Fat	Soft Tissue	Bone	Metal

FIGURE 11-3 Various exposed film densities. Air is the least dense (most radiotransluscent), resulting in film exposure, whereas metal is the most dense (thus, the most radiopaque) and absorbs more x-rays, allowing fewer x-rays to penetrate the film. (Courtesy Heidi Anthony.) (From Sirois M: Principles and practice of veterinary technology, ed 3, St Louis, 2011, Mosby.)

when the interfaces between tissues and organs are sharp. Many factors can affect the detail on a radiograph; the most common are patient motion and the **penumbra effect**. The penumbra effect causes a loss of detail and results in collimation (limitation) of the x-ray beam. The fuzziness caused by stray x-rays is known as the penumbra effect. The smallest focal spot size should be used whenever possible to prevent this effect.

Another factor that affects the amount of penumbra is the source-image distance, which is the distance between the source of the x-ray and the film. The term *source-image distance* (**SID**) is preferred, but **film–focal distance (FFD)** and SID are used interchangeably.

The penumbra effect can be decreased by increasing the SID (Fig. 11-4). There is a limit to how much the SID can be increased because of what is stated in the inverse square law. According to this law, the intensity decreases at a rate inverse to the square of the distance. In simpler terms, if the SID is doubled, the mAs must increase by a factor of 4 to maintain the same radiographic density. In most cases, this is not practical because the shortest possible exposure times are necessary to counteract patient motion. An SID of 36 to 40 inches is sufficient to minimize the penumbra effect.

The third factor that affects penumbra is the object-image distance (OID). This is the distance from the object being imaged to the film or image receptor. The penumbra is decreased by keeping the OID as short as possible (Fig. 11-5). Using a combination of these factors, the penumbra can be minimized and good radiographic detail achieved.

Patient motion causes loss of detail because of blurred interfaces. A blurred image is generally a result of long exposure time combined with motion of the patient. This can be controlled by using the shortest possible exposure. If the image remains blurred, the patient should be sedated.

CRITICAL CONCEPT

Patient motion and the penumbra effect have the greatest influence on radiographic detail.

DISTORTION

Foreshortening occurs when the object is not parallel to the recording surface. This distorts size by shortening the length of the object. This occurs mainly when imaging the long bones, such as the humerus or femur. If one end of the bone is farther from the recording surface than the other, the bone appears shorter. The object being radiographed must be parallel to the recording surface and the OID kept as short as possible. Increasing the OID increases the penumbra and greatly magnifies the size of the object. The degree of magnification increases as the distance to the recording surface becomes greater.

It is important to project areas between a series of radiodense and radiolucent objects accurately. The vertebral column is a good example. The vertebrae must be parallel to the recording surface. When radiographing the cervical vertebrae in lateral recumbency, if the patient is allowed to lie naturally, the midcervical vertebrae tend to sag. This produces false narrowing of the intervertebral spaces. A small amount of padding beneath the patient brings the vertebral column parallel to the recording surface. Care must be taken not to use too much padding because this can elevate the spinal column, also producing a false narrowing of the intervertebral spaces.

Distortion can also occur when the x-ray beam is not perpendicular to the recording surface. X-rays in the center of the primary beam penetrate perpendicular to the intervertebral spaces. As the distance from the center of the primary beam increases, the x-rays strike the intervertebral spaces at an increasing angle. False narrowing of the intervertebral space occurs because of this increase in distance from the center of the primary beam (Fig. 11-6). To combat such distortion, it is sometimes necessary to make multiple images of the vertebral column, centering the primary beam over multiple areas. This type of distortion is also apparent when radiographing complex joints, such as the stifle and elbow. When imaging these areas, be sure the center of the primary beam is directly over the joint.

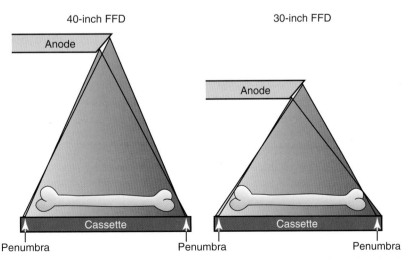

FIGURE 11-4 Increasing the SID decreases the amount of penumbra, increasing the radiographic detail. (From Sirois M: *Principles and practice of veterinary technology*, ed 3, St Louis, 2011, Mosby.)

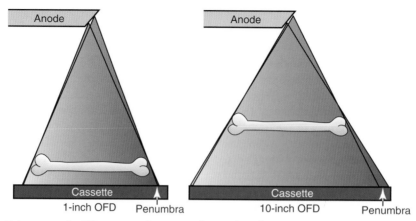

FIGURE 11-5 Increasing the OID increases the amount of penumbra, decreasing the radiographic detail. (From Sirois M: Principles and practice of veterinary technology, ed 3, St Louis, 2011, Mosby.)

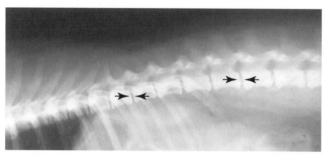

FIGURE 11-6 The intervertebral spaces appear narrow toward the edges of the radiograph *(arrows)* as compared with the spaces in the center of the radiograph. (From Sirois M: Principles and practice of veterinary technology, ed 3, St Louis, 2011, Mosby.)

> **CRITICAL CONCEPT**
>
> Distortion occurs when the x-ray beam is not perpendicular to the recording surface.

SCATTER RADIATION

When an x-ray photon strikes an object, it can do one of three things: it can pass through the object, be absorbed by the object, or produce scatter radiation (secondary radiation). Scatter radiation fogs the film, greatly decreasing the contrast. It also is a safety hazard to patients and personnel. Scatter radiation is projected in all directions. Exposure techniques that use a high kVp produce more scatter radiation. Body parts measuring 10 cm or larger produce enough scatter radiation to significantly decrease detail on the radiograph. Beam-limiting devices are commonly used to decrease scatter radiation by confining the primary beam to the area being examined. Several types of beam-limiting devices are available. Cones are lead cylinders placed over the collimator on the x-ray tube head. This restricts the primary beam to the size of the cone used. However, these are no longer in common use. Diaphragms are sheets of lead with a rectangular, square, or circular opening that limits the size of the primary beam to the size of the diaphragm used. **Collimators** consist of adjustable lead shutters installed in the tube head of the x-ray machine. Finally, filters are used to absorb the less penetrating or soft x-rays as they leave the tube head. Filters are made of a thin sheet of aluminum and are placed over the tube window.

> **CRITICAL CONCEPT**
>
> The collimator in the x-ray tube head is used to limit the size of the primary beam, thus reducing scatter radiation.

GRIDS. Grids are used to decrease scatter radiation and increase the contrast on the radiograph. As the thickness of the area being imaged increases, the amount of kVp required also increases. As the kVp increases, more scatter radiation is produced. To minimize scatter radiation, grids are necessary when radiographing areas 10 cm or more in thickness.

A grid is a series of thin, linear strips made of alternating radiodense and radiolucent material. The radiodense strips are made of lead, whereas the radiolucent spacers are plastic, aluminum, or fiber. The grid is placed within or under the table between the patient and imaging receptor. X-rays that penetrate the patient and pass in perfect alignment between the lead strips expose the film. Scatter radiation diverges in all directions and is more likely to be absorbed by one of the lead strips.

The grid also absorbs a portion of the usable x-rays. To compensate for this loss, the number of x-rays generated must be increased by increasing the mAs. Depending on the type of grid used, the increase may be up to 6.6 times the mAs required for the tabletop exposure.

Grids are manufactured with parallel or focused lead strips arranged in a crossed or linear configuration. Parallel grids have the lead strips placed perpendicular to the grid surface. X-rays and scatter radiation that interact with the lead strips are absorbed, whereas those that interact with the spacers pass through to expose the film. A disadvantage of a parallel grid is that the x-ray beam diverges at increasing angles and is absorbed at the periphery of the grid. This decreases the number of x-rays reaching the film near the grid edges, commonly called grid cutoff. **Focused grids** have the lead strips placed at progressively increasing angles to match the divergence of the x-ray beam. By angling the lead strips, cutoff of the primary beam is eliminated and radiographic density is uniform. The grid manufacturer supplies a list of distances, called the grid focal distance; setting the SID out of the grid focal distance results in primary beam cutoff on the periphery of the radiograph (Fig. 11-7). Cutoff of the primary beam also occurs if the grid is not perpendicular to or centered with the x-ray tube (Fig. 11-8).

Grids produce thin white lines on the finished radiograph. Visibility of the grid lines can be decreased in three ways. First, the lead strips can be made as thin as possible while retaining the ability to absorb scatter radiation effectively. The thinner the lead, the thinner is the white line that it produces on the radiograph.

The second way is to increase the number of grid lines per inch, making the individual lines less visible. To increase the grid lines per inch and keep the thickness of the lead the same, the width of the radiolucent strips must be decreased. This produces a grid with more lead in it, which absorbs more of the primary beam and requires higher mAs. A grid

with 80 to 100 lines/inch is sufficient to make the grid lines less visible.

The third way is by using a Potter-Bucky diaphragm, also called a **Bucky**. This device puts the grid in motion as the x-rays are generated, blurring the white grid lines on the radiograph. The Bucky is placed in a cabinet beneath the x-ray table, with a tray to hold the cassette. When a grid is used in combination with a Bucky, fewer lines per inch are necessary. This allows for the use of lower mAs. One disadvantage of using a Bucky mechanism in veterinary medicine is the noise and vibration that it produces. Some animals may object to this and struggle or move during the x-ray exposure.

EXPOSURE VARIABLES

Four exposure factors control radiographic density, contrast, and detail—mAs, kVp, FFD, and OFD. Changing one of these factors usually requires adjustments in another factor to maintain the same radiographic density.

MILLIAMPERAGE AND EXPOSURE TIME

The mAs is a product of the milliamperage and exposure time. The milliamperage controls the number of electrons in the electron cloud generated at the filament of the cathode. This is done by controlling the temperature of the cathode filament. When the mA is increased, the temperature of the filament is increased, producing more electrons to form the electron cloud. Increasing the mA increases the amount of radiographic density because more x-rays are generated.

The other factor is the time during which the electrons are allowed to flow from the cathode to the anode. By varying the exposure time, the number of x-rays generated is controlled. Using a longer exposure time allows the electrons more time to cross from the cathode to the anode, thus generating more x-rays.

Exposure time and mA are inversely related. As mA increases, the exposure time required to maintain the desired

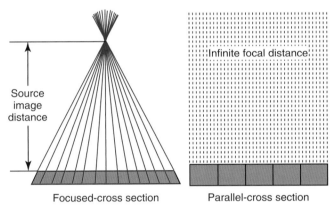

FIGURE 11-7 The focused grid has lead strips angled so that the lines are drawn through each lead continuing out of the grid. They will intersect at a grid focus point. The grid is termed a parallel grid when the strips are not angulated but are located at 90 degrees to the grid surface. (From Sirois M: Principles and practice of veterinary technology, ed 3, St Louis, 2011, Mosby.)

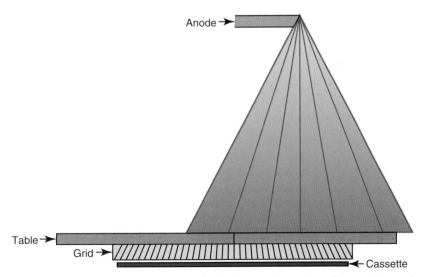

FIGURE 11-8 Grid cutoff. When the grid is not centered with the x-ray tube, grid cutoff occurs. This produces visible grid lines more prominently on one end of the film and an overall decrease in radiographic density. (From Sirois M: Principles and practice of veterinary technology, ed 3, St Louis, 2011, Mosby.)

number of x-rays generated decreases. Many different combinations of mA and time can be used to produce the same mAs. For example, consider the following:

$$300 \text{ mAat } ^1\!/_{60} \sec = 5 \text{ mAs}$$

$$200 \text{ mAat } ^1\!/_{40} \sec = 5 \text{ mAs}$$

$$100 \text{ mAat } ^1\!/_{20} \sec = 5 \text{ mAs}$$

When faced with a choice of which mAs to use, always choose the one with the fastest exposure time to allow less effect of movement on the film. The mAs can be used to adjust the radiographic density by following these rules:
- To double the radiographic density, double the mAs.
- To halve the radiographic density, halve the mAs.

KILOVOLTAGE PEAK

The kVp is the voltage applied between the cathode and the anode. It is used to accelerate electrons flowing from the cathode toward the anode side. Increasing the kVp causes the electrons to move faster, increasing the force of the collision with the target, which produces an x-ray beam with a shorter wavelength and more penetrating power. The correct kVp setting is determined by the thickness of the part being imaged; thus, the thicker the part, the higher the kVp setting, because more penetration is needed. As with mAs, there are rules when changing the radiographic density with kVp:
- To double the radiographic density, increase the kVp by 20%.
- To halve the radiographic density, decrease the kVp by 16%.

SOURCE-IMAGE DISTANCE

The SID is the distance from the target to the recording surface (film). For most radiographic procedures, this distance is held constant, at approximately 36 to 40 inches. In some situations, the SID must be changed. This requires changing one of the other factors to maintain radiographic density. As noted, the inverse square law states that the intensity of the x-ray beam is inversely proportional to the square of the distance from the source of the x-ray. If the SID is doubled, the mAs must be increased by a factor of 4 to maintain radiographic density. The same number of x-rays must diverge to cover an area that is four times as large. Changing the SID does not affect the penetrating power of the beam, so the kVp remains constant.

> **CRITICAL CONCEPT**
>
> The higher the mA setting on the x-ray machine, the greater is the number of x-rays produced. The higher the kVp, the greater is the penetrating power of the x-rays.

OBJECT-IMAGE DISTANCE

The OID (also called the **object-film distance [OFD]**; with digital imaging, the term *object-image distance* is now being used) is the distance from the object being imaged to the recording surface (film or digital recording plate). This distance should be as short as possible to minimize the penumbra effect and the magnification that occurs with a long OID.

RADIOGRAPHIC FILM

X-ray film consists of three layers—a thin protective layer, an emulsion containing silver halide crystals, and a polyester film base. The first layer is a thin, clear gelatin that acts as a protective coating. This protective material helps protect the sensitive film emulsion. The second layer is the emulsion, which contains finely precipitated silver halide crystals in a gelatin base.

The emulsion coats both sides of the film base. When placed in the developing chemicals, the emulsion swells, allowing the chemicals to act on the exposed or sensitized crystals without losing the crystals. Once the emulsion is dry, it hardens again, trapping the black metallic silver. The film base is in the center of the film, giving it support. It does not produce a visible light pattern or absorb the light.

When the silver halide crystals are exposed to electromagnetic radiation, they become more sensitive to chemical change. These sensitized crystals are what make up the **latent image**. When the film is placed into the developer, the latent image is reduced to black metallic silver. The remaining silver halide crystals are removed in the fixer. This produces varying shades of black metallic silver and the clear film base.

Film is sensitive to all types of electromagnetic radiation. These include gamma radiation, particulate radiation (alpha and beta), x-rays, heat, and light. Film is also sensitive to excessive pressure, so care must be taken when handling and storing radiographic film.

> **CRITICAL CONCEPT**
>
> X-ray film is sensitive to heat, light, and pressure in addition to x-rays and other forms of radiation.

The two types of film used in veterinary radiography are screen-type film and direct exposure film. Screen-type film is more sensitive to the light produced by intensifying screens. Two screen-type films are blue-sensitive and green-sensitive films. Blue-sensitive film is more sensitive to light emitted from screens containing blue light–emitting phosphors. Calcium tungstate and some rare earth phosphors are the most common blue light–emitting phosphors. They emit light in the ultraviolet, violet, and blue light range. Green-sensitive film is most sensitive to light from green light–emitting phosphors. Rare earth phosphors are the most common green light–emitting phosphors. **Direct exposure film** is more sensitive to direct x-rays than it is to light. Because it does not use the intensifying effect of the screens, it requires higher mAs than screen film. General anesthesia or heavy sedation may be necessary to prevent patient motion and blurring on the radiograph because of the higher mAs. Direct exposure film is mainly used to image the extremities or rostral mandible or maxilla, where good detail is needed. It is often used for imaging exotic animals and in dental radiology studies. It is packaged in a paper folder enclosed in a stout lightproof envelope. Take care when handling this film because it is protected only by paper. Pressure artifacts can easily occur. Some direct exposure film can only be processed manually because of the thickness of the emulsion. However, some types of direct exposure film can be processed in an automatic developer.

Film speeds are rated as high (regular or fast), average (par), and slow (detail). The faster the film, the more sensitive it is and the lower mAs it requires. Average-speed (par) film is used for most veterinary radiography applications.

Another important feature in x-ray film is **film latitude**. This is the film's inherent ability to produce shades of gray. Film with a long or increased latitude can produce images with a long scale of contrast (many shades of gray). Longer-latitude film is desirable because it allows for greater exposure errors but still produces a diagnostic radiograph.

Proper storage and handling of the film are important to ensure a good diagnostic radiograph. Unexposed film should be stored in a cool, dry place, away from strong chemical fumes. A base fog can develop if film is stored under adverse conditions over a long period. Film is pressure-sensitive, so it should be stored on end and not laid flat on its side.

INTENSIFYING SCREENS

Intensifying screens contain fluorescent crystals bound to a cardboard or plastic base. When exposed to x-rays, they emit foci of light. Placing radiographic film in direct contact with the screens accurately records any x-rays that penetrate the patient. Approximately 95% of the film's radiographic density results from fluorescence of the intensifying screens and only 5% is the result of direct x-ray exposure. For each x-ray photon the screen absorbs, it emits 1000 light photons, amplifying the photographic effect of the x-rays. The film is sandwiched between two screens mounted inside a lightproof cassette. The cassette holds the film in close, uniform contact with the screens (Fig. 11-9).

The screens are supported by a plastic or cardboard base. Next to the base is a thin reflecting layer, which reflects the light back toward the film side or front of the screen. The third is the phosphor layer. The most common phosphor used today consists of rare earth elements such as lanthanum oxybromide and gadolinium oxysulfide, which emit green light. Rare earth screens allow shorter exposure time. A thin waterproof protective coating that prevents static during cassette loading and unloading is over the phosphor layer. It also provides physical protection and is a surface that can be cleaned.

Intensifying screens are available in three different speeds—high (regular), par (medium), and slow (detail or fine). High-speed screens require less exposure time as compared with the par or slow speed, but detail is decreased. When changing from a high-speed screen to a par-speed screen, the mAs must be increased two times. When changing from high speed to slow speed, the mAs must be increased four times to maintain radiographic density.

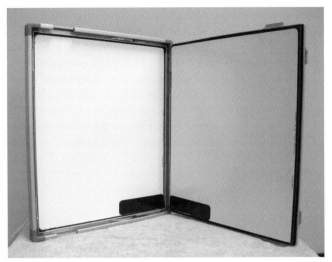

FIGURE 11-9 Cassette with intensifying screens. (From Sirois M: Principles and practice of veterinary technology, ed 3, St Louis, 2011, Mosby.)

Proper care of intensifying screens is important. Routine cleaning is necessary to ensure that the screens are free from dirt and foreign materials. These can block the light emitted from the screens, leaving parts of the film unexposed. The result is a white area on the film that resembles the foreign material. Identifying the cassettes inside on the intensifying screen and also on the outside of the cassette enables the dirty cassette to be retrieved and cleaned. Processing chemicals can cause permanent damage if the screen surface is not cleaned promptly. The screens should be cleaned with a soft, lint-free cloth and screen-cleaning solution. If a commercial cleaner is not available, warm water is acceptable. Do not use denatured alcohol or abrasive products because they can damage the protective coating and phosphor layer. Be sure to allow the screen to completely dry before reloading.

Cassettes are precision instruments and should be handled that way. Do not drop them or set heavy objects on them. This can result in poor film-screen contact and blurring of one area of the image. To check the film-screen contact of your screens, place paper clips over the surface of the cassette. Use enough to cover every area completely. Expose the cassette using 50 to 60 kVp and half the mAs that you would use for a nongrid extremity. Process the film and view it dry. Any areas with poor film-screen contact are indicated by a blurred image of the paper clips.

X-RAY EQUIPMENT

There are many factors to consider when choosing x-ray equipment. The needs of individual practices will vary depending on the species to be radiographed, caseload, and type of technology desired. There are three basic types of x-ray equipment—portable, mobile, and stationary units. A portable unit can be carried to the animal. These machines generally have a fixed mA set by the manufacturer at 15 to 30 mA, a variable kVp ranging from 40 to 90, and exposure times as short as 1/120 second (Fig. 11-10). Because the mA is fixed, the exposure time is changed to increase the radiographic density. For this reason, motion can be a problem with some animals because of the prolonged exposure times.

The mobile unit can be transported to the patient. However, because of its large size, it is limited to in-hospital use, such as in the treatment room or perhaps in a driveway (Fig. 11-11). These units generally produce a maximum 300 mA, 125 kVp, and a 1/120-second exposure. The tube head on a mobile unit can be suspended above a table for small animal radiography.

Stationary units are those that are installed in a room with proper leaded wall shielding for radiography. These units have many different exposure capabilities, depending on the quality desired. A general small animal practice that does mainly routine radiographic examinations may be well served by a machine with 300 mA, 125 kVp, and at least a 1/120-second output (Fig. 11-12). However, practices that provide specialty services, such as internal medicine or surgery referrals, will require higher-output equipment.

The caseload should be taken into account when choosing x-ray equipment. If a practice has an average of one to two cases requiring radiographs per week, with a majority of large animal extremities and an occasional small animal film, a portable unit would probably be considered appropriate. If a practice has an average of 3 to 15 radiography cases/week, with a mixture of large and small animals, a mobile unit may be considered. A high-volume practice that radiographs an average of more than 16 cases/week will benefit from a stationary unit.

Accessory equipment used depends on the type of x-ray machine needed. Basic equipment requirements for a stationary x-ray machine include the x-ray generator system, collimator, grid, table, tube stand, and positioning aids. Because most large animal extremity radiographs are made with portable or low-output x-ray machines, tube stands and cassette holders must be used. These pieces of accessory equipment allow personnel to be positioned farther from the primary beam, thus decreasing personal exposure. Cassettes and x-ray tubes should never be handheld.

DIGITAL X-RAY IMAGING

The analog or film-screen system remains the most widely used system in veterinary clinical settings. However, the increased availability and affordability of digital radiography

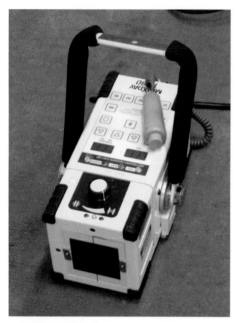

FIGURE 11-10 Portable x-ray unit. (From Sirois M: Principles and practice of veterinary technology, ed 3, St Louis, 2011, Mosby.)

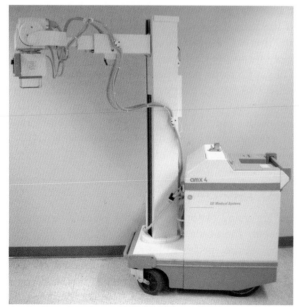

FIGURE 11-11 Mobile x-ray unit. (From Sirois M: Principles and practice of veterinary technology, ed 3, St Louis, 2011, Mosby.)

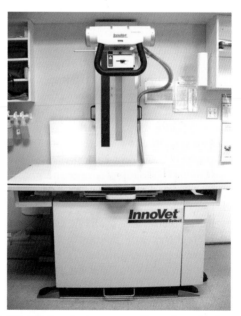

FIGURE 11-12 Standard x-ray unit. (From Sirois M: Principles and practice of veterinary technology, ed 3, St Louis, 2011, Mosby.)

has made replacing analog systems much easier and digital systems are becoming much more common. Digital radiography refers to the process whereby images are obtained and displayed on appropriate computer monitors in a grayscale digital display. There are three main types of digital systems currently available. These include computed radiography (CR), digital radiography (DR), and charge-coupled device (CCD) technologies. An advantage of the use of digital systems is that the digitized image can then be enhanced and viewed by using computer software that enables contrast, brightness, zoom, and pan adjustments, as well as measurement of various anatomic structures.

> **CRITICAL CONCEPT**
>
> Digital radiographic images can be manipulated to enhance contrast and brightness and to allow for enlargement and measurement of anatomic structures.

Other advantages of digital radiography include elimination of the need for film, processing chemicals, and screens. Existing x-ray machines can be retrofitted for DR use, or standard CR systems will be accepted without any changes being made to the grid cabinet or Bucky mechanism. With CCD systems, however, a brand new radiology generator and table will need to be purchased. However, current CCD systems are competitively priced as compared with CR and DR systems. DR systems may reduce the amount of repeat radiographs needed caused by inappropriate exposure settings or chemical processing errors.

It should be noted that a hard copy film can still be made from digital radiographs. There are a number of manufacturers of dry laser printers for printing images, if necessary.

COMPUTED RADIOGRAPHY

CR uses a cassette system not unlike conventional film-screen systems. Instead of having two screens and a film within the cassette, there is an imaging plate (IP) that contains a photostimulable phosphor, which can store the radiation level received at each point on the plate. This eliminates the need for film as a medium for viewing radiographs. Instead of chemical processing, the cassette is run through a computer scanner that uses a scanning laser beam. This causes the electrons to relax to a lower energy level, which emits light. These light measurements are proportional to the amount of radiation reaching and being absorbed by the IP in a given area. This light is measured, and the digital image created. The imaging plate is then erased by fluorescent light in the reader, and the IP is reloaded into the cassette for reuse. The imaging plate can be reused thousands of times.

DIGITAL RADIOGRAPHY

DR also uses an imaging plate comprised of an array of detectors. These detectors translate or convert the x-rays into an electrical signal or pulse that is then digitalized by the computer to an image. This imaging plate is connected directly to a computer dedicated to that function, thereby eliminating the need for a cassette such as that used in a CR system. This plate can be permanently placed in an x-ray table or can be portable, depending on the user's needs.

DIGITAL RADIOGRAPHY STORAGE

Digital radiography (and other modalities, such as CT, MRI, ultrasound, and NM) uses a DICOM (*d*igital *i*maging and *co*mmunications in *m*edicine) format, which is the universally accepted format for the dispersion and storing of medical information. Each DICOM file includes the pertinent information associated with the patient, such as modality, date and time of examination, and patient identification and number. DICOM files are encrypted so that patient and image data are kept secure and tamper-proof.

> **CRITICAL CONCEPT**
>
> Digital radiography, CT, MRI, and ultrasound images are stored using a universally accepted format known as DICOM.

Storage of these DICOM files can be as simple as archiving to a compact disc (CD), digital video disc (DVD), or magnetic optical disc (MOD), or it can be managed through a picture archiving and communication system (PACS). This greatly reduces the amount of space needed for storage. A PACS has the advantage of storing multiple patients and making images available to multiple computers within a hospital or network of hospitals. It is capable of handling multiple modalities and enhances communication among clinicians. A typical setup for PACS is a dedicated computer workstation, monitor, and server.

Fluoroscopy is used for those patients for whom the visualization of dynamic structures is of importance. Using an x-ray tube, a beam is directed through a patient onto a fluorescent screen or image intensifier to form an image. This is commonly referred to as real-time imaging because it is a continuous stream of images. The image is then transferred to a monitor and can be recorded on spot film or videotape, or digitized by computer. Fluoroscopy is generally used for gastrointestinal (GI) studies (e.g., barium studies, gastrograms, upper GI studies), angiography (cardiac catheterizations), and myelography. Fluoroscopy is not a commonly used modality in the general clinical setting because of economic limitations. However, referral clinics and most university veterinary hospitals have one or have access to one.

RADIATION SAFETY

Ionizing radiation can be a difficult concept to grasp, because at diagnostic levels it cannot be seen, felt, or heard by the patient or operators. Why is radiation safety important? Radiation ionizes intracellular water. This releases toxic products, which can damage critical components of the cell, such as DNA. When radiation comes into contact with the cells of living tissue, it can do the following:

- Pass through the cells with no effect.
- Produce cell damage that is reparable.

- Produce cell damage that is not reparable.
- Kill the cells.

Radiation damages the body in several ways. It may have carcinogenic effects, which means that cancer may develop in body tissues. Effects on the body may be genetic, occurring in future generations. Tissues that are most sensitive to ionizing radiation are those with rapidly growing or reproducing cells. The reproductive organs may suffer from temporary or permanent infertility, decreased hormone production, or mutations. The hematopoietic (blood-forming) cells are relatively sensitive to ionizing radiation. The lymphocytic blood cells are most sensitive. Damage to blood cells can reduce resistance to infection and cause clotting disorders. The thyroid gland, intestinal epithelium, and lens of the eye are also radiosensitive. There may be an increased incidence of squamous cell carcinoma with chronic, low-level skin exposure. Radiodermatitis (reddened, dry skin) can result from excessive, chronic, low-level radiation exposure.

The developing fetus is sensitive to the effects of ionizing radiation. The degree of sensitivity depends on the stage of pregnancy and the dose received. The preimplantation period (0 to 9 days) is the most critical time for the embryo. The period of organogenesis (10 days to 6 weeks) carries the greatest risk of congenital malformation in the fetus, because this is the critical development period for fetal organs. The fetus may have skeletal or dental malformations. Other abnormalities include microphthalmia (small eyes) and overall growth retardation. A fetal dose greater than 25 rad (0.25 gray [Gy]) is recognized as the threshold for significant damage to the fetus (for an explanation of these units of measure, see later, "Terminology"). The fetal period (6 weeks to term) is the least sensitive time for the fetus; however, growth may be affected and mental retardation may occur. Irradiation after 30 weeks is less likely to cause abnormalities because the sensitivity of the fetus approaches that of the adult.

TERMINOLOGY

Rem stands for roentgen equivalent in man. Rem units are used to express the dose equivalent that results from exposure to ionizing radiation. Rem takes into account the quality of radiation, so doses of different types of radiation can be compared. The **sievert (SV)** is the current terminology used to define a rem (1 SV = 100 rem). A millirem (mrem) is equal to 0.001 rem or 1/1000 rem. A rad is the radiation absorbed dose. Current terminology is Gy (1 Gy = 100 rad). This chapter discusses x-rays only and not other types of radiation, so 1 rad can be considered to be equivalent to 1 rem. Other types of radiation must have a quality factor figured in to determine the dose. MPD is the **maximum permissible dose**. The National Council on Radiation Protection and Measurements recommends that the dose for occupationally exposed persons not exceed 5 rem/year. An occupationally exposed individual is one who normally performs his or her work in a restricted access area and has duties that involve exposure to radiation. **ALARA** stands for *as low as reasonably attainable*. The MPD for nonoccupational persons is

10% of the MPD for occupationally exposed persons, or 0.5 rem/year. This is known as the ALARA MPD. Also, a fetus should not receive more than 0.5 rem during the entire gestation period. A pregnant employee who chooses to continue working around radiation-producing devices should wear an additional badge at waist level, underneath the lead gown, to monitor the fetal dose. This should not exceed 0.05 rem/month.

There are three important ways to minimize occupational exposure to radiation. The first is lead shielding. Lead shielding should be a requirement for all personnel remaining in the room while an exposure is made. Lead gowns, gloves, and thyroid shields (Fig. 11-13) should all contain at least 0.5 mm of lead. Lead-based glasses can also be worn to protect the lens of the eye. Lead apparel is expensive, so it should be handled appropriately. Lead aprons should be draped over a rounded surface, without folds or wrinkles, to prevent cracks in the lead. Lead gloves can be stored with open-ended soup cans inserted to prevent cracks and provide air circulation to the liners. Lead gloves should be radiographed every 6 months to check for damaged areas. Lead gowns should be checked every 12 months to screen for holes and cracks in the lead. Check gloves and gowns for damage by radiographing them using 5 mAs and 80 kVp. This can be adjusted as needed to attain the proper density in the radiographs.

Non-leaded protective aprons have recently become available and provide the same protection as standard lead apparel. The non-leaded apparel is much lighter in weight.

Lead mittens and hand shields are also available. These are not generally recommended since part of the hand may be exposed to scatter radiation.

Another method for decreasing personnel exposure is by increasing the distance from the primary beam. If the animal cannot be sedated or anesthetized, personnel restraining the animal should try to remain as far as possible from the x-ray source during exposure. During exposure, if restraining an animal, one should use tape and sandbags and/or other types of mechanical restraints to extend the distance of the

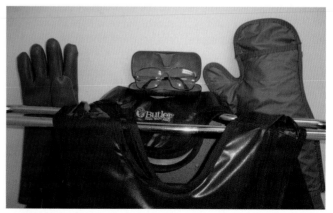

FIGURE 11-13 Lead gloves, gowns, thyroid shield, and lead-based glasses must be properly used and stored. (From Sirois M: Principles and practice of veterinary technology, ed 3, St Louis, 2011, Mosby.)

gloved hands from the collimated area (Fig. 11-14). Employees should take care to wear protective apparel properly to obtain full protection. Placing a glove on top of a hand for protection does not protect the hand from scatter radiation. The scatter can come from any direction, including from under the tabletop.

Using the fastest film-screen combinations allows reduced exposure time for the patient and personnel by using less mAs. Proper darkroom practices and technique charts allow for the consistent production of high-quality films, which reduces the number of repeat radiographs. It is important to collimate the primary beam down to the area of interest because this reduces the exposure of personnel to scatter (secondary) radiation. A 2-mm Al filter is used at the tube window to filter out soft rays that are too weak to penetrate the patient. If these rays are not filtered out, they scatter about the room, fogging the film and striking personnel.

Each clinic should have a radiation protection supervisor. A veterinary technician can fill this role. Responsibilities include educating personnel on radiation safety, monitoring safety practices, and maintaining a radiologic badge system. The supervisor also maintains x-ray equipment, darkroom facilities, and radiographic records. A good radiation control program consists of safe x-ray equipment, low-exposure techniques, use of positioning aids, proper measuring of patients, proper positioning methods, shielding, and monitoring personal radiation exposure (Box 11-1). The x-ray equipment is usually under the control of the state government (e.g., state board of health). Regulations vary among states, so check with your state government about their policy regarding radiation-producing devices.

> **CRITICAL CONCEPT**
>
> Methods to reduce occupational exposure to ionizing radiation include the use of lead shielding and the proper use of patient positioning aids.

DARKROOM TECHNIQUES

Along with a good technique chart, proper darkroom techniques should be followed to ensure consistent production of high-quality radiographs. Properly exposed radiographs can quickly become nondiagnostic with poor film handling and darkroom techniques.

DARKROOM SETUP

For most veterinary practices, the darkroom does not need to be large or fancy, as long as the layout is designed for efficiency. The room must be just large enough to provide a dry bench area away from the wet bench area (Fig. 11-15). The

BOX 11-1	General Radiation Safety Rules

- Always wear lead gloves and apron as well as lead thyroid shield when remaining in the room during radiography or fluoroscopy. Lead protective shielding must be worn by all individuals involved in restraint of the animal.
- Always wear a radiation-monitoring device on your collar outside the apron or on the edge of the glove when working around x-ray equipment. **Note:** Badges should not be exposed to sunlight, dampness, or extreme temperatures. This could cause falsely high readings.
- Never allow any part of your body to be exposed to the primary beam. Lead clothing does not protect against primary beam exposure.
- Wear lead-based glasses to protect the lens of the eye.
- Using mechanical restraints such as tape and sandbags; distance will aid in minimizing exposure.
- Use alternative methods of restraint (e.g., drugs, tape, sandbags) when using high-exposure radiographic techniques.
- Pregnant women and persons < 18 yr should not be involved in radiographic procedures. Use proper safety precautions.
- Only those required for restraint should remain in the room when an exposure is made.

Adapted from Sirois M: *Principles and practice of veterinary technology,* ed 3, St Louis, 2011, Mosby.

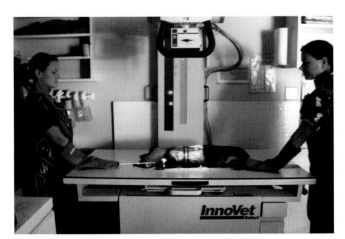

FIGURE 11-14 The restrainers have increased their distance from the primary beam by using mechanical devices (sandbags and tape) and are wearing proper protective gear. (From Sirois M: *Principles and practice of veterinary technology,* ed 3, St Louis, 2011, Mosby.)

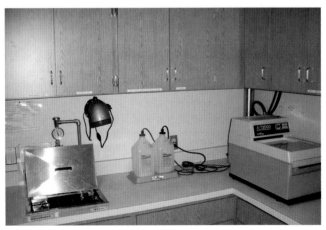

FIGURE 11-15 Darkroom processing area. Note that the dry and wet preparation areas are well separated. (From Sirois M: *Principles and practice of veterinary technology,* ed 3, St Louis, 2011, Mosby.)

dry bench area is for unloading and loading cassettes and film storage. The wet bench area is for film processing and drying. These areas must be separated to prevent processing chemical splashes from damaging the dry films or sensitive intensifying screens. In a small room, this can be achieved by placing a partition between the two areas. Sufficient electrical outlets should be available to power the safelights, view boxes, and labeling equipment.

The most important feature of a darkroom is that it be light-tight. White light that leaks around the door, through a blackened window, or around ventilation fans can fog the film. Film is more sensitive after it has been exposed to x-rays, so even low-grade light leaks decrease the quality of the finished radiograph. When checking for light leaks, stand in the darkroom for at least 5 minutes to allow your eyes to adjust to the darkness. Look around the door frame, ventilation fan, or blackened windows for any signs of white light. When performing this test, vary the intensity of light outside the door. Because work in the darkroom is done with a limited amount of light, painting the walls and ceiling a light color that reflects the available light helps greatly.

The darkroom should have adequate ventilation to prevent volatile chemical fumes from accumulating in the room. These fumes can cause fogging of the film, damage to electrical equipment, and health problems for personnel. A light-tight ventilation fan installed in the ceiling helps remove the fumes and also controls the temperature and humidity in the room. The exhaust from automatic processors and film dryers should also be vented away from the darkroom, because they contain volatile chemical fumes.

Cleanliness is important in the darkroom because intensifying screens and the film are handled in this area. Dirt and hair on countertops can fall into cassettes, causing white artifacts on subsequent radiographs from that cassette. Chemical spills also cause artifacts on the radiographs and damage the intensifying screens. Keeping wet and dry areas of the darkroom clean prevents these problems. Film hangers for manual processing should also be cleaned regularly. Chemicals that remain on the hanger clips could drip down the next film to be processed, causing an artifact.

FILM IDENTIFICATION

Permanent labeling is necessary for all radiographs. Each film must be identified before the film is processed for legal purposes and for certification organizations. The labeling can be done during or after the exposure, but it must be done before the film is processed. The label should include the clinic name, date, owner's name, address, patient's name, and some patient data, such as age and breed.

There are several methods for film identification. One method is the photo labeler, which uses a cassette containing a leaded window that protects a small area of the film during exposure. During identification, the window slides back from the protected area to expose the information on a card. This forms a latent image of the information on the film. Manual printers are similar to photo labelers, except that they use a flash of light through an information card to produce a latent

image on the film. The manual printer is placed in the darkroom, and the film is taken out of the cassette to be identified. Another method uses lead letters or radiopaque tape. These are placed on the cassette during exposure of the radiograph.

CRITICAL CONCEPT

X-rays must be labeled with the clinic name and location, date that the x-ray was taken, owner's name, and patient's name.

SAFELIGHTS

Safelight illuminators are important for darkroom processing. A safelight provides sufficient light to work in the room but does not cause fogging of the film. Safelights can be mounted to provide light directly or indirectly. With direct lighting, the safelight is mounted at least 48 inches above the workbench and directed toward the workbench. Indirect lighting has the safelight directed toward the ceiling and uses the reflected light to illuminate the room. With indirect lighting, the safelight can be mounted closer to the bench but should be as high as possible (Fig. 11-16).

Many types of safelight filters are available to filter out light in different areas of the light spectrum. The type of film used dictates which filter is necessary. Film that is blue light–sensitive requires a safelight that filters out blue and ultraviolet light. Film that is green light–sensitive requires a safelight to filter both green and blue light. This filter can also be used with blue light–sensitive film. A red light bulb should never be used to replace a safelight filter. It does not filter the light; it only colors it. A white, frosted, 7½- to 10-watt bulb is recommended for most safelight filters.

Periodically check the safelight filter. First, make a moderate exposure on a film using approximately 1 to 2 mAs and 40 to 50 kVp. Film that has been exposed to x-rays is more sensitive to low-grade light, producing an overall fogged appearance. Cover two thirds of the film with black paper or cardboard, and allow the remaining third to be exposed to the safelight for 30 seconds. This is a little longer than it should take to place the film in an automatic processor or to place the film on a hanger and into the manual tanks. After 30 seconds,

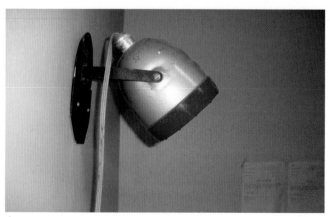

FIGURE 11-16 Direct safelight illumination. (From Sirois M: *Principles and practice of veterinary technology,* ed 3, St Louis, 2011, Mosby.)

uncover another third of the film and wait 30 more seconds. Repeat the process for the final third and develop the film. This test exposes portions of the film to the safelight for 30, 60, and 90 seconds and then it is processed. When the film is dry, look for areas of increased film density. If an increase in density is detected, a close check of the darkroom is necessary. Improper safelight distance, a cracked safelight filter, and light leaking around the filter can all cause film fogging.

FILM PROCESSING

CHEMISTRY

DEVELOPER. The developer's main function is to convert the sensitized silver halide crystals into black metallic silver. Sensitized silver halide crystals are those that have been exposed to electromagnetic radiation, making them susceptible to chemical change. The developer contains five ingredients—a solvent, reducing agents, restrainer, activator, and preservative.

Water is used as the solvent to keep all the ingredients in solution. It also causes the film emulsion to swell so that the reducing agents can penetrate the sensitized crystals. Reducing agents change the sensitized silver halide crystals into black metallic silver. Restrainers are used to protect the unexposed silver halide crystals by preventing the reducing agents from affecting the unsensitized crystals. Activators help soften and swell the film's emulsion so that the reducing agents can work effectively. Preservatives prevent the solution from oxidizing rapidly. Developing chemicals are manufactured in two forms, liquid and powder. The liquid form may be a concentrate that requires dilution with water. Working-strength liquid solutions that do not require dilution are also available. The powder form should never be mixed in the darkroom because the chemical dust contaminates unprotected film, causing artifacts. Always mix the powder in a bucket outside the darkroom and then finish the dilution in the darkroom.

FIXER. The fixer removes the unchanged silver halide crystals from the film emulsion, leaving the black metallic silver. It also hardens the film emulsion, decreasing the susceptibility to scratches. The fixer contains five ingredients—solvent, fixing agent, acidifier, hardener, and preservative.

As with the developer, the solvent for the fixer is water. It keeps the ingredients in solution and causes the film emulsion to swell, allowing the fixing agents to reach the unexposed crystals. The fixing agent clears the remaining silver halide crystals from the film emulsion. The acidifier is used to neutralize any alkaline developer remaining on the film. The hardener prevents excessive swelling of the film emulsion, shortening the drying time. The final ingredient is the preservative, used to prevent decomposition of the fixing agents.

Fixer chemicals are manufactured in two forms, liquid and powder. The liquid form may be a concentrate that requires dilution with water. Working-strength liquid solutions that do not require dilution are also available. The powder form requires dissolving and mixing to get it into solution. It should never be mixed in the darkroom because the chemical dust can contaminate unprotected film, causing artifacts. Always mix the powder in a bucket outside the darkroom and then finish the dilution in the darkroom. Also, the powder form requires a longer clearing time than the liquid form.

EQUIPMENT

MANUAL PROCESSING. With the ready availability of reasonably priced automatic processors, few veterinary clinics now use manual methods. However, there are still some locations in which these are present. Manual processing is sometimes used for dental radiographs and other nonscreen films used for exotic animal radiography. Manual processing tanks are usually made from stainless steel and are large enough to accept 14- by 17-inch film hangers. Tanks with a 5-gallon capacity are sufficient. Plastic or wooden lids are needed to cover the developer and fixer tanks, which reduces the rate of evaporation and oxidation of the chemicals. Separate stirring rods for the developer and fixer are used to mix the chemicals before processing. Also, an accurate timer and floating thermometer should be available.

Developing x-ray film is a chemical process that depends on the duration of immersion in the chemicals and the temperature of the chemicals. Manufacturers generally recommend a temperature for the chemicals they produce. Most use 68° F (20° C), with 5 minutes of developing time. For some cases, this may not be possible, so the time can be adjusted to compensate for the increase or decrease in temperature. The time can be decreased by 30 seconds for every 2°-F increase in developer temperature, or the time can be increased by 30 seconds for every 2°-F decrease in developer temperature. This applies only between 65° F (18° C) and 74° F (23° C).

The rinse bath removes developer from the film, preventing carryover into the fixer tank. Agitating the film in the running water bath for 30 seconds removes the developer adequately. The rinse water should be continually exchanged to prevent accumulation of developer. The temperature of the incoming rinse water can often be used to regulate the temperature of the developer and fixer tanks.

The fixing process is also dependent on immersion time and temperature of the chemicals. The standard temperature is 68° F (20° C), and the fixing time is double the developing time. The temperature affects the time that the film is left in the fixer. The warmer the chemicals, the shorter the fixing time. The film can be removed from the fixer after 30 seconds and viewed with white light. However, it must be placed back into the fixer for the remainder of the time. The clearing time increases as the thickness of the emulsion increases. Direct exposure film has a thicker emulsion and requires a longer time in the fixer.

The final wash rinses away the processing chemicals. Failure to rinse the film completely results in a film that eventually becomes faded and brown. This is caused by oxidation of the chemicals remaining in the film emulsion. The wash tank should have fresh circulating water to decrease the time needed for the final wash. Generally, the wash time is at least 30 minutes.

MAINTENANCE. There are two methods for maintaining manual processing tanks. The first is the exhausted method. With this method, allow the chemicals to drain back into their respective tanks and not into the wash tank. This permits the exhausted chemicals to remain in the tank, maintaining the chemical levels. The second method is the replenishing method. Do not allow the chemicals to drain back into their respective tanks, but place them in the wash tank. The chemical levels are maintained by replenishing with chemicals that are more concentrated than those in the initial solution. In this way, the potency and levels of the chemicals can be preserved. With either method, the chemicals should be changed every 3 months.

AUTOMATIC PROCESSING. Use of an automatic processor has some advantages over manual processing. Automatic processors can develop film more quickly; they can process and dry a film in 90 to 120 seconds. Also, automatic processors consistently provide high-quality radiographs. This eliminates the need for repeat radiographs because of processing errors.

Automatic processors move the film through the developer, fixer wash bath, and dryers at a uniform rate of speed. Chemicals and film are specially manufactured to withstand the high temperatures involved in automatic processing. The chemicals are kept at temperatures of approximately 95° F (35° C), depending on the type of film and equipment used. The emulsion on film designed for automatic processing is harder than on film designed for manual processing, preventing scratches from the roller. This film can also be manually processed in case of mechanical problems with the automatic processor.

MAINTENANCE. Small tabletop automatic processors are easily maintained in most veterinary practices. The equipment should be completely cleaned every 3 months. This includes draining and cleaning the tanks. A 1:32 solution of laundry bleach (e.g., Clorox) helps reduce algae and remove chemical buildup. The rollers can be cleaned with a mild detergent and soft sponge. When any cleaning solution is applied to the tanks

or rollers, they should be rinsed thoroughly before replacing the chemicals. Also, check the springs and gears for signs of wear and replace if necessary. Wipe the feed tray and top rollers with a clean, soft sponge every day. This helps remove dirt, debris, and chemical residue between episodes of routine maintenance.

SILVER RECOVERY

When an exposed film is placed in the developer, the exposed silver halide crystals are converted to black metallic silver. The remaining silver halide crystals are removed from the film in the fixer. Over time, the fixer solution becomes rich with silver that can be reclaimed. Silver recovery systems can be attached to automatic processors to filter and store the silver that would normally be discarded down the drain. The black metallic silver in the processed radiographs can also be recovered.

The manual processing fixer solution, silver recovery systems, and old radiographs can be sold to companies that reclaim the silver. These companies are usually listed in the Yellow Pages under the heading "Gold and Silver Refiners and Dealers."

RADIOGRAPHIC ARTIFACTS

An artifact is any unwanted density in the form of blemishes caused by improper handling, exposure, processing, or housekeeping. Artifacts can mimic or mask a disease process or distract from the overall quality of the film.

Before radiographing an animal, check for external debris, wet hair, or any lumps or bumps on the patient. Remove any dirt or mats from the coat. If the coat is wet, dry it as much as possible. Remove any collars, leashes, or halters. Bandage material is visible on radiographs, so remove it, if feasible. Boxes 11-2 and 11-3 list common artifact problems.

BOX 11-2 | Causes of Common Radiographic Artifacts That Occur Before Processing

Fogged Film
- Film exposed to excessive scatter radiation. A grid is necessary when radiographing areas ≥ 10 cm (overall gray appearance).
- Film exposed to radiation during storage
- Film stored in an area that was too hot or humid
- Film exposed to a safelight filter that was cracked or inappropriate for the type of film used
- Film exposed to a low-grade light leak in darkroom
- Film expired

Black Crescents or Lines
- Rough handling of film before or after exposure (Fig. 1)

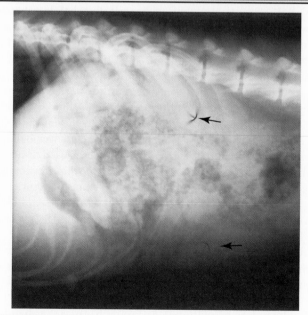

FIGURE 1 Black crescent from rough handling of the film before or after exposure.

BOX 11-2 | Causes of Common Radiographic Artifacts That Occur Before Processingg—cont'd

- Static electricity caused by low humidity
- Scratched film surface before or after exposure
- Fingerprints from excessive pressure before or after exposure

Black Areas

- Black, irregular border on one end of film caused by light exposure while still in the box or film bin
- Black, irregular border on multiple sides of the film caused by felt damage in the cassette

White Areas

- Foreign material between the film and screen (Fig. 2)

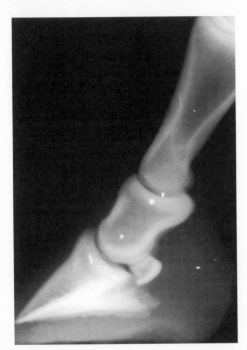

FIGURE 2 Foreign material between the film and screen blocks light from exposing the film and creating white areas.

- Chemical spill on the screen, causing permanent damage to the phosphor layer
- Contrast medium on the patient, table, or cassette
- White fingerprints on film from oil or fixer on fingers before processing
- Visible grid lines
- Grid lines on the entire film from FFD outside the range of the grid's focus
- Grid lines more visible on one end of the film and overall decrease in radiographic density caused by the grid's not being centered in the primary beam
- Grid lines on the entire film caused by the grid's not being perpendicular to the center of the primary beam
- Grid lines more visible in some areas than others from grid damage

Decreased Detail

- Patient motion
- Poor film-screen contact
- Increased object-film distance
- Decreased FFD

Adapted from Sirois M: Principles and practice of veterinary technology, ed 3, St Louis, 2011, Mosby.

BOX 11-3 | Causes of Common Radiographic Artifacts That Occur During Manual or Automatic Processing

Increased Radiographic Density With Poor Contrast

- Film overdeveloped (longer than manufacturer recommendation)
- Film developed in hot chemicals; correct temperature for manual tanks is 68° F (20° C); for automatic processors, 95° F (35° C)
- Film overexposed

Decreased Radiographic Density With Poor Contrast

- Film underdeveloped (shorter than manufacturer recommendation)
- Film developed in cold chemicals; correct temperature for manual tanks is 68° F (20° C), for automatic processors, 95° F (35° C)
- Film processed in old or exhausted chemicals

- Film underexposed

Uneven Development

- Lack of stirring, allowing chemicals to settle to tank bottom
- Repeated withdrawal of film from tank to check on development results
- Uneven chemical levels

Black Areas, Spots, or Streaks

- Identical black areas on two films processed together from films stuck to one another in fixer and not cleared properly
- Black area on only one film from film sticking to side of tank
- Well-defined spots or streaks from developer splash before processing
- Black lines along full length of the film and equal distance apart from pressure of rollers in the processor

Defined Areas of Decreased Radiographic Density

- Identical light areas on two films processed together from sticking together in the developer
- Light area on one film from film sticking to the side of the tank during development (Fig. 1)
- Air bubbles clinging to the film during development
- Well-defined spots or streaks from fixer splash before processing

Clear Areas or Spots

- Streaks where emulsion scratched away
- Large clear areas from leaving film in final wash too long and emulsion sliding off film base

Entire Film Clear

- No exposure
- Film placed in fixer before developer

Film Turns Brown

- Improper final wash

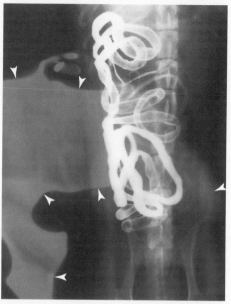

FIGURE 1 This radiograph stuck to the side of the manual tank while in the developer. The arrows outline the artifact. A light image can still be seen, because the file has emulsion on both sides of the film base. One side developed normally.

Adapted from Sirois M: Principles and practice of veterinary technology, ed 3, St Louis, 2011, Mosby.

RADIOGRAPHIC POSITIONING AND TERMINOLOGY

Proper patient positioning is as important as the radiograph itself. Misinterpretations can result from inaccurate positioning. A basic knowledge of directional terminology is essential when describing radiographic projections. The American College of Veterinary Radiology (ACVR) has standardized the nomenclature for radiographic projections by using currently accepted veterinary anatomic terms. The projections are described by the direction at which the central ray enters and exits the part being imaged (Fig. 11-17):

- Ventral (V): Body area situated toward the underside of quadrupeds
- Dorsal (D): Body area situated toward the back or topline of quadrupeds; opposite of ventral
- Medial (M): Body area situated toward the median plane or midline
- Lateral (L): Body area situated away from the median plane or midline
- Cranial (Cr): Structures or areas situated toward the head (formerly anterior)
- Caudal (Cd): Structures or areas situated toward the tail (formerly posterior)
- Rostral (R): Areas on the head situated toward the nose
- Palmar (Pa): Situated on the caudal aspect of the front limb, distal to the antebrachiocarpal joint
- Plantar (Pl): Situated on the caudal aspect of the rear limb, distal to the tarsocrural joint

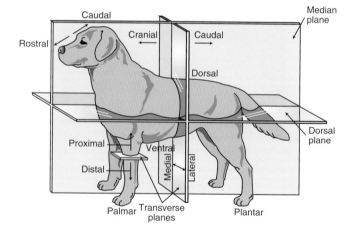

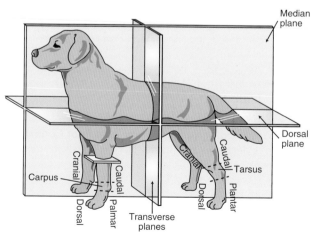

FIGURE 11-17 Anatomic planes of reference and directional terms. (From Colville TP, Bassert JM: Clinical anatomy and physiology for veterinary technicians, ed 2, St Louis, 2008, Mosby.)

- Proximal (Pr): Situated closer to the point of attachment or origin
- Distal (Di): Situated away from the point of attachment or origin

OBLIQUE PROJECTIONS

Oblique projections are used to set off an area that normally would be superimposed over another area (Fig. 11-18). Some rules should be followed when deciding which type of oblique projection is needed and how it is to be identified:

- The area of interest should be as close to the cassette as possible. This decreases magnification and increases detail.
- Place a marker on the cassette or near the anatomy within the primary beam during exposure to indicate the direction of entry and exit of the primary beam.

Table 11-1 shows the landmarks used to produce radiographs of various body parts. For most small animal patients, abdominal and thoracic radiographs required a VD (Fig. 11-19) and lateral projection.

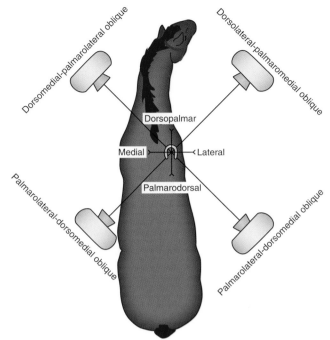

FIGURE 11-18 Correct anatomic directional terms for oblique views. (From Brown M, Brown L: Lavin's radiography for veterinary technicians, ed 5, St Louis, 2014, Saunders.)

TABLE 11-1	Landmarks Used in Producing Radiographs of Various Body Areas			
BODY PART	**CRANIAL OR PROXIMAL LANDMARK**	**CAUDAL OR DISTAL LANDMARK**	**CENTER LANDMARK**	**COMMENTS**
Thorax	Manubrium sterni	Halfway between xiphoid and last rib	Caudal border of the scapula	Expose at peak inspiration
Abdomen	Halfway between xiphoid and caudal border of the scapula	Greater trochanter	Last rib	Expose at peak expiration
Shoulder	Midbody scapula	Midshaft humerus	Over joint space	
Humerus	Shoulder joint	Elbow joint	Midshaft	
Elbow	Midshaft humerus	Midshaft radius	Over joint space	
Radius, ulna	Elbow joint	Carpal joint	Midshaft	
Carpus	Midshaft radius	Midshaft metacarpus	Over joint space	
Metacarpus	Carpal joint	Include digits	Midshaft	
Pelvis	Wings of ilium	Ischium		
Pelvis ventrodorsal (VD), flexed	Wings of ilium	Ischium		Pushes stifles cranially
Pelvis VD, extended	Wings of ilium	Stifle joint		Femora parallel to each other and table
Femur	Coxofemoral joint	Stifle joint	Midshaft	
Stifle	Midshaft femur	Midshaft tibia	Over joint space	
Tibia, fibula	Stifle joint	Tarsal joint	Midshaft	
Tarsus	Midshaft tibia	Midshaft metatarsal	Over joint space	
Metatarsus	Tarsal joint	Include digits	Midshaft	
Cervical vertebrae	Base of skull	Spine of scapula		Extend front limbs caudally; collimate width of beam to increase detail.
Thoracic vertebrae	Spine of scapula		Halfway between xiphoid and last rib	Collimate width of beam to increase detail.
Thoracolumbar vertebrae			Halfway between to increase detail	Collimate width of beam xiphoid and last rib.
Lumbar vertebrae	Halfway between xiphoid and last rib	Wings of ilium		Collimate width of beam to increase detail.

Adapted from Sirois M: Principles and practice of veterinary technology, ed 3, St Louis, 2011, Mosby.

CONTRAST STUDIES

The purpose of a contrast study is to delineate an organ or area against surrounding soft tissues. They are useful for determining the size, shape, position, location, and function of an organ. The information obtained from a contrast study complements or confirms findings of the survey radiographs. A contrast study should never replace survey radiographs.

With contrast studies, tissues of interest appear radiopaque or radiolucent on the finished radiograph. Areas that are radiopaque appear white. Positive contrast agents are radiopaque on a radiograph. Radiolucent areas on the finished radiograph appear black. Negative contrast agents produce radiolucent areas on a radiograph.

Obtaining survey radiographs before doing a contrast study establishes proper exposure technique and proper patient preparation. In addition, a diagnosis may be achieved from survey radiographs, eliminating the need for the contrast study. Because most contrast studies require multiple images, it is important to label each film with the time and sequence. Always record the amount, type, and administration route of the contrast agent.

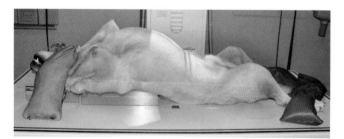

FIGURE 11-19 Patient lying in ventrodorsal recumbency. The beam enters the abdomen and exits out the back. (From Brown M, Brown L: Lavin's radiography for veterinary technicians, ed 5, St Louis, 2014, Saunders.)

POSITIVE CONTRAST MEDIA

Positive contrast media contain elements with a high atomic number; elements with a high atomic number absorb more x-rays. Thus, fewer x-rays penetrate the patient and expose the film, creating a white area on the radiograph. Two common types of positive contrast agents are barium sulfate and water-soluble organic iodides. Barium sulfate is commonly used for positive contrast studies of the GI tract. It is insoluble and is not affected by gastric secretions. Therefore, it provides good mucosal detail on the radiograph. Barium sulfate preparations are relatively inexpensive and are manufactured in the form of powders, colloid suspensions, or pastes. A disadvantage of using barium sulfate is that it can take 3 hours or longer to travel from the stomach to the colon. Also, it can be harmful to the peritoneum, so it should never be used when GI perforations are suspected. Barium is insoluble and the body cannot eliminate it, resulting in granulomatous reactions in the abdominal cavity. While administering barium orally, take care to prevent the patient from aspirating barium into the lungs. Aspiration of large amounts can be fatal. Barium sulfate may also aggravate an already obstructed bowel by causing further impactions. A product that consists of barium-impregnated polyethylene spheres is also available and may present less risk of peritonitis when GI perforation is present (Fig. 11-20).

Water-soluble organic iodides in ionic form are also used for positive contrast procedures. Different forms of the water-soluble organic iodides can be administered intravenously, orally, or by infusion into a hollow organ or into the subarachnoid space. Because they are water soluble, they are absorbed into the bloodstream and excreted by the kidneys. These agents may be used to perform contrast studies of the GI tract when perforation is suspected.

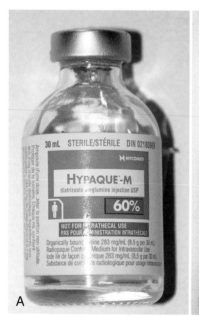
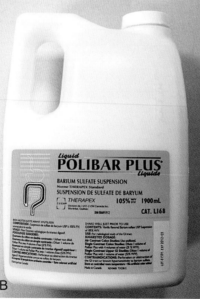
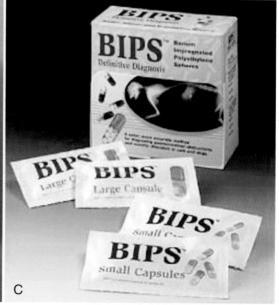

FIGURE 11-20 Positive contrast media. **A,** Iodine. **B,** Barium. **C,** Barium-impregnated polyurethane spheres (BIPS). (From Brown M, Brown L: Lavin's radiography for veterinary technicians, ed 5, St Louis, 2014, Saunders.)

Ionic water-soluble organic iodides for IV use are prepared in various combinations of meglumine and sodium diatrizoate. Diatrizoate can also be infused into hollow organs, such as the urinary bladder, or into fistulous tracts. Ionic water-soluble organic iodides cannot be used for myelography because they are irritating to the brain and spinal cord.

Nonionic water-soluble organic iodides are used for myelography and can be used intravenously. Because of their low osmolarity and chemical nature, they cause fewer adverse effects when placed in the subarachnoid space.

NEGATIVE CONTRAST MEDIA

Negative contrast agents include air, oxygen, and carbon dioxide. They all have a low atomic number, appearing radiolucent on the finished radiograph.

DOUBLE-CONTRAST PROCEDURE

Double-contrast procedures use both positive and negative contrast media to image an organ or area. The most common organs imaged with double contrast are the urinary bladder, stomach, and colon. In most cases, the negative contrast medium is added first and then the positive contrast medium. Mixing a negative contrast medium with a positive contrast medium can cause air bubbles to form, which might be misinterpreted as lesions.

DIAGNOSTIC ULTRASOUND

Diagnostic ultrasound (**ultrasonography**) is a noninvasive method of imaging soft tissues. A transducer sends low-intensity, high-frequency sound waves into the soft tissues, where they interact with tissue interfaces. Some of the sound waves are reflected back to the transducer, and some are transmitted into deeper tissues. The sound waves that are reflected back to the transducer (echoes) are then analyzed by the computer to produce a grayscale image. Use of ultrasound in conjunction with radiography gives the veterinarian an excellent diagnostic tool. Radiographs demonstrate the size, shape, and position of the organs. Ultrasound displays the findings found on the radiographs as well as the soft tissue textures and dynamics of some organs (e.g., motility of the bowel).

> ### CRITICAL CONCEPT
> Ultrasound imaging is ideal for displaying the characteristics of soft tissues.

TRANSDUCERS

Ultrasound transducers emit a series of sound pulses and receive the returning echoes. A weak electrical current applied to the piezoelectric crystals incorporated in the transducer causes the crystals to vibrate and produce sound waves. After sending a series of pulses, the crystals are dampened to stop further vibrations. When struck by the returning echoes, the crystals vibrate again and these echoes are converted into electrical energy.

Transducers are available in different configurations, mechanical or electronic. The scan plane can be a sector scan (pie-shaped image) or a linear array scan (rectangular image). A mechanically driven sector scan can be produced by a belt and pulley used to wobble a single crystal or rotate multiple crystals across a scan plane. Another method of producing a sector scan is with the use of a phased array or annular array configuration. With a phased array configuration, the crystals are pulsed sequentially with a built-in delay to create a so-called pseudosector scan plane. **Annular array** arranges the crystals in concentric rings. By using electronic phasing of the many crystals, annular array transducers produce a two-dimensional image by steering the entire array through a sector arc.

The frequency of the transducer determines the amount of detail or resolution of the image. As frequency increases, the wavelength gets shorter. The shorter the wavelength, the better will be the resolution of the image.

Transducers are expensive and the most fragile part of ultrasound equipment. Care must be taken when handling them. Avoid hard impacts that can severely damage the sensitive crystals. Prevent exposure to extreme temperature changes. Some transducers are sensitive to certain types of cleaning agents. Always refer to the manufacturer's instructions for appropriate cleaning products.

TERMINOLOGY DESCRIBING ECHOTEXTURE

The terminology used to describe tissue texture in an ultrasound image is simple. Echogenic or **echoic** means that most of the sound is reflected back to the transducer. Echogenic areas appear white on the screen. **Sonolucent** means that most of the sound is transmitted to the deeper tissues, with only a few echoes reflected back to the transducer. Sonolucent areas appear dark on the screen. **Anechoic** is used to describe tissue that transmits all the sound through to deeper tissues, reflecting none of the sound back to the transducer. Anechoic areas appear black on the screen and are generally fluid-filled structures.

Soft tissues are represented not only as black or white but also as many shades of gray. Additional terminology has been established to describe these areas. **Hyperechoic** is used to describe tissues that reflect more sound back to the transducer than surrounding tissues. Hyperechoic areas appear brighter than surrounding tissues. **Hypoechoic** is used to describe tissues that reflect less sound back to the transducer than surrounding tissues. Hypoechoic areas appear darker than surrounding tissues. **Isoechoic** is used to describe tissue that appears to have the same echotexture on the screen as surrounding tissues.

Terminology has been established to describe areas displayed on the monitor screen. The screen is divided into nine zones, with each zone having its own label. In this way, the sonographer can verbally indicate the area of interest, such as midfield right or near-field left.

PATIENT PREPARATION

To achieve an optimal acoustic window and produce the best-quality image, the transducer head must be placed into close contact with the skin. The animal's hair must be clipped and, in some cases, shaved before the study. Occasionally, thin-coated animals can be imaged with minimal preparation. An acoustic coupling gel is used on the patient's skin to eliminate the air interface and improve the acoustic window. Before applying the acoustic coupling gel, wipe the area with alcohol or generous amounts of soapy water to remove any loose hairs, dirt, and skin oils.

Fasting of small animals before abdominal ultrasound examination is recommended. Ingesta and gas in the bowel decrease the amount of the abdomen that can be visualized.

INSTRUMENT CONTROLS

Ultrasound equipment has many controls for adjusting the quality of the image. Improper adjustment of any of these can greatly decrease the quality of the image. Controls include those for brightness and contrast, depth, gain and power, and time gain compensation.

ARTIFACTS

Artifacts can occur during any ultrasound study. Proper identification of these artifacts is important to prevent confusion or misinterpretation. Some are beneficial when making a diagnosis. Two such artifacts include acoustic shadowing and **distance enhancement**. Others, if not readily identified, can be confused as part of the anatomy or a disease process.

Acoustic shadowing occurs when the sound is attenuated or reflected at an acoustic interface. This prevents the sound from being transmitted to the deeper tissues, resulting in no echoes or fewer echoes returning from those areas. Structures that can cause acoustic shadowing include bone, calculi, mineralized tissues and, occasionally, fat. Distance enhancement occurs when the sound beam traverses a cystic structure. Tissues deep to the cystic structure appear brighter than surrounding tissues. The enhancement occurs because the sound that travels through the fluid-filled areas is less attenuated than the sound in surrounding tissues. This artifact is useful in establishing that an anechoic or hypoechoic structure is actually fluid filled.

Many artifacts have no diagnostic use, although if not identified as artifacts, they can lead to confusion. One of these is the **slice thickness** artifact. This artifact occurs when the transducer receives echoes with different amplitudes from the same area at the same depth. Reverberation occurs when sound is reflected off a highly reflective interface (e.g., soft tissues to air or soft tissues to bone or metal) and then reflected back into the tissues by the surface of the transducer. This bouncing back and forth can continue until the sound energy has completely attenuated. Each time the sound returns to the transducer, it produces an image at a location on the screen proportional to the time of travel between the transducer and reflective interface. This creates a series of lines that are of equal distance apart on the screen.

The **mirror image** artifact creates the illusion of the liver on the thoracic side of the diaphragm or the appearance of a second heart beyond the lung interface. This artifact can be produced in areas with strongly reflective interfaces. Sound transmitted into the liver is reflected off the diaphragm. Some of these echoes are not reflected directly toward the transducer but back into the liver. In the liver, some of the misdirected echoes are reflected back to the diaphragm and then to the transducer. The computer sees the misdirected echoes as being reflected from the other side of the diaphragm. One way that this artifact can be minimized is by decreasing the depth to include only the area of interest.

ENDOSCOPY

Endoscopy is an essential tool for diagnosing many conditions and diseases. The opportunity to examine and obtain tissue samples without the invasiveness of surgery makes endoscopy one of the best methods for evaluating the digestive system. Responsibilities of veterinary staff members assisting with endoscopy include selection, care, and maintenance of the endoscopes and care and positioning of the patient.

> **CRITICAL CONCEPT**
> Endoscopic imaging can be used to diagnose disease as well as collect tissue samples for analysis.

TYPES OF ENDOSCOPES

Rigid endoscopes are commonly used for rhinoscopy, female cystoscopy, laparoscopy, arthroscopy, vaginoscopy, and thoroscopy. Flexible endoscopes are used for GI endoscopy, male cystoscopy, and bronchoscopy examinations. Flexible endoscopes are also used for percutaneous placement of gastrostomy tubes in small animals (Fig. 11-21).

RIGID ENDOSCOPES

Rigid endoscopes are composed of a metal tube, lenses, and glass rods (Fig. 11-22). They vary in size and characteristics; however, all are composed of a hollow tube containing no fiber bundles. Rigid endoscopes tend to be less expensive than flexible endoscopes, but their uses tend to be limited to those for which they were designed.

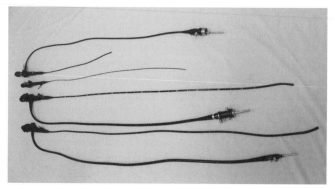

FIGURE 11-21 *Variety of endoscopes. Top to bottom, Storz, Olympus, cystoscope, and bronchoscope. (From Sirois M: Principles and practice of veterinary technology, ed 3, St Louis, 2011, Mosby.)*

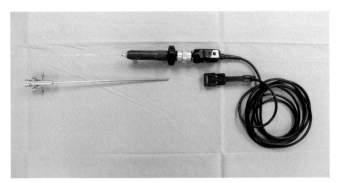

FIGURE 11-22 Rigid endoscope with camera. (From Sirois M: Principles and practice of veterinary technology, ed 3, St Louis, 2011, Mosby.)

Rigid endoscopes should be held by the eyepiece and not by the rod. Even slight bending of the rod section could change the angle of deflection, decreasing the degree of visualization. Rigid endoscopes should never be handled in bunches or piled on top of one another.

FLEXIBLE ENDOSCOPES

There are two types of flexible endoscopes, fiberoptic and video. Fiberoptic endoscopes use glass fiber bundles for the transmission of images. These bundles transmit light from the light source to the distal tip of the endoscope. Fiberoptic glass fiber bundles are fragile and can be damaged easily. Broken fibers show up on the monitor screen as black dots. Too many of these black dots (many broken fiber bundles) can significantly reduce the field of view. For this reason, fiberoptic endoscopes must be handled carefully and never bent at a sharp angle.

Video endoscopes contain a microchip located at the distal end that records and transmits the image to a computer and then to a monitor screen. The image can be recorded on a VCR; pictures can be recorded to show the owner and can be included in the patient's record. Many operators find the video endoscope to be more ergonomically pleasing because the controls are held at the waist and not near the face.

ENDOSCOPY ROOM

In an ideal situation, all endoscopic examinations are performed in the same room. This room should preferably be out of the way of hospital traffic. Because the lights are usually dimmed during endoscopic examination to reduce glare on the viewing monitor, a room with curtains or shades is ideal. The room should never be so dark, however, that proper anesthetic monitoring is inhibited.

A sturdy cart with three or four shelves can conveniently store the light source, suction unit, endoscope, and any accessory equipment until ready for use. All necessary equipment should be located near this endoscopy unit so that it can be reached quickly if needed during endoscopy. These items should be meticulously organized. The assisting staff must be able to locate any necessary equipment quickly during a procedure.

To avoid complications and delays, the procedure room should be well stocked before the endoscopic examination begins. All anesthetic equipment must be ready before the

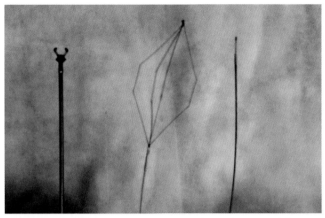

FIGURE 11-23 Accessory equipment. Left to right, Rat tooth forceps, basket foreign body retrieval forceps, cytology brush. (From Sirois M: Principles and practice of veterinary technology, ed 3, St Louis, 2011, Mosby.)

procedure begins. Procedure cards or checklists are excellent ways to ensure that each type of endoscopic examination starts with the proper equipment.

ACCESSORY INSTRUMENTS

Accessory instruments can be passed through the working channel of the flexible endoscope and directed to a specific area. The most basic instruments include biopsy forceps, foreign body removal forceps, and a cytology brush (Fig. 11-23).

Endoscopes are fragile and expensive, so personnel must be instructed about their proper care, use, and maintenance before endoscope use. Before each endoscopic examination, be sure that each piece of ancillary equipment is functioning properly and anticipate the need for these pieces of equipment. They should be cleaned as soon as possible after use or the jaws of the forceps may become locked in the closed position. If this occurs, soaking the tip of the biopsy forceps in warm water for 10 to 15 minutes helps loosen the debris around the jaws.

All personnel involved with endoscopic procedures should wear latex examination gloves. This protects the animal from contamination and also protects the clinician and staff. The endoscope should not be allowed to contact the video accessories or any other potentially conductive object directly; wearing latex gloves offers added protection against electrical shock.

CARE OF ENDOSCOPES
CLEANING A FLEXIBLE ENDOSCOPE

All endoscopy equipment should be thoroughly cleaned as soon as possible after the procedure. The manufacturer's specific cleaning instructions should be closely followed. Endoscopes must be handled carefully during cleaning and never placed where they could fall or be bumped. It is also a good idea for the person cleaning the endoscope to wear latex examination gloves. Gather the following supplies:
- Latex examination gloves
- Cleaning solution
- Two large basins for cleaning solution and distilled water

- Distilled water
- Methyl alcohol
- Lint-free gauze pads
- Cotton-tipped applicators
- Channel-cleaning brush

Immediately after the procedure, flush water and then air through the air-water channel of the flexible endoscope. Gently wipe off the insertion tube with soft gauze or a cloth that has been soaked in an approved detergent solution. Do not squeeze the flexible section. Place the distal end of the endoscope in detergent-water mixture and suction a small amount through. Alternately suction water and then air a few times. Remove the air-water valve, suction valve, and biopsy cap and place them in a small amount of cleaning solution to soak. Pass the channel-cleaning brush through the biopsy channel and suction the channel repeatedly until the brush comes out clean. Clean the brush each time it is passed through the channel.

If the endoscope has a suction cleaning tube, it should then be placed on the biopsy port. Place the end of the suction cleaning tube and the end of the endoscope into a mixture of detergent and water. Cover the suction valve hole with your finger and suction soapy water, distilled water, and then air to dry the endoscope. Remove the suction cleaning tube and carefully clean the valve holes with a cotton-tipped swab. Clean and rinse the air-water valve, suction valve, and biopsy cap and replace them on the endoscope.

It is a good preventive measure to lubricate the air-water and suction valves lightly periodically to prevent cracking. Wipe off the outside of the endoscope with an alcohol-soaked gauze pad. Clean the lenses with an approved lens cleaner by applying some lens cleaner onto a soft gauze pad and rubbing the lens; then rub with a clean gauze pad. Replace any lens caps, light source insertion bar covers, and ETO caps before placing the endoscope back into the cabinet. For proper drying of the biopsy channel, leave the biopsy port in an open position.

Biopsy instruments should be immersed in soapy water, brushed carefully with a cleaning brush, and then rinsed. Check to be sure that the jaws of biopsy instruments are not sticking by opening and closing them carefully.

STORING AN ENDOSCOPE

The ideal way to store a flexible endoscope is in a hanging position in a well-ventilated cabinet. This allows the endoscope to drain completely after cleaning and permits better air movement through the channels. The padded case in which the endoscope was supplied by the manufacturer is another possible storage area; however, little air circulates in these containers and moisture in the channels of the endoscope offers an environment for bacterial growth. Rigid endoscopes are best stored in their original carrying case.

GASTROINTESTINAL ENDOSCOPY
PATIENT PREPARATION

For GI endoscopy, the patient should be fasted for 12 to 24 hours. A longer period of fasting may be required in patients with delayed gastric emptying. An IV catheter should be placed and fluid administration started. Endotracheal intubation and proper endotracheal tube cuff inflation are needed to avoid aspiration of gastric contents in the event of regurgitation. For colonoscopy, all feces should be removed from the colon before endoscopic examination; however, this is not always possible. Food should be withheld from the patient for at least 36 hours. For rigid colonoscopy, a warm water enema (10 to 20 mL/kg) the evening before the procedure, another enema the following morning, and a final enema 1 hour before the examination usually provide enough cleansing.

COMPUTED TOMOGRAPHY

Using x-rays and a bank of detectors, a CT scan provides a cross-sectional image of all tissue types of the body region scanned based on the physical density of the tissue compared with water. Within the CT scanner, there are an x-ray tube and multiple detectors on a slip ring device that allows the tube to move freely in a circular motion around a patient. The patient is stationary on a table that is passed through the rotating x-ray beam. The images are then reconstructed into thin slices through the patient, similar to a slice from a loaf of bread. The raw data from the image acquisition can be reprocessed using a dedicated computer for soft tissue or edge-enhanced display or reformatted into other imaging planes, such as dorsal and sagittal planes, from the original data that were acquired in a transverse plane. This form of imaging, tomography, provides the radiologist with much more information about the patient than conventional radiography.

CT is frequently used for imaging many disease processes, such as cancer, fractures, lung disease, and vascular anomalies. CT also provides invaluable information for surgical and radiation treatment planning. Unlike radiography and ultrasound, tomographic imaging frequently requires the patient to be anesthetized.

CRITICAL CONCEPT

A CT scanner produces cross-sectional images by placing the patient on a table that is passed through a rotating x-ray beam.

MAGNETIC RESONANCE IMAGING

MRI uses a high-strength external magnetic field, a variety of radiofrequency excitation pulses, and the natural resonance (normal circular motion of the atom) of protons (hydrogen ions) in the body to visualize the structure and function of organs. MRI is primarily used to examine the internal organs; it is noninvasive and superior to other modalities for imaging soft tissue. The primary examinations performed using MRI include imaging of the brain, spinal cord and intervertebral disc areas, tumor localization and extension within soft tissues, tendon and muscle injury, vascular and arterial anomalies or disease, and thoracic and abdominal organs.

The principles of MRI imaging are complex. Many types of magnets are used, but they can be summarized as being low- and high-field strengths depending on the strength of the magnetic field, which is measured in tesla (T). Low-strength field are 0.3 T or less and high-strength field magnets are 0.6 T and higher. The patient is placed in this external, strong magnetic field, and the magnetic field is then manipulated by small increments as a specific radiofrequency (RF) is transmitted into the patient to cause certain changes in the orientation and speed with which the protons resonate. All the protons then relax, based on the immediate interactions of the protons and the type of tissue of which the protons are a part. This relaxation produces weak RF signals, which are detected by coils surrounding the area of interest in the patient. These signals are then processed through a computer and converted into images of the patient.

Depending on the MRI scan performed, contrast medium may or may not be administered. Gadolinium is the most common contrast medium used for enhancement of tissues in MRI. Given IV, it enhances or brightens tissues such as vessels and tumors.

Serious safety concerns apply when housing and operating an MRI unit. It is prudent to remember that for super-conducting magnets of high-field strength, the magnet is always on. No ferromagnetic object can be taken into the room in which the magnet is kept. The magnet will forcibly pull any ferromagnetic objects into the magnet. This could cause serious damage to the MRI machine, patient, or operator who might be within its path. A few examples of ferrous objects include gas anesthesia machines, collars, watches, glasses, hairpins, ink pens, clipboards, IV poles, and cell phones. Certain metallic surgical implants may also be of concern. It is necessary to know the type of implant and manufacturer of the implant to make sure that it contains no ferromagnetic component. Microchips do not seem to cause any issues other than magnetic susceptibility artifacts in the image. Keep a small magnet outside the room and test objects for their magnetism when there is any doubt. Because general anesthesia is required for MRI, the use of an IV injectable agent is the most common route of anesthesia. However, there are MRI-compatible gas anesthetic machines and monitoring equipment available. Although MRI units are uncommon in general veterinary practices, most university veterinary hospitals and referral hospitals have MRI units or access to one for diagnostic imaging.

CRITICAL CONCEPT

Nuclear scintigraphy and MRI imaging modalities are commonly performed at veterinary teaching hospitals and some large veterinary referral practices.

NUCLEAR MEDICINE

Nuclear medicine, also called scintigraphy, is an imaging modality that uses radionuclides and a gamma camera for detection of the decay of gamma radiation emitted from the radionuclide within the patient. This allows for imaging of anatomic, physiologic, or metabolic processes that occur within the patient. The most common radionuclide used for imaging is technetium-99m (^{99m}Tc). ^{99m}Tc has a low-energy gamma ray (140 keV), with a short physical half-life of 6 hours. ^{99m}Tc is typically bound to a specific pharmaceutical that then targets the organ of interest after IV administration. The most common nuclear medicine studies performed in veterinary medicine are thyroid scans, bone scans, renal function testing with calculation of the glomerular filtration rate (GFR), and hepatobiliary scans. The most common therapeutic nuclear medicine application in veterinary medicine is radioactive iodine (^{131}I). ^{131}I is used for the treatment of hyperthyroidism and thyroid tumors.

Because of the potential for radioactive contamination, latex gloves and laboratory coats are worn at all times when handling any radionuclide or radioactive patient. Special housing considerations are a factor for the radioactive patient after the study because technetium is primarily excreted in the urine and feces. Each state or locality has strict release criteria for patients that are imaged with radionuclides. Special holding areas are required to isolate the radioactive patient to prevent contamination of other areas of the hospital and personnel. Patients treated with ^{131}I require an isolated and well-ventilated area because of the potential for the aerosolization of iodine. Radioactive iodine may be excreted in saliva, feces, and urine. Because ^{131}I has a longer physical half-life (2.82 days) than ^{99m}Tc (6 hours), patients are required to stay in the isolation area longer than patients undergoing a ^{99m}Tc radiopharmaceutical study.

RECOMMENDED READINGS

Barr F: *Diagnostic ultrasound in the dog and cat*, London, 1990, Blackwell Scientific.

Brearley MJ, Cooper JE: *A colour atlas of small animal endoscopy*, St Louis, 1991, Mosby.

Brown M, Brown L: *Lavin's radiography in veterinary technology*, ed 5, St Louis, 2014, Saunders.

Burk RL, Ackerman N: *Small animal radiology and ultrasonography*, ed 3, St Louis, 2003, Saunders.

Curry TS, Dowdey JE, Murry RC: *Christensen's physics of diagnostic radiology*, ed 4, Philadelphia, 1990, Lea & Febiger.

Han CM, Hurd CD: *Practical diagnostic imaging for the veterinary technician*, ed 3, St Louis, 2000, Mosby.

Nyland TG, Mattoon JS: *Small animal diagnostic ultrasound*, ed 2, St Louis, 2003, Saunders.

Sirois M, Anthony E, Mauragis D: *Handbook of radiographic positioning for veterinary technicians*, Clifton Park, NY, 2010, Delmar Cengage.

Tams T: *Small animal endoscopy*, ed 2, St Louis, 1999, Mosby.

Thrall DE: *Textbook of veterinary diagnostic radiology*, ed 5, St Louis, 2007, Saunders.

Traub-Dargatz JL, Brown CM: *Equine endoscopy*, ed 2, St Louis, 1997, Mosby.

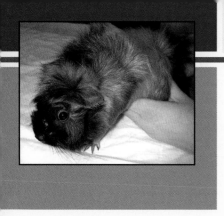

Avian and Exotic Animal Care and Nursing[1]

OUTLINE

Small Mammals, 361
Housing, 361
Nutrition, 362
General Nursing Care of Small Mammals, 370
Diagnostic and Treatment Techniques, 370
Birds, 372
Avian Anatomy, 373
Basic Pet Bird Behavior, 378
Client Education, 380
Housing and Husbandry, 380
Beak, Wing, and Nail Trimming, 381
Determination of Gender, 382
Microchipping, 382
Physical Examination, 383
Diagnostic Sampling Techniques, 386
Imaging, 387
Nursing Care, 389

Common Diseases and Conditions, 393
Ethical Euthanasia Techniques, 398
Reptiles and Amphibians, 398
Reptile Biology, 398
Husbandry, 399
Housing, 399
Water Quality, 400
Feeding, 400
Taking a History, 400
Capture, Restraint, and Handling, 401
Diagnostic Techniques, 404
Force Feeding, 405
Administration of Fluids and Medications, 406
Common Diseases and Presentations, 406
Emergency and Critical Care, 406
Euthanasia, 407

LEARNING OBJECTIVES

After reviewing this chapter, the reader will be able to:

1. State the general characteristics of mice, rats, hamsters, gerbils, guinea pigs, chinchillas, rabbits, and ferrets.
2. Discuss husbandry and principles of sanitation for small mammals.
3. Describe techniques for general nursing care of rodents, rabbits, and ferrets.
4. Describe techniques used for diagnosing and treating disease in small mammals.
5. Describe the unique features of the anatomy of birds and basic biology of common reptile species.
6. Discuss the basic behavior of birds, reptiles, and amphibians.

7. Discuss the basics of client education, husbandry, and nutrition for avian, reptile, and amphibian species.
8. Describe how to obtain a complete and thorough history of avian, reptile, and amphibian patients.
9. Explain the different capture and restraint techniques used for birds, reptiles, and amphibians.
10. Identify methods of sample collection for laboratory analysis.
11. Describe how to obtain quality diagnostic images of avian reptile and amphibian patients.
12. Discuss nursing care and supportive therapy techniques for avian, reptile, and amphibian patients.
13. Identify and discuss some common diseases of avian, reptile, and amphibian patients in the veterinary clinic.

[1]Elsevier and the author acknowledge and appreciate the original contributions from Sirois M: Principles and practice of veterinary technology, ed 3, St Louis, 2011, Mosby, and Sheldon CC, Sonsthagen TF, Topel JA: Animal restraint for veterinary professionals, St Louis, 2006, Mosby, whose work forms the heart of this chapter.

KEY TERMS

Anisodactyl	Contour feathers	Malocclusion	Rodents
Barbering	Coprodeum	Molting	Sow
Boar	Coverts	Mouthing	Syrinx
Buck	Crop	Murine	Urates
Bumblefoot	Doe	Nocturnal species	Urodeum
Cavy	Down feathers	Operculum	Uropygial gland
Cere	Flight feathers	Passerines	Vent
Choana	Hobs	Pneumatized	Ventriculus
Cloaca	Jill	Proctodeum	
Coelom	Keel	Proventriculus	
Columella	Lagomorphs	Psittacines	

SMALL MAMMALS

Small mammals are popular pets. These so-called pocket pets include ferrets, rabbits, mice, rats, hamsters, gerbils, guinea pigs, and chinchillas. Although small mammals are relatively easy to care for, they require care that is different from that of dogs and cats. Prospective owners should be encouraged to read about a species they have never cared for before. Sometimes, success or failure in raising an animal will depend on the knowledge that an owner has about the pet.

Small mammals are often purchased as first pets for children. Small mammals can make acceptable pets for children, but children should always be supervised when handling these delicate creatures. Small mammals can bite, and children should be made aware of this and told that these pets are real live creatures and not stuffed animals. All pets should be handled with care. Small mammals should not be allowed free run of the house because this can prove fatal to them. Because the life span of most small mammals is only 2 to 4 years, children should be counseled so that an early death is not unexpected. Allergies to animal dander, saliva, and urinary proteins occur commonly in humans. Cutaneous and upper respiratory allergies to small mammals, especially rats and guinea pigs, are common.

HOUSING

Caging must be escape-proof to prevent injury or fatality. **Rodents** can be housed in plastic or metal cages with slotted bars or wire mesh lids. Shoebox-type cages made of plastic materials are popular for housing rodents (Fig. 12-1). Cage flooring can be a solid bottom or wire mesh. Solid flooring with bedding material is generally preferred. If mesh flooring is used, care must be taken to prevent foot injury and loss of neonates through the flooring. Aquariums are adequate to house pet rodents but should have a screen-type top with a locking device. This type of housing unit allows easy access to the pet; however, it is heavy and can be difficult to clean. Aquariums generally need more frequent cleaning to prevent ammonia build up within the cage. When aquariums are used for housing, care should be taken to ensure that

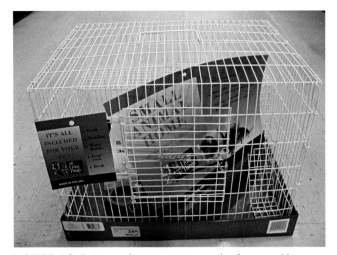

FIGURE 12-1 A typical mouse cage is made of wire and has room for a hide box and exercise wheel. (From Mitchell M, Tully TN, Jr: Manual of exotic pet practice, St Louis, 2008, Saunders.)

rodents have access to food and water. Conventional cages such as those purchased from pet stores should have a large door to facilitate easy removal of the animal and should be easy to disassemble and clean. Rabbits, chinchillas, and ferrets can be housed in wire or front-opening cages with catch pans to collect urine and feces. Pet ferrets and rabbits can also be housed in large cat or dog carriers with a litter box. Some owners build rather elaborate housing for their pet rabbits and ferrets. Rabbits and ferrets can be housed outdoors, but care must be taken to prevent heat stroke, myiasis, and dog and cat attacks. Animals maintained outdoors should be provided with shelter from direct sunlight, rain, snow, and wind.

Animals should be housed in caging that is appropriate for the animal's size and weight. Some animals, such as chinchillas, are acrobatic and active and should be provided with a large cage to allow for exercise. Cage height should allow an animal to make normal postural adjustments. For example, gerbils frequently sit upright, so the height of their caging should allow them to do so. The cage should be located in an area protected from climatic extremes. Care should be taken not to house pet rodent cages in direct sunlight because they will overheat. Changes in temperature and humidity and/or drafty conditions should be avoided because these can be stressful and predispose the animal to disease. The recommended housing temperature for mice, rats, hamsters, gerbils, and guinea pigs is 18° to 26° C (65° to 79° F); for rabbits and chinchillas it is 16° to 22° C (61° to 72° F); and for ferrets it is 4° to 18° C (39° to 64° F). The acceptable range of relative humidity is 30% to 70%.

Albino rodents are susceptible to phototoxicity, so care should be taken to ensure safe illumination levels in their housing area. Noise should be minimized in animal housing areas because excessive sound exposure can be stressful and produce untoward effects. It is important to remember that many species can hear frequencies of sound that are inaudible to humans and some rodents are prone to sound-induced seizures.

Bedding used for solid-bottom caging should be absorbent, comfortable, non-nutritive, nontoxic, and disposable. A variety of bedding material can be used, including paper, sawdust and soft pine, aspen, cedar, corncob, and hardwood chips. Cedar and soft pine shavings are frequently used for pet rodent bedding because of their pleasant aroma. However, these are not recommended because they emit aromatic hydrocarbons that can induce liver changes and cytotoxicity. Burrowing rodents such as the rat and gerbil should be provided with deeper bedding to allow for this behavior.

Cage toys can provide psychological stimulation as well as exercise for small mammals. Tubes, mazes, and exercise wheels are popular. Timid animals such as guinea pigs and chinchillas are more comfortable if they are given a place to hide. Polyvinyl chloride (PVC) plumbing pipes, especially elbows and Y and T sections, make ideal hiding places. These pipes can be sanitized in the dishwasher. Cardboard tubes, softwood pieces, and small Nylabones can be given to rodents to gnaw on. Paper tissues or towels can be given to rodents who build nests, such as mice, gerbils, and hamsters. Metallic items such as washers can be suspended in a rabbit's cage to encourage nudging, playing, and investigative behaviors. Paper bags, hard plastic or metal toys, or cloth toys made for cats or babies are safe for ferrets. Ferrets love to run through cylindrical objects such as large mailing tubes and dryer vent tubing. Latex rubber toys that are intended for dogs or cats should not be given to ferrets.

NUTRITION

The rat and mouse are omnivorous, whereas the guinea pig, rabbit, chinchilla, and gerbil are herbivorous. The hamster is primarily granivorous. Ferrets are carnivorous and depend on meat proteins and fats for their dietary requirements. Animals should be fed a clean, wholesome, and nutritious diet ad libitum (ad lib, free choice). It is important to feed a balanced diet, freshly milled and formulated for that particular species. Pelleted foods are available commercially. These diets are complete and do not require supplementation. Block-style pellets work well for rodents such as mice, rats, hamsters, and gerbils. Many types of the rodent feed found

in pet stores and sold as seed mixes or treats are inadequate in protein for these species. Smaller pelleted foods work well for guinea pigs, chinchillas, and rabbits. Rabbits should be fed a high-fiber rabbit chow to prevent obesity and hairball formation. Rabbits, guinea pigs, and chinchillas can be fed small amounts of grass or alfalfa hay. Hay not only provides them with fiber but helps reduce boredom. Ferrets can be fed ferret chow or commercial cat food. As with dogs and cats, periodontal disease is common in ferrets. Feeding dry food can help reduce tartar accumulation. In most cases, the food should be placed in a feeder hung in the animal's cage. This prevents soiling of the food with urine and feces, keeping it dry and clean. If vegetables or fruit are offered to supplement the diet, they should be fresh and washed before feeding them. Any uneaten vegetables or fruits should be removed daily. Supplements should not make up more than 10% of the animal's daily food ration. Animals should always have access to fresh water.

RABBITS

The domestic rabbit, or European rabbit (*Oryctolagus cuniculus*), still exists on the European continent in three forms—wild, feral, and domestic. In North America, only feral and domestic rabbits exist. The Flemish Giant is a large breed of rabbit weighing 6 to 7 kg, the New Zealand and Californian are medium-size breeds weighing 2 to 5 kg, and the Dutch and Polish are small breeds weighing 1 to 2 kg. The albino New Zealand is popularly used for meat production. The smaller breeds are kept as pets. Rabbits make good pets. They are mild tempered, seldom bite, and can be litter box trained.

Rabbits are **lagomorphs**, differentiated from rodents by the presence of two upper pairs of incisors that continuously grow. The second set of upper incisors is smaller and are found behind the large front incisors. They are called peg teeth or wolf teeth. The rabbit has a life span of 5 to 6 years or longer, a body temperature of 38.5° to 40° C (101° to 104° F), heart rate of 130 to 325 beats/min, and respiratory rate of 30 to 60 breaths/min. Rabbits have a wide field of vision, can readily detect motion, and see well in dim light. Their ears are highly vascular and function in heat regulation.

Rabbits have several unusual features in their intestinal tract, including a sacculus rotundus located at the terminal end of the ileum, a large cecum that terminates in a vermiform process or appendix, and a colon with regular sacculations called haustra. Rabbits are coprophagic, a term which refers to eating of feces, and pass two types of feces. Soft, moist, night feces are rich in vitamins and protein and are eaten directly from the anus. Firm dry pellets are passed during the daytime. Hairballs can be a serious, potentially fatal problem in rabbits because they cannot vomit. The addition of proteolytic enzymes such as those found in unpasteurized papaya or pineapple-type products helps prevent this condition. High-fiber diets are of value in trying to prevent hairballs and also tend to prevent obesity, hair chewing, and enteritis. The color of rabbit urine varies from orange-red to brown; the pH is higher than 8 and therefore very basic.

A small amount of protein in the urine is normal. Crystals of calcium carbonate and magnesium phosphate can be expected to be found in rabbit urine.

Male rabbits are called **bucks** and female rabbits are called **does**. Determining gender can be accomplished by gently pressing the skin back from the genital opening. Females have an elongated vulva, with a slit opening; males have a rounded, protruding penile sheath. The dewlap, a heavy fold of skin at the throat, is more prominent in females.

Rabbits have a small skeletal mass compared with similar-sized animals and large hindquarter muscles that make them prone to back fractures. Back fractures are considered incurable, and the animal must be euthanized. Most fractures of the spinal column result from poor handling techniques. When carrying a rabbit for a longer distance, its head should be tucked into the crook of the arm that is supporting the hindquarters (Fig. 12-2). Rabbits that are incorrectly handled may injure themselves by struggling and can also scratch their handler with their powerful hind legs. A towel wrapped around the rabbit works well for restraint, especially if the eyes are covered. Mechanical devices made of plastic or metal are frequently used for restraint during minor procedures, such as blood collection from an ear vein,

IV injections, or treatments. The restraining device holds the head in place and has a sliding partition that fits snugly against the rabbit's rump (Fig. 12-3). Rabbits should never be lifted or restrained by grabbing their ears because their ears are sensitive and fragile. When returning a rabbit to its cage, place it in the cage rump first to prevent injury to the rabbit or handler. A rabbit has a tendency to leap toward the cage if allowed to enter the cage headfirst.

Malocclusion can result in overgrown incisors that may need to be trimmed every 2 to 3 weeks. Ear mite infections with *Psoroptes* spp. are common in pet rabbits. The mites characteristically cause a dry, brown, crusty material to accumulate on the inner surface of the ears. Pododermatitis, a pressure necrosis of the plantar surface of the metatarsal area commonly called sore hocks or **Bumblefoot,** is seen in heavy, obese rabbits. Rabbits are susceptible to infection with *Pasteurella multocida*. Several clinical forms of the disease occur; the most common are rhinitis (snuffles) and pneumonia. Stressed or recently weaned rabbits are frequently infected with coccidia.

FERRETS

The domestic ferret *(Mustela putorius furo)* belongs to the same family as weasels, mink, otter, and skunks. Ferrets were initially used as hunting animals for the control of rabbits and rodents and raised for their pelts. They have become popular pets because of their small size, ease of care, and comical and engaging personalities. Keeping domestic ferrets as pets is not legal in all states and/or cities. Thus, it is

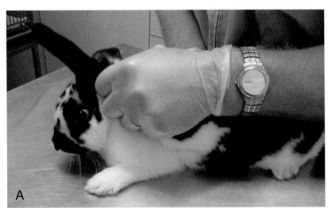

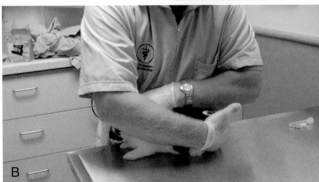
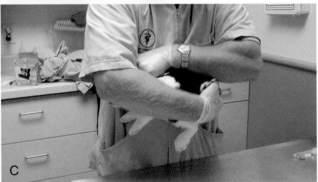

FIGURE 12-2 A, To get control of the rabbit initially, scruff it just behind its ears. Grab the scruff into the palm of your hand while keeping your arm along the rabbit's body. **B,** Reach over the rabbit to support its body by pushing it against your body and supporting its hindquarters. **C,** Lift the rabbit while supporting its hindquarters against your body. (Sheldon CC, Sonsthagen TF, Topel JA: Animal restraint for veterinary professionals, St Louis, 2006, Mosby.)

important to be aware of legislation in your area regarding the keeping of ferrets as pets. The natural color of ferrets is fitch, also known as sable. Fitch-colored ferrets have black guard hair with a cream-colored undercoat, black feet and tail, and a black mask on the face. Two other natural colors that are seen are albino and cinnamon. In addition, more than 30 color variations are recognized. Ferrets have long, tubular bodies with short legs and flexible spines. This allows them to get into small openings and turn around easily. Ferrets leap and jump, and can climb. Pet owners need to keep a ferret in a secure, escape-proof cage. If a ferret is allowed to run loose in the house, it should be ferret-proofed to close up any holes or areas from which a ferret cannot be retrieved.

CRITICAL CONCEPT

Ferrets are susceptible to canine distemper and require vaccinations against it.

Ferrets that are neutered early weigh from 0.8 to 1.2 kg when adult. Unneutered animals are larger, especially males. The ferret has a life span of 5 to 8 years, body temperature of 37.8° to 40° C (100° to 104° F), heart rate of 180 to 250 beats/min, and respiratory rate of 33 to 36 breaths/min. A ferret's skin is remarkably thick, especially over the neck and shoulders. Ferrets experience a seasonal change in body fat, losing weight in the summer and gaining it back in the winter. They also molt in the spring and fall. Ferrets do not have sweat glands in their skin and thus are prone to heat stroke. Their claws are not retractable, as in cats, and need to be trimmed. The canine teeth are prominent, as they are in other carnivorous animals. Ferrets have a simple stomach and short small intestine. They do not have a cecum. Ferrets have well-developed anal glands that produce a foul-smelling liquid when they are frightened. The anal gland secretion, however, is not responsible for the musky body odor of ferrets. The sebaceous secretions of their skin produce the animals' odor. Ferrets originating from large breeding farms are routinely descented and neutered when they are 5 to 6 weeks of age before entering the pet market.

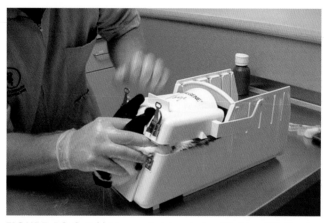

FIGURE 12-3 Rabbit in a restraining device. (Sheldon CC, Sonsthagen TF, Topel JA: Animal restraint for veterinary professionals, St Louis, 2006, Mosby.)

Female ferrets are called **jills** and males are called **hobs**. Young are called kits. A neutered female is called a sprite and a neutered male a gib. It is easy to determine the gender of a ferret. The preputial opening in male ferrets is located on the ventral abdomen, as in male dogs, and the os penis is readily palpable. The urogenital opening in female ferrets is located in the perineal region ventral to the anus.

Most ferrets are docile and can be easily examined without undue restraint. Assistance is usually needed to give medications. Tractable ferrets can be lightly restrained on the examination table. An active ferret can be restrained by scruffing the loose skin on the back of the neck and suspending it off the table. Many animals can be distracted by feeding Nutri-Cal with a syringe or placing a small amount of it on their fur for them to lick (Fig. 12-4).

Ferrets are highly susceptible to canine distemper. They must be vaccinated against this virus because canine distemper is typically a fatal disease in ferrets. Ear mites are common in ferrets. Ferrets are susceptible to human influenza virus. Influenza causes upper respiratory disease in ferrets, as it does in humans. Adrenal gland disease and insulinomas are common conditions seen in older pet ferrets. If female ferrets are not spayed, they frequently remain in estrus if they are not bred. They can develop estrogen toxicity with bone marrow suppression and severe anemia.

RODENTS

Mice, rats, gerbils, hamsters, guinea pigs, and chinchillas are rodents. The word *rodent* is derived from a Latin verb that means to gnaw. Rodents have four continuously erupting, chisel-like incisors and powerful jaw muscles that account for their gnawing ability. They are nocturnal for the most part, being more active at night rather than during the day. The gender of most rodents can be determined by evaluating anogenital distance; this is longer in males and shorter in females (Fig. 12-5). Rodents are usually prolific breeders. Pet owners need to be aware of the potential for overpopulation when housing animals of the opposite sex together. The term *murine* specifically refers to mice and rats. Guinea pigs and chinchillas are hystricomorph, or hedgehog-like, rodents related to porcupines.

Although rodents do not require annual vaccinations, an annual examination is recommended to ensure good health and husbandry. Owners should be encouraged to bring their new pet in for a visit to the veterinarian. The pet can be examined to ensure health, maintain the health guarantee that might accompany the purchase, and allow the veterinary team to educate the owner on proper feeding, housing, and handling of the species.

MICE. The mouse *(Mus musculus)* is a small rodent, easily housed and handled and relatively inexpensive to purchase and maintain as a pet. Mice may live up to 3 years. They weigh 20 to 40 g and have a rapid heart rate (≈500 to 600 beats/min), rapid respiration rate, and body temperature of 36.5° to 38° C. Mice have a high metabolic rate and are constantly active. They spend much of their time grooming and keeping their environment organized. Mice can be caught and safely picked up by grasping the scruff of the neck with forceps or by grasping the base of the tail with the fingers (Fig. 12-6). For manipulation or examination, the animal is caught by the base of the tail and placed on a surface that it can grasp, such as the cage lid. The scruff of the neck is then grasped by the thumb and forefinger (Fig. 12-7), and the mouse is inverted to lie on its back with its tail positioned between the palm of your hand and little finger. Clear plastic restraint devices can also be used for restraint and manipulation (Fig. 12-8).

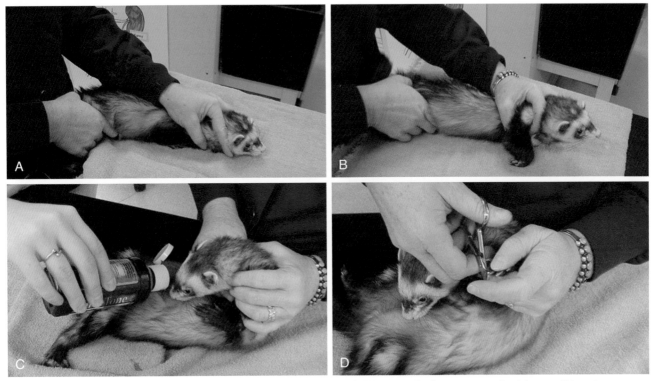

FIGURE 12-4 **A,** Good head control can be accomplished by placing your index finger on one side of the mandible with your middle finger on the other. **B,** You can then place your thumb and ring finger around the ferret's front limbs and support it by its armpits. **C,** Add a small amount of laxatone or ferret supplement to the fur on the animal's ventral abdomen. **D,** The ferret will be occupied by licking off its abdomen while you carry out this procedure. (Sheldon CC, Sonsthagen TF, Topel JA: Animal restraint for veterinary professionals, St Louis, 2006, Mosby.)

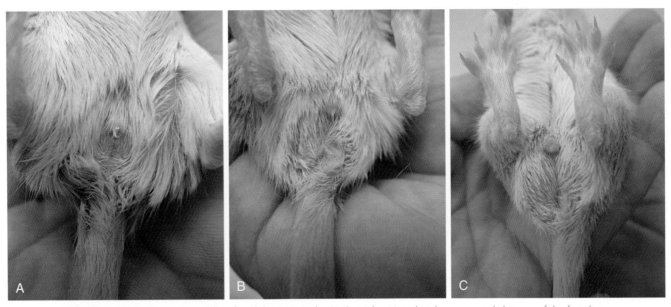

FIGURE 12-5 External genitalia of gerbils. **A,** Female. **B, C,** Male. Note that the anogenital distance of the female is shorter than that of the male. The adult male can also be determined by the presence of testicles in the scrotum **(C)**, but the frightened gerbil may retract the testicles from the scrotum **(B)**. (From Mitchell M, Tully TN, Jr: Manual of exotic pet practice, St Louis, 2008, Saunders.)

A dominant mouse sometimes chews the fur off a subordinate mouse in the facial area. This harmless behavior is called **barbering**. Unlike female mice, male mice housed together frequently fight. Bite wounds are inflicted on the back and rump.

RATS. The common rat *(Rattus norvegicus)* found in pet stores was developed from the wild brown Norway rat. Rats are easily maintained and make excellent pets if handled gently. They are burrowers and communal critters. The life

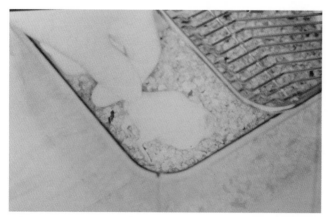

FIGURE 12-6 Proper technique for removal of a mouse from its cage. (From Sirois M: Principles and practice of veterinary technology, ed 3, St Louis, 2011, Mosby.)

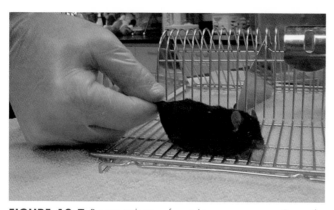

FIGURE 12-7 Proper technique for picking up a mouse. Grasp the loose skin over the back of the neck when the animal grabs the bars of the wire cage lid. (Sheldon CC, Sonsthagen TF, Topel JA: Animal restraint for veterinary professionals, St Louis, 2006, Mosby.)

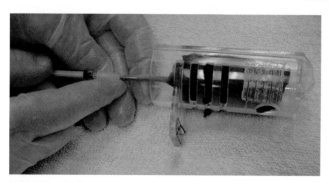

FIGURE 12-8 Mouse restraining device. (Sheldon CC, Sonsthagen TF, Topel JA: Animal restraint for veterinary professionals, St Louis, 2006, Mosby.)

span of the rat is 2.5 to 3.5 years. Rats weigh 250 to 500 g, with females being smaller than males. Their body temperature is 36° to 37.5° C (97° to 100° F). Rats have continuously erupting incisors and cheeks that close into the diastema, a space that separates the incisors from the oral cavity. They have no gallbladder. The Harderian gland, a lacrimal gland located caudal to the eyeball, secretes a red, porphyrin-rich secretion that lubricates the eye. In times of stress or illness, red tears overflow and stain the face and nose.

CRITICAL CONCEPT

Most rodents' incisors grow continuously, so they need hard food to prevent overgrowth.

Rats can be caught and safely picked up by grasping the base of the tail to transport them a short distance, such as when changing cages. When rats are held upside down, they are more interested in righting themselves than in biting the handler. To restrain for manipulation or examination, pick up the rat by placing your hand firmly over the back and rib cage and restraining the rat's head and shoulders with your thumb and forefinger (Fig. 12-9). If additional control is needed, the base of the tail may be restrained with the other hand. An alternative method is to pin the rat with your free hand while pulling on the base of the tail. Position your index and third fingers to grasp either side of the rat's neck caudal to the mandible firmly; the thumb and other fingers are used to restrain the chest gently.

HAMSTERS. The Syrian or golden hamster *(Mesocricetus auratus)* originated in the Middle East. It is the most common species of hamster in the pet trade and in research. It is noted for its ease of taming, low waste production, and lack of odor. The golden hamster is stocky and short tailed, weighs approximately 120 g, and has a reddish–golden brown body color with a gray ventrum. Other color varieties, such as cinnamon, cream, white, piebald, albino, and long-haired teddy bears, are popular as pets. The Chinese or striped hamster *(Cricetulus griseus)* is gray-brown with a dark stripe down its back and is smaller than the golden hamster, weighing 35 g. It tends to be more difficult to handle and

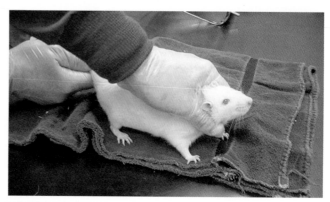

FIGURE 12-9 Restraining a rat. (Sheldon CC, Sonsthagen TF, Topel JA: Animal restraint for veterinary professionals, St Louis, 2006, Mosby.)

thus is not as popular as a pet. Female Chinese hamsters are belligerent and must be housed individually. Caging should be selected with the knowledge that hamsters are adept cage chewers and escape artists. Plastic tubes frequently sold as cage extensions are easily chewed through. Hamsters do seem to enjoy running on exercise wheels placed in their cages.

Hamsters usually have a life span of 1.5 to 2 years. Females are usually larger than males and, unlike most mammals, tend to fight more readily and are generally more aggressive. Males, therefore, live longer than females. On occasion, hamsters are cannibalistic. They have cheek pouches that can transport an amazing amount of food and bedding. A female hamster sometimes packs her whole newborn litter in her pouches to move them to another location. The hamster's cheek pouches are considered an immunologically privileged site; therefore, they have been used in research settings for the study of transplanted tumors. Hamsters have extremely loose skin. Marking glands, called flank or hip glands, are located in the skin of both flanks and are more prominent in males. Hamsters are permissive hibernators, so when temperatures fall below 8° C (46° F), some hamsters become inactive for periods of 2 to 3 days. During this transient state of hibernation, they have a reduced body temperature and reduced heart and respiratory rates. Hamsters have some control over whether they will hibernate. When hamsters are group-housed, the nonhibernating hamsters will on occasion cannibalize the sleeping hamsters.

> **CRITICAL CONCEPT**
>
> Hamsters have cheek pouches and they can hibernate in very cold weather.

Hamsters are sound sleepers and, on casual observation, may appear dead. An important point to remember when handling a hamster is to avoid surprising it. Make sure that the hamster is awake and knows that the handler intends to pick it up. Startled or awakened hamsters often bite. Hamsters are most easily moved by grasping the loose skin across the shoulders or using your hands as a scoop to transfer the hamster from one cage to another. They can also be picked up in a small can or cup. To restrain a hamster, gently grasp the loose skin across the back by curling your fingers and thumb around opposite sides of the animal to gather in as much loose skin as possible. Grasp the skin, not the body, of the hamster (Fig. 12-10). An alternative method is to reverse your hand so that your thumb and forefinger hold the skin at the base of the tail.

GERBILS. The Mongolian gerbil *(Meriones unguiculatus)* is a native to desert regions of Mongolia and northeastern China. It is an active, burrowing, social animal that tends to be more exploratory than other rodents. The gerbil is clean and produces little waste, making it one of the simplest animals to maintain. It is relatively odorless, nonaggressive, and easy to handle, making it a good pocket pet. The agouti

or mixed-brown gerbil is the color variety most commonly seen, but black and other colors, such as piebald, white, and cinnamon, are available.

The gerbil, or jird, as it is sometimes referred to, has an average life span of 3 years and weighs less than 100 g when mature. It has long hindlimbs adapted for leaping and, unlike most other rodents, has a hair-covered tail. When threatened or excited, gerbils will drum their hind legs on the cage flooring. They have large adrenal glands, adaptive mechanisms for temperature extremes, and a unique ability to conserve water. Gerbils have a high cholesterol level and lipemic serum. These can be accentuated by feeding sunflower seeds. Both sexes have a distinct dark orange midventral sebaceous gland, which is used for territorial marking.

A gerbil can be safely picked up by cupping both hands under it or by grasping the base of the tail to lift it from its cage. To restrain the gerbil for examination or injection, the loose skin at the nape of the neck is grasped with one hand and the base of the tail is grasped with the other hand (Fig. 12-11). Extreme care must be taken not to grasp the tip of the tail because the skin may tear and slip off, exposing the underlying muscle and vertebrae. Alternatively, an over-the-back grip can be used. Gerbils resist being placed on their back.

GUINEA PIGS. The guinea pig *(Cavia porcellus)*, often referred to as a **cavy**, is a tailless rodent with a compact, stocky body and short legs. They originated in South America and are a hystricomorph rodent related to chinchillas and porcupines. The guinea pig makes a nice children's pet because it is docile and seldom bites or scratches. Guinea pigs have a variety of vocalizations and frequently whistle and squeak when a caregiver approaches their cage. They are messy housekeepers and commonly scatter food and bedding. Guinea pigs can be

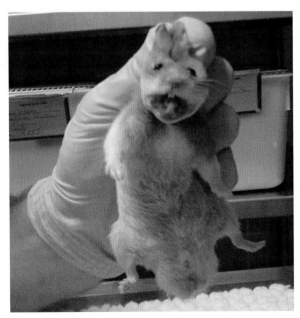

FIGURE 12-10 Holding the hamster. (Sheldon CC, Sonsthagen TF, Topel JA: Animal restraint for veterinary professionals, St Louis, 2006, Mosby.)

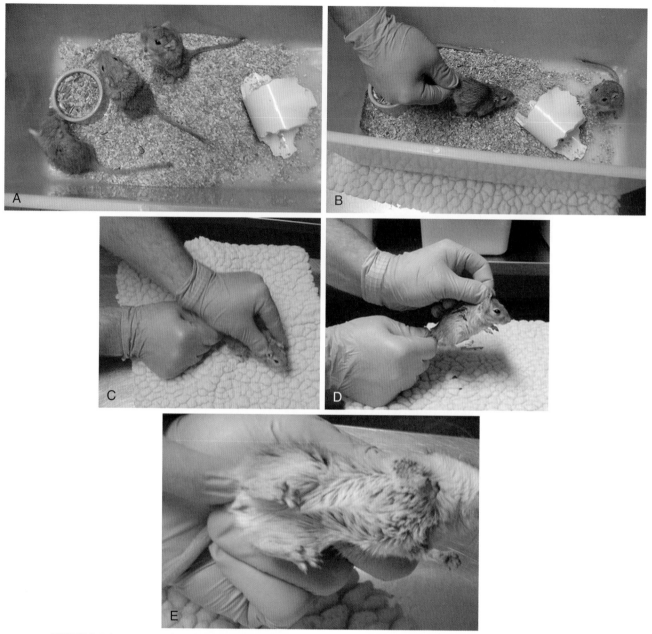

FIGURE 12-11 **A,** Gerbils should take an active interest in you as you approach. **B,** When retrieving the gerbil, reach into its enclosure, bringing your hand from over its head to grasp its tail firmly at the base. **C,** Firmly hold the base of the animal's tail while you scruff the animal with your other hand. **D,** You can then pick the animal up. **E,** Once you have a good hold of the animal's scruff, you can transfer the base of its tail to your little finger on the hand with which you are scruffing so that the animal rests in the palm of your hand. (Sheldon CC, Sonsthagen TF, Topel JA: Animal restraint for veterinary professionals, St Louis, 2006, Mosby.)

monocolored, bicolored, or tricolored. The most common pet variety is the English, American, or short-haired guinea pig (Fig. 12-12). The Abyssinian has short, rough hair arranged in whorls or rosettes; the Peruvian or rag mop variety has long, silky hair (Fig. 12-13).

The guinea pig weighs 700 to 1200 g as an adult. It has a normal body temperature of 37.2° to 39.5° C (99° to 103° F) and a life span of 4 to 5 years. Guinea pigs have four digits on their front limbs and three digits on their hind limbs. All teeth are open rooted and erupt continuously. They have a large cecum and a long colon. Guinea pigs are actively coprophagic. Their urine is normally opaque and creamy yellow and contains crystals. Marking glands are located around the anus and on the rump. Both male and female guinea pigs have inguinal nipples. Sexing is difficult because, unlike other rodents, there is little difference in the anogenital distance in males and females. The female has a Y-shaped anogenital opening and vaginal membrane that remains intact and closed, except during the few days of estrus and at parturition. Males have scrotal pouches lateral to the anogenital line and a penis that can be protruded by manual pressure. The guinea pig usually responds to danger in one of two ways, either by becoming immobile for up to 20 minutes or by the scatter response, in which they run for their lives.

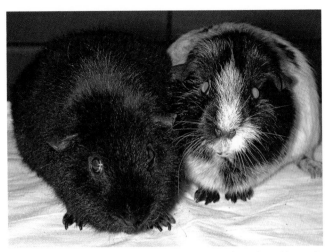

FIGURE 12-12 Two common guinea pig breeds. *Left,* Teddy. *Right,* American. (From Mitchell M, Tully TN, Jr: Manual of exotic pet practice, St Louis, 2008, Saunders.)

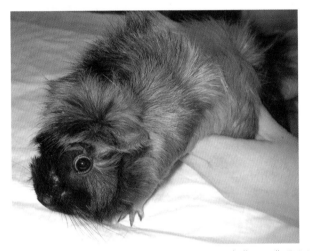

FIGURE 12-13 Abyssinian guinea pig. (From Mitchell M, Tully TN, Jr: Manual of exotic pet practice, St Louis, 2008, Saunders.)

Female guinea pigs are called **sows,** males are called **boars,** and the act of giving birth is called farrowing. The sow is polyestrous throughout the year and has an estrous cycle of 15 to 17 days. A sow should be bred for the first time before 6 months of age, before fusion of the pubic bones, to prevent dystocia. The gestation period is lengthy, averaging 68 days. Larger litters have shorter gestation periods. Neonates are precocious and almost self-sufficient. They are born fully furred, with eyes and ears open and teeth erupted. Young guinea pigs eat solid food within the first few days postpartum and can be weaned at 14 to 21 days.

Guinea pigs have rigid eating habits, and any change in food or water may cause them to stop eating. Dietary vitamin C must be provided to guinea pigs because, like primates, they cannot synthesize their own vitamin C. Lack of vitamin C causes scurvy.

To restrain a guinea pig, lift the animal by grasping under the trunk with one hand while supporting the rear quarters with your other hand (Fig. 12-14). It is especially important to use a two-hand support method with adult and pregnant

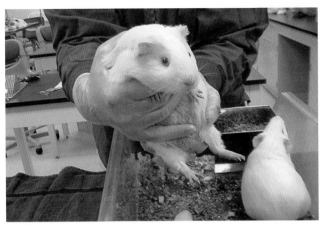

FIGURE 12-14 Remove the guinea pig from its cage by lifting it up while supporting its body with your hand. (Sheldon CC, Sonsthagen TF, Topel JA: Animal restraint for veterinary professionals, St Louis, 2006, Mosby.)

animals. An alternative method is to place one hand over the shoulder area, with your thumb and forefingers just caudal to the front legs, while the other hand supports the rear quarters. Use care not to compress the chest too much with this method.

CHINCHILLAS. The chinchilla *(Chinchilla laniger)* has a compact body, delicate limbs, large eyes, large round ears, long whiskers, and a bushy tail. It has a soft, very dense hair coat that is normally bluish-gray, with yellow-white underparts. It originated in South America like its relative the guinea pig. Chinchillas are quiet, shy animals that adapt well to humans when handled at a young age. They rarely bite and are almost odorless. Chinchillas are very active, agile, and like to climb and jump. They require a larger cage than guinea pigs, who tend to be less active.

The chinchilla weighs 400 to 600 g as an adult. It has a normal body temperature of 37° to 38° C (99° to 100 ° F) and a life span of 10 years. Its life span is much longer than that of other pet rodents. Chinchillas have four toes on their front and rear feet. Like the guinea pig, all their teeth are open rooted and ever growing. They have a long gastrointestinal (GI) tract and are coprophagic. The female has a vaginal closure membrane that remains intact and closed except during a few days of estrus and at parturition. The anogenital distance is the best criterion for sexing. The female has a large urinary papilla that can be confused with a penis. The penis can be protruded by manual pressure to confirm the sex. Males do not have a true scrotum. The testes are contained within the open inguinal canal or abdomen.

A tamed chinchilla will willingly come out of its cage. To restrain it, place one hand under the abdomen or around the scruff of the neck and hold it by the base of the tail with your other hand. If the chinchilla escapes from its cage, you must be fast to catch it. Use care because a frightened chinchilla can lose a patch of fur where it is grasped. This condition is called fur slip and is a predator avoidance mechanism. It takes 6 to 8 weeks for the hairless patch to fill in.

Access to a dust bath should be provided for 1 hour daily to prevent matted fur (Fig. 12-15). Commercial chinchilla dust or a mixture of silver sand and Fuller's earth can be used. One inch of dust is placed in a pan big enough for the chinchilla to roll around in and fluff its fur. Chinchillas are susceptible to many of the same bacterial diseases as guinea pigs. The bones of chinchillas are thin and fragile. It is common to see traumatic fractures. The tibia is particularly fragile, being longer than the femur, and has little soft tissue covering it. Chinchillas are prone to heat stroke at an environmental temperature in excess of 28° to 30° C (82° to 86° F), especially when coupled with high humidity.

GENERAL NURSING CARE OF SMALL MAMMALS

Because of the cost involved in hospitalization and intensive care, most pet rodents are treated on an outpatient basis, whereas rabbits and ferrets are often hospitalized. As with any other sick pet, proper nursing care is vital to maximize the pet's chances for full recovery.

Pet rodents that must be hospitalized are usually critically ill. Fluid therapy, antibiotics, nutritional support, and proper environment are important. These patients should be handled as little as possible. The proper ambient temperature must be maintained. Incubators serve this function well; however, care must be taken not to overheat small mammals. The temperature should be kept no warmer than 80° F (25° C). Temperatures above this often result in death from heat stroke. When necessary, oxygen can be supplemented through a port on the incubator. Food and water should be offered, even if forced feeding is needed.

When possible, small mammals should be isolated from other hospitalized animals, not only because of the

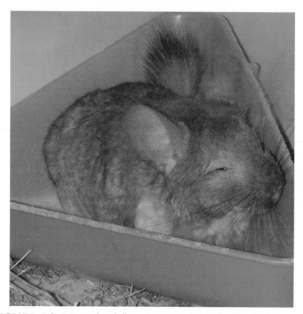

FIGURE 12-15 A chinchilla enjoying a dust bath. Dust baths are essential for chinchillas' skin maintenance and coat health. (From Mitchell M, Tully TN, Jr: Manual of exotic pet practice, St Louis, 2008, Saunders; courtesy Dr. M.G. Hawkins.)

risk of disease spread (e.g., *Bordetella* spp. passed from dogs, cats, or rabbits to guinea pigs), but also because these sick pets are extremely stressed. Remember that most small mammals are prey in the wild. Housing them near a natural predator such as a dog or cat may increase their stress level.

DIAGNOSTIC AND TREATMENT TECHNIQUES

Techniques used to diagnose disease in companion and food animals are used in small mammals. Some techniques such as skin scrapings can be more challenging in rodents because they are very mobile and can be difficult to restrain. Diagnostic testing is important because many of these pets are presented with vague complaints such as lethargy and lack of appetite. Although certain syndromes are more common in certain species, diagnostic testing can help determine a definitive diagnosis and proper treatment plan. Unfortunately, many owners of some less expensive small mammals, particularly rodents, may not allow diagnostic testing because of the cost involved. In addition, the small size of these animals makes it more difficult to obtain adequate laboratory samples. In the research setting, the health status of the rodent colony is often more important that the health status of an individual animal. Health status is frequently monitored by serologic testing of sentinel animals that are placed in the colony.

VENIPUNCTURE

Venipuncture is a technique commonly used for ferrets and rabbits but infrequently used for pet rodents. Venipuncture is used for withdrawing blood for hematologic and biochemical analysis, administration of certain medications, and catheterization for administration of fluids. Anesthesia may be required when performing venipuncture on small mammals. Although each diagnostic laboratory has specific requirements for the volume of blood required for various tests, most laboratories can perform a minibattery of tests (e.g., complete blood count [CBC], chemistries, electrolytes) on 0.5 mL of blood collected in a green-topped (lithium heparin) tube. Special blood collection tubes (e.g., Microvette), which hold a maximum of 0.3 mL, are commercially available. These are particularly useful when collecting samples from small rodents.

RODENTS. Small blood samples can be collected from rodents by superficial venipuncture. The lateral saphenous vein is a good superficial vessel to use. Other superficial vessels that can be used include the cephalic vein, jugular vein, and tail vessels in rodents that have long tails (Fig. 12-16). The central vena cava of guinea pigs is easily accessible, but they must be anesthetized first. The orbital sinus is frequently used to collect blood from anesthetized rodents. Cardiac puncture can also be used in an anesthetized rodent, but is not recommended except for collection before euthanasia.

RABBITS. The marginal ear veins and central ear artery of the rabbit are easily visualized and can be used to collect blood (Fig. 12-17). Blood can be collected with a syringe and needle or by cannulating the vessel and collecting the blood in a blood tube or heparinized microhematocrit tube as it drips freely from the vessel. Jugular venipuncture is also fairly easy and is collected in a manner similar to that used for dogs and cats. The veterinary assistant will restrain the rabbit in ventral recumbency. The cephalic vein tends to be a more difficult vessel from which to collect blood.

FERRETS. The cephalic vein, jugular vein, cranial vena cava, and lateral saphenous vein can be used to collect blood samples in ferrets (Fig. 12-18). Venipuncture is most easily performed under isoflurane anesthesia maintained by face mask. When obtaining a jugular sample, the ferret is placed in dorsal recumbency, with the legs pulled caudally while the head and neck are extended dorsally. Venipuncture can be done in an awake, cooperative ferret. Obtaining small volumes of blood from larger ferrets is possible using the central artery of the tail.

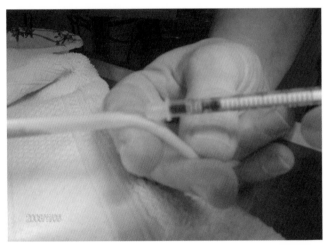

FIGURE 12-16 Blood collection from the tail vein of a rat. (From Sirois M: Principles and practice of veterinary technology, ed 3, St Louis, 2011, Mosby.)

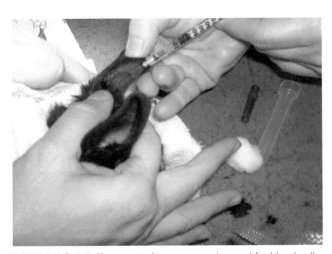

FIGURE 12-17 The marginal ear vein can be used for blood collection or small-volume IV injections in rabbits. (From Sirois M: Principles and practice of veterinary technology, ed 3, St Louis, 2011, Mosby.)

FORCE FEEDING

Many small mammals are presented for veterinary care because of anorexia and lethargy. In addition to the need for rehydration, nutritional supplementation is often required but overlooked. Small mammals such as rodents have high metabolic rates and thus high energy requirements. Animals that are not eating are in a catabolic state. Decreased food intake results in the breakdown of protein and fat for energy. This can contribute to hepatic lipidosis (especially in rabbits), acidosis, azotemia, muscle wasting, impaired GI function, and decreased immunity. To prevent or correct these complications, supplementation with food is important. Force feeding can be done in the hospital or by the owner at home if the pet will be treated on an outpatient basis.

High-energy paste supplements such as Nutri-Cal can be given to all small mammals on a short-term basis. Sick rabbits often eat hay or greens, such as carrot tops and parsley, even if they refuse pellets. These can be offered free choice. Apples and yogurt can also be used. A nasogastric or gastric tube can be used to deliver a mixture of powdered pellets and water. Rodents' diets can be supplemented with apples and peanut butter. Sweetened condensed milk is also a favorite. Pedialyte or Gatorade can be fed via a small syringe for hydration, along with water. Hospitalized ferrets can be force fed any of the diets suitable for cats, including Hill's a/d or Abbott's Clini-Care. Meat-based baby foods can also be used. The food can be offered to the ferret to eat voluntarily or via syringe or tube. Warming the food slightly may increase the appetite of ferrets.

ADMINISTRATION OF MEDICATIONS

With the exception of ferrets, small mammals are difficult to medicate with pills. Liquid oral medication given by eye

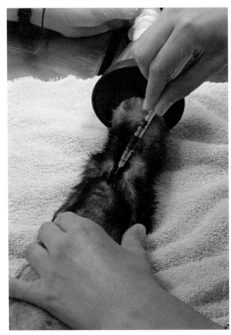

FIGURE 12-18 With the anesthetized ferret in dorsal recumbency, the anterior vena cava can safely be sampled. (From Mitchell M, Tully TN, Jr: Manual of exotic pet practice, St Louis, 2008, Saunders.)

dropper or small syringe is generally better accepted by the pet. Because of the small size of rodents, medications usually have to be diluted. For increased accuracy of dosing, it is important to have an accurate body weight and use a tuberculin syringe. Medication can also be administered orally by mixing the medication in the water or feed and by gavage needle. Rodents often do not drink medicated water because of its unpleasant taste.

Injectable medications are usually preferred over oral medications in hospitalized small mammals. Extremely ill pets may have reduced intestinal function, making absorption of oral medication erratic and unpredictable. Using the parenteral rather than the oral route of drug administration also decreases the possibility of GI problems in these small mammals.

The standard routes of injection (intravenous [IV], intramuscular [IM], subcutaneous [SC], intradermal [ID], intraperitoneal [IP]) are used for small mammals. Rodents have few readily accessible veins, making it difficult to administer drugs IV. Tail veins can be used in the mouse and rat. The margin ear veins, located on the lateral sides of the pinna in the rabbit, are accessible and can be used for IV injections. Because it is difficult to carry out venous catheterization in small mammals, some doctors and technicians prefer intraosseous catheterization to administer fluids to critically ill exotic pets. The SC route is frequently used for fluid supplementation. SC fluids are given over the dorsal neck, back, and flank of small mammals. Fluids can also be given IP in rodents, although this is least desirable because of the risk of peritonitis and laceration of internal organs. The small muscle mass of rodents makes it difficult to inject drugs IM. For this reason, the IP route is more commonly used in rodents. When giving IP injections, it is best to use the caudal left abdominal quadrant and tilt the animal's head and forequarters ventrally. This helps avoid accidental puncture of the internal organs in these animals (Fig. 12-19).

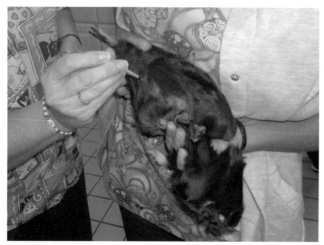

FIGURE 12-19 The guinea pig should be held with its body tilted downward when administering an IP injection. (From Sirois M: Principles and practice of veterinary technology, ed 3, St Louis, 2011, Mosby.)

ANTIBIOTICS. Caution must be used when administering antibiotics to rodents and rabbits. These animals have a predominantly gram-positive GI flora and are sensitive to antibiotics that change the balance of the flora. Guinea pigs and rabbits are particularly prone to antibiotic-associated enterotoxemia. Drugs such as ampicillin and penicillin will destroy susceptible gram-positive organisms and allow for the overgrowth of *Clostridium difficile* and production of its toxin. Safe antibacterials for use in rabbits and rodents include enrofloxacin, ciprofloxacin, trimethoprim-sulfamethoxazole, and chloramphenicol. If diarrhea develops, drug administration should be stopped immediately and the animal examined. Ferrets can be treated safely with most antibacterials used for cats.

VACCINES. Rodents and rabbits do not currently require annual vaccines. Ferrets must be vaccinated against canine distemper virus with an appropriate vaccine. Never use canine combination vaccines or vaccines of ferret cell origin because of the possibility of vaccine-induced disease. Give ferrets a series of vaccines at 6 to 8, 10 to 12, and 14 weeks of age, and then annually. Vaccination against rabies is highly recommended for ferrets, especially in rabies-endemic areas. An inactivated rabies vaccine approved for use in ferrets should be given SC at 3 months of age and annually.

FECAL ANALYSIS

Microscopic fecal analysis is used to evaluate animals with diarrhea and any nonspecific complaint. The method is similar to that used for dogs and cats. A fresh fecal smear and flotation test should be performed. A cellophane tape test can be used on the anal region to check for the presence of pinworms in rodents.

URINALYSIS

Urine samples can be obtained by gentle manual expression of the bladder or cystocentesis. Rodents can be placed on a cold surface or in a cooled plastic bag until urine is voided.

BIRDS

The common companion birds seen in a small animal veterinary hospital are typically members of the psittacine or passerine family (Box 12-1). These are distinguished by a number of physical characteristics. **Psittacines**, or parrots, make up the majority of avian patients. The psittacines are known as hookbills because of their curved upper beak. Their feet are shaped with the second and third toes facing forward and the first and fourth toes directed backward. This is referred to as zygodactyl. **Passerines** are usually small birds with a pointed or slightly curved beak. Their feet are **anisodactyl**—three toes point forward and one toe points to the rear. Many of these birds are very active and tend to hop or fly about their cage. Most are not trained to sit on their owner's hand and remain inside their cages. Canaries and finches are the most frequently kept passerines.

BOX 12-1	Common Companion Species Seen in an Avian Practice

Psittacines
- Macaw
- Cockatoo
- Amazon
- African Grey
- Love bird
- Conure
- Parakeet (budgerigar)
- Cockatiel
- Caique
- Lori
- Lorikeet

Passerines
- Finches
- Canaries

From Sirois M: Principles and practice of veterinary technology, ed 3, St Louis, 2011, Mosby.

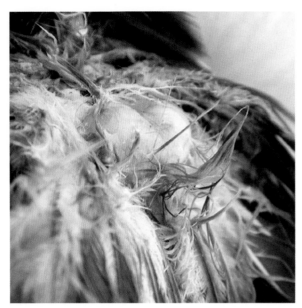

FIGURE 12-20 Uropygial gland of a Meyers parrot located at the base of the tail. (From Sirois M: Principles and practice of veterinary technology, ed 3, St Louis, 2011, Mosby.)

AVIAN ANATOMY
INTEGUMENT

The integument is the largest and most extensive organ system of the body. It protects the underlying structures and forms a physical barrier between the body and external world.

The body of a bird is covered by skin and its derivatives, the beak, claws, and feathers. The skin is delicate and has a dry, slightly wrinkled appearance. Underlying muscles and blood give the skin a reddish appearance in some areas. The skin on the legs resembles the scales of reptiles. The **cere**, or the area around the nostrils, the beak, and the nails, are all modified skin.

CRITICAL CONCEPT

The cere is the fleshy structure around the nares in some birds. In parakeets (budgerigars), the cere is generally blue or pink and smooth in males and brown and lumpy in females.

Sweat glands are absent in birds. The one major skin gland that most birds possess is the **uropygial gland** (Fig. 12-20). This gland has one duct that empties into a lone papilla, found dorsally at the base of the tail. It secretes a fatty sebaceous material that is spread over feathers during preening to help with waterproofing. This gland is absent in the ostrich, emu, cassowaries, bustards, frogmouth, many pigeons, woodpeckers, and Amazon parrots.

Feathers are necessary for flight; they protect the skin from trauma and exposure and assist in thermoregulation, camouflage, and communication. Feather follicles are located in specific tracts over the surface of the body called pterylae. These tracts are separated by nonfeathered areas of skin called apteria. These tracts overlap each other to give the bird a fully feathered look.

Birds have several types of feathers (Fig. 12-21). The **contour feathers** cover the body and wings and are identified as **flight feathers** or body feathers. The large, primary flight feathers (remiges) are found on the outer end of the wing. The secondary flight feathers are located on the wing between the body and the primaries. Body feathers, also known as **coverts**, provide surface coverage over most of the rest of the bird. **Down feathers** insulate the bird and have a soft, fluffy appearance. Cockatoos, cockatiels, and African Greys have powder down, which breaks down to produce a white, dusty powder. A healthy bird of these species will have a fine layer of this powder over most of its body, most noticeably on the beak. Birds spend several hours a day preening, or rearranging and conditioning their feathers. **Molting** occurs in all species and results in the periodic replacement of old feathers. A new, growing feather has a vascular supply until it reaches full size. The shafts of these so-called blood feathers appear dark and bleed profusely if broken, possibly leading to the death of the bird.

MUSCULOSKELETAL SYSTEM

The skeleton of birds is highly modified. Some bones are **pneumatized**, or contain air, which results in a lighter skeleton. The bones have thin walls, which makes them lighter but also more fragile. The skull bones are fused, which strengthens the beak structure. The vertebrae of the neck are shaped so as to create a long, flexible neck. The large sternum, or **keel**, supports the pectoral muscles, which are needed for flight. A large portion of the caudal vertebrae is fused to form the synsacrum, which stabilizes the back during flight.

The largest muscles in the body are the pectorals, which account for approximately 20% of the bird's weight. Because of their mass, they are used to determine the body condition of the bird and are ideal for IM injections.

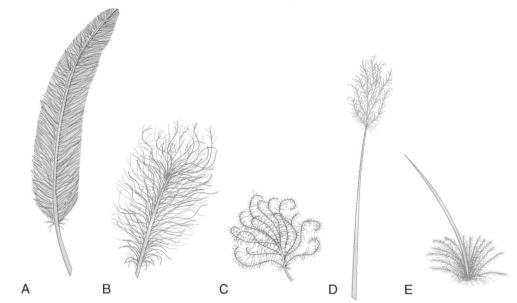

FIGURE 12-21 Types of feathers. **A,** Contour. **B,** Semiplume. **C,** Down. **D,** Filoplume. **E,** Bristle. (From Colville T, Bassert JM: Clinical anatomy and physiology for veterinary technicians, ed 2, St Louis, 2008, Mosby.)

RESPIRATORY SYSTEM

Birds possess a highly specialized and efficient respiratory system (Fig. 12-22). Air enters the respiratory system through the nares and continues over an **operculum**, which is a cornified flap of tissue located immediately behind the nares in the nasal cavity. Air then travels through the many sinuses in the head and then enters the oral cavity through the slitlike opening in the roof of the mouth known as the **choana**. The choana is a V-shaped notch in the roof of the bird's mouth that directs air from the mouth and nasal cavities to the glottis. The choana closes during swallowing. This structure should be surrounded by many sharp papillae. Blunted or absent papillae may be indicate disease or malnutrition.

Birds lack an epiglottis, so air travels through the glottis at the base of the tongue and down the trachea. The trachea is located on the left side of the cervical area, is mobile the entire length of the neck, and consists of complete cartilaginous rings that cannot expand. At the caudal portion of the trachea lies the **syrinx**, the voice box of birds. Birds produce vocalizations by forcing air over the syrinx and vibrating membranes during the expiratory phase of respiration. The complexity of a bird's vocalizations depends on the species and number of muscles in the syrinx.

The air continues into the small lungs located dorsally near the spine, where air exchange takes place. There are no lobes or alveoli, so the lungs do not inflate. Inspiration of air occurs by extension of the intracostal joints, drawing in inspired air with a bellows-like action into the caudal air sacs. The **coelom** of a bird is a triangle-shaped cavity that allows for the bellows-like action during breathing. Both inspiration and expiration require active muscle contraction.

> ### CRITICAL CONCEPT
> Birds require the movement of their keel to achieve air exchange. If the keel is not allowed to expand (e.g., as with aggressive restraint), the bird cannot breathe and will go into respiratory and then cardiac arrest.

Air flows into the air sacs, which are thin-walled hollow spaces that are lightly vascularized membranes found throughout the bird's body. There are a total of nine air sacs, consisting of one unpaired interclavicular air sac, located in the thoracic inlet between the clavicles, and four paired air sacs—cranial thoracic, caudal thoracic, cervical, and abdominal. Normal respiratory effort in the bird should not be noticeable, and the beak should remain closed. In some cases, there may be increased head and tail movements and increased abdominal effort after exercise. The bird should return to normal within a few minutes.

DIGESTIVE SYSTEM

The high metabolism of birds requires the ingestion of large amounts of food. The beak will vary with the diet and foraging strategies. Generally, the beak is used to grasp food and crush it with the aid of the tongue. Birds do not have teeth. The mouth consists of a hard upper palate, soft lower plate, distinctive tongue, and scattered taste buds and salivary glands. The mouth is relatively dry because little saliva is produced.

When food is swallowed, it travels through the esophagus, a somewhat muscular tube that extends from the pharynx to the stomach along the right side of the neck. In several species, the esophagus expands into the interclavicular space to create a **crop**. The crop anatomy varies among species and can be a dilation of the esophagus, a single pouch, or

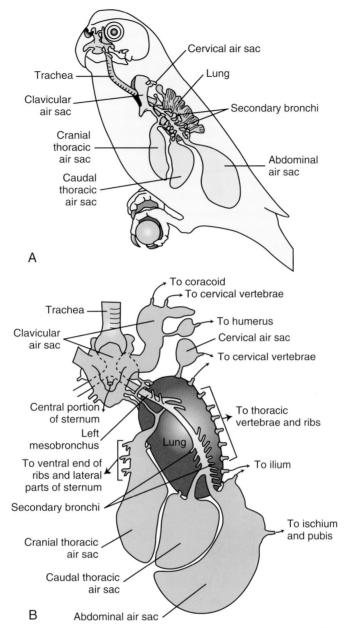

FIGURE 12-22 Diagram of the avian respiratory system. **A,** Lateral view. **B,** Ventral view. (From Colville T, Bassert JM: Clinical anatomy and physiology for veterinary technicians, ed 2, St Louis, 2008, Mosby.)

a double pouch. It softens food and allows continuous passage of small amounts of food to the **proventriculus**, or true stomach. The proventriculus is unique to birds; however, it is comparable to the stomach of mammals, containing digestive acid and enzymes.

The food next passes into the **ventriculus**, or gizzard. This is a thickly muscled organ that grinds food into smaller particles. Historically, it was thought that companion birds need grit, or small pieces of gravel, in the gizzard to break down hard foods. However, this is not true, and companion birds do not need to be given grit. Grit can be problematic in some birds and they may develop an impaction if they have access to it.

The intestinal tract is comparable to that of mammals (Fig. 12-23). Birds have a pancreas, which is a relatively large gland that rests in the loop of the duodenum. The liver is

bilobed, with the right side usually larger than the left. The gallbladder is absent in most parrots but is found in many other avian species. The duodenum or small intestine varies in length and diameter, depending on the species, and is the major organ responsible for digestion and absorption of nutrients. The large intestine is the segment that extends from the end of the small intestine and terminates at the cloaca.

The **cloaca** is the common terminal chamber of the GI, urinary, and reproductive systems. The cloaca is divided in to three compartments—the coprodeum, urodeum, and proctodeum. The **coprodeum** is the cranial portion of the cloaca that receives feces from the rectum. The **urodeum** is the middle part of the cloaca into which the ureters enter dorsolaterally on both sides; in males, the ductus deferens enters near the ureters, and in females a single oviduct enters

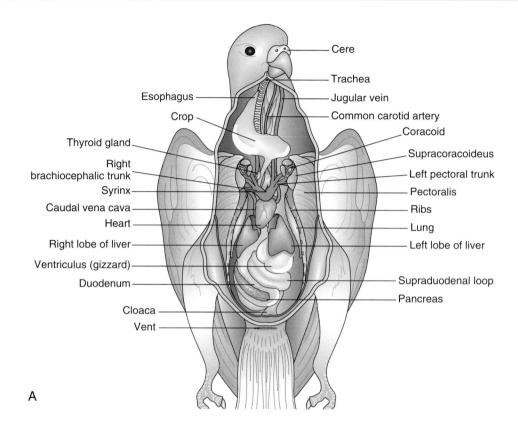

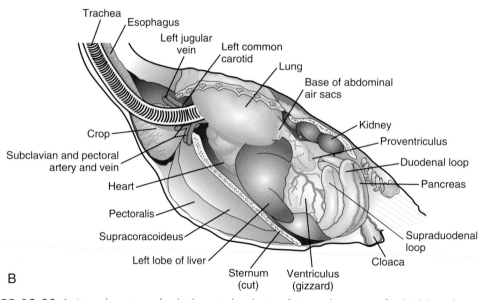

FIGURE 12-23 A, Internal anatomy of a bird, ventrodorsal view. B, Internal anatomy of a bird, lateral view. (From O'Malley B: Clinical anatomy and physiology of exotic species, Oxford, England, 2005, Saunders.)

the urodeum dorsolaterally on the left side. The **proctodeum** is the caudal part of the cloaca; if a phallus is present, it would be located on the floor of the proctodeum. Psittacines do not have a phallus but it is found in many other avian species.

The external opening of the cloaca is called the **vent**, from which the droppings are passed. In most species, the vent is horizontally flattened, rather than circumferential, as in mammals. Normal bird droppings have three

distinct components—liquid urine, semisolid white or cream **urates**, and feces. The droppings will vary in consistency, depending on the diet.

URINARY SYSTEM

The paired kidneys of birds are closely attached to the vertebrae (see Fig. 12-23B). They empty into the ureters, which carry the liquid urine and semisolid urates to the cloaca. Urine is not concentrated in the kidneys; rather, urine moves into the coprodeum and rectum, where the resorption of water, sodium, and chloride takes place. Urates are the major excretion product in birds and compose the white portion of the droppings. Birds do not have a urinary bladder.

> **CRITICAL CONCEPT**
>
> A suddenly stressed bird, such as an avian patient on presentation after transport or an examination, may have an increased urine component to its droppings because the droppings pass before lower intestinal water resorption occurs; these are known as stress droppings.

REPRODUCTIVE SYSTEM

In the female bird, only the left side of the reproductive tract develops fully. As in mammals, an ovary, oviduct, and vagina are present. Various regions of the oviduct produce the egg white and eggshell. The entire process from ovulation to egg laying takes approximately 15 hours. The female lays eggs even if no male is present.

The male bird has paired testes located internally near the kidneys. During periods of active breeding, they enlarge dramatically. Sperm cells travel to the cloaca through the epididymis and then the ductus deferens. Most birds do not have a penis or phallus, and mating takes place when the vents of the male and female birds come into contact.

CIRCULATORY SYSTEM

The heart of birds closely resembles that of mammals, but it is proportionally about 1.5 times larger. The heart rate ranges from 250 to 350 beats/min in large parrots and up to 1400 beats/min in the very small species. Blood pressure in birds is typically higher than in mammals.

The circulatory system of birds differs from that of mammals in several ways. The red blood cells of birds are oval and contain a nucleus. Birds do not have lymph nodes and the lymphatic system is less extensive.

SPECIAL SENSES

As with mammals, birds have the traditional five senses—seeing, hearing, feeling, smelling, and tasting. The brain of a bird is large in proportion to its body size. The location and control centers within the brain that receive and process stimuli from the senses are comparable to those of mammals, with several exceptions. In birds, the control centers for vision and hearing are larger than those for taste, touch, and smell.

Vision is highly developed in the avian species. The eyes of birds are relatively large, and a significant part of the avian skull is devoted to housing and protecting the eyes (Fig. 12-24). The shape of the eyes is determined by the orbits. Bird eyes can be round, flat, or tubular, depending on the species. Diurnal birds, birds that forage or hunt in the daytime, have round or relatively flat eyes, whereas **nocturnal species**, those that forage and hunt at night, have tubular eyes. Tubular eyes have a pupil with a larger diameter than the retina, allowing more light into the eye.

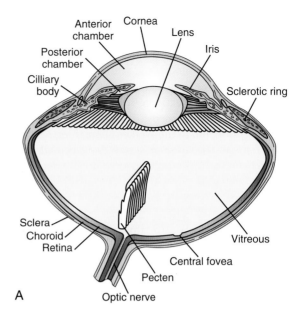

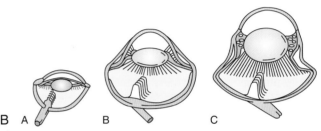

FIGURE 12-24 A, The avian eye, transverse section. B, Shapes of the avian eye. A, Flat. B, Round. C, Tubular. (From Colville T, Bassert JM: Clinical anatomy and physiology for veterinary technicians, ed 2, St Louis, 2008, Mosby.)

The lens and anterior chamber of the avian eye are comparable to those of mammals, with the exception of the presence of a highly vascular, ribbonlike structure called the pecten. The pecten is believed to provide nutrition to the eye.

Bird vision is acute, and they can perceive color. Birds often look closely at something with one eye, tilting their head for a better view. In many species, the color of the iris is darker in young birds. The iris contains striated muscles that allow voluntary control over the size of the pupils. Thus, the pupillary light response is not a good diagnostic indicator in birds; however, this should always be part of a thorough physical examination. Blinking is done using the nictitating membrane, or third eyelid. This structure is mostly transparent. Most birds close their eyes completely when they sleep.

The avian ear is simpler than that of mammals but has exceptional acoustic ability. Located on the sides of the head and slightly below the eyes, the ears of birds are hidden from view by feathers that protect the ear during flight and yet allow sound to pass through. The external auditory canal funnels sound to the middle ear and tympanic membrane. There is a single bone in the middle ear called the **columella**, in contrast to the three bones in mammals, and it connects to the inner ear. The inner ear is comparable to that in mammals. It consists of a membranous labyrinth that helps maintain balance and equilibrium and converts sounds into nerve impulses that are sent to the brain.

Birds have fewer taste buds than most mammals; these are located on the roof of the mouth and scattered over the soft palate. Many birds enjoy eating highly spiced or sweet foods. The sense of smell varies greatly in birds. In a few species, such as the turkey vulture, the sense of smell is highly developed for locating food, but in the average companion species it is thought that the sense of smell is poorly developed. The sense of touch is an important sense in many species for finding food and for defense. The skin of birds contains sensory nerve endings that respond to pain, heat, cold, and touch. Some are responsive to the slightest feather movement, and some birds will respond when the tips of their feathers are touched.

BASIC PET BIRD BEHAVIOR

Veterinary clinics that provide care for companion birds must also be prepared to assist clients with behavior complaints. Many birds are needlessly abused, ignored, abandoned at shelters or rescue societies, put up for adoption, or euthanized because the client has a lack of understanding of natural or adapted bird behaviors. Birds have been kept as companions for hundreds of years but are far from domestic. They are genetically close to their wild ancestors and retain many of the characteristics of their wild relatives. Most birds have a higher than average intelligence, resulting in a patient that is both entertaining and challenging to alter behaviors. The veterinary clinic should be the client's first credible authority for correcting behavior problems, not the local pet or feed store personnel. The veterinary clinic staff must know the basics of bird behavior and be prepared to assist clients or refer problem cases to avian behaviorists.

COMMON BEHAVIORS

Many of the behaviors that owners wish to modify are the result of instinctive avian reactions or related to the stresses of captivity. To have an understanding of the problem behaviors that birds exhibit in captivity, you must have a clear understanding of normal psittacine behavior.

Many parrots use their agile feet to hold food while they eat or manipulate objects that they are interested in exploring (Fig. 12-25). They tend to be good climbers, often moving around their cage using a combination of beak and feet. Birds will wag their tail back and forth when happy and relaxed. Birds grind their beak when they are comfortable and ready to fall asleep. Some birds will regurgitate food for those to which they are closely bonded, whether it is the owner or another bird. The typical behavior that indicates defecation in a calm bird is a slight wiggle of the tail, followed by a squat and an uplifted tail. All birds defecate frequently and more often when afraid or stressed.

Fear is a common behavior when the bird is in the clinic; personnel should be aware of this and take appropriate measures to reduce the stress involved with the visit. When a bird is frightened, it may fling itself about the cage, struggle violently, flap its wings, scream loudly, or take flight in response to sudden movements or unfamiliar sights or sounds (Fig. 12-26). This is common during capture and restraint. Birds may easily be injured in their efforts to get away. Clients often seek help with problems such as biting, chewing, screaming, or destructive feather behavior.

CHEWING. **Mouthing** is a term used to describe a juvenile parrot that uses its tongue to explore surfaces. Juvenile parrots pass through an innocent beaking phase, in which they attempt to taste or chew almost anything, somewhat like puppies. Contrary to puppies, birds do not grow out of this behavior (Fig. 12-27). Clients should be counseled to supervise the parrot when out of its cage and provide the pet with safe, well-designed toys that can be destroyed. Toys that are safe to destroy, such as paper-based manufactured, homemade, or natural wood toys embedded with nuts, provide much needed enrichment for these intelligent confined creatures.

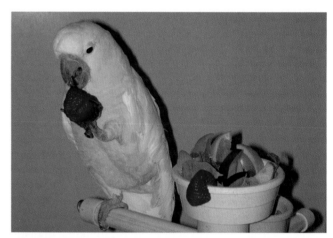

FIGURE 12-25 Birds are very agile and use their feet as utensils for eating. (From Sirois M: Principles and practice of veterinary technology, ed 3, St Louis, 2011, Mosby.)

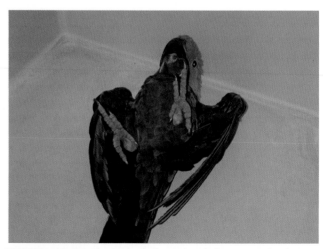

FIGURE 12-26 This bird is frightened and objecting to the clinic visit by throwing itself on its back, flapping and screaming to avoid capture. (From Sirois M: Principles and practice of veterinary technology, ed 3, St Louis, 2011, Mosby.)

BITING. Birds bite to exhibit dominance, express fear, or exhibit jealousy, or as a result of hormonal fluctuations during puberty or the breeding season. Biting may not be an instinctual behavior but rather one that captive birds have developed in confinement. In the wild, the beak is used primarily for eating, preening, and communication. If a conflict arises, most birds generally fly away rather than using their beak as a weapon. Some protective birds may bite the owner in an effort to communicate with the person to move away from perceived danger. It is important for the owner to realize that the bird must not be allowed to bite as a way of controlling a situation. Mature parrots are more likely to bite during handling as a method of defense.

The larger psittacines, such as macaws, can exert up to 300 pounds pressure per square inch (psi), inflicting deep bruises and lacerations. Birds such as cockatiels and parakeets have the potential to draw blood with their bites. Biting is a common behavior problem; identifying why the bird is biting is the first step to a resolution.

DOMINANCE. Psittacines may attempt to become dominant over their flock, and in the captive companion bird world, the flock is their human family. It is important that the owner and other household members use certain techniques to maintain the dominant position in the home. Birds should be taught consistently to step up on or down from the owner's hand when asked. Clipping the bird's wings to limit its flying ability can diminish dominance behaviors, such as flying down from a curtain rod to attack members of the household. When holding the bird, keep it at midchest level. Never allowing it to sit on the head or shoulders keeps it from attaining the highest perch, a position of great power. Situating the cage or perches so that the bird is below eye level also discourages dominant behavior.

VOCALIZATION. Parrots are naturally loud creatures and vocalize for many reasons, such as communication, entertainment, exercise, and in response to discomfort or restraint. Birds tend to be noisy at dawn and dusk and at feeding time. Noise levels vary among species. Parrots can scream loudly enough to damage human hearing, so hearing protection is recommended when working with companion birds. Some of these birds have the ability to repeat what they hear; some will recite any unsavory word or derogatory phrase and bodily function sounds if these scenarios are repetitive. Vocalizations may become a problem in some insecure or dependent birds that call constantly to their owner. Some species are relatively quiet, but all birds make a certain amount of noise. Owners may inadvertently encourage the bird to make more noise by responding to the bird's loud calls with anger or shouting in an effort to quiet the bird.

SELF-MUTILATION AND FEATHER DESTRUCTIVE BEHAVIOR. Feather destructive behavior, also called feather picking or plucking, is a well-known but poorly understood condition. The bird uses its beak to chew on and pull out any feathers that are accessible, including any that start to grow back. Some birds remove all but the feathers on their heads, and some may damage muscle as well as skin (Fig. 12-28). Some affected birds may have an underlying medical condition that initiates plucking, but some healthy birds respond to stress with self-mutilation (Fig. 12-29). Stresses can be in the form of separation anxiety from the owner, a change in the cage location, or the addition of a new pet or family member. This is a difficult problem to solve and may become a chronic condition. It is most common in cockatoo species and African Grey Parrots (Fig. 12-30).

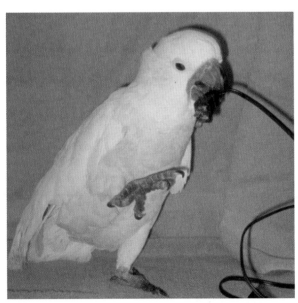

FIGURE 12-27 Birds are naturally curious and will chew on almost anything. (From Sirois M: Principles and practice of veterinary technology, ed 3, St Louis, 2011, Mosby.)

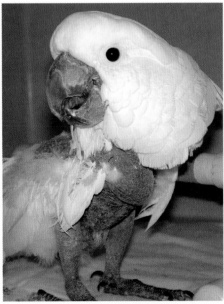

FIGURE 12-28 Some birds will remove all the feathers that they can reach, such as this cockatoo with a featherless body and fully feathered head. (From Sirois M: Principles and practice of veterinary technology, ed 3, St Louis, 2011, Mosby.)

The most important first step in correcting this behavior is a thorough medical workup to rule out any underlying pathologic conditions. Once a medical condition has been ruled out or treated, behavior modification and training can be implemented. Once feather destructive behavior has been established, behavior modification and training may decrease the severity of the disorder but will rarely stop the habit completely.

INAPPROPRIATE BONDING. Some owners will unintentionally allow a parrot to form a sexual bond with them by

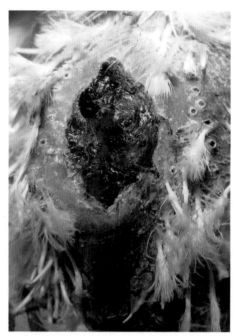

FIGURE 12-29 Cervical self-mutilation wound on a cockatoo. Feather mutilation and plucking can often go a step further; the bird can start to destroy the skin and muscle and, eventually, internal structures. (From Sirois M: Principles and practice of veterinary technology, ed 3, St Louis, 2011, Mosby.)

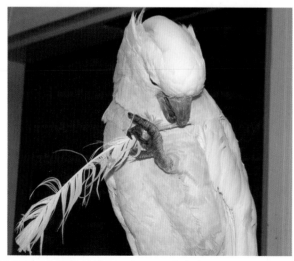

FIGURE 12-30 Feather mutilation and plucking is a common behavior in cockatoos. (From Sirois M: Principles and practice of veterinary technology, ed 3, St Louis, 2011, Mosby.)

inappropriate petting. Petting the bird repeatedly over its back and tail sends a message to that bird that is comparable to courtship behaviors performed in the wild. Cuddling and feeding the bird warm foods by hand or mouth can have similar inappropriate bonding results. The bird may pant and masturbate; this is especially common in cockatoos. Chronic masturbation can lead to medical problems that may require corrective surgery.

Correction of behavior problems takes time, an understanding of the underlying cause, and judicious use of behavior modification. Prolonged physical or mental isolation of the bird, withholding food or water, and physical punishment are totally unacceptable methods of dealing with these problems. All may result in permanent emotional or physical damage to the bird.

CLIENT EDUCATION

Client education is a vital service that you must provide to ensure the well-being of your avian patients. Most birds that present to your clinic for the first time will have medical problems related to improper diet and husbandry provided by ill-educated clients. Client education needs to be available for a vast range of topics, including proper cages and perch dimensions, substrate, safe transport, nutrition, and disease prevention. Handouts are easy to create about these topics, and appointments can be made with the knowledgeable veterinary technicians on the staff to discuss these topics and address any problem areas.

HOUSING AND HUSBANDRY

Enclosures for birds come in many shapes and sizes designed to appeal to the client but that may fail to address the needs of the bird. The enclosure should be spacious; the minimum size would allow the bird to spread its wings without touching the sides of the cage. It should be easy to clean and disinfect regularly and be constructed of a durable, nontoxic material. Newspapers or paper towels are inexpensive, safe substrates for birds and do not promote the growth of pathogens as do other organic substrates such as wood shavings and corncob bedding. Some of the latter substrates can also be ingested and create a gastrointestinal (GI) foreign body with the possibility of obstruction. The position of the enclosure should be in a draft-free area, partially out of direct sunlight, and in an area of the house in which the family routinely congregates.

Perches should be made from branches of clean, nontoxic hardwood trees and shrubs free of pesticides, mold, or wood rot. Birds need varying sizes, textures, and irregularly shaped perches to decrease the pressure placed on any one point of the foot and decrease the potential for pododermatitis.

Food dishes, toys, mirrors and other accessories should be provided without overcrowding the bird. If there is insufficient room to move about, the bird may not exercise appropriately and become entrapped in parts of the accessories or toys and be injured. Toys should be made of nontoxic substances and of an appropriate size for the bird so as not to allow for ingestion of the pieces.

Nutrition is an important subject and requires a handout for routine inquiries. Fresh water should be provided at all times. The water dish should be placed high in the bird's cage and not below any perches to decrease the possibility of fecal contamination. Birds should be offered fresh food on a daily basis. The optimal diet consists of a variety of pellets (70%) and fresh fruits and vegetables (30%). Feeding the bird at the dinner table and from the client's mouth should be discouraged because some human foods are too high in salts and sugars and some can be toxic to the bird, such as chocolate and avocado. Conversion from seeds to pellets is encouraged; clients may need assistance with this task in the form of a handout and face to face or telephone consultations.

CRITICAL CONCEPT

For birds on an all-seed diet, the hospital stay is not the time to convert from seeds to pellets. If the patient is ill and will eat only seeds, do not force the issue; let the patient get well first. It is a good idea to try a healthier diet with fortified pellets; you may be pleasantly surprised, and the patient may instantly take a liking to the pellets or even some fresh fruits and vegetables.

BEAK, WING, AND NAIL TRIMMING
BEAK TRIMMING

Overgrowth of the beak in psittacines is a common deformity (Fig. 12-31). It is important that you know (or have a reference for) the normal lengths of the beaks of various species. It is also important to try to determine why the beak is overgrown. In some cases, overgrowth results from malocclusion, resulting in insufficient wear on the beak; liver disease can be another cause. Any patient presenting for beak overgrowth should be required to have a complete workup to determine the cause.

Reducing the length and grooming the beak can be done with a Dremel Moto Tool (Dremel, Racine, WI). Cone-shaped aluminum oxide grinding stones work well on beaks and toenails. To prevent the spread of disease, it is best to have a separate grinding stone for each patient, which you can sell to the owner and the owner can bring to each visit. To perform this procedure, the restrainer holds the bird in an upright position. The person performing the trim holds the beak closed with one hand and applies the Dremel with the other (Fig. 12-32). Care should be taken not to cover the nares as you hold the beak shut. Monitor the patient closely for hypoxia and hyperthermia. Once you have achieved the desired length or shape, a small amount of mineral oil can be applied to remove the dust and make the beak aesthetically pleasing.

WING TRIMMING

Trimming a bird's wings is one method to decrease the bird's ability to fly. This is done by selectively trimming some of the primary and secondary feathers. The flight feathers are numbered 1 through 10 from the inside out. There is a natural break in the direction of the feathers, with the feathers of the manus (primaries, P-1 to P-10) angled out and the feathers on the brachium and antibrachium (secondaries, S-1 to S-10) angled in.

It is important to question the client to determine how much flight is needed and how aesthetically pleasing he or she wants the trim. A nice, aesthetically pleasing trim leaves the distal two primary feathers intact, trimming only four to eight feathers on each wing. The recommendation is to trim both wings evenly for balance. The general rule of wing trim is that the heavier bodied is a bird, the fewer feathers are removed.

The trim is done up high under the coverts, so that the jagged edges of the cut feathers are not showing. Evaluate

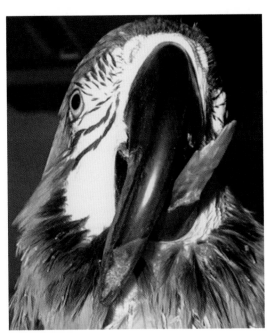

FIGURE 12-31 The need for a beak trim will be obvious in some patients. (From Sirois M: Principles and practice of veterinary technology, ed 3, St Louis, 2011, Mosby.)

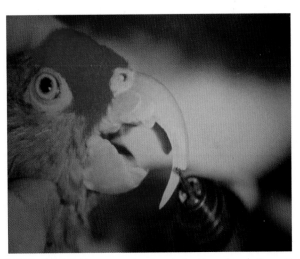

FIGURE 12-32 Trimming a beak with the Dremel tool. (From Sirois M: Principles and practice of veterinary technology, ed 3, St Louis, 2011, Mosby.)

the feather to be trimmed and ensure that it is not a blood feather; these should be avoided. If one is located, the mature feather on either side should be left as support. Flying ability should be tested in the clinic before the bird is sent home. Flight distance should be limited to less than 25 feet and lift to less than 2 feet. Additional feathers can be trimmed after a flight test if necessary.

Various instruments are used to perform wing trimming; these include suture scissors, cat nail trimmers, wire cutters, and sharp-sharp scissors. Prevent the spread of disease by sterilizing the trimmers after each use.

> ### CRITICAL CONCEPT
> Always test the bird's flying ability in the clinic after trimming flight feathers.

NAIL TRIMMING

A regularly requested service is trimming of long or sharp nails. Nail trimming is an important preventive care procedure. Excessive nail length can result in improper perching and the nail could be traumatically avulsed. An overgrown nail could get caught in the grate commonly found in the bottom of most bird cages or on the carpet as the bird wanders around the house. Untrimmed nails can grow into the pad of the foot, causing cellulitis or abscess formation. The size and temperament of the bird determines the number of people required to perform the trim (Fig. 12-33). Towel restraint is commonly used.

The most common tools used for nail trims include Resco trimmers (Tecla, Walled Lake, MI), the Dremel (motorized) tool, files, nail scissors, fingernail trimmers, and cautery instruments. These should be disinfected or sterilized after use to help prevent the spread of disease between birds. The Dremel tool, typically used on large birds, uses a grinding tip to blunt the tips of the nails. This handheld motorized tool is noisy and can overheat nail tissues if applied too long. Flat or rounded fine-toothed files are preferred by some for trimming the nails of birds of any size. This method slowly

blunts the nail tips, causing some birds to become impatient and struggle. Clients can be trained to do this at home if the pet and owner are willing. Some veterinarians use electrocautery instruments to trim nails and prevent bleeding at the same time. Many birds exhibit pain reactions to this procedure, presumably related to the high heat of the instrument. This method of nail trimming should be done primarily on anesthetized animals.

Any blood loss in birds should be considered serious. In very small birds, loss of what appears to be a minute amount of blood is potentially fatal. When bleeding is noticed, a hemostatic powder must be pressed immediately onto the nail.

DETERMINATION OF GENDER

Pet birds often have spectacularly colorful plumage. However, it is important to realize that it is almost impossible to determine the gender of most companion birds by appearance because males and females of each species look identical. The major exception to this rule is the eclectus parrot, in which the female is a deep reddish color, with a dark beak, and the male is bright green, with an orange beak (Fig. 12-34). The gender of a bird can be determined by endoscopy; however, DNA sexing is a safer alternative to the surgical approach and is available through some labs around the country. With a very small amount of whole blood (1 or 2 drops), the gender of a bird can be determined within a few days. DNA sexing uses the polymerase chain reaction (PCR) assay to analyze the DNA from the sex chromosomes of the bird.

MICROCHIPPING

Microchipping is an identification method that uses a tiny computer chip with an identification number programmed into it that is encapsulated in a biocompatible material. The whole device is small enough to fit inside a hypodermic needle and can be simply injected IM, where it will stay for the life of the bird. This provides a permanent positive identification that cannot be lost, altered, or intentionally removed.

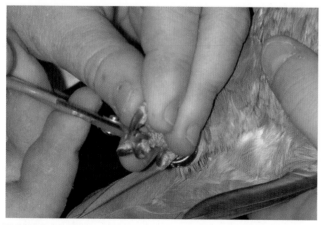

FIGURE 12-33 Grasp one toe at a time, keeping the other toes safely away from the trimmer so that the other toes or toenails will not be cut by mistake. (From Sirois M: Principles and practice of veterinary technology, ed 3, St Louis, 2011, Mosby.)

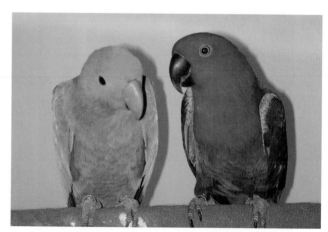

FIGURE 12-34 A pair of eclectus parrots demonstrate sexual dimorphism. Determining the sex of the average psittacine seen in an avian practice is not that easy. DNA sexing is an available and reliable blood test that requires only one drop of blood, and the results are rapid. (From Sirois M: Principles and practice of veterinary technology, ed 3, St Louis, 2011, Mosby.)

Microchip devices are sold as a disposable syringe and large-needle unit for one-time use. Before anesthetizing the bird for placement of a microchip, it is best to scan the patient to verify that there is not already a chip present. Also scan the chip to ensure that it works. The bird should be anesthetized for the procedure because the microchip is injected into the pectoral muscle via a 15-gauge needle, which can be a painful and stressful procedure. The site should be aseptically prepared. After the chip has been inserted, scan the bird to verify that the chip is functioning correctly.

PHYSICAL EXAMINATION

HISTORY

The physical examination occurs in three unique steps. The first is a thorough history combined with a brief visual examination, followed by the complete, hands-on physical examination. One of the most important first steps when evaluating an avian patient is to obtain a detailed history (Fig. 12-35). Husbandry-related problems are common findings with the first visit to an avian practitioner. Many medical conditions can be directly related to poor diet and husbandry.

PROCEDURE BEFORE CAPTURE AND RESTRAINT

The physical examination starts with observing the bird's behavior and physical appearance before capture and restraint. Companion birds are commonly a prey species with survival instincts and frequently alter their behavior when they are in a stressful environment, such as a clinic. Birds will mask their symptoms so as not to stand out in their flock, so they will not be eliminated by a predator or members of their own flock. The respiratory rate should be smooth and regular; a healthy bird should show no signs of increased effort. If the bird is exhibiting a tail bob, forward movement of the head, or open beak breathing, this could be a sign of respiratory distress and may need immediate attention. If the is bird trying to sleep, is droopy-eyed, wobbling, or barely hanging on to the perch, immediate medical attention may be necessary.

When a bird is stressed or excited, its droppings may be mostly urine. Seed eaters will have drier droppings than those with a diet supplemented with fruits. If the bird is anorexic, the droppings will be fewer. Blood, parasites, or undigested seeds may be seen in the droppings. The feces may be green or light brown and may vary in consistency among species and according to diet. The color of the droppings can be affected by the color of the food consumed. The urine should be clear, and the urates can appear white to a pale tan. In addition to the species and any disease considerations, water intake and diet influence the appearance of droppings.

CAPTURE AND RESTRAINT

Restraint is often required for the safety of the patient and those working with the bird. You must learn how to capture and restrain the avian patient safely and confidently to perform various procedures, such as a thorough physical examination and many different diagnostic and therapeutic procedures.

Competent knowledge about birds and handling of the avian patient in the clinic will inspire confidence in your client.

Capturing a bird needs to be done in a room that can be sealed and has no escape route or hiding places for the bird to access. Close and lock the door, close the window blinds or shades, turn off any fans, and remove any cage accessories. Darkening the room may help reduce the stress of capture in some cases—mainly for smaller birds that otherwise try to fly around in their cages.

A terry cloth towel is often useful when capturing and restraining birds that range in size from cockatiels or conures to the largest parrots (Fig. 12-36). Paper is sometimes used when restraining parakeets, cockatiels, or conures. The bird should be allowed to chew on the towel if it wishes, which keeps its beak busy and makes it less likely for the holder to be bitten. The use of a towel to capture a bird helps keep the bird from developing a fear of hands. When the animal returns home after being captured by a human hand, the bird may have a fear of its owner's hands, possibly creating a dissatisfied client. The use of gloves is discouraged because this also will create a fear of hands. Gloves also reduces the handler's tactile sensation and ability to feel the patient's most subtle movements and reactions to the stress of restraint.

Small pet birds such as finches, canaries, and parakeets are sometimes transported to the veterinarian in their own cage. They must be safely and gently removed for a hands-on physical examination. Slow and deliberate movements minimize stress to the bird, accompanied by a quiet tone of voice for reassurance. Place the towel over the patient, gain control of the head, pin the wings to the body, and pick the patient up.

Larger parrots may be caught in the cage, in the carrier, on the floor, or from a tabletop. Never capture a bird from the owner's shoulder. This is dangerous because the bird might bite the owner. As with small birds, a slow and deliberate approach works best. A quiet, soothing tone of voice should be used when approaching the bird. In most cases, a towel is used during capture to avoid injury to the bird or handler. It is extremely important to exhibit confidence in the approach to large birds, because they may become aggressive when they detect uncertainty.

Once the bird is captured, the towel can be wrapped around the bird to form a so-called birdy burrito to control the wings and the legs. With or without a towel, the body of the bird can be tucked under your arm once you have control of the head. This will aid in restraint of the wings. As with all methods of restraint, you must monitor the patient carefully for stress, hypoxia, and hyperthermia.

The restrainer is the primary person monitoring the bird's condition and stress level during the examination. This allows the person performing the physical examination to proceed in a timely fashion. The restrainer should keep the bird from injuring itself and others and should assist the person performing the physical examination by readjusting his or her hands to allow access to the bird.

In some practices, a restraint board is used for procedures that require the awake (unanesthetized) bird to remain

AVIAN HISTORY FORM

General History

Bird's Name_____ Sex: M_____ F_____UNK_____

How was bird sexed?   Blood Test_____   Surgical?_____

Any specific Identification? (i.e. tattoo, band, microchip)_____

If bird is female, has she produced eggs in the past? (if yes, please describe)_____

Bird is a : Pet_____ Breeder_____

How did you acquire the bird?   Store_____Breeder_____Other (describe)_____

Date acquired? _____

Do you have any other pets? Y_____ N_____

If yes, please specify including ages and when acquired_____

Housing

Is this bird kept: Indoors_____ Outdoors _____ Both _____ (if both, please specify % time in each)
_____

Is the bird housed alone? Y_____ N _____ If no, describe _____

If bird is caged, what type of cage? _____

What do use on the bottom of the cage? _____

How often is the cage cleaned? _____

Method/ frequency of cleaning food/ water dishes _____

Any toys in the cage? Y_____ N _____ If yes, describe _____

Has the bird's environment changed recently? Y_____ N_____ If yes, describe_____

At night, do you cover the bird? Y_____ N_____

How many hours of darkness does the bird have each day? _____

Diet:

What foods are offered to your bird/ in what total percentages? (i.e. 50% seed, etc.)_____

What percentages of these foods do you remove from the cage at night? _____

Any supplements offered? Brand name? _____

Any treats offered? Type? How often?_____

Any recent diet changes or new foods? Y_____ N_____ If yes, describe _____

How is water offered? (i.e. sipper bottle, bowl)_____

Reason For Today's Visit:

What signs have you noticed that prompted today's visit? _____

How long have you noticed the problem?_____

Has your bird been sick previously? _____

Has the bird ever been seen by any other veterinarian? Y_____ N_____ If yes, when/ why?
_____

Have any tests been performed previously on your bird? Please circle all that apply:

Psittacosis; CBC; Psittacine Beak and Feather Disease; Polyoma Disease;   Parasites;Other bloodwork;

Other (please describe) _____

Additional comments (your comments regarding the reason for this visit):

FIGURE 12-35 Avian history form filled out by clients annually or as needed. (From Sirois M: Principles and practice of veterinary technology, ed 3, St Louis, 2011, Mosby.)

completely still, such as for radiographs or implantation of microchips for identification, or in other situations in which both hands may be needed to perform complicated tasks. Restraint boards should not be used except for radiographs, and only for heavily sedated or anesthetized companion birds. Proper handheld restraint allows for better observation of the bird's condition and a faster reaction time to return the bird to its cage or carrier if the patient is becoming too stressed during restraint (Fig. 12-37).

Restraint can be a stressful experience for a bird. It is not unusual for the bird to show signs of extreme distress when released. The bird will typically pant and exhibit open beak breathing, have hot feet, hold its wings away from its body, and fluff its feathers to allow air to cool the skin. Birds with areas of featherless areas on the face, such as African Greys and macaws, will blush occasionally. One restraint method that may be useful involves gripping the bird around the cervical region while extending its neck. This prevents the bird from dropping its head down and biting your fingers. This may look like a choke hold, but it is a helpful way to restrain macaws or other birds that have fragile facial skin that bruises easily with traditional restraint methods. With the other hand, keep the wings pinned to the sides of the body (Fig. 12-38). After restraint, these birds may develop bruises in the featherless areas on the face.

PERFORMING THE PHYSICAL EXAMINATION

Table 12-1 presents physiologic data for common avian species. When performing the physical examination, you should be systematic and proceed in a timely manner. A typical physical examination involves examination of the eyes, external auditory canals (or ears), nares, beak, and oral cavity. The crop and esophagus, neck, pectoral region, coelom and pelvic region, wings, legs, feet, and back are all palpated. Feather quality is evaluated, and the preen gland is checked. The heart, air sacs, lungs, and sinuses are auscultated. The cloaca is examined and the mucosa everted to examine for lesions. The restrainer may need to assist with opening the beak so that the oral examination can be performed. The bird should be in an upright position and the oral cavity exposed by using gauze or tape strips to gently fatigue the powerful muscles controlling the beak (Fig. 12-39). In smaller birds, you can use a small speculum such as a hemostat, paper clips, or small tape strips. When restraining the bird

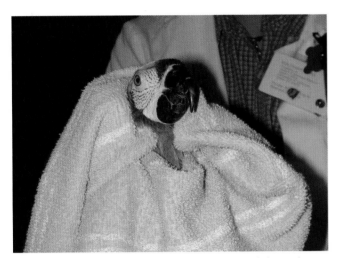

FIGURE 12-36 Small macaw captured by a terry cloth towel. (From Sirois M: Principles and practice of veterinary technology, ed 3, St Louis, 2011, Mosby.)

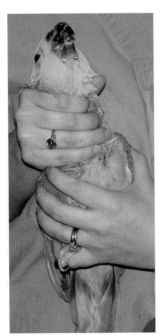

FIGURE 12-37 Improper method of restraint. The restrainer is compressing the keel, and the patient is unable to breathe properly. (From Sirois M: Principles and practice of veterinary technology, ed 3, St Louis, 2011, Mosby.)

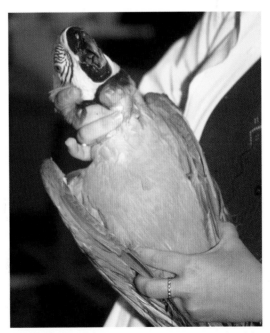

FIGURE 12-38 Choke hold restraint of a blue and gold macaw. (From Sirois M: Principles and practice of veterinary technology, ed 3, St Louis, 2011, Mosby.)

during examination of the wings, take care to curve the wing in the direction of the body at all times.

WEIGHING THE PATIENT. It is important to obtain an accurate weight of your patient at every visit. Some birds will sit on the scale nicely, but others may require that you place them in a box or small cage to weigh them (Fig. 12-40). Weigh the patient every time it comes into the clinic, even if the bird is not sick.

DIAGNOSTIC SAMPLING TECHNIQUES
BLOOD COLLECTION

Obtaining blood from a severely trimmed toenail is not acceptable. This is painful, stressful, and can yield abnormal cell distributions and cellular artifacts. A venous blood sample should be obtained. The medial metatarsal vein or leg vein is the vessel of choice for collecting blood in medium-to-large birds (Fig. 12-41). You must restrain the bird securely during blood collection. The person taking the blood will grasp the leg and syringe in one hand while collecting the sample; this will provide more control if the patient moves. The jugular vein is the method of choice for small birds such as parakeets and lovebirds (Fig. 12-42) because the other vessels are usually too small. Birds have two jugular veins; however, the

TABLE 12-1	Physiologic Data for Common Avian Species				
BIRD	**AVERAGE WEIGHT (G)**	**HEART RATE (BEATS/MIN)**	**RESPIRATORY RATE (BREATHS/MIN)**	**SEXUAL MATURITY**	**AVERAGE CAPTIVE LIFE SPAN (YR)**
Parakeets	30	500-600	60-70	6 mo	6
Love birds	38-56	400-600	60-80	8-12 mo	4
Cockatiels	75-125	400-500	40-50	6-12 mo	6
Conures	80-100	500-600	60-70	1-3 yr	10
Lories	100-300	300-500	35-50	2-3 yr	3
Cockatoos	300-1100	150-350	20-30	1-6 yr (species dependent)	15
Eclectus parrots	380-450	160-300	20-30	3-6 yr	8
Amazon parrots	350-1000	160-300	20-30	4-6 yr	15
Macaws	200-1500	120-300	15-32	4-7 yr (species-dependent)	15
African Greys	400-550	200-350	25-30	4-6 yr	15

Adapted from Sirois M: Principles and practice of veterinary technology, ed 3, St Louis, 2011, Mosby.

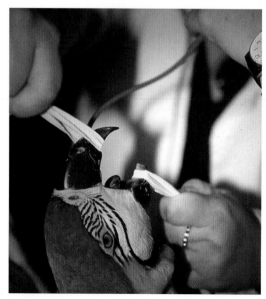

FIGURE 12-39 Oral examination method. (From Sirois M: Principles and practice of veterinary technology, ed 3, St Louis, 2011, Mosby.)

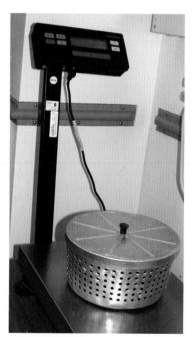

FIGURE 12-40 Weighing your patients is a vital part of monitoring the health status of hospitalized patients during the physical examination. The scale should be able to read to ±1 g. (From Sirois M: Principles and practice of veterinary technology, ed 3, St Louis, 2011, Mosby.)

right jugular is more prominent than the left. The restrainer should hold the bird in left lateral recumbency. The phlebotomist should arch and extend the neck, part the feathers, lightly wet them with alcohol, and find the featherless track and the jugular. Once the sample is collected, pressure must be applied by the restrainer; this is crucial to prevent large hematomas and possible bleeding out.

With appropriate restraint, the ulnar or basilic vein (also referred to as the wing vein) is an easily accessible vessel for venipuncture (Fig. 12-43). Because of the severity of the complications that can occur, it is recommended that this be attempted only on anesthetized patients.

FECAL EXAMINATIONS

The examination of feces requires a fresh sample, with little to no contaminants. A direct smear of the feces is the method for the detection of protozoa. Fecal flotation is needed to detect helminths. Gram staining should be included in any workup to detect yeast and bacteria. Grain- and fruit-eating Psittaciformes should have a gram-positive bacterial flora,

with potentially some yeast. A few yeasts or gram-negative bacteria per high-power field (HPF) could be considered normal, but budding yeasts are not normal. Carnivorous or insectivorous Passeriformes, raptors, Galliformes, and Anseriformes will have some gram-negative bacteria in their cloaca. A fecal occult blood test can also be performed.

IMAGING
RADIOGRAPHY

The diagnostic value of a radiograph is dependent on the quality of the technique and positioning of the patient. Most companion psittacine birds will require anesthesia or heavy sedation for diagnostic radiographs. If digital radiology is not available, high-detail rare earth cassettes with single-emulsion film provide desired results. Mammography film will produce even better detail but does require a higher kilovolt potential (kVP) and milliamperage (mA). The positioning of the patient is crucial for a diagnostic radiograph. The standard whole-body views are ventrodorsal (VD) and right lateral views. It is vital always to take both views. Plexiglas restraint boards that assist with patient positioning can be used and usually provide excellent results (Fig. 12-44). For the VD view, place the bird on its back, legs stretched down to expose the coelomic cavity, wings stretched out symmetrically to the sides, and two pieces of masking tape or paper tape in the form of an X across each carpus. Palpate the keel to ensure that it is in line with the backbone. A patient that is not positioned correctly can cause misinterpretation of the x-ray because of the superimposition of tissues and organs.

Positioning for the lateral view has the patient placed in right lateral recumbency, legs stretched downward, and wings pulled back together. Paper or masking tape is placed across the carpus to keep the wings back, and tape or gauze is used to keep the legs stretched downward. Once the plain films are reviewed, it may be necessary to isolate limbs for an individual shot or perform a contrast study of the GI system or an ultrasound.

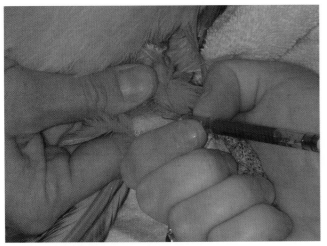

FIGURE 12-41 Venipuncture of the medial metatarsal vein. (From Sirois M: Principles and practice of veterinary technology, ed 3, St Louis, 2011, Mosby.)

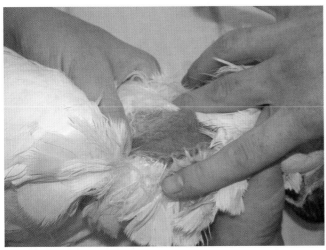

FIGURE 12-42 Jugular venipuncture. (From Sirois M: Principles and practice of veterinary technology, ed 3, St Louis, 2011, Mosby.)

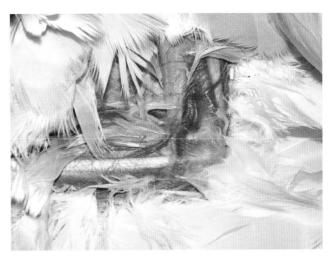

FIGURE 12-43 The ulnar or basilic vein should not be used routinely for blood collection because of hemostasis and traumatic injury concerns. (From Sirois M: Principles and practice of veterinary technology, ed 3, St Louis, 2011, Mosby.)

The VD and lateral views reveal the same lateral view of the wing. When two views are necessary, a posteroanterior (PA) view needs to be obtained. The PA can be obtained by placing the bird in a dive-bombing position—head on the plate, body up in the air. Extend the wing out as close to the plate as possible and collimate to the desired area (Fig. 12-45).

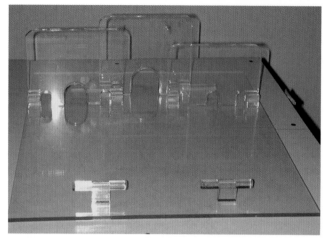

FIGURE 12-44 Avian restraint boards are used to assist with proper positioning for a radiograph. Most companion birds do not tolerate placement on such a device without heavy sedation or anesthesia. (From Sirois M: Principles and practice of veterinary technology, ed 3, St Louis, 2011, Mosby.)

STANDING RADIOGRAPH. The critically ill bird or one in respiratory distress may not be able to survive the stress of restraint required for a routine diagnostic radiograph. The bird can be placed in a cardboard box or induction chamber or allowed to stand on a low perch to obtain a standing radiograph. If your machine has horizontal beam capabilities, you can obtain a lateral standing view as well. These views are useful to evaluate for heavy metal densities, radiopaque foreign bodies, and bone density.

GASTROINTESTINAL CONTRAST STUDY

Contrast studies are often done when abnormalities are indicated on the plain films. These are done with the exact positioning as mentioned earlier for plain films, with the addition of barium. The barium is administered via a gavage tube into the crop. An immediate radiograph is taken, with subsequent views taken at 15, 30, 60, and 90-minute intervals. To reduce the risk of aspiration of barium from the crop, the patient can be elevated on the restraint board during positioning (Fig. 12-46). The board can be placed level for the radiograph and then elevated again for patient repositioning.

CRITICAL CONCEPT

To help prevent passive reflux of barium into the mouth during a GI contrast study, place a small Vet Wrap bandage around the bird's neck, close to the mandible.

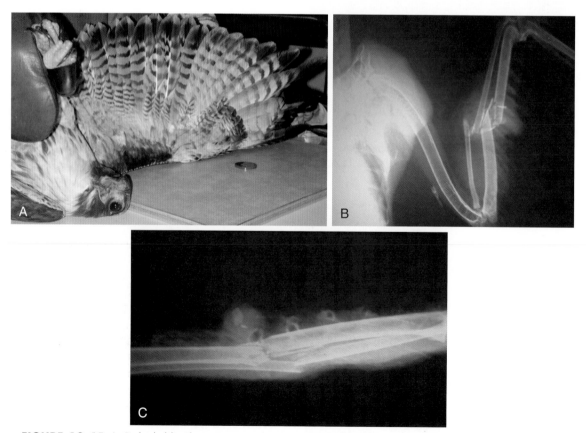

FIGURE 12-45 A, Red-tailed hawk in posteroanterior wing position for radiographs. B, Lateral view of the wing with a fracture. C, Posteroanterior view of the wing with the same fracture. (From Sirois M: Principles and practice of veterinary technology, ed 3, St Louis, 2011, Mosby.)

ENDOSCOPY

Endoscopes are fiberoptic probes that use magnification that can provide direct visualization of body structures. Many veterinarians use the 2.7-mm rigid fiberoptic endoscope because it can be successfully used for birds of almost any size (Fig. 12-47). Most endoscopic procedures are minimally invasive, and patient recovery time is more rapid than with exploratory surgery. Endoscopy can be used for the visual examination of any part of the body that has an orifice large enough to allow the insertion of the instrument. Laparoscopy, tracheoscopy, rhinoscopy, and cloacaloscopy are common diagnostic procedures. Using endoscopy, the veterinarian can obtain tissue biopsies and apply interlesional and topical treatments and surgical interventions, in addition to the sexing of nondimorphic species.

Proper positioning of the bird for the procedure is important. The organs or system to be studied determine whether the right or left side will be the site of entry for the endoscope. The bird will need to be anesthetized and the endoscope insertion site aseptically prepped and draped. The standard approach for diagnostic evaluation of the internal organs is right lateral recumbency. There are two approaches that can be used, one with the left leg pulled caudally and the other with the left leg pulled cranially. The specific position depends on the clinician's preference. A small incision is made in the skin, and the muscle layer is bluntly dissected with forceps. The endoscope and cannula are introduced into the incision through the cranial thoracic or abdominal air sac, and the organs can be viewed. The lungs, reproductive organs, kidneys, adrenal glands, ventriculus, and other organs will typically be visualized during this examination. Once the endoscopy is complete, the area will need to be sutured.

The endoscope is delicate and must be picked up by the eyepiece. Endoscope maintenance is essential. Proper cleaning and disinfecting will not only provide higher-quality diagnostics but also increase the longevity of the endoscope. Make sure to read the manual and follow the manufacturer's instructions for the proper care of each endoscope.

NURSING CARE

HOSPITALIZATION

Housing the avian patient can be a challenge if you have a small clinic. A separate room is needed for birds. The room should have its own thermostat and be able to maintain a room temperature of 85° to 90° F (29° to 32° C). The cages and perches should be easy to disinfect, and you should have a way to isolate patients suspected of carrying infectious diseases (Fig. 12-48).

For the patient with special requirements such as oxygen, supplemental humidity, or nebulization, you may need to get creative. Heat lamps and water-circulating heating pads are helpful for providing extra heat to the debilitated patient, but the enclosure needs to be monitored closely so that the patient does not become overheated or destroy the pads.

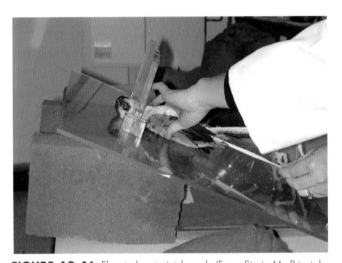

FIGURE 12-46 Elevated restraint board. (From Sirois M: Principles and practice of veterinary technology, ed 3, St Louis, 2011, Mosby.)

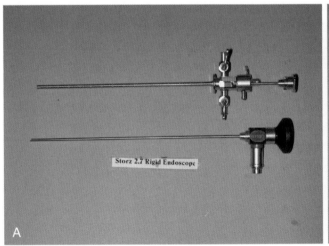
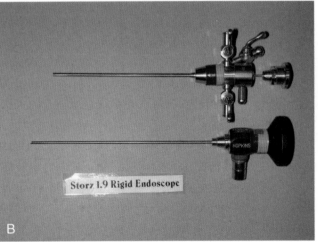

FIGURE 12-47 Common rigid endoscopes in an avian practice. **A,** The most valuable type for the avian practitioner is the 2.7-mm rigid endoscope. **B,** The 1.9-mm Storz rigid endoscope. (From Sirois M: Principles and practice of veterinary technology, ed 3, St Louis, 2011, Mosby.)

An investment in incubator-oxygen cages is recommended (Fig. 12-49). These cages can supply heat, humidity, and oxygen and are easy to disinfect.

Avian patients are extremely intelligent and, when hospitalized, can become bored and stressed. Patient enrichment is an important part of the patient's road to recovery. This can be achieved by providing the patient with nontoxic, safe disposable toys and mirrors or playing a radio or television for the patient to enjoy. If the patient is willing and receptive, you can spend a little time talking quietly and hand-feeding the bird in its hospital cage.

INFECTIOUS DISEASE AND ZOONOSES. Infectious and zoonotic diseases are critical problems for bird owners and veterinarians (Box 12-2). These can be caused by a variety of viruses or bacteria. Vaccines are available to protect pet birds against some of these diseases.

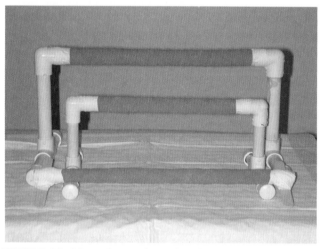

FIGURE 12-48 Perches can be made with inexpensive PVC pipe in a variety of sizes and heights. Padding can be added as needed for each patient. (From Sirois M: *Principles and practice of veterinary technology,* ed 3, St Louis, 2011, Mosby.)

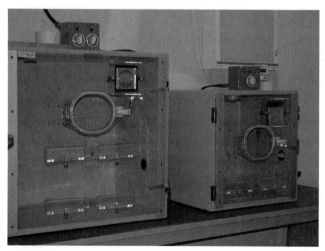

FIGURE 12-49 An oxygen cage is a valuable part of the avian practice. (From Sirois M: *Principles and practice of veterinary technology,* ed 3, St Louis, 2011, Mosby.)

The West Nile virus is a mosquito-borne disease that primarily infects horses, humans, and birds. It has spread rapidly throughout the United States in the past few years. Psittacines appear to be somewhat resistant because only a few cases have been reported from endemic areas. However, keeping pet birds inside or in screened areas is suggested to prevent exposure. No avian vaccine is available. Chlamydiosis is caused by the obligate intracellular bacterium, *Chlamydophila psittaci.* This is a zoonotic disease that causes psittacosis in humans and avian chlamydiosis in avian species.

Preventing the Spread of Disease in the Clinic. Patients suspected of having infectious diseases must be isolated from other patients. Isolation areas must be out of the mainstream of the clinic, where there is minimal foot traffic. Ideally, the isolation room should have a ventilation system separate from that of the main clinic. Disposable protective shoe covers or foot baths must be used when exiting this room to prevent carrying any infectious agent out of the isolation area.

All veterinary team members who handle animals suspected of having a zoonotic or any infectious disease must wear personal protective equipment, not only to protect themselves against infection but also to prevent transmission to others. Personal protective equipment includes disposable outer garments, laboratory coats or coveralls, disposable head or hair covers and gloves, safety goggles, and disposable particulate respirators approved by the National Institute for Occupational Safety and Health. Disposable equipment should be considered contaminated and properly disposed of after use. Nondisposable items such as laboratory coats and goggles should be cleaned and disinfected between uses. When removing contaminated protective equipment, personnel should first remove their outer garments, except for gloves, and discard them. They should then remove their gloves, wash their hands with soap and water, remove their goggles and particulate respirators, and immediately wash

---

BOX 12-2 | Infectious and Zoonotic Diseases of Birds

- Adenoviruses
- Avian influenza
- Avian polyoma virus (APV)
- *Chlamydophila psittaci* (zoonotic)
- Eastern equine encephalitis (EEE)
- Exotic Newcastle disease virus
- Fungal infections such as *Aspergillus* spp.
- *Mycobacterium* spp. (zoonotic)
- Papillomaviruses
- Paramyxovirus-3 (PMV-3)
- Poxviruses
- Psittacid herpesviruses (PsHVs), Pacheco's disease
- Psittacine beak and feather disease virus (PBFDV), circovirus
- Psittacine proventricular dilation disease (PDD)
- West Nile virus (WNV)

From Sirois M: *Principles and practice of veterinary technology,* ed 3, St Louis, 2011, Mosby.

their hands again. If soap and water are not available, an alcohol-based hand gel is sufficient. **NOTE:** Washing your hands is the primary and best way to prevent the spread of disease, so do it between each patient, regardless of whether the patient is suspected of carrying an infectious disease. Using these protective measures will help prevent the spread of disease in your clinic and protect those working with the patients. A number of websites are available that provide reliable, accurate, and timely information about infectious diseases and personal protection (Box 12-3).

PREPAREDNESS WHILE PROVIDING SUPPORTIVE CARE.

Preparation and efficiency are essential when providing supportive care to the avian patient. Try to develop a systematic routine that is followed consistently. Before capturing and restraining any patient, determine exactly what needs to be done and which patients you should start with. Prepare each patient's medications, fluids, and food before capture. Make sure to treat infectious disease suspects last, wear disposable attire (or change your laboratory coat or scrub top after handling), and wash your hands well after handling all patients to prevent the spread of disease.

ORAL ADMINISTRATION.

Medication and fluids may be administered to birds orally if the patient is alert and active. Primary regurgitation or vomiting, poor patient reflexes or recumbency, and oral and upper GI trauma may exclude this method. This route of administering medication is almost stress-free if the patient is tolerant. Some birds will love the attention of being hand-fed and medicated. Medications mixed in mashed banana or fruit baby foods are often well accepted.

Medication of feed and water is unreliable for most of the patients that you will see in practice. This method should not be used for pet birds. However, this is the major method of administering drugs to poultry and others in large flock situations.

GAVAGE FEEDING.

Fluid therapy, nutritional support, and medication administration can be provided by gavage or tube feeding. Limiting factors may include patients with crops stasis, ileus, GI impactions, or other GI abnormalities that reduce motility or absorption. A variety of flexible and rigid feeding needles and tubes are available (Fig. 12-50).

Gavage feeding will require a number of people for larger birds, but with smaller birds a skilled person can usually do it alone (Fig. 12-51). In larger birds, one person holds the patient in an upright position, another opens the mouth, and another person advances the tube into place and administers the medications and food. Care must be taken so that the patient does not bite the tube and ingest it. The tube can be palpated in the crop to verify correct placement. While administering the medications or food, watch the back of the bird's mouth. If food or liquid material appears in the oral cavity, the bird should be placed back into its enclosure immediately without further handling to prevent the risk of regurgitation and potential aspiration.

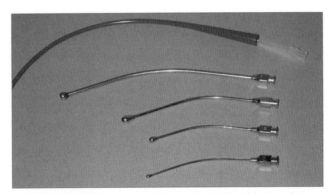

FIGURE 12-50 Gavage needles and red rubber feeding tubes can be used to provide fluid nutritional support and medications to hospitalized birds. (From Sirois M: Principles and practice of veterinary technology, ed 3, St Louis, 2011, Mosby.)

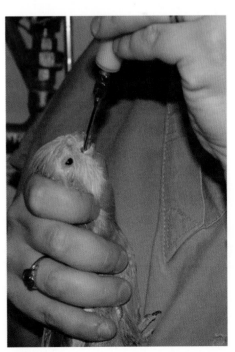

FIGURE 12-51 This experienced technician is able to gavage-feed this cockatiel alone, which is the standard accepted method. (From Sirois M: Principles and practice of veterinary technology, ed 3, St Louis, 2011, Mosby.)

BOX 12-3	Resources for Information on Infectious Diseases

- Centers for Disease Control and Prevention (http://www.cdc.gov)
- World Health Organization (http://www.who.int)
- National Institute of Allergy and Infectious Diseases (http://www3.niaid.nih.gov)
- Occupational Safety and Health Administration (http://www.osha.gov)

From Sirois M: Principles and practice of veterinary technology, ed 3, St Louis, 2011, Mosby.

SUBCUTANEOUS INJECTION SITES. Subcutaneous sites are found in the inguinal, axillary, and dorsal regions. The inguinal region is the preferred site to administer SC fluids and medications (Fig. 12-52). The patient is restrained in dorsal recumbency and the legs pulled straight down. A small amount of alcohol is applied to the medial side of the most proximal portion of the leg, parting the feathers. A small-gauge needle is inserted just under the skin. Similar administration techniques are used for the axillary and dorsal regions; however, you cannot get as much fluid into these areas.

INTRAMUSCULAR INJECTIONS. For IM injections, the pectoral muscles are generally used. These represent the largest muscle mass on the bird and are found on both sides of the keel (Fig. 12-53). A small-gauge needle is used to reduce the amount of muscle damage, and a different area of the muscle is used for any subsequent injections. The patient

is restrained in an upright position. The technician will then wet the feathers slightly to visualize the skin.

BANDAGING. The figure-of-eight bandage is used when a patient is presented with fractures or soft tissue injuries distal to the elbow, or when you need to stabilize a wing with an intraosseous catheter. Soft roll gauze followed by a layer of self-adherent bandage material will provide the best results. Restrain the bird with the wing in a flexed position. The bandage is started at the carpus and the gauze wrapped around the carpus, thus creating the top of the eight in the figure eight. The gauze is rolled toward the elbow and wrapped around the area proximal to the elbow. This will create the lower end of the figure eight.

A body wrap is added in addition to the figure-of-eight bandage when the patient has a humeral or pectoral girdle fracture. When placing a body wrap, care must be taken not to place tension on the keel, which can cause inadequate breathing. The body wrap is placed directly over the keel without putting pressure on the crop or coelomic cavity or interfering with the movement of the legs. Once the bandage is in place, the bird should be monitored for increased stress, dyspnea, and chewing or destroying the bandage. An Elizabethan collar or sedative may be necessary in some cases.

ELIZABETHAN COLLAR PLACEMENT. Elizabethan collars (E collars) and other mechanical barriers are placed for many reasons, including prevention of self-trauma such as feather picking and self-mutilation or protection of a bandage or wound (Fig. 12-54). You can make these collars out of old x-ray film or insulation pipe found at the hardware store, or you can purchase small versions of the ones used for canine and feline patients. If you make a collar, the edges must be padded to prevent sores from forming and ensure that the bird cannot chew at the outside rim of the collar. Crib-type collars have an attachable disc. This collar prevents the bird from dropping its head far enough to pick at the upper and

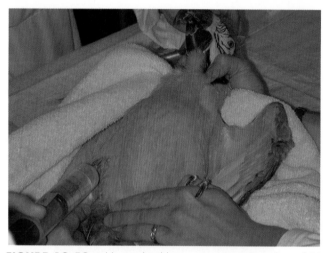

FIGURE 12-52 A blue and gold macaw is receiving a dose of SC fluids in the right inguinal region. (From Sirois M: Principles and practice of veterinary technology, ed 3, St Louis, 2011, Mosby.)

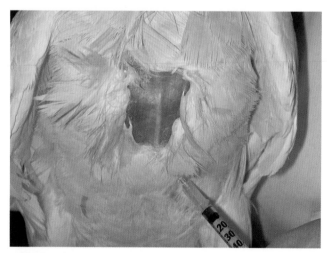

FIGURE 12-53 The pectoral muscles are the optimal site for IM injections in birds. (From Sirois M: Principles and practice of veterinary technology, ed 3, St Louis, 2011, Mosby.)

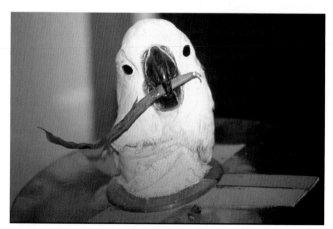

FIGURE 12-54 Some birds adapt very well to life in an E-collar. Every bird will need to be monitored for proper hydration and ability to eat. (From Sirois M: Principles and practice of veterinary technology, ed 3, St Louis, 2011, Mosby.)

lower portions of the body. In some cases, the bird can still reach the area just below the lower rim of the crib collar and the tips of the wings. The disc can be added to prevent any picking altogether; however, you should monitor the bird closely to ensure that it can still eat and drink. Commercially available bubble-style E collars can be used but may not be as effective at keeping the bird from reaching the back half of its body (Fig. 12-55).

When a collar is first placed on the bird, sedation and cage padding may be required until the collar is accepted. Some birds are highly stressed after the collar is placed and begin flipping in all different directions, along with flapping uncontrollably and screaming. Once the bird has adjusted to the collar, you can return the bird to its owner, provided that you counsel the owner about possible complications with use of the collar. These include trouble eating and drinking, trouble with balance and navigating around its normal environment, and pressure sores or abrasions from the collar.

COMMON DISEASES AND CONDITIONS

An emergency can be defined as a sudden or unforeseen situation that requires immediate action (Box 12-4). Emergency care of the avian patient can be challenging. Birds are primarily species that are preyed on and tend to mask signs of illness as a means of self-preservation. Instinctively, birds hide these symptoms so that they will not be killed by members of their own flock or by a predator for being the weakest in the flock. By hiding their illnesses,

birds can be in an advanced state of debilitation by the time they are brought into the clinic. In some cases, handling for examination can be contraindicated, and supportive therapy should be considered a priority. The bird that is having trouble perching or is fluffed may be very ill and should be considered an emergency. Fluffing—elevating the body feathers to trap warm air near the body—is a bird's response to loss of body heat (Fig. 12-56). Birds are often presented with nonspecific signs such as being fluffed up, sitting on the cage bottom, loss of appetite, untidy appearance, lethargy or weakness, droopy eyelids, and loss of interest in its surroundings. The bird that is simply not doing well is a challenge. Patient size often limits the diagnostic and treatment options.

A bird in respiratory distress can present to your clinic for a variety of reasons, including inhaled toxins, space-occupying masses in the coelomic cavity, foreign body aspiration, tumors or other growths in the airway, or respiratory disease. Normal respiratory patterns should be slow and regular and, in the healthy bird, almost unnoticeable (Box 12-5). The respiratory rate can vary from 10 to 40 breaths/min, depending on the size of the bird. Upper airway emergencies can result from aspirated foreign bodies such as seeds, splinters from wooden

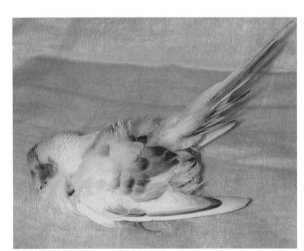

FIGURE 12-56 When a bird is cold or does not feel well, it will elevate its body feathers to trap warm air near the body to conserve energy for other vital functions, such as metabolic functions. (From Sirois M: Principles and practice of veterinary technology, ed 3, St Louis, 2011, Mosby.)

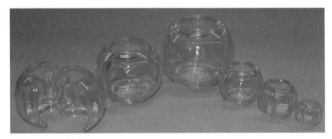

FIGURE 12-55 Commercially available bubble-style E-collars. (From Sirois M: Principles and practice of veterinary technology, ed 3, St Louis, 2011, Mosby.)

BOX 12-4	Avian Emergencies

Dyspnea, gasping for air
Bleeding
Generalized weakness
Sudden depression
Fluffed bird
Trauma
Trouble perching
Regurgitation, vomiting, inappetence
Coelomic distention
Prolapsed cloaca

From Sirois M: Principles and practice of veterinary technology, ed 3, St Louis, 2011, Mosby.

BOX 12-5	Signs of Respiratory Distress

- Tachypnea
- Labored respiration
- Open mouth respiration
- Audible respirations
- Change in vocalizations
- Tail bobbing
- Collapse

From Sirois M: Principles and practice of veterinary technology, ed 3, St Louis, 2011, Mosby.

toys, or other pieces from toys in the cage. Any condition that results in tracheal obstruction can lead to an upper airway emergency (Box 12-6).

RESPIRATORY EMERGENCIES

LOWER AIRWAY. Airborne toxins are dangerous to birds. They may die within a few minutes of exposure or develop chronic problems. Examples include overheated polytetrafluoroethylene (Teflon) pans, hairspray, tobacco smoke, paint fumes, strong cleaning chemicals, carbon monoxide, and dust from lead-containing paint (Box 12-7).

Treatment for aerosol toxicity includes removing the source of the toxin and removing the bird from the toxic environment. Once in the clinic, the patient should be placed in an oxygen cage. In these situations, the lungs may have been compromised or damaged, so an air sac tube may have little to no effect. These cases are best managed with minimal stress or restraint of the patient, with supportive care such as nutritional, fluid, and oxygen therapy with nebulization.

SPACE-OCCUPYING MASSES. Some respiratory emergencies may be caused by a space-occupying mass in the coelomic cavity. This can be the result of egg stasis, tumors, organ enlargement, or fluid buildup in the coelom (Fig. 12-57). Birds need air to move through their air sacs to breathe, so if a space-occupying mass is putting pressure on the air sacs, the bird will present in respiratory distress. Obese birds will often present in respiratory distress because their adipose tissue is compressing the air sacs, causing difficulty breathing.

BLEEDING EMERGENCIES

A variety of conditions may cause bleeding emergencies (Box 12-8). Broken blood feathers will often be the result of a traumatic fall or injury to the bird. The bird may be covered in blood from flapping, or there may be an area covered with matted, bloody feathers. Immediately locate the broken blood feather. You may need to clean the site with saline or water while trying to locate the feather in question. If the bird is stable, apply direct pressure, with or without styptic powder, to stop the bleeding and try to save the feather from removal. If the bleeding will not stop, remove the feather using hemostats or needle-nosed pliers. With one hand, hold the wing stable and pull in the same direction that the feather is growing. Apply direct pressure to the feather follicle if bleeding continues.

EGG STASIS OR BINDING

Egg retention is defined as the failure of an egg to pass through the oviduct at a normal rate. This is a commonly seen emergency in parakeets, canaries, cockatiels, finches, and lovebirds. These birds typically have been laying eggs for some time, thus depleting their calcium stores. This causes decreased muscle activity in the oviduct, and the egg becomes trapped. Signs can include abdominal distention and straining, lack of droppings, depression, sitting on the cage bottom, tail wagging, and walking with widespread legs.

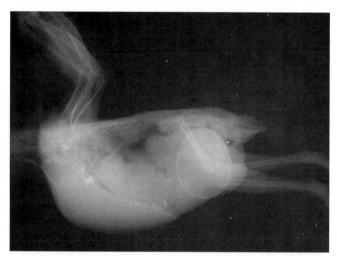

FIGURE 12-57 Space-occupying masses, such as the egg in the bird, can displace air sacs needed for air exchange. This can cause a bird to present to your clinic in respiratory distress. (From Sirois M: Principles and practice of veterinary technology, ed 3, St Louis, 2011, Mosby.)

BOX 12-6	Upper Airway Emergencies

Tracheal obstructions with:
- Tumors
- Papillomas
- Granulomas
- Transtracheal membranes

From Sirois M: Principles and practice of veterinary technology, ed 3, St Louis, 2011, Mosby.

BOX 12-7	Causes of Lower Airway Avian Emergencies

- Cigarette smoke
- Overheated polytetrafluoroethylene
- Pesticides
- Paint fumes
- Carpet-cleaning solutions
- Wood-burning stoves
- Hairspray and perfume
- Scented candles

From Sirois M: Principles and practice of veterinary technology, ed 3, St Louis, 2011, Mosby.

BOX 12-8	Avian Bleeding Emergencies

- Broken blood feathers
- Broken toe nails
- Wounds, big cat–little bird syndrome
- Open fractures

From Sirois M: Principles and practice of veterinary technology, ed 3, St Louis, 2011, Mosby.

In some cases, the bird may be limping because of the pressure placed on the pelvic plexus.

PROLAPSED CLOACA

Occasionally, birds will present to your clinic with a prolapsed cloaca (Fig. 12-58). The most important immediate therapy is to keep the prolapsed tissue moist and clean. If the patient is too stressed to restrain, you can place the patient in a cage lined with clean towels or gauze moistened with sterile saline. There are many aliments that can lead to a prolapsed cloaca, such as egg stasis, papillomas, chronic masturbation, and coelomic masses. It is important to determine the cause of the prolapse to ensure that it will not be a recurring problem.

ANIMAL BITES

This accident normally occurs when a larger animal attacks the smaller bird, and in some cases, birds versus bird (Fig. 12-59). Mammal bites are usually from a pet dog or cat

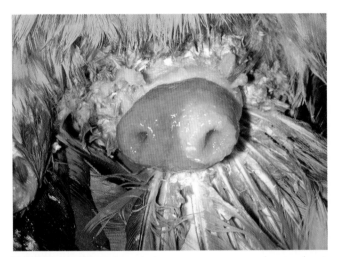

FIGURE 12-58 Prolapsed cloaca may occur secondary to chronic straining from egg laying, space-occupying masses, inappropriate social behavior, and masturbation. (From Sirois M: Principles and practice of veterinary technology, ed 3, St Louis, 2011, Mosby.)

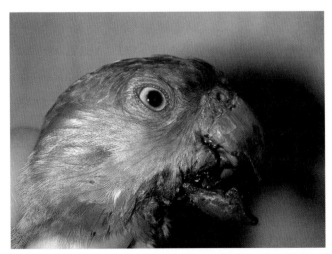

FIGURE 12-59 This Meyers parrot was attacked by a large bird and has severe trauma to the lower beak. (From Sirois M: Principles and practice of veterinary technology, ed 3, St Louis, 2011, Mosby.)

and are true emergencies. Pathogenic oral bacteria from such an animal can be detrimental to the avian patient. When a wound is located, it will need to be cleaned up. Remove any surrounding feathers by plucking. Be careful when attempting to flush while cleaning the wound because of the possibility that the puncture may communicate with an air sac. When in doubt, clean the wound but do not flush.

BEAK INJURIES AND REPAIR

Some birds inflict severe injuries to other birds if given the opportunity. They may destroy the upper or lower beak of their victim. Fractures of the mandible may occur. Even seemingly minor injuries may lead to permanent damage. After hemorrhage is controlled, the patient is evaluated for the type of repair that will be required.

FOREIGN BODIES

Foreign bodies are often ingested by a curious bird that has been roaming and chewing, a scenario similar to that found with mammals. Potential ingested foreign materials are toys or parts of toys, bedding, metallic items (e.g., wire, hairpins), string, fish bones, splinters, and tough plant fibers. A thorough physical examination and radiographs often determine the problem, but specialized studies may be required. Endoscopic techniques and/or surgical removal may be required to retrieve the objects.

FRACTURES

Birds are commonly presented with a number of different scenarios resulting in a fracture. These include being attacked by a larger animal, caught in its cage or cage toys, leg band entrapped in toys or other objects, flying into a window or ceiling fan, or being stepped or sat on. When this type of patient presents to your hospital, place the patient in a quiet, dark, well-padded environment until stable enough to restrain. Provide analgesics and determine the best method to stabilize the fracture.

Bandages and splints are used when some support of the fracture is all that is necessary (Fig. 12-60). This method

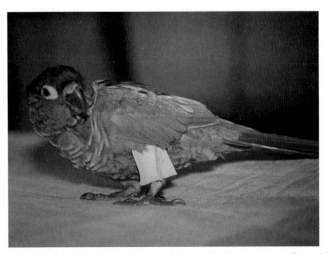

FIGURE 12-60 Tape splints are a lightweight alternative to traditional bulkier bandages for smaller birds. (From Sirois M: Principles and practice of veterinary technology, ed 3, St Louis, 2011, Mosby.)

will make the bird more comfortable but may not allow proper healing and return to full function. Fractures commonly stabilized with this treatment are some wing and foot breaks. Alternatively, there are many different surgical methods and approaches to fracture repair that will be case dependent. In extreme cases, a traumatized leg or wing cannot be salvaged. In this case, amputation may be the only choice. Most psittacines do well after losing a leg because they can use their beaks to move around. Most birds will perch comfortably but do run the risk of developing pododermatitis (Fig. 12-61) on the remaining foot. In pet birds, removal of a wing may cause some loss of balance, but most seem to manage rather well. Most birds are not troubled by toe amputations.

LEG AND WING FRACTURES. Fractures of the wing usually are immobilized with a figure-of-eight bandage. This holds the flexed wing snug against the body. If the humerus is fractured, a body wrap is also applied. An open fracture should also be cleaned and flushed, using caution because of the pneumatic bones of birds; flushing could introduce fluid into the airway. Appropriate supportive, antimicrobial, and analgesic therapies should be implemented as soon as possible. Most broken wings will need to be bandaged for 3 to 5 weeks, with routine changes. The bandage should be removed as soon as healing is complete. Complications include stiffness, muscle atrophy from disuse, and loss of flight feathers. Physical therapy will help the bird become limber and recover muscle mass.

Some lower leg fractures are stabilized with a splint until healing occurs, usually in 4 to 6 weeks. Because of the bird's anatomy, splints will often worsen fractures of the femur and upper tibiotarsus. These often require prompt surgical repair. Toe fractures can be treated in large birds by taping the broken toe to the neighboring intact toe. An open fracture should also be cleaned and flushed with caution because of the pneumatic bones of birds; flushing could introduce fluid into the airway.

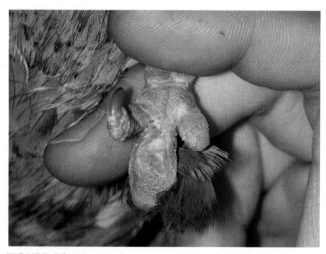

FIGURE 12-61 Pododermatitis on the foot of a bird. (From Sirois M: Principles and practice of veterinary technology, ed 3, St Louis, 2011, Mosby.)

The Schroeder-Thomas splint can be used to treat fractures of the lower third of the tibiotarsus and the entire tarsometatarsus. The bandage is changed every 1 to 3 weeks and is accompanied by passive physical therapy. A Robert Jones bandage can be used for simple lower leg fractures. Although these are heavily padded, additional splinting materials such as tongue depressors may be needed. The bandage needs to be changed at least every 2 weeks. A ball bandage is used for broken toes or pododermatitis. A ball formed of gauze sponges is placed so that the toes curl around it. The foot is covered with cotton padding and wrapped with stretchy, self-adherent bandaging. Very small birds can be difficult to splint. Materials such as pipe cleaners, toothpicks, paperclips, and wooden applicator sticks can be used to stabilize their fractures.

With all splints, it is necessary to assess circulation in the foot. Look for swelling of the toes, blue coloration, and coldness. The bandage will need to be changed if any of these occur. Bandages need to be checked often for signs of chewing or moisture. Clients should be advised to bring the bird in to the clinic for a bandage change. Removal of leg bands is advised because they may cause fractures when they become caught on the cage or other objects.

HEAD TRAUMA

Head trauma cases in which the bird flies into a window or a ceiling fan require immediate supportive therapy and evaluation. Place the patient in a dark, quiet, and (contrary to other situations) a cool environment to prevent vasodilation of the intracranial vessels. Provide supportive care as needed.

BURNS

Burns on birds commonly occur on the feet and legs. Birds that are left to fly freely through the house can run the risk of landing in a pot of boiling hot liquid or the burners of the stove, causing severe burns to the legs and feet. Burns to the oral cavity and tongue may occur if the bird bites an electrical cord. Treatments for burns is comparable to treating burns in other patients. Flush areas with copious amounts of cool water or saline and remove the surrounding feathers. Do not use greasy or oily medications because these can accumulate in the feathers and have an effect on thermoregulation. Silver sulfadiazine applied topically has antibacterial, antifungal, and analgesic effects.

CROP BURN AND CROP TRAUMA

Owners or breeders may bring in a baby bird that seems to have food leaking from its chest. A crop burn is normally caused by poorly mixed microwaved foods that are fed to neonates. Once the burn has occurred, normally in the right ventral portion of the crop, the crop and skin necrose, forming a fistula (Fig. 12-62). Food will leak from this fistula, creating an alarming situation for the client and maybe an emergency. If the bird cannot retain enough food or water, there is a risk of dehydration and starvation. This will require anesthesia and a surgical closure, but recovery

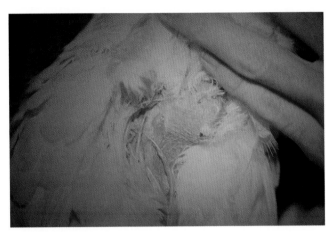

FIGURE 12-62 Crop fistula leaking food in a hand-fed juvenile cockatoo. (From Sirois M: Principles and practice of veterinary technology, ed 3, St Louis, 2011, Mosby.)

is usually fairly quick. Client education on how to heat the food properly is essential to prevent future crop burns.

HEAVY METAL TOXICOSIS

Birds are naturally curious and like to investigate unfamiliar objects with their mouths. When this behavior is combined with the bird being given free run of the house, the potential for ingesting foreign objects is increased. Unfortunately, this poses numerous hazards, one of which is heavy metal toxicosis. Some materials used for the cage or toys are made of zinc or lead. Because there is no quality control for toys manufactured for birds, the toys themselves can be made from toxic materials, and the client is generally unaware of this. Client education is a necessity.

Lead and zinc are the two most common heavy metal poisonings that you will encounter with avian patients. Typically, ingestion of curtain weights, lead clappers from bells, old-style solder, lead-based paints, plaster, foil from wine bottles, and calcium-rich dolomite or bone meal can cause lead poisoning. Galvanized cage wire is the usual source of ingested zinc. Treatment for lead and zinc toxicosis is supportive; it may include chelation therapy with calcium EDTA (ethylenediaminetetraacetic acid) and removal of the foreign body, if possible.

Diagnosis may be based on signs and radiographic findings of heavy metal densities within the body (Box 12-9). Whole-blood samples can be sent to an outside laboratory for heavy metal analysis. Consult with your laboratory about sample testing requirements. Some laboratories use serum or heparinized plasma for the zinc evaluation, and a separate sample is submitted in lithium EDTA for lead evaluation.

INGESTED POISONS

As noted, birds often explore new items by mouthing them and feeling their texture with their tongues. This exposes them to possible poisoning, with lethal effects. It is imperative to prevent contact of the pet bird with common household items that are poisonous and other potentially lethal

substances. Cleaning products can cause skin eruptions, GI upset (including vomiting and diarrhea), respiratory tract irritation, and esophageal damage. Hydrocarbon-based compounds such as furniture polish and other petroleum products can cause central nervous system effects such as disorientation and depression, pneumonia, GI upset, kidney and liver damage, and mucous membrane and skin damage. Perfumes and deodorants may cause damage to the skin and mucous membranes, respiratory tract, kidneys, liver, and central nervous system. Shampoos lead to irritation of the eyes and diarrhea. Small amounts of tobacco products can result in vomiting, diarrhea, convulsions, and sudden death. Eating fireworks or matches can result in vomiting, diarrhea, blood in the stools, and increased respiration. Cyanosis may also occur.

The client must be advised to bring the bird and container (if any) of the item ingested in for evaluation as soon as possible. To ascertain the correct treatment, consult a pharmacology reference book and call the poison control center.

POISONOUS PLANTS. Many plants have been blamed for illness in birds, but plant poisoning is actually rare. Birds often will tear leaves without eating them, decreasing the amount ingested. The avian GI tract empties quickly, further reducing the chance of poisoning. Owners may unintentionally expose their birds to poisonous plant materials through feeding, use of poisonous plants for perches, or certain house plants (Box 12-10).

If owners call the clinic with a bird showing unusual signs after exposure to any plant, they should be asked to bring the bird in for evaluation. Clients should be advised that poisonings can be lethal without prompt intervention. The offending plant or a sample should be brought to the clinic. The client should try to estimate the amount ingested.

BOX 12-9	Signs of Heavy Metal Toxicosis

- Lethargy
- Depression
- Anorexia
- Weakness
- Weight loss
- Anemia
- Regurgitation
- Polyuria
- Polydipsia
- Diarrhea
- Emaciation
- Ataxia
- Convulsions, paresis, paralysis
- Regenerative anemia
  Amazon parrots are the only species that will develop hematuria in acute cases. Eclectus will characteristically show biliverdinuria (greenish staining of urine). Other parrots have no urinary color changes.

From Sirois M: Principles and practice of veterinary technology, ed 3, St Louis, 2011, Mosby.

ETHICAL EUTHANASIA TECHNIQUES

Euthanasia is sometimes necessary to alleviate patient suffering and should be done in a humane manner. Having to make the decision to end a pet's life is never easy. Many people do not want to talk about it until they have to, and then it becomes a decision made under emotional stress. It is important to have the ability to discuss this issue with compassion and explain the details of the procedure with empathy.

Acceptable methods should include anesthesia to create an environment in which the patient is unaware of the injection. In some cases, the patient may be incoherent enough that only heavy sedation is necessary and, in others, gas anesthesia is required. When the patient is unconscious, a commercially available euthanasia solution can be administered. Routes of administration are IV, intracardiac, or IP. The patient must be anesthetized if an intracardiac or IP routes is to be used, and in all cases the patient must be monitored until its heart stops. If the client is present, you must make them aware that some patients may experience agonal breaths, muscle twitching, or vocalizations, the eyes may not close, and GI contents may release through the cloaca. In most cases, the patient will have a peaceful release of tension, as if going to sleep. Because of the animal's individual level of health and stress, each euthanasia procedure will be an individual experience.

REPTILES AND AMPHIBIANS

Reptiles and amphibians are a diverse group of animals that have become popular pets. The class Reptilia contains four orders, of which only two are commonly seen in the private clinical setting. These two orders include Squamata (snakes and lizards) and Testudines (turtles and tortoises). The most common lizards kept as pets in North America include iguanas, bearded dragon, geckos, chameleons, monitors, and water dragons. The most common snakes kept as pets in North America include boas, pythons, king snakes, rat snakes, corn snakes, and gopher snakes. The most common chelonians kept as pets in North America include box turtles, red-eared sliders and other water turtles, and various tortoises. It is important to remember that these are unique animals and not just small dogs and cats. If the veterinary hospital decides to treat reptiles, the staff must become knowledgeable about proper capture, restraint, diagnostic techniques and procedures, anesthesia, husbandry, and common diseases. The veterinary staff must be properly trained to handle reptiles because this can prevent injuries to the staff and patient. The class Amphibia contains three orders, which include Anura (frogs and toads), Caudata (salamanders, newts, and sirens), and Gymnophiona (caecilians). Although there are over 4000 species alive today, only a few are commonly seen in most clinical practices.

REPTILE BIOLOGY

Reptiles are ectothermic, meaning they cannot generate their own body heat. Instead, heat is obtained from the environment. Reptiles are able to regulate their body heat by moving in and out of the heat or shade. Each species has a specific temperature range at which it thrives. Reptiles have a protective layer of keratinous scales covering the skin. The outermost layer of the skin is shed on a regular basis. Species such as snakes shed their skin all at once. Just before the shed, the skin becomes sensitive and turns an opaque color (Fig. 12-63). It is suggested that the snake not be handled during this time unless absolutely necessary. The snake may become aggressive and anorexic just before and during the shed.

> ### CRITICAL CONCEPT
> Handling snakes should be kept to a minimum approximately 1 week before and during a shed because the skin is delicate and can be easily damaged.

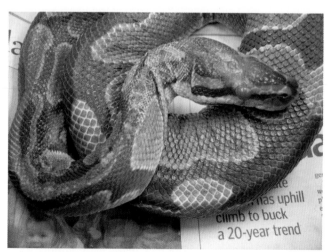

FIGURE 12-63 Just before shedding, the snake's skin and eyes turn an opaque blue color. The snake should not be handled just before and during the shed because this can damage the delicate new skin. (From Sirois M: Principles and practice of veterinary technology, ed 3, St Louis, 2011, Mosby.)

BOX 12-10	Toxic Plants

- Avocado
- Black locust*
- Clematis
- Crown vetch
- Dieffenbachia
- Foxglove
- Lily of the valley
- Lupine
- Oak*
- Oleander*
- Philodendron
- Poinsettia
- Rhododendron*
- Yew

*Should not be used for perches.
From Sirois M: Principles and practice of veterinary technology, ed 3, St Louis, 2011, Mosby.

Unlike snakes, lizards and chelonians shed their skin in pieces. Some reptiles will have problems shedding the skin. This is called dysecdysis. If the patient is having problems shedding the skin, the humidity in the cage should be increased or the animal can be soaked in a warm water bath (Fig. 12-64). You should always examine the toes of lizards such as leopard geckos if they are having problems shedding their skin because the skin can become wrapped around the digits, cutting off circulation and causing necrosis.

Like birds, reptiles lack a diaphragm to separate the thoracic and abdominal cavities. They have one visceral cavity called the coelom. Reptile excrement includes three components—urine, urates, and feces. This is similar to birds. The cloaca is the common opening through which the urinary, digestive, and reproductive systems empty.

HUSBANDRY

One of the most common reasons for a reptile patient being brought to the veterinary hospital is illness caused by poor husbandry and diet. It is therefore extremely important that clients be properly educated. The veterinary hospital should provide the client with accurate educational handouts or information.

HOUSING

Many pet reptiles can be housed in a simple terrarium. The cage should be appropriately sized for the animal; in most cases, the larger the better. The terrarium should be easy to clean and disinfect. Appropriate cage furniture should also be placed in the terrarium. Cage furniture will vary based on the species but includes items such as logs, plants, hide boxes, and rocks. Cage furniture is often used by animals to help them shed. The terrarium setup for amphibians will vary based on the species of amphibian with which you are working and whether it is aquatic or terrestrial. A terrestrial amphibian cage may consist of mosses, various plants, rocks, logs, and a small amount of water in the cage. An aquatic cage will have a completely different set of criteria. If the

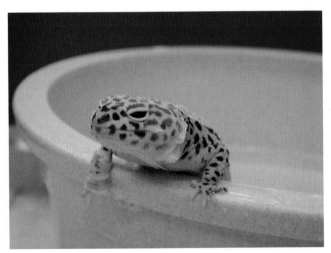

FIGURE 12-64 This leopard gecko has dysecdysis and is being soaked to help shed its skin. (From Sirois M: Principles and practice of veterinary technology, ed 3, St Louis, 2011, Mosby.)

amphibian is arboreal, you must provide height in the cage so that it can climb into a planted canopy. Regardless of the type of enclosure or species, the native habitat should be mimicked whenever possible.

> ### CRITICAL CONCEPT
> Placing appropriate cage furniture in the reptile's enclosure is important not only for providing hiding places and visual barriers, but also to help the animal shed. Reptiles rub against cage furniture such as logs, rocks, and plants to loosen their skin.

It is important to choose the appropriate bedding or substrate for the cage bottom. The substrate should be easy to remove for cleaning and replacement. Indoor-outdoor carpet is easy to clean and inexpensive enough to throw away when necessary. Other appropriate substrates include newspaper, butcher paper, hay, and commercial recycled newspaper bedding. Some people use wood chips and sand, but these can cause intestinal foreign bodies if eaten by the animal. Shavings should not be used because they can cause irritation to the respiratory tract.

Appropriate lighting is important for reptiles. Without the proper ultraviolet (UV) lighting, many species of reptiles cannot metabolize nutrients or synthesize vitamin D adequately. The light should be full spectrum with the light source being approximately 18 to 24 inches from the animal. UV bulbs need to be changed approximately every 6 months, even if they are not burnt out, because the UV portion of the light does not usually last longer than 6 months. Light cycles will vary by species.

Proper heating is critical for reptiles because they are ectothermic. Because reptiles thermoregulate using their surrounding environment, a basking spot (using various types of bulbs) providing increased heat should be provided, as well as a nonheated spot. The reptile will move between the two spots to regulate its own body temperature. The basking spot should be positioned so that the animal cannot come in contact with it. Hot rocks or sizzle stones should not be used to provide heat because they often have uncontrolled hot spots that can cause thermal burns (Fig. 12-65). Under-tank heaters can be useful in providing additional heat to the cage, but they should be used under only half of the cage so that the animal can escape the heat if necessary. Under-tank heaters can cause thermal burns if not used properly.

> ### CRITICAL CONCEPT
> Hot rocks and sizzle stones can cause thermal burns and should never be used in reptile enclosures.

Humidity requirements vary among different species of reptiles. Some tropical species such as the green iguana (*Iguana iguana*) require extremely high levels of humidity to stay healthy. This is difficult to provide in captivity, especially in dry areas of the United States. Many species of amphibians also need a temperature and humidity gradient in the cage.

Proper sanitation of the enclosure is important. The cage should be cleaned thoroughly and disinfected on a routine basis. Excrement should be picked up daily. Owners should be aware that all reptiles have the ability to shed *Salmonella* spp. if they are positive carriers of the bacteria. Owners should take precautions by wearing examination gloves during cleaning and handling of the pet. Handling the animal and cleaning of the enclosure should never take place near areas where food for human consumption is prepared or stored.

WATER QUALITY

Water quality and care is one of the most important aspects of caring for amphibious pets. Amphibians are sensitive to poisoning from nitrogenous waste buildup and disinfectant residues. Frequent water changes and having a good filtration system on the terrarium will help keep water parameters under control. There are several parameters that should be checked on a regular basis, including temperature, pH, salinity, water hardness, alkalinity, dissolved oxygen, carbon dioxide, nonionized ammonia, nitrite, nitrate, and chlorine.

FEEDING

Improper diet and nutrition is a common cause of disease in exotic animals. Diets are generally species-specific and are beyond the scope of this chapter. Commercial diets are available for some reptile species but are generally not recommended. Reptiles must have water available at all times and the water changed daily because reptiles often defecate in the dish. There is no simple commercial diet available for owners to feed amphibious pets. Most amphibians are carnivorous or insectivorous as adults. The key to providing a healthy diet is offering a variety of different types of food.

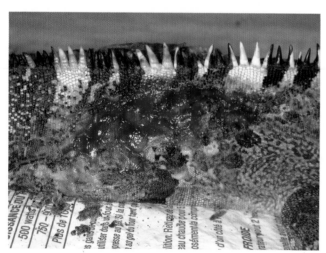

FIGURE 12-65 This lizard has a thermal burn caused by a light in the cage. (From Sirois M: Principles and practice of veterinary technology, ed 3, St Louis, 2011, Mosby.)

SNAKES

All snakes are carnivores and feed on whole prey items. The digestive system of snakes has evolved to digest whole prey and defecate the parts of the prey that are not digested, such as fur. Ingesting the entire carcass provides added nutrients such as calcium from bone. Further supplementation is not needed when feeding whole prey. Common whole prey items include rats, mice, rabbits, and guinea pigs. It is never appropriate to feed meat such as chicken breast, hot dogs, or raw beef because this does not provide a complete diet.

It is suggested that prekilled or stunned food be offered to snakes so that they will not be harmed by the prey item. Prekilled food can be ordered frozen from several companies. If frozen mice or rats are offered, they must be thawed before being offered as food.

LIZARDS

Feeding requirements vary with different species of lizards. Herbivores should be fed various types of dark, leafy greens and vegetables. Proper leafy greens include, but are not limited to, kale, chard, turnip greens, and escarole. Most insectivores can eat worms and insects such as mealworms, silkworms, and crickets. Carnivorous lizards should be fed whole prey. Whole prey includes all the bones, GI contents, muscle, and fur. Whole prey items include mice, rats, and fish, depending on the species that you are feeding. Omnivores should be offered a variety of dark, leafy greens and, in most cases, insects. The quality and variety of food offered are important. Animals should not be fed the same food day after day.

CHELONIANS

Most aquatic turtles are omnivorous; they generally consume food such as fish, invertebrates, algae, and leafy greens. Commercial diets are acceptable to feed in moderation, but it is important to make sure that they contain essential nutrients needed to maintain good health. Tortoises are herbivores. They eat a variety of food such as leaves, grasses, and flowers in the wild. In captivity, a healthy diet includes dark, leafy greens, rose petals, hay, and vegetables. Commercial diets can be fed in moderation and should be appropriate for herbivores. Do not feed dog food, tofu, monkey biscuits, or anything that has animal protein in it.

TAKING A HISTORY

A thorough history should be taken from the owner before the physical examination is performed. The owner should be asked to bring in pictures of the patient's regular enclosure. This will give the veterinary staff a good idea of which type of husbandry practices are being used.

> **CRITICAL CONCEPT**
>
> Reptiles can intermittently shed *Salmonella* spp. if they are carriers of the bacteria. Vinyl or latex examination gloves should be worn anytime you are working with reptiles to help prevent spread of *Salmonella* spp.

CAPTURE, RESTRAINT, AND HANDLING
SNAKES

Most snakes can be easily captured directly out of the carrier or cage that they are in. When dealing with nonaggressive snakes, the restrainer can simply pick the animal up and pull it out of the cage. If the snake is aggressive, it may be necessary to use a towel along with leather gloves to capture it safely. In these cases, it is easiest to toss the towel over the snake gently and find the head. Once the head has been isolated and restrained, the snake can be safely taken out of the enclosure. If the snake is extremely aggressive or if it is a venomous snake, a snake hook should be used to pin down the head of the snake long enough to grasp its head and body safely. Improper use of the snake hook can cause trauma to the patient, so extreme caution should be taken.

Snakes are commonly brought into the clinic in a pillowcase (Fig. 12-66). It is important that the veterinarian or staff does not just open the pillowcase and pull the snake out quickly, especially if unfamiliar with the patient. To remove the snake from the pillowcase safely, first find the snake's head and gently grasp it from the outside of the pillowcase. Once the snake is restrained, the restrainer should put his or her free hand into the pillowcase and transfer the head to the free hand. After this is accomplished, it should now be safe to take the entire snake out of the pillowcase. It is important to hold the snake gently, directly behind the head, with one hand (so it cannot turn around and bite) and support the body with the other hand (Fig. 12-67). If the snake is large, more than one person may be needed to restrain it. A good rule of thumb is one person per 3 feet of snake.

CHELONIANS

Although chelonians are usually the easiest to capture, they are the hardest to restrain. Unless working with extremely large tortoises, most chelonians can just be picked up with both hands and placed on the examination table. When examining large tortoises (i.e., several kilograms), it is easiest to set up an examination area within the animal's enclosure or on the floor in the clinic's examination area. Because there is a great deal of variation in size and strength, restraint techniques may vary between small and large chelonians. Once the animal's body is under control, it is imperative that the head be properly restrained. Although this is relatively easy when the animal is sick, it can be difficult on strong, healthy chelonians, especially large tortoises and box turtles.

There are several ways that the restrainer can gain control of the animal's head. Many turtles and tortoises are curious. If they are set down on the table or the ground, they may just start walking around to check things out. If this is the case, the restrainer can just walk up to them and grasp the head with one hand while restraining the body with the other hand. To keep control of the head, it is best to position your thumb on one side of the cranial portion of the neck and position the rest of your fingers (or just the index finger, for smaller species) on the other side of the neck, just behind the base of the skull (Fig. 12-68). Healthy chelonians are strong, so it may take much constant but gentle force to keep the turtle or tortoise's head out of the shell. If the animal is extremely active, another person may be necessary to help restrain the limbs and body.

Another way to gain control of the head is by trying to coax the animal out of its shell. Many chelonians will extend their head out of the shell if food is offered to them or if they are placed in a container of shallow warm water. When the head is extended, the same techniques mentioned earlier can be used to gain and keep control of the animal's head. If these techniques fail, it may be possible to slip a small, blunt, ear curette or spay hook under the horny portion of the upper beak, known as the rhinotheca. Once the probe has been placed, it can be gently pulled back to extend the neck to a position for the restrainer to grasp. It is important to note that this technique can be dangerous. The beak can be chipped or broken if the animal struggles or is in poor health. If a spay hook is the tool of choice, it may be a good

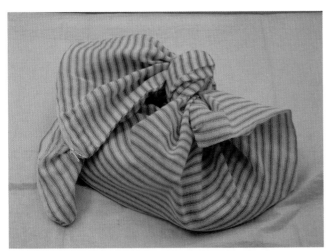

FIGURE 12-66 Snakes are commonly transported to the veterinary hospital in a pillowcase. (From Sirois M: Principles and practice of veterinary technology, ed 3, St Louis, 2011, Mosby.)

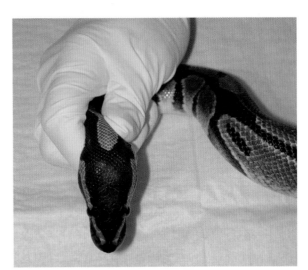

FIGURE 12-67 The snake's head is restrained by placing your hand behind the base of the skull. This will keep the snake from turning around and biting you. (From Sirois M: Principles and practice of veterinary technology, ed 3, St Louis, 2011, Mosby.)

idea to pad the hooked portion of the instrument. Padding can consist simply of tape or an elastic wrap cut to the appropriate size. Caution should be taken when dealing with any aquatic turtle, especially snapping turtles. These species of turtles have a tendency to bite, and many of the larger turtles can cause serious bodily harm to the people working with them.

Box turtles can be the most challenging chelonians to restrain properly. Because box turtles have a hinge on their plastron, many species are able to tuck themselves completely into their shells. The easiest way to extend their head is to prop open the cranial portion of the carapace (upper shell) and the plastron (lower shell) gently. Extreme care must be taken when trying to prop the shell open. It is suggested that a well-padded object be used when attempting this. This will help avoid traumatizing or fracturing the shell. Another way to extend a box turtle's head is to grasp one of the forelimbs, keeping the leg extended out of the shell until the head can be successfully pulled out and properly restrained. This method works well because once the leg is extended, the turtle will usually not close its shell down on its own leg. It is important to remember that any of these capture and restraint techniques can potentially cause some stress to the turtle or tortoise. If initial attempts at capture and restraint are not successful, chemical restraint may be necessary for any reptile, especially large tortoises and box turtles.

LIZARDS

Smaller lizards are generally easy to capture but can be difficult to restrain because they tend to wiggle and squirm while they are being held. Most small lizards can simply be picked up with both hands and taken out of the enclosure. This is also true of the larger lizard species. However, some of the larger lizards can be difficult to capture and restrain, especially if they are aggressive. If the lizard is aggressive, a

towel or blanket, along with leather restraint gloves, should be used. It is important to remember that lizards can scratch and bite when they are scared or nervous. Therefore, it is a good idea to wear long sleeves when possible and always keep track of where the head is. Long-necked lizards such as monitors can easily turn around and bite if their head is not properly restrained during capture. Keeping one hand on the neck, just behind the base of skull, will help prevent getting bitten (Fig. 12-69). Many species of lizards have a natural predatory response to drop or autotomize their tail voluntarily in an attempt to escape predation. Therefore, it is a good rule of thumb never to capture any species of lizard by the tail.

Generally, lizards can be restrained by placing one hand around the neck and pectoral girdle region while the other hand can be used to support the body near the pelvis (Fig. 12-70). Although it is sometimes difficult, try to avoid pressing down and damaging the dorsal spines of lizards

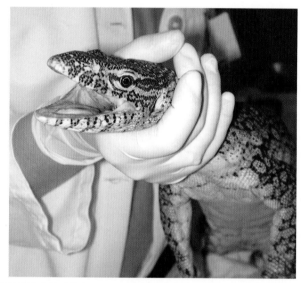

FIGURE 12-69 Long-necked lizards such as monitors should be restrained by placing one hand behind the base of the skull and the other hand supporting the body. Placing your hand behind the skull base will help keep the animal from biting you. (From Sirois M: Principles and practice of veterinary technology, ed 3, St Louis, 2011, Mosby.)

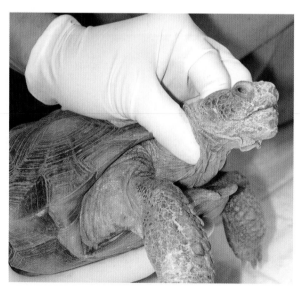

FIGURE 12-68 The tortoise is restrained by placing one hand behind the base of the skull to help keep the head and neck extended. The other hand should be used to support the body. (From Sirois M: Principles and practice of veterinary technology, ed 3, St Louis, 2011, Mosby.)

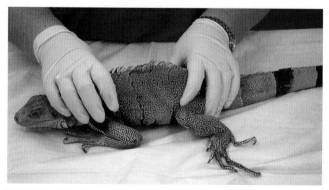

FIGURE 12-70 Restraint of a large lizard, with one hand around the pectoral girdle and the other hand around the pelvic girdle. (From Sirois M: Principles and practice of veterinary technology, ed 3, St Louis, 2011, Mosby.)

such as iguanas when they are being restrained. It is also important to remember that not all lizards have durable and tough skin. Some lizards, such as geckos, have extremely delicate skin that can easily be damaged by capture and restraint. Make sure that only soft towels are used on geckos.

AMPHIBIANS

Amphibians can be challenging animals to capture and restrain. It is important to keep stress to a minimum; therefore, the patient should be handled only when necessary. You should always wear nonpowdered gloves when handling an amphibian and keep the patient moist to avoid dehydration. This will protect both you and the patient. Some amphibians can release toxins from their skin that cause irritation or illness in humans; also, amphibians can absorb substances through their skin, so anything on your hands can be potentially harmful to the patient.

Generally, amphibians can be restrained by placing one hand around the neck and pectoral girdle region while the other hand can be used to support the body near the pelvis. In some cases, the patient may need to be anesthetized to perform a physical examination. This is especially true with aggressive or extremely stressed animals.

CRITICAL CONCEPT

Nonpowdered latex or vinyl examination gloves should always be worn when working with amphibian patients.

NORMAL PHYSIOLOGIC VALUES

Generally, normal physiologic values in reptiles have an extremely large range. Many reptiles can have a heart rate that ranges from approximately 10 to 80 or more beats/min. Heart rates and respiratory rates can vary depending on ambient temperature, age, species, and health status. The respiratory rate may range from 2 or 3 breaths/min to 20 breaths/min or more, depending on the factors mentioned earlier. The body weight of the patient will also vary depending on age, nutritional status, species, and sometimes sex. Patients' weight can range from as little as a few grams to several kilograms. A scale that weighs to the nearest gram should always be used to obtain an accurate weight on the patient. Body condition scoring is also performed on reptiles and follows the same guidelines used in mammalian medicine. The scale ranges from 1 to 9, with 1 being emaciated and 9 being grossly obese.

DETERMINING GENDER

It is relatively easy to determine gender in many species of reptiles. For example, male iguanas and bearded dragons have very large femoral pores compared with females (Fig. 12-71). Many species of male tortoises have a concave plastron, making it easier to mount the female. Several male water turtles have elongated nails, which are used to dangle in front of the female to impress her. Some species

of male box turtles have brilliant red eyes. These are just a few examples.

To determine gender in snakes, a well-lubricated metal or plastic probe is inserted into the cloaca and then directed caudolaterally (Fig. 12-72). In male snakes, the probe will enter the cavity in which the inverted hemipenis—one of the two reproductive organs—is located. In female snakes, the probe will enter a blind diverticula. Once the probe has been inserted, it is advanced slowly and gently until it will not advance any farther. Your thumb should be placed on the scale where the end of the probe is located. You can now pull the probe out and count the number of scales from the cloacal opening to your thumb. If the number is more than 7, it is a male; if it is less than 5, it is a female. If the number is in between, it is very hard to say whether the animal is a male or female.

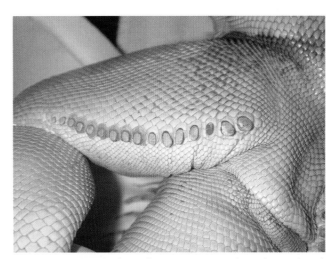

FIGURE 12-71 The femoral pores are commonly used to sex lizards such as iguanas and bearded dragons. The males (pictured) have large femoral pores, whereas females have tiny femoral pores. (From Sirois M: Principles and practice of veterinary technology, ed 3, St Louis, 2011, Mosby.)

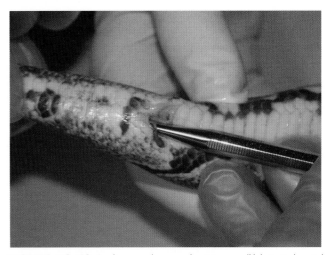

FIGURE 12-72 Snakes can be sexed using a well-lubricated metal or plastic probe inserted into the cloaca. (From Sirois M: Principles and practice of veterinary technology, ed 3, St Louis, 2011, Mosby.)

DIAGNOSTIC TECHNIQUES
REPTILE VENIPUNCTURE

Venipuncture sites vary with different species (Table 12-2). Clipping toenails to obtain a blood sample is a method that some veterinary professionals may use on very small lizards or when attempts to access other venipuncture sites have failed. Cutting toenails to the point of bleeding should not be used as a means for obtaining a blood sample. This can be painful for the animal and may introduce infection. Blood from a clipped toenail also has the potential to skew blood chemistry levels (e.g., uric acid).

SNAKES. There are two common venipuncture sites in snakes, which include the caudal tail vein and heart. The palatine vessels are not appropriate for drawing blood samples in snakes. Drawing blood from the tail vein is best accomplished in large snakes; it can be difficult in small snakes because of the size of the vessel. The same method used to draw blood from the ventral midline in lizards is also used in snakes. Obtaining a blood sample from the heart (also called cardiocentesis) is generally the quickest method and will yield a large amount of blood. The snake should be placed in dorsal recumbency. The heart can then be located in the cranial third of the body.

CHELONIANS. The radiohumoral plexus (brachial plexus sinus), subcarapacial venous sinus, dorsal venous sinus (coccygeal vein), and jugular vein are the major sites from which blood can be obtained from a turtle or tortoise. The venipuncture site will depend on the size and species of the patient and the preference of the phlebotomist. If blood is drawn from the jugular vein, the turtle or tortoise should be placed in lateral recumbency. The head and neck should be pulled away from the shell. To obtain the sample, the phlebotomist will hold the head while the restrainer will keep the patient in lateral recumbency. The subcarapacial venous sinus is generally used when jugular venipuncture is not an option (Fig. 12-73). The radiohumoral plexus sinus is generally used in larger chelonians. When drawing blood from the dorsal venous sinus, the patient should be placed in sternal recumbency. The tail should be held as straight as possible, and the needle should be inserted in the midline.

LIZARDS. The cephalic, jugular, and ventral abdominal vessels can be used to obtain a blood sample from various species of lizards that may be encountered in your clinic. However, these vessels are not commonly used for several reasons. The cephalic vein is usually extremely small, and the ventral abdominal vein is not generally used (especially in awake animals) because of the inability to properly restrain the animal and control hemorrhage. Finally, the jugular vein is not commonly used because in many species it is a blind stick and may require a surgical cut-down to access the vessel. Lymphatic fluid contamination is also common when performing venipuncture from the jugular vein. The most common vessel used for lizard venipuncture is the caudal tail vein, also called the ventral coccygeal vein. Lizards usually struggle when they are placed on their backs, making it difficult to draw blood from them. Therefore, it is important to keep the animal in sternal recumbency while obtaining the blood sample. During the blood draw, it is also important that the phlebotomist gently restrain the caudal portion of the tail with one hand and obtain the blood sample with the other.

AMPHIBIANS. Blood collection can be challenging in amphibians. Alcohol should not be used to clean the venipuncture site. This can irritate and/or desiccate the patient's skin. A 1:40 diluted 2% chlorhexidine solution should be used to cleanse the site instead. The caudal tail vein is generally used for venipuncture in salamanders . The vessel is very small and can collapse easily, so do not place a large amount of negative pressure on the syringe during collection. Venipuncture sites in frogs and toads include the femoral vein, ventral abdominal vein, and lingual vein. The femoral and lingual veins are rarely used. The ventral abdominal vein is the easiest vessel from which to obtain a blood sample. The frog or toad is gently positioned on its back with the restrainer holding the pectoral girdle. The person drawing blood can hold the pelvic girdle with one hand and draw blood with the other hand. Some amphibians will need to be anesthetized for venipuncture.

TABLE 12-2	Common Venipuncture Sites in Reptiles
SPECIES	**VENIPUNCTURE SITES**
Chelonians	Radiohumoral plexus sinus (brachial sinus)
	Dorsal venous sinus (coccygeal vein)
	Jugular vein
	Subcarapacial venous sinus
	Femoral vein
Lizards	Ventral and lateral aspects of the caudal tail vein
Snakes	Heart
	Ventral aspect of the caudal tail vein

From Sirois M: Principles and practice of veterinary technology, ed 3, St Louis, 2011, Mosby.

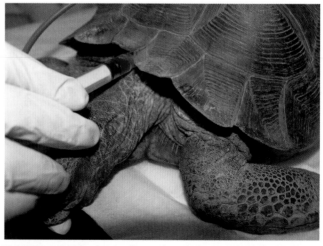

FIGURE 12-73 Blood collection from the subcarapacial venous sinus. (From Sirois M: Principles and practice of veterinary technology, ed 3, St Louis, 2011, Mosby.)

PARASITOLOGY

Reptiles and amphibians can be affected by a wide variety of parasites. There are several different ways to check for parasite load, including direct fecal examination, fecal flotation, and cloacal wash. The direct fecal examination and flotation are done in the same manner as for a dog or cat. The cloacal wash is done by inserting a soft rubber feeding tube attached to a syringe into the cloaca. Saline is then flushed into the cloaca and suctioned out, obtaining a diagnostic sample.

RADIOLOGY

Good radiographs are an important tool used as part of the diagnostic workup. The diagnostic value of a radiograph depends on the quality of the technique and positioning of the patient. Digital radiology will yield the best results. However, if digital radiology is not available in your hospital, high-detail rare earth cassettes with single-emulsion film provide desired results. Mammography film will produce even better detail but does require a higher kVp and mA.

AMPHIBIANS. Two views are normally taken, dorsoventral (DV) and horizontal lateral (Fig. 12-74). A horizontal beam is essential to obtain good radiographs. In most cases, the patient will just sit there while the radiographs are being taken.

SNAKES. Two views are normally taken, a DV or VD and lateral views. Radiographs are taken in sections from head to tail and labeled with numbered lead markers to delineate each section. In most cases, the snake will need to be heavily sedated or anesthetized to obtain good radiographs, unless the snake is very sick. A plastic snake tube can be used to obtain radiographs, but often diagnostic films are not produced unless the snake cannot move within the tube and remains completely straight.

CHELONIANS. Three views are normally taken—DV, horizontal lateral, and horizontal craniocaudal views. The craniocaudal view is taken to evaluate the left and right lung fields. A horizontal beam is essential to obtain good radiographs. Because chelonians do not have a diaphragm, placing them in lateral recumbency shifts the organs into the lung cavity, which leads to poor radiographs. Most chelonians do not need to be sedated for radiographs, but chemical restraint can be used if necessary. In most cases, the patient will just sit there or it can be placed on a plastic dish with its feet hanging in the air.

LIZARDS. Two views are normally taken, DV and horizontal lateral views. A horizontal beam is essential to obtain good radiographs. Because reptiles do not have a diaphragm, placing them in lateral recumbency shifts the organs into the lung cavity, which leads to poor radiographs. Most lizards do not need to be sedated for radiographs, but chemical restraint can be used if necessary. In most cases, the patient will just sit there while the radiographs are being taken. You can also use vagal stimulation or the vagal response to calm the patient, if needed. The vagal response in iguanas and other medium-to-large lizard species can be induced by gently applying digital pressure to both eyes for a few seconds to a few minutes. The patient will usually respond with a decrease in heart rate and blood pressure. The vagal response can also be induced by placing cotton balls over their eyes (Fig. 12-75). The vagal response induces a short-term trancelike state, allowing time to take radiographs and, in some cases, even draw blood.

FORCE FEEDING

Patients often present to the veterinary hospital because of anorexia or lethargy. Nutritional supplementation and fluid therapy are often required. Patients that are not eating on their own will need to be tube- or syringe-fed. Syringe feeding is relatively easy. Tube feeding is comparable to that in birds. The mouth is opened with a speculum, such as a plastic spatula. The tube is premeasured to estimate the location of the stomach before inserting it into the patient. Unlike metal

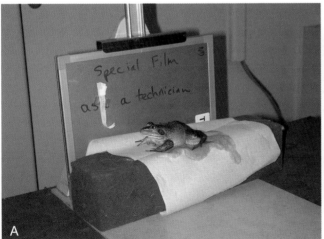
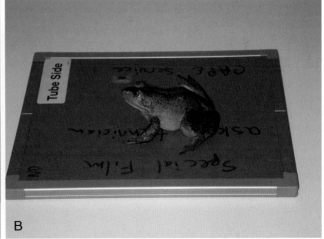

FIGURE 12-74 **A,** The horizontal lateral view is preferred over a traditional lateral view because the patient does not generally have to be anesthetized. It will often just sit on the plate. **B,** A DV view is also part of a complete radiographic series taken of amphibians. In some cases, the animal will need to be anesthetized. It is important to keep the animal moist during this time. (From Sirois M: *Principles and practice of veterinary technology,* ed 3, St Louis, 2011, Mosby.)

tubes that are generally used in birds, a red rubber feeding tube is typically used for most reptile and amphibian species (Fig. 12-76).

It is important to use proper syringe-feeding diets such as Carnivore Care (Oxbow Murdock, NE) for carnivores or Critical Care (Oxbow) for herbivores. Omnivorous animals can have a mixture of the two. Other diets can be used as well, as long as they are complete and balanced. Insectivores can be fed an appropriate meat-based baby food.

ADMINISTRATION OF FLUIDS AND MEDICATIONS

The IM and SC routes are most commonly used for the administration of medications in reptiles. The IV route is rarely used, but administration of fluids and some medications can be given into the caudal tail vein in reptiles or the jugular vein in chelonians (Table 12-3). This can be accomplished

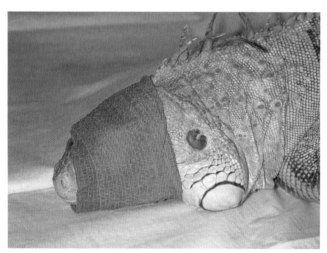

FIGURE 12-75 To induce the vagal response, place cotton balls over the eyes and lightly wrap elastic wrap around the head. This wrap takes the place of digital pressure. (From Sirois M: Principles and practice of veterinary technology, ed 3, St Louis, 2011, Mosby.)

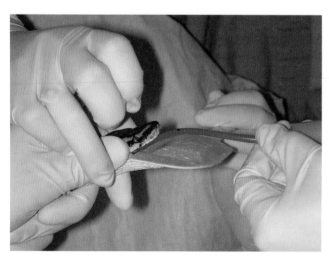

FIGURE 12-76 Tube feeding is best accomplished by opening the mouth with a soft plastic spatula, plastic card, or tape stirrups. (From Sirois M: Principles and practice of veterinary technology, ed 3, St Louis, 2011, Mosby.)

by a single injection or by placing an indwelling catheter. Intraosseous fluids can be given in many lizard species.

COMMON DISEASES AND PRESENTATIONS

There is a myriad of diseases commonly seen in clinical practice (Box 12-11). It is beyond our scope here to discuss each disease. It is suggested that a reptile and amphibian medicine textbook be consulted for details about common disease processes.

EMERGENCY AND CRITICAL CARE

Chelonians, lizards, and snakes commonly present in emergency situations for traumatic injuries. Common emergencies include being hit by a car, attacked by another animal, stepped on or dropped, and thermal burns (Fig. 12-77). Wounds are treated with the same medical techniques used to treat small mammals. Wound care, fluid therapy, nutritional support, and pain medications should be provided as necessary.

TABLE 12-3	Common Intravenous Catheter Sites in Reptiles
SPECIES	**CATHETER SITES**
Chelonians	Jugular vein
Lizards	Ventral and lateral aspects of the caudal tail vein
Snakes	Ventral aspect of the caudal tail vein

From Sirois M: Principles and practice of veterinary technology, ed 3, St Louis, 2011, Mosby.

BOX 12-11	Common Diseases and Conditions of Reptiles and Amphibians

- Cutaneous bacterial infection (red leg)
- Egg binding
- Foreign body obstruction
- Gout
- Hypocalcemia
- Hypovitaminosis A*
- Metabolic bone disease
- Mycobacteriosis
- Parasitic infestations
- Poor husbandry and diet
- Reproductive organ prolapse
- Respiratory disease
- Shell rot*
- Stomatitis
- Thermal burns
- Toxin exposure
- Trauma
- Ulcerative dermatitis
- Variety of bacterial, viral, and fungal infections
- Various bacterial and fungal infections

*Chelonians only.
Adapted from Sirois M: Principles and practice of veterinary technology, ed 3, St Louis, 2011, Mosby.

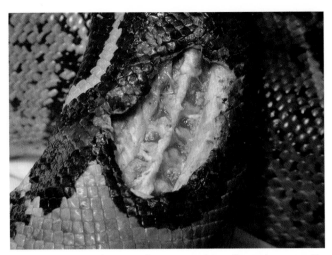

FIGURE 12-77 This wound was caused by offering live prey. The snake did not eat the rat and was left alone with it for a few days. When the owner returned, the rat had caused severe damage to the snake's flesh and vertebrae. (From Sirois M: Principles and practice of veterinary technology, ed 3, St Louis, 2011, Mosby.)

EUTHANASIA

Euthanasia can be difficult because it can sometimes be hard to access a vessel. For reptile patients, euthanasia barbiturate solution can be given into any vessel, the heart, or the coelomic cavity. If injecting into the heart, the patient must be anesthetized before the injection. Amphibian patients can be given ketamine for sedation or placed into a bath of tricaine methanesulfonate (MS-222, Argent Chemical Laboratories, Redmond, WA) to anesthetize the animal before injecting the euthanasia solution. Euthanasia solution can be given into any vessel or the coelomic cavity. The heart may take several minutes to several hours to stop completely, even though the patient may be clinically dead. Doppler ultrasound can be used to check for a heartbeat. The patient should be kept in the clinic for several hours or overnight to ensure that the patient has been properly euthanized before sending it home with the owner if that is the owner's preference.

RECOMMENDED READINGS

Small Mammals

Harkness JE, Turner PV, VandeWoude S, Wheler CL: *Harkness and Wagner's the biology and medicine of rabbits and rodents*, ed 5, Ames, IA, 2010, Wiley-Blackwell.

Hrapkiewicz K, Medina L, Homes D: *Clinical laboratory animal medicine: An introduction*, ed 3, Ames, IA, 2006, Wiley-Blackwell.

Quesenberry KE, Carpenter JW: *Ferrets, rabbits, rodents: Clinical medicine and surgery*, ed 3, St Louis, 2012, Saunders.

Sirois M: *Laboratory animal medicine: Principles and procedures*, St Louis, 2005, Mosby.

Companion Birds

Altman RB, Clubb SL, Dorrestein GM: *Avian medicine and surgery*, Philadelphia, 1997, WB Saunders.

Carpenter JW: *Exotic animal formulary*, ed 3, St Louis, 2005, Saunders.

Companion Parrot Online Magazine (https://companionparrotonline.com).

Harcourt-Brown C, Chitty J, editors: *BSAVA manual of psittacine birds*, Gloucester, England, 2005, British Small Animal Veterinary Association.

Harrison G, Lightfoot T: *Clinical avian medicine*, vols. 1 and 2. Palm Beach, FL, 2006, Spix.

Johnson-Delaney CA: *Exotic companion medicine handbook for veterinarians*, Lake Worth, FL, 1996, Wingers.

Mitchell M, Tully T: *Manual of exotic pet practice*, St Louis, 2009, Saunders.

O'Malley B: *Clinical anatomy and physiology of exotic species*, Oxford, England, 2005, Elsevier Saunders.

Ritchie BW: *Avian viruses*, Lake Worth, FL, 1995, Wingers.

Ritchie BW, Harrision GJ, Harrison LR: *Avian medicine: Principles and application*, Lake Worth, FL, 1994, Wingers.

Silverman S, Tell LA: *Radiology of birds: An atlas of normal anatomy and positioning*, St Louis, 2010, Saunders.

Reptiles and Amphibians

Ballard B, Cheek R: *Exotic animal medicine for the veterinary technician*, ed 2, Ames, IA, 2010, Wiley-Blackwell.

Carpenter JW: *Exotic animal formulary*, ed 3, St Louis, 2005, Saunders.

Fowler M: *Zoo and wild animal medicine*, ed 5, St Louis, 2004, Saunders.

Hatfield III JW: *Green iguana: The ultimate owner's manual*, ed 2, Ashland, OR, 2004, Dunthorpe Press.

Mader D: *Reptile medicine and surgery*, St Louis, 2006, Saunders.

Miller RA, Fowler M: *Fowler's zoo and wild animal medicine current therapy*, vol. 7, St Louis, 2011, Saunders.

Mitchell M, Tully T: *Manual of exotic pet practice*, St Louis, 2009, Saunders.

O'Malley B: *Clinical anatomy and physiology of exotic species*, Oxford, England, 2005, Elsevier Saunders.

West G, Heard D, Caulkett N: *Zoo animal and wildlife immobilization and anesthesia*, Ames, IA, 2007, Blackwell.

Wright KM, Whitaker BR: *Amphibian medicine and captive husbandry*, Malabar, FL, 2001, Krieger.

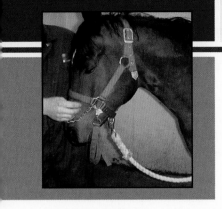

OUTLINE

Livestock Nutrition, *409*
Feedstuffs, *409*
Feed Analysis, *411*
Feeding Management of Livestock, *411*
Dairy Cattle, *411*
Beef Cattle, *412*
Nutrition in the Debilitated Calf, *412*
Horses, *414*
Pigs, *414*
Sheep, *415*
Goats, *415*
Livestock Clinical Nutrition, *415*
General Care of Horses, *416*
Bedding, *416*
Fly Control, *416*
Exercise, *416*
Grooming, *417*
Hoof Picking, *417*
Care of Cattle (Bovine), *418*
Care of Sheep (Ovine), *419*
Care of Goats (Caprine), *419*
Care of Swine (Porcine), *420*
Horse Handling and Restraint, *420*
Approaching and Capturing a Horse, *421*
Leading a Horse, *423*
Tying a Horse, *423*
Restraint of the Head, *424*
Distraction Techniques, *425*
Twitches, *425*
Tail Tying, *428*

Hobbles, *428*
Restraint of Foals, *428*
Cattle Restraint, *429*
Mechanical Devices, *430*
Sheep Restraint, *432*
Goat Restraint, *432*
Swine Handling and Restraint, *433*
Driving and Catching, *433*
Directing a Single Pig, *433*
Hog Snare, *433*
Restraining Piglets, *433*
Restraining Potbellied Pigs, *434*
Common Procedures in Livestock, *434*
Hoof Trimming, *434*
Crutching (or Tagging), *434*
Tail Docking and Castrating, *434*
Clipping Teeth, *435*
Umbilical Cord Clipping, *435*
Monitoring Hospitalized Patients, *436*
Care of Recumbent Horses, *436*
Bandaging, *437*
Foot Wraps, *438*
Tail Bandages, *438*
Sample Collection, *438*
Urine Collection, *438*
Blood Collection, *439*
Administration of Medication, *440*
Oral Administration, *440*
Parenteral Injections, *442*
Eye Medication, *445*

[1]Elsevier and the author acknowledge and appreciate the original contributions from Sheldon, CC, Sonsthagen TF, Topel J: Animal restraint for veterinary professionals, St Louis, 2006, Mosby; Holtgrew-Bohling K: Large animal clinical procedures for veterinary technicians, ed 2, St Louis, 2012, Mosby; and Brotherton, Teeple, Sonsthagen P&P, whose work forms the heart of this chapter.

LEARNING OBJECTIVES

After reviewing this chapter, the reader will be able to:

1. Describe the general husbandry needs of large animals.
2. Describe restraint methods used with large animals.
3. Explain and demonstrate routine procedures used in grooming and foot care.
4. Discuss the techniques used in general nursing care of large animals.
5. Discuss the methods of sample collection for laboratory analysis.
6. Compare and contrast various routes of administration of medication in large animals.
7. Identify and describe various methods of sample collection for laboratory analysis.

KEY TERMS

Agammaglobulinemic	Crutched	Frick's speculum	Orogastric administration
Body condition score	Decubital ulcers	Gestation	Perivascular
Boluses	Diastema	Gilts	Proximate analysis
Byproduct feeds	Drenching	Hay	Silage
Chain twitch	Ensiling	Hog snare	Spoilage
Colostrometer	Farrowing	Humane twitch	Squeeze chute
Commissure	Feed analysis	Laminitis	Thrush
Concentrates	Feedstuff	Needle teeth	Wether
Cross tying	Forages	Nonnutritive feed additives	Withdrawal time

LIVESTOCK NUTRITION

Livestock species (cattle, horses, pigs, sheep, goats) require certain essential nutrients to meet metabolic and physiologic needs. Essential nutrients include water, energy, amino acids (proteins), fatty acids, minerals, and vitamins; these are discussed in the first part of this chapter.

There is a unique feature to protein nutrition in ruminants (cattle, sheep, goats). As a result of their pregastric fermentation system, nonprotein nitrogen (e.g., urea), in addition to rumen-degradable dietary protein, can be used by the resident microbes as a nitrogen source of synthesis of microbial proteins. Microbial protein then passes into the abomasum (true stomach) and is digested like any other dietary protein. Microbial protein can account for a significant amount of dietary protein in ruminants.

Dietary fiber is required to maintain adequate gastrointestinal function in herbivores (plant-eating animals) with active microbial fermentation chambers. These include ruminants and hind gut–fermenting animals (horses). Therefore, gastrointestinal anatomy has a very critical role in the animal's ability to derive essential nutrients from the feedstuffs available. Domestic livestock extract essential nutrients from plant materials. The plant material consumed by livestock species contains cellulose, hemicellulose, pectin, and lignin compounds that are indigestible by people and carnivorous predators. Microbes within the gut use these plant compounds, and the animal uses the end products of microbial fermentation. Animals have evolved in many ways to take advantage of microbial fermentation in their digestive process.

The alimentary tract includes the mouth and associated structures, esophagus, stomach, small intestine, cecum, and colon (large intestine). The rumen of cattle, sheep, and goats functions as a pregastric fermentation vat (Fig. 13-1). This allows ruminants to efficiently derive nutrients from plant material. In hind gut fermenters, such as horses, a greatly enlarged colon serves as a fermentation vat. These animals can also digest plant material, but not to the same extent as ruminants. As a result of differences in their anatomy, ruminants digest prefermented feed material, whereas hind gut herbivores ferment predigested feed material. Pigs are considered omnivores, which means that they can digest materials of both plant and animal origin, although they are primarily fed less bulky plant materials. Pigs have some microbial fermentation capacity in their enlarged, sacculated colon, but not to the extent of hind gut fermenters or ruminants.

FEEDSTUFFS

A **feedstuff** is any dietary component that provides some essential nutrient or serves some other function. Nonnutritive feedstuffs may provide bulk, flavor, odor, or color, or act as an antioxidant to protect other dietary components. More than 2000 different feedstuffs have been fed to domestic livestock throughout the world. The variety of feedstuffs available for use in a given geographic area depends on the crops grown locally. Potential feedstuffs must be matched with the appropriate livestock species, based on nutrient requirements and gastrointestinal tract capabilities. Feedstuffs may be divided into a number of categories, based on their source and nutrient concentration. General categories include forages (roughages), concentrates, byproducts, mineral and vitamin supplements, and nonnutritive additives.

Forages are feeds made up of most or all of the plant. Forages generally have large amounts of fiber, low energy

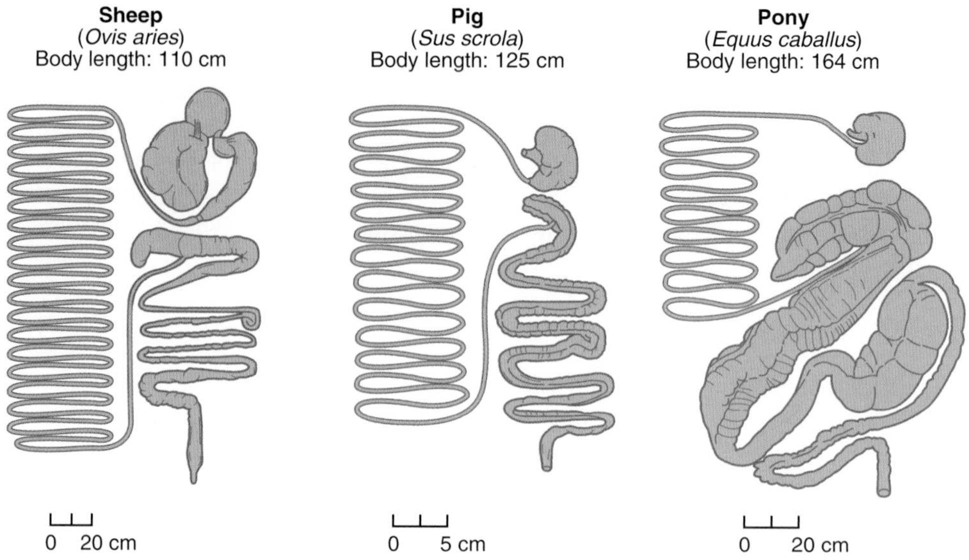

Sheep
(*Ovis aries*)
Body length: 110 cm

Pig
(*Sus scrola*)
Body length: 125 cm

Pony
(*Equus caballus*)
Body length: 164 cm

FIGURE 13-1 Schematic diagrams comparing the gastrointestinal tract of ruminants (sheep), horses, and pigs. (From Sirois M: Principles and practice of veterinary technology, ed 3, St Louis, 2011, Mosby.)

density, and high bulk (low weight per unit volume). This is a direct result of the amount of plant cell wall material present. Plant cell walls are composed of cellulose, hemicelluose, lignin, and other compounds. A forager's protein content depends on the type of plant and stage at harvesting. For example, alfalfa hay has much higher protein levels than grass hays at a comparable stage of plant growth. Within plant species, there is an increase in fiber content and a decrease in protein content, energy content, and overall digestibility with advancing maturity of the plant. The decrease in digestibility with maturity is because of increasing lignin content of the plant. Lignin is an inert compound that increases rigidity of the plant cell wall. Straw represents the most mature and indigestible form of forages.

Forages fed to livestock belong to either the legume or grass plant families. Legumes commonly used for forage production include alfalfa, red and white clover, bird's foot trefoil, and vetch. Grasses offer more variety for forage production and include Bahia grass, Bermuda grass, bluegrass, bromegrass, fescue, timothy, orchard grass, reed canary grass, ryegrass, and Sudan grass. Other grass forages that can be used for cereal grain production include corn, wheat, rye, oats, and sorghum. Of these, corn is the most important forage and cereal grain product grown for livestock.

Forage products are harvested and stored for livestock feeding purposes in a number of ways. Livestock may graze grasses, legumes, and other broadleaf vegetation (forbs and browse). Allowing livestock to harvest forage avoids costs incurred in mechanical harvesting and storage. However, forage quality and quantity can be extremely variable, depending on plant maturity and environmental conditions. A more controlled method of grazing, called intensive rotational grazing, is being adopted. In this method, animals are allowed to graze restricted areas of forage for limited periods and are then moved to another area; the forage in the grazed area is allowed to regrow until the animals are returned for grazing. With highly managed rotational grazing, forage quality can be maintained at a very high level.

Forage crops can also be mechanically harvested, stored, and fed using various methods. Green chop or **spoilage** represents forage harvested at a given stage of development and fed directly. Green chop contains a high water content (75% to 85%) and available nutrients; however, it must be harvested daily to avoid rapid deterioration with storage.

Ensiling is a harvesting process by which forage is chopped and placed into a storage unit (e.g., silo) that excludes oxygen. As the forage ferments, lactic acid is produced and the pH decreases. This effectively "pickles" the forage to a partially fermented state called **silage**. Good-quality silage can be stored indefinitely in upright silos, bunker silos, or plastic bags, the important feature being exclusion of oxygen. Silage has an intermediate water content (55% to 75%) and has the least loss of nutrients from harvesting and storage. Grass, legume, and corn silages are the most common ensiled forages fed to livestock.

Hay is forage that is cut and allowed to dry before being collected into bales for storage. Hay should have less than 15% water to be stable in storage. Harvesting losses are high in hay making, but storage losses are usually minimal if it is properly dried.

CRITICAL CONCEPT

Feedstuff types include forages (roughages), concentrates, byproducts, mineral and vitamin supplements, and nonnutritive additives.

Concentrates are generally low in fiber and high in energy and/or protein. Cereal grains, such as barley, corn, millet, oats, rye, sorghum, and wheat, are the seeds of many of the grass species. Corn is the most common grain fed to livestock and the standard with which others are compared. Cereal grains contain large amounts of energy in the form of starch and are added to diets to increase energy density. Other feed products used as energy concentrates include molasses, root crops (e.g., turnips, beets, carrots), and potatoes. Fats and oils of plant or animal origin contain 2.25 times the energy density of carbohydrates and are also used as energy concentrates.

Concentrate feeds that contain more than 20% crude protein are subclassified as protein supplements. Protein supplements may be of plant or animal origin, including marine fish. Plant-based protein products are derived from oilseed crops such as soybean, canola, cottonseed, sunflower, and peanut seed meals. Of these, soybean meal is by far the most common oilseed meal fed to livestock. Oil from the seeds is harvested for a variety of industrial and nutritional uses; the remaining seed contains more than 40% crude protein. Animal-based protein supplements are derived from rendered animal or fish tissues or from dried-milk products. Animal proteins generally range from more than 50% crude protein to 90% crude protein. As compared with plant-based protein sources, animal protein sources have a better amino acid composition relative to requirements. However, there is much variability in the quality of animal-based products and the way in which they are manufactured.

Byproduct feeds are residues of the feed-processing industry and span a wide array of feedstuffs. Examples of byproduct feeds include sugar beet pulp, bakery waste, blood, bone meal, brewer's grains, tallow, and whey. Many byproduct feeds contain substantial amounts of fermentable fiber, energy, and protein.

Mineral and vitamin supplements are sources of individual minerals or a combination of minerals, with or without vitamins. Fat-soluble vitamins are supplemented primarily in the form of premixes. Fat-soluble vitamins are sensitive to oxidation, sunlight, heat, and fungal growth. Certain water-soluble vitamins may be supplemented in swine and horse diets; they are not routinely supplemented in ruminant diets. Yeast cultures are good sources of B complex vitamins and are commonly added to livestock diets.

Nonnutritive feed additives can include buffers, hormones, binders, and medications. Feed medications may include antibiotics, antifungals, anthelmintics, antiparasitics, and ionophores (antibiotics with growth-promoting effects). Their use is regulated by the Food and Drug Administration in an effort to prevent tissue residues. Nonnutritive additives are used to stimulate animal performance, improve feed efficiency, and improve animal health or metabolic status.

FEED ANALYSIS

Different classes of feedstuffs contribute variable amounts of the essential nutrients (Table 13-1). Even within certain feed groups, such as forages, nutrient composition can vary tremendously. **Feed analysis** is a procedure by which chemical analysis determines the proportion of specific components of a feedstuff. The **proximate analysis** includes determinations of dry matter (DM), crude protein (CP), ether extract (EE, crude fat), crude fiber (CF), and ash. The nonfiber carbohydrate portion of the feed is termed nitrogen-free extract (NFE). More recently crude fiber analysis has been replaced with neutral and acid detergent fiber analysis, improving our estimate of cell wall components and their availability. Feed analysis should be routinely completed in any nutritional diagnostic problem.

FEEDING MANAGEMENT OF LIVESTOCK

The goal of any livestock feeding management program is to provide sufficient daily amounts of the essential nutrients for optimal (cost-effective) productivity. Because feed costs account for the greatest amount of total production costs in the livestock industry, we must minimize feed costs to ensure profitability. Byproduct feeds are widely used when available because they usually are of lower cost.

DAIRY CATTLE

Dairy cattle are segregated and housed by production stages and fed according to specific nutrient requirements. Typical

TABLE 13-1	Relative Nutrient Content of Various Feedstuffs for Livestock						
	RELATIVE NUTRIENT CONTENT						
FEEDSTUFF GROUP	**PROTEIN**	**ENERGY**	**MINERALS**		**VITAMINS**		**FIBER**
			Macro	Micro	Fat-Sol	B-Complex	
High-quality roughage	+++	++	++	++	+++	+	+++
Low-quality roughage	+	+	+	+	−	−	++++
Cereal grains	++	+++	+	+	+	+	+
Grain mill feeds	++	++	++	++	+	++	++
Fats and oils	−	++++	−	−	−	−	−
Molasses	+	+++	++	++	−	+	−
Fermentation products	+++	++	+	++	−	++++	±
Oil seed proteins	++++	+++	++	++	+	++	+
Animal proteins	++++	+++	+++	+++	++	+++	+

+ to ++++: low to very high content.
±: may or may not be present in significant amounts.
−: not present.
(From Sirois M: Principles and practice of veterinary technology, ed 3, St Louis, 2011, Mosby.)

feeding groups on a dairy farm include milk-fed calves, growing replacement heifers, nonlactating pregnant cows (dry cows), and lactation groups. Lactation groups are usually based on level of milk production, parity (first lactation versus older cows), days in milk, or a combination of these factors.

Feeding systems and housing facilities vary among dairy farms, depending on prevailing environmental conditions. Smaller family dairies with fewer than 100 cows generally have individual tie stalls, and cows are fed individually. The amount of forage and concentrates are fed according to production level and **body condition score** (Table 13-2). These farms are predominantly found in the northeastern and midwestern United States as a result of the cold winters. In larger dairies cows are generally housed in free-stall barns or in open drylots, depending on environmental conditions. Drylots are found primarily in the southern and western United States, whereas free-stall barns are found anywhere in the United States. In larger dairy management systems, cattle are fed in groups at a common feedbunk, rather than individually. Feedbunks may be located within the free-stall facility or along one side of the drylot.

Although feeding management of dairy cattle depends on the type of facility available, there are some options as to how feed is delivered to the animals. Forage (hay, silage) may be fed separately from concentrates in any of the feeding management systems described. Concentrates may be fed separately in the milking parlor or from computerized feeders. Parlor grain feeding and computerized feeding are becoming more common with current interest in pasture-grazing management systems. In large dairies, the most common method of feed delivery is by total mixed ration (TMR). In this system, all individual feed ingredients are mechanically mixed in a feed wagon and presented as a single mixture to the cows. This allows cows to consume the same blend of nutrients in each bite and minimizes selectivity. Some dairies feed what might be termed a partial TMR in that dry hay is fed separate from the rest of the diet.

BEEF CATTLE

Beef cattle management can be divided into cow-calf and cattle feeding (feedlot) operations. Cow-calf enterprises produce calves that enter the breeding herd or are sent to cattle-feeding operations (feedlots). Forage use is the basis of cow-calf enterprises. Feed costs account for more than 60% of production costs and therefore must be minimized. Cows are allowed to graze pasture or range land, depending on availability, and then are supplemented with energy, protein, and vitamin-mineral supplements as necessary to meet specific nutritional requirements. Depending on geographic location and season, pasture grazing may be replaced with feeding of dry hay or silage. Supplementation programs depend on prevailing forage quality relative to nutrient requirements of the various production units. Cow-calf operations may have feeding groups for bulls, replacement heifers, growing calves, maintenance, and pregnant or lactating cattle.

Cattle-feeding enterprises involve feeding calves from weaning to slaughter and include backgrounding, stocker, and feedlot systems. In backgrounding and stocker feeding systems, weanling calves are placed on low-cost pasture and supplementation feeding programs to gain weight at a moderate rate and then sold to feedlot operations. The goal of a feedlot enterprise is to maximize rate of gain and feed conversion efficiency for the lowest cost. New arrivals at the feedlot are initially fed a high-forage, low-concentrate diet to acclimate the animal to the operation. The proportion of forage is gradually reduced and concentrate increased to facilitate the desired rate of gain. To minimize feeding costs, a wide variety of byproduct feeds and grain products is fed. To ensure animal health with high-grain feeding, ionophores, buffers, and antimicrobial agents are incorporated into the feedlot diet. Generally, the feedlot diet is fed as a TMR similar to the method for dairy cattle.

NUTRITION IN THE DEBILITATED CALF
FEEDING COLOSTRUM

Because calves are born essentially **agammaglobulinemic** (without immunoglobulins), provision of colostrum shortly

TABLE 13-2	Body Condition Scoring Classifications for Livestock
BODY CONDITION SCORING SCALE*		**GENERALIZED ANIMAL DESCRIPTION†**
1.0	1	*Emaciated.* All bones obviously protruding; no subcutaneous fat evident
1.5	2	*Very thin.* Bones visible and easily palpated; minimal subcutaneous fat
2.0	3	*Thin.* Thin, flat musculature; prominent ribs, pelvic bones, and spinal processes
2.5	4	*Moderately thin.* Minimal subcutaneous fat; individual ribs not obvious
3.0	5	*Moderate.* Smooth musculature; bones not visible but palpable
3.5	6	*Moderately fleshy.* Fat palpable; soft fat over ribs and covering pelvis
4.0	7	*Fleshy.* Fat visible; ribs barely visible; spinal processes buried in fat
4.5	8	*Fat.* Thick neck; ribs difficult to palpate; rounded appearance to pelvis
5.0	9	*Grossly obese.* Bulging fat all over; patchy fat pads around tailhead

*The body condition scoring scale used depends on the species. Dairy cattle, sheep, pigs, and goats are typically scored on a scale of 1 to 5, whereas beef cattle and horses are scored on a scale of 1 to 9.
†When determining body condition score, evaluate for the presence or absence of fatty tissue over the neck, ribs, spine, and pelvis, independent of animal body weight and frame size.
From Sirois M: Principles and practice of veterinary technology, ed 3, St Louis, 2011, Mosby.

after birth is critically important for the calf to obtain passive maternal antibodies. As a rule of thumb, beef calves should be fed all of the dam's first-milking colostrum as soon as they develop a suckle reflex. If dairy cow colostrum is used, be sure that the colostrum is of sufficient quality. The quality of colostrum is a rough measure of the concentration of immunoglobulin. This is most easily determined by use of a **colostrometer**, a simple tool that measures the specific gravity of the colostrum.

> ### CRITICAL CONCEPT
> Administration of colostrum shortly after birth is critically important for the calf to obtain passive maternal antibodies.

Dairy cows produce much more colostrum than beef cows do, but generally the quality and the concentration of immunoglobulin is lower. As a general rule, if calves are provided with dairy cow colostrum, it can be administered orally at 10% of body weight over the first 24 hours of life. Absorption of maternal colostral immunoglobulin by the calf's intestine usually begins to decrease after the first feeding of colostrum or at about 8 hours of age. Therefore, it is important that the first feeding of colostrum is usually of fairly large magnitude. If the calf has a vigorous suckle reflex, allow the calf to nurse all of the dam's colostrum that it will consume. If more colostrum is available, continue to feed it throughout the first 24 hours, offering it at 2-hour intervals and allowing the calf to suckle. If the calf does not have a suckle reflex, continue to offer the colostrum frequently, looking for development of a suckle reflex up to about 6 hours of age. If the calf has not developed a suckle response at that time, intubate the calf and give all of the colostrum from a beef heifer or 5% of the calf's body weight in colostrum from a dairy cow.

For administration of colostrum or milk, allowing the calf to suckle versus intubating is an important question. If the calf has already been nursing the dam and is presented for treatment beyond the first several days of age, it is common for the calf to refuse a rubber nipple feeder. It may be worthwhile to reintroduce the calf to the dam because it may then suckle the dam quite readily. On the other hand, if it is a newborn calf that has not yet suckled the dam, it will usually suckle from a nipple feeder as readily as from the dam's teats.

Development of a suckle reflex is a very important indicator of the calf's status. Calves with a variety of problems, including hypoxemia, hypoglycemia, hypothermia, or acidosis resulting from dystocia, frequently do not develop the reflex until these problems are corrected. Therefore, lack of a suckle reflex is a good indicator of one or more of these problems. In some cases if these problems are present, the calf may not absorb immunoglobulin, even if colostrum is provided via intubation.

Development of a suckle reflex usually suggests improvement in an underlying condition. Further, when other problems are present, the calf's gastrointestinal tract may not be fully functional. Therefore, repeated intubation of newborn calves or calves of older ages suffering from similar problems may result in large accumulations of fluid in the forestomachs or abomasum. If you resort to intubation to supply the calf with oral fluids or milk, carefully monitor the calf for fecal production and palpate its abdomen, looking for evidence that the fluid administered is sequestering in the gastrointestinal tract, rather than proceeding on through and being absorbed. If the calf will not suckle and there is evidence that fluid has accumulated in the gastrointestinal tract, continue to offer fluids frequently via nipple feeder but discontinue orogastric intubation.

Stimulation of the calf to develop a suckle reflex is another important function of the dam. Most calves are very responsive to stroking or rubbing along the back, especially near the tailhead. If the calf is not suckling well, such rubbing stimulation can often provide very rewarding results. If the calf has been sleeping or is compromised by one of the aforementioned problems, it may require several minutes before it begins to suckle. Therefore, it is worthwhile to repeatedly introduce the nipple into the calf's mouth and try to deliver a small amount of milk before giving up and assuming the calf does not have a suckle reflex.

Newborn ruminants, such as calves and lambs, essentially function as monogastric animals while they are nursing. Fermentation of the swallowed milk in the rumen and reticulum would likely result in digestive upsets. Closure of a structure called the esophageal groove enables the swallowed milk to bypass the rumen and reticulum and pass directly into the omasum and abomasum. Closure of the groove is stimulated by the act of nursing and by the presence of milk. When the maturing animal begins eating solid foods, the groove does not close, and the swallowed food enters the rumen and reticulum for microbial fermentation, as in adult animals.

FEEDING MILK

Beyond colostral feeding, provision of milk as nutrition is obviously of critical importance. Although dairy calves are often raised with the provision of only 10% of body weight per day as fluid milk, this practice should not be mistakenly construed as providing optimal nutrition. The strategy of providing 10% of body weight per day is geared to enhancing intake of solid feeds so that dairy calves can be weaned at an early age. Most calves, if given the opportunity, freely consume between 20% and 30% of their body weight in milk per day. Although sick calves may not have a very hearty appetite, a recovering calf or premature calf commonly has an exaggerated appetite. For these reasons provide a calf with up to 3% of its body weight per feeding and offer milk feedings at approximately 2-hour intervals. With this regimen some calves consume more than 30% of their body weight in milk per day.

FEEDING ELECTROLYTES

For calves with fluid loss because of neonatal enteritis, oral electrolyte solutions are commonly offered as a means to provide additional fluid therapy. Calves with mild to moderate dehydration may respond adequately with only oral fluid supplementation, whereas calves with severe dehydration require intravenous fluid support. It has been a common practice to withhold milk from calves with enteritis. You do not have to hold to that practice, but rather offer milk via nipple feeder if the calf will accept it. Because milk alone will not provide the electrolytes that have been lost through the gastrointestinal tract, provide oral electrolyte solutions at alternate feedings with the milk. The electrolyte fluids and milk or milk replacer should not be mixed because this adversely influences normal milk digestion. Offer milk at 2% to 3% of body weight maximum, alternating with oral fluid feedings offered at 5% of body weight per feeding, with the alternate feedings at 2-hour intervals. Many calves refuse the milk feedings but eagerly suckle the electrolyte. With this regimen, even when calves do refuse the milk, they can be provided as much as 30% of body weight per day in additional oral electrolyte fluids.

HORSES

Horse feeding management is primarily designed to meet the nutritional requirements of individual horses. Although horses are not ruminants, they require a substantial amount of dietary fiber, in the form of forage, to maintain a healthy digestive tract. Forages fed to horses are primarily hay and pasture. Silage is not commonly fed to horses because of their sensitivity to the molds and mycotoxins potentially found in silage. Many varieties of grasses and legumes can be suitable forages for horses. The need for energy, protein, and mineral-vitamin supplementation depends on forage quality and nutrient requirements of the horse. Corn, barley, and oats are common grain supplements fed to horses for added energy. Recently, fat supplementation has been advocated to provide energy for growing, lactating, and working horses. Protein sources such as linseed, canola, and soybean meal are commonly used. Byproducts containing fermentable fiber, such as rice bran and beet pulp, are becoming more popular.

> **CRITICAL CONCEPT**
>
> Horses are not ruminants, but they do require a substantial amount of dietary fiber, in the form of forage, to maintain a healthy digestive tract.

Many commercial horse feeds are available to horse owners. These range from complete feeds (no supplementation required) to specific vitamin-mineral supplements. Various grain supplements containing energy, protein, minerals, and vitamins are available. These commercial grain supplements may be formulated specifically for growing foals, lactating mares, or geriatric horses, or they may be more generic in purpose. Horse owners should match the concentrate to their forage relative to energy, protein, mineral, and vitamin requirements. A proper horse-feeding program would provide adequate amounts of water and provide sufficient energy to achieve and maintain proper body condition. The diet must then be balanced for protein, minerals, and vitamins according to the National Research Council recommendations. Appropriate dental care and parasite management programs should accompany all horse-feeding systems.

FEEDING AND WATERING HOSPITALIZED HORSES

Hospitalized horses often have special dietary needs. Their diseases can often create a catabolic state. The horse may require extra calories to maintain its weight. Horses that can chew and swallow normally should be fed their usual diet if their disease permits. Good-quality alfalfa or grass hay, such as timothy hay, can be fed. Good-quality oat hay is also a suitable feed. Horses with gastrointestinal disturbances, such as colic or diarrhea, need special consideration. Horses recovering from impactions may need more laxative feeds, such as alfalfa hay, grass pasture, and even bran mashes. Horses with diarrhea or those that have been operated on for colic may benefit from a diet that is not so rich, such as timothy or oat hay. Hay pellets or cubes that contain alfalfa or a mixture of alfalfa and Bermuda or oat hay can also be used. If added carbohydrate is needed, a pelleted feed that also contains grains may be fed.

Pelleted feed produces less dust and may be better for horses recovering from respiratory allergies or pneumonia. Horses recovering from gastrointestinal ulceration may also need to be fed a pelleted ration because the increased fiber and stem in hay may irritate and exacerbate certain kinds of ulcers. Pellets soaked to make gruel can be fed to horses with oral lesions, facial fractures, dental problems, or recurrent episodes of choke. Feed softened in this manner is easier for the animal to chew and swallow. Horses with neuromuscular disorders such as botulism may be unable to chew and swallow normally. A pelleted ration that has been soaked may be the only feed the animal can eat.

Fresh water should always be available. Some horses may not know how to use an automatic waterer if it requires the horse to push on a lever to fill the water cup. Water buckets or tubs should always be provided in these cases. Salt may need to be provided topically on the feed or in the form of a salt lick during hot weather, or for horses that have diseases that create a sodium deficiency, such as colitis.

PIGS

Pig feeding management is similar to beef cattle management in that there are breeding-farrowing (reproductive) and growing enterprises. The farrowing unit produces baby pigs as reproductive replacements or to enter the growing unit for feeding to slaughter weight. The pig industry is one of the most intensively managed agricultural enterprises. Current pig production units are moving to total confinement farrow-to-finish operations containing many animals. Within these operations, feeding groups are segregated according to nutrient requirements, with diets for lactating and gestating sows and gilts, boars, nursery pigs, and growing pigs. For the most part, animals in the farrowing unit are housed and fed as individuals to better control body weight and condition. Within the feeding operation, starting with the nursery pigs, all animals are group-housed and fed according to age and moved between groups as an entire unit.

As omnivores, pigs have a digestive tract that can accommodate a certain level of dietary fiber. Given the economics of rate of gain from forages versus grains, pig diets consist primarily of concentrates, along with energy, protein, mineral, and vitamin supplements. All feed ingredients are thoroughly mixed and provided as a single diet, like the TMR for cattle. Dietary ingredients depend on the nutritional requirements of the specific group of animals being fed. The classic pig diet consists of corn grain and soybean meal, with a vitamin-mineral premix. Learning more about the specific nutrient requirements of pigs has resulted in more sophisticated diets for pigs. Crystalline amino acids, high-quality animal byproduct protein meals, fiber sources, and vitamin-mineral supplements have been incorporated into specific pig diets to improve growth efficiency.

CRITICAL CONCEPT

Pig diets consist primarily of concentrates, along with energy, protein, mineral, and vitamin supplements.

SHEEP

Sheep are managed similarly to beef cattle in that there are reproductive and lamb-growing enterprises. Sheep are raised under a wide variety of conditions, ranging from large flocks on western rangelands to small flocks in confinement. The basis of any sheep production system is forage. The advantage of feeding sheep is their ability to selectively graze. This allows sheep to consume a diet of higher nutritional value than the quality of the total forage. A variety of forage types including harvested and stored forages can be used for feeding sheep. As ruminants, sheep can also use a wide variety of byproduct feeds efficiently.

For the most part, sheep diets consist of vitamin-mineral supplements added to the base forage. The composition of the vitamin-mineral supplement depends on the forage. Grazing sheep are provided with minerals as a block (salt lick) or loose from a feeder. Additional energy and protein supplementation may be used for late gestation, lactation, and growing diets. A wide variety of feed sources may be used, with cost being of primary concern. These supplements may be top-dressed on (spread on top of) the forage or fed by themselves in a feed bunk. Commercial concentrate pellets are also available for ewes and growing lamb diets. Growing lambs may be sent to slaughter directly from grazing high-quality forage or after feeding in a feedlot. Lamb feedlots are similar in organization and feeding practices to beef feedlots. Lambs are acclimated from a high-forage to high-concentrate TMR diet to increase grain and feed efficiency.

GOATS

Goats are managed similarly to dairy cattle because of their milk production. However, some breeds of goats are primarily used for mohair (wool) or meat production. Forage is the primary component of goat-feeding programs. Like sheep, goats can selectively graze the more nutritious parts of plants. Goats raised for mohair and meat are managed with grazing or browsing rangeland or pasture and appropriate energy and protein supplementation when necessary. Dairy goats are managed more intensively because of their higher nutritional requirements for milk production.

Dairy goats are usually housed in smaller areas and fed stored forages, such as dry hay. Pasture grazing alone cannot support milk production, so supplements are necessary. The energy and protein feed supplements for goats are similar to those of dairy cattle. Many commercial concentrate products used for horses, sheep, and dairy cattle can also be fed to goats. The amount and nutrient composition of the supplement depend on the nutrient requirements of the animal being fed and on forage quality. Lactating goats require substantial energy supplementation and should be fed the highest-quality forages. Supplements may be top-dressed on forage in a feedbunk or provided in the milking parlor.

LIVESTOCK CLINICAL NUTRITION

A basic understanding of nutrition can be applied to medical management of livestock. The most important part of clinical nutrition is obtaining an appropriate nutritional history. This is used to determine the potential role of nutrition in a medical problem. Questions one should ask in obtaining a nutritional history are outlined in Table 13-3.

Following the history taking, assess the nutritional status of the animal through physical assessment and via blood chemistry determinations. Physical assessment of the animal involves obtaining an accurate body weight, height measurement, and body condition score. Body height at the shoulders (withers) can be used to assess frame size and growth. Body weight and height measurements can be compared with those in standardized growth charts to assess growth performance.

Body condition scoring is a method of subjectively quantifying subcutaneous body fat reserves. Animals are scored on a scale of 1 to 5 or 1 to 9, with the low and high scores representing emaciated and obese animals, respectively. Changes in body condition score represent either a positive (increased) or negative (decreased) energy balance. A negative energy balance suggests that the diet contains insufficient energy to meet needs and that body fat reserves are being mobilized.

Beyond this quantitative measure, physical assessment of the animal may include observations of hair coat, hoof quality, hydration status, manure consistency, and attitude. Assess these factors and record them in the animal's records daily for hospitalized patients. Indirect measures of nutritional status may be evaluated through metabolite concentrations in blood.

TABLE 13-3	Nutritional History in Livestock (Specific Information Depends on the Species of Livestock)
GENERAL CATEGORIES OF INFORMATION	**SPECIFIC INFORMATION**
Identify the people involved	Names and telephone numbers of the owner, herdsman, veterinarian, nutritionist, others
Owner's primary concern	Pertaining to the presenting problem
Historical information about the agribusiness	Ask questions relating to years of ownership, number of hired hands, new animal purchases, acreage, other farms, etc.
Herd information	Function, breeds, average weights, and age distribution of animals on the farm
Production information	Level of performance (milk production, weaning weights, litter size, etc.) in the herd over time; use production record systems if available
Housing facilities	Type of housing, stall surfaces, and bedding used for each group of animals; adequacy of ventilation
Feeding system	Feed storage facilities, feeding system used, feed and water availability, bunk space per animal, number of times fed per day, etc.
Dietary information	Feed ingredients and their nutrient analyses, specific feeds for each feeding group; obtain feed samples if feed analysis or feed tag information is unavailable
Herd disease information	Disease prevalence for pertinent disease problems, animal culling and mortality rates over the past month, 6 months, and year
Reproductive information	Measures of fertility, pregnancy losses, etc.
Preventive medicine practices	Vaccinations, treatments, and dewormings administered and when; ask if routine herd health visits are made by the veterinarian

From Sirois M: Principles and practice of veterinary technology, ed 3, St Louis, 2011, Mosby.

GENERAL CARE OF HORSES

BEDDING

Horses can be bedded on a variety of materials. It is important that the bedding be clean, as dust free as possible, and relatively deep. Another important consideration when choosing bedding is its usefulness as a fertilizer after composting. Pine shavings are adequate for most patients, but they tend to be very dusty. This may not be acceptable for horses with open wounds or respiratory disorders. Pine shavings with minimal dust or shredded paper bedding is preferable for horses with severe respiratory problems. It is best to obtain wood shavings from a known source to prevent accidental exposure to black walnut shavings, which can cause **laminitis** when the horse stands in the shavings. Black walnut wood is darker than pine but can be difficult to recognize if the bedding is soiled or if multiple types of wood chips have been mixed. Straw bedding is often used for mares with newborn foals. Bedding should always be deep unless the horse has a problem that necessitates a firmer surface for standing. Regardless of the type of bedding used, it should be kept very clean by removing soiled bedding at least once daily. The use of rubber stall mats has also reduced the amount of bedding that has to be used.

Recumbent adult horses must have very deep bedding to help prevent formation of **decubital ulcers** (pressure sores). Alternatively, large mattresses or specially designed water beds can be used. Critically ill foals can be kept on mattresses with waterproof covers and fleece pads to keep them clean and dry. It may be necessary to clean the stall or change the bedding each time the horse or foal urinates or defecates if the animal is recumbent. Strategically placed diapers or absorbent mats may help reduce the number of bedding changes needed with a recumbent foal.

FLY CONTROL

The best method of fly control is to maintain a clean barn with frequent manure removal. Various topical fly sprays are available. Those containing permethrins, pyrethrins, or citronella sprays are the safest for sick horses. Overhead fly systems that release fly repellents at regular intervals can also minimize the fly population. A soft cloth can be used to apply fly repellent to the horse's face, taking care to apply the repellent around the eyes without getting any into the eyes. Fly masks are available for the face and the ears of sensitive patients, and a fly sheet can also be used to cover most of the body, except the distal parts of the legs.

> **CRITICAL CONCEPT**
>
> Fly repellents containing organophosphates should not be applied to debilitated horses or foals.

EXERCISE

Adult horses and foals should have some form of exercise daily unless their medical problem requires stall rest. Walking on soft dirt or grass surfaces is preferable to walking on concrete or asphalt. Foals may be allowed to run freely alongside the mare if they do not have a condition that warrants more restricted activity, and if the area is properly fenced with no hazards, such as drains or moving vehicles. If the foal's activity must be controlled, the foal can be walked using a halter and a rope around the foal's hindquarters in the area of the semimembranosus and semitendinosus muscles. Good judgment and caution are needed to prevent the foal from rearing and flipping over backward. Neonates whose exercise must be limited can be walked by placing one arm in front of the foal's chest and one arm behind the foal to cradle it while walking. Alternatively, an adult horse halter can be used over the foal's body like a harness, with the nose piece around the foal's neck, the buckle strapped around the ventral thorax, and the rope clip located on the caudodorsal portion of the foal's back. The hind end of the foal may still need to be supported.

GROOMING

Equine patients should be groomed daily, unless the horse has a condition whereby vigorous grooming would be painful or damaging (e.g., severe skin infections, cutaneous burns). A rubber curry comb (Fig. 13-2) should be used in a circular motion to remove dried sweat or mud. Next, a stiff-bristled brush can be used to remove dirt and loose hair. If stiff brushes and rubber curry combs are used on the horse's face and distal limbs, they should be used gently because overly vigorous grooming may be uncomfortable for the animal. Metal curry combs should not be used on the horse's head or distal limbs. A soft brush can be used to finish removing loose hair and dirt. If needed, a damp or dry cloth can be used to remove the remaining dust from the horse's coat. A stiff brush, hair brush, or metal mane comb should be used on the tail and mane.

HOOF PICKING

A horse's hooves should be picked clean daily. Stand facing the back of the horse, run your hand down the horse's near front leg, and ask it to pick up its foot or say, "Give me your foot." As the horse allows you to pick up its foot, be sure to hold the hoof and not the fetlock or pastern because that kind of hold puts pressure on that joint and can make the horse uncomfortable. When the horse has lifted its foot, balance the hoof on your knee. To clean, hold the hoof with your left hand and the hoof pick with your right hand. The hoof is then cleaned with a hoof pick by removing debris from the lateral and central sulci, starting at the heel and working toward the toe, and then from the rest of the hoof (Fig. 13-3).

To lift the rear foot, stand facing the back of the horse, fairly close to the side of its hindquarters. Run your hand down the horse's near leg and ask it to give you its foot as you get to just above the pastern. As the horse gives you its foot, move forward a bit to stretch its leg out while you place its hoof on your thigh (Figure 13-4). If the horse starts to pull the foot away, grasp it with both hands to steady it on your knee. To clean the hoof out again, move the pick from heal to the toe.

A degenerative condition called **thrush** is common in feet that are infrequently cleaned, or if the horse stands for long periods in damp bedding or muddy soil. Thrush may occur secondary to a bacterial infection and appears as black, malodorous material in the region of the frog. A 10% sodium hypochlorite (bleach) solution or 2% iodine solution can be applied to the lateral and central sulci to dry the foot and kill the bacteria. Commercial formulations

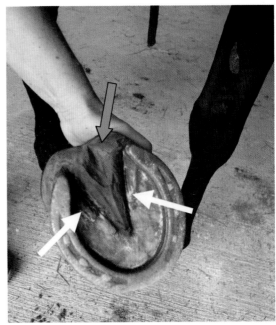

FIGURE 13-3 Central sulcus *(green arrow)* and lateral sulci *(white arrows)* of the frog. (From Sirois M: Principles and practice of veterinary technology, ed 3, St Louis, 2011, Mosby.)

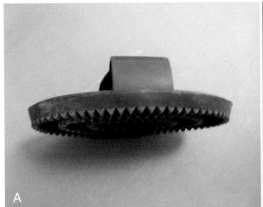
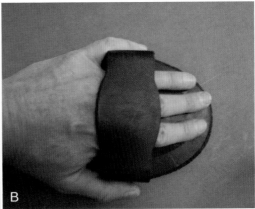

FIGURE 13-2 Grooming using a curry comb. **A,** Curry comb. **B,** Holding the curry comb. (From Sirois M: Principles and practice of veterinary technology, ed 3, St Louis, 2011, Mosby.)

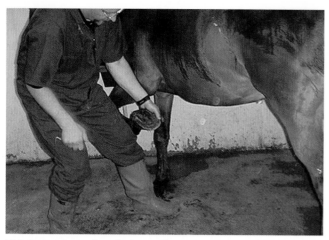

FIGURE 13-4 Lifting the horse's foot. As the horse gives you its foot, move forward a bit to stretch its leg out while you place the hoof on your thigh. (From Sheldon CC, Topel J, Sonsthagen BS: Animal restraint for veterinary professionals, St Louis, 2006, Mosby.)

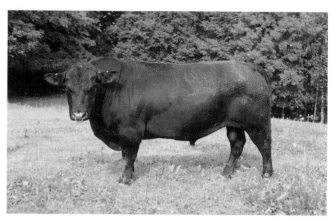

FIGURE 13-5 Angus. (From Holtgrew-Bohling K: Large animal clinical procedures for veterinary technicians, ed 2, St Louis, 2012, Mosby.)

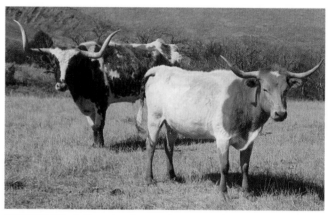

FIGURE 13-6 Texas longhorn cattle. (From Holtgrew-Bohling K: Large animal clinical procedures for veterinary technicians, ed 2, St Louis, 2012, Mosby.)

containing formaldehyde or copper sulfate can also be used. Care must always be used to avoid spilling caustic solutions on the coronary band or other parts of the horse's leg. The technician and assistant should wear gloves tfor protection from the solutions. Some animals with severe thrush require foot trimming to remove diseased hoof tissue and wraps to help keep the foot clean and dry during the length of the treatment program.

CARE OF CATTLE (BOVINE)

The cattle industry can be divided into two distinctly different areas; each with its own set of production goals and management techniques. The beef industry uses heavily muscled breeds of cattle that are capable of efficient conversion of hay and grain into skeletal muscle mass for maximum meat production. Common breeds of beef cattle include the Angus (Fig. 13-5), Texas Longhorn (Fig. 13-6), Brahman (Fig. 13-7), and Hereford (Fig. 13-8). The dairy industry uses other breeds of cattle that are more efficient in converting cattle food into the production of large volumes of saleable milk as the main production goal. Dairy cattle breeds include Guernsey (Fig. 13-9), Jersey (Fig. 13-10), and Holstein (Fig. 13-11). Labor expenses in the beef industry are mainly centered on processing and moving the cattle with additional demands around calving time. The labor involved with milking cows in the dairy industry is essentially an all-day, 365 days a year event.

Breeding in the beef industry still occurs by allowing bulls (intact males) to roam the pastures with cows (adult females) seeking those who are "in heat" (estrus); however, many operations are now using artificial insemination (AI) with frozen bull semen as common method of breeding. The dairy industry uses AI almost exclusively as the preferred method of breeding. The **gestation** period (pregnancy length) for cattle is about 9 months. The female calf is called a heifer (until she has had a calf) and the male calf

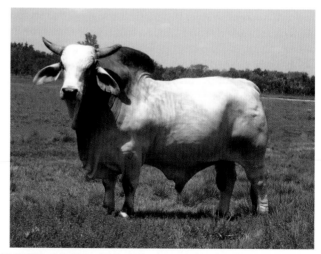

FIGURE 13-7 Brahman bull. (From Holtgrew-Bohling K: Large animal clinical procedures for veterinary technicians, ed 2, St Louis, 2012, Mosby.)

is called a bull calf until he is castrated (at which time he is called a steer).

All cattle require various vaccinations and/or blood tests before being sold or transported between states. Some of the vaccinations and tests must be done by an accredited

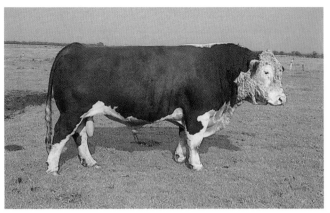

FIGURE 13-8 Hereford beef bull. (From Holtgrew-Bohling K: Large animal clinical procedures for veterinary technicians, ed 2, St Louis, 2012, Mosby.)

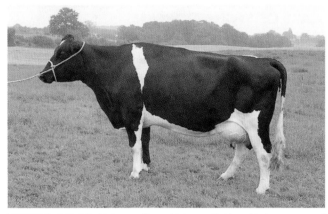

FIGURE 13-11 Holstein. (From Holtgrew-Bohling K: Large animal clinical procedures for veterinary technicians, ed 2, St Louis, 2012, Mosby.)

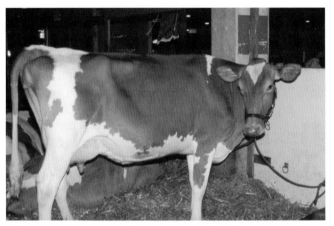

FIGURE 13-9 Guernsey. (From Holtgrew-Bohling K: Large animal clinical procedures for veterinary technicians, ed 2, St Louis, 2012, Mosby.)

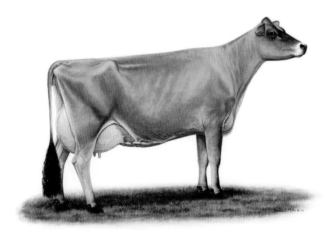

FIGURE 13-10 Jersey. (From Holtgrew-Bohling K: Large animal clinical procedures for veterinary technicians, ed 2, St Louis, 2012, Mosby.)

veterinarian on behalf of state or federal regulatory departments that require the procedure. Private practice veterinarians can become accredited by learning the required laws and rules and by passing a test to demonstrate that knowledge.

Veterinary personnel who deliver or prescribe any medications to any food-producing animal must inform the farm manager about the proper **withdrawal time** for that medication. The withdrawal time refers to the minimum length of time that must pass from the last administration of the medicine until the time that the animal is slaughtered for food or the milk is collected for human consumption. Failure to do so can lead to serious legal repercussions for the prescribing veterinarian.

CARE OF SHEEP (OVINE)

Sheep are raised for meat and wool. There are particular breeds that are selected to do one or the other specifically. However, all sheep have wool of some type; it just may not be very much or of as good quality as from sheep raised specifically for wool.

Some husbandry terms related to the sheep industry include the following: The ewe (adult female) gives birth to one to three lambs (lambing) that are called ram lambs (male) or ewe lambs (female). The gestation for sheep is about 5 months, and breeding usually occurs in the fall of the year resulting in spring lambs. The buck or ram is the name of intact adult male, and a castrated male is called a **wether**.

CARE OF GOATS (CAPRINE)

Goats are rising in popularity as an alternative farming enterprise and as pets. They are also used in many teaching and research institutions as models for animal or human diseases. The rise in popularity of goats has increased the need for veterinary team members to familiarize themselves with the nursing care and treatment techniques applicable to goats.

The adult female (doe) gives birth to kids (kidding) following a 5-month gestation. An intact adult male is called a billy or ram, and castrated males are called wethers. The kids are castrated at a young age with an elastrator. The billy goats have a strong, musky smell that is attractive to the females; however, it permeates through the entire farm as well. Although there is some demand for goat meat, the major use of goats today is milk production for milk or cheese. Goat fiber (mohair) is also marketed in the United States.

CARE OF SWINE (PORCINE)

The present trend in swine production is the use of confinement rearing facilities. However, total confinement operations have received some criticism from organizations concerned with the lack of natural environments being available for the swine under these conditions. Confinement housing facilities allow producers to raise more pigs per farm and to market pigs in 5 to 6 months. The increase in pig density raises concerns in regard to prevention of disease. If a disease occurs, the entire herd can be affected, and the economic loss can be devastating. Pigs become unhealthy because of disease transmission from adjacent pigs or infections from outside sources (e.g., trucking, feed personnel, wind, other species of animals). Therefore, it is imperative when visiting a confinement swine unit that you follow their rules for dress and foot coverings. Never enter a unit without their personnel present. Disease is best prevented by ensuring good health status, nutrition, housing, management, and husbandry.

The adult female (sow) gives birth to piglets (an act called **farrowing**) after a gestation of 3 months, 3 weeks, and 3 days (about 114 days). The intact adult male is a boar, and the castrated male is called a barrow. Young females are called **gilts** until they farrow.

Sows enter the farrowing room a few days before expected parturition. The use of traditional farrowing crates limits the movement of the sows and provides an area for the piglets to avoid being laid on and stay warm and dry. Litter sizes range from 7 to 12, and the average birth weight is approximately 1.5 kg. Hypothermia is a problem in newborn piglets. The piglet's body temperature at birth is 39° C but decreases to 37° C within a few hours. Over the next 24 hours the piglet's body temperature returns to 39° C. An environmental temperature of 30° to 35° C should be maintained with heat lamps and heat mats during this time of relative hypothermia.

> **CRITICAL CONCEPT**
>
> Be aware that some postfarrowing sows can become very aggressive toward handlers when you are handling their newborn piglets.

HORSE HANDLING AND RESTRAINT

The size, speed, strength, and personality of horses make them potentially dangerous animals to restrain. Horses are suspicious creatures and are quick to detect nervousness in handlers. Most horses are not vicious, and most submit to properly applied restraint procedures. Most horses you will work with have a close working relationship with humans. Because they are companion animals, it is important to always talk to them in a calm, low voice. This helps to keep them calm and lets them know where you are. However, even cooperative horses can cause fatal injures if they are suddenly frightened or hurt.

Because they are herd animals, horses find comfort in being with other horses and will react if other horses around them spook or get startled. Horses are also prey animals that have evolved a great sense of flight or fight. If frightened or threatened, a horse's natural instinct is to run away. If a horse cannot get away, it will fight to get away. This often causes injury to the handler or the horse.

Horses have keen eyesight for seeing movement at great distances, but they do not see well up close, nor do they see just below their noses or directly behind themselves. Never walk directly behind a horse unless you stay close and talk to the horse so that it knows you are there. Never walk under a horse's neck. The horse cannot see you there and may throw its head, raise a front leg and knock you down, or rear up and come down on you. Horses will run over the top of you if you are between them and freedom or if they perceive you have cornered them.

Horses will kick as a means of protection. They can kick with either back hoof directly behind themselves as well as out to the sides. They can kick with both back legs at once by rocking their weight to their front legs. They can strike with one front leg at a time or rock all their weight onto their back legs and rear up and strike with both front legs. Horses toss their heads, which can cause serious injury if you are not cautious. Never stand directly in front of a horse; it may strike you with its front leg or its head. Horses also bite. They have both upper and lower incisors that pinch, and they can lock their jaws together making it very difficult to get your body part out from between the jaws. Horses use biting as a means of communication. Horses use nips and outright bites to teach youngsters their place in the herd. However, a horse that bites people should be disciplined quickly and without hesitation.

Horses have elaborate body language that is learned from birth through adulthood. This body language can tell you if the horse is paying attention, and if it is upset, angry, or in pain. The most expressive parts of the horse are the ears. An alert horse has its ears pricked forward. This shows it is aware of your approach and is curious. A nervous or uncertain horse constantly flicks its ears back and forth, especially if there is activity behind it. An angry or fearful horse often pins its ears back. Do not confuse this sign with the laid-back ears of a horse that is concentrating on a difficult task, such as calf roping or barrel racing.

The tail also indicates a horse's attitude. A wringing or circling tail indicates nervousness. A tail held straight down indicates pain or sleeping. A tail that is clamped tight indicates fear.

The mouth and tongue can also indicate what the horse is thinking or how it is feeling. Yawning or grimacing may indicate pain. When asking a horse to do something new to the horse, you know the horse understands the new task when it smacks its lips or its tongue licks in and out. Trainers often use this behavior as a guide to determine when the horse understands what the trainer has asked it to do.

The horse's eyes can also tell you what it is feeling. If you can see the whites all around its eyes with its head held up and its ears working furiously, the horse is probably very frightened. If the horse's eyelids are droopy or half-closed, the horse may be in pain or exhausted.

Horses can be calmed by an even tone of voice, and most cooperate if handled quietly and decisively. Many horses are easily bribed with lumps of sugar, horse biscuits, or grain. Scratching behind its ears, across its eye ridges, and along its neck also helps to convince a horse that you mean it no harm and want to be friends.

When properly restrained, you can give a horse injections, draw blood, auscultate its lungs and heart, take its temperature, administer oral medications, or perform other examinations safely and efficiently. If you are consistent and firm, but not brutal, the horse will respond to you and try to do what you ask.

APPROACHING AND CAPTURING A HORSE

Horses should be approached from the front and slightly to the near (left) side. The reason for approaching from the near side is that horses are accustomed to being handled from that side. They are trained to be saddled and mounted from the near side (Fig. 13-12). The animal may become nervous if you approach or work on the far (right) side. You also need to stay within the horse's range of vision. Each eye is placed on the very edge of its head, allowing the horse to see straight forward and around to its hindquarter almost in a perfect half circle. A horse does not see directly in front of it where it would have to cross or directly behind its hindquarters.

As you approach the horse, watch it carefully. Determine the animal's behavior by looking at its body language and the positions of the ears, tail, and legs. Check out the escape routes within the stall in case the horse becomes frightened or aggressive. If it starts to move away, stop and talk to it, and maybe offer it some oats. If you keep moving toward the horse, it may think it is in danger and try to flee. Move slowly and without sudden movements because horses are easily startled.

Once close enough to touch the animal, it is often best to scratch it behind the ears and on the side of the neck before applying a halter. After this introduction, slip the lead rope over the horse's neck and catch the end as it comes into your reach; tie a single overhand knot to keep the rope from slipping off (Fig. 13-13). Most horses believe they are caught and stand peacefully, but be alert for the possibility that something may frighten the horse, causing it to bolt. If this happens, a quick hand on the rope looped around the horse's neck and some gentle talking should calm it down. If the horse panics and begins resisting restraint, it is better to let it go than to be injured trying to restrain it.

Some horses quickly learn that a rope or halter slung over a human's shoulder means they must go to work, and these horses will not allow you to catch them. For these horses, it is best to keep the ropes hidden from view until you are up close. Baling twine or a small rope works well with these horses because it is more easily concealed and need not be very strong; once the horse is caught, it usually submits quietly. More nervous horses must be enclosed in a smaller pen to catch them. Luring them into the pen with grain is much better than chasing them in because they are then less agitated.

If all else fails, try to rope the horse. Again, it is better to have the horse in a fairly small pen for this. Keep your movements slow and deliberate. Do not swing the rope around your head like you are going to rope a calf. It is best to use a low, backhand technique. Hold the rope at waist height and make a large loop that just brushes the ground. The major portion of the rope should be coiled and held loosely in your left hand so it can peel off after you catch the horse. Hold the loop in your right hand on the left side of your body, palm facing toward you, then situate yourself 8 to 10 feet from the fence on your right side.

Have another person drive the horse between you and the fence; as it goes by, you can toss the loop up so the horse runs into it. Keeping the horse along the fence prevents it from dodging away from the rope as you toss it, so the person driving the horse between you and the fence must keep it moving. The rope can be snubbed around a post to take up the

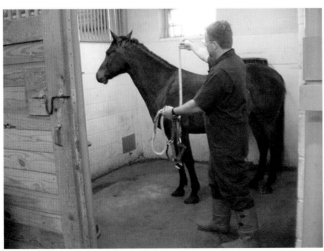

FIGURE 13-12 Horses are trained to be saddled and mounted from the near side. (From Holtgrew-Bohling K: Large animal clinical procedures for veterinary technicians, ed 2, St Louis, 2012, Mosby.)

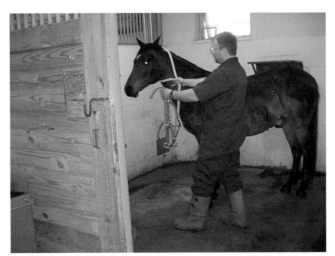

FIGURE 13-13 Slip the lead rope over the horse's neck and catch the end as it comes into your reach; tie a single overhand knot to keep the rope from slipping off. (From Sheldon CC, Topel J, Sonsthagen BS: Animal restraint for veterinary professionals, St Louis, 2006, Mosby.)

slack when the horse is caught. Because the roped horse may resist violently, it is wise to wear gloves to protect your hands from rope burns. Never wrap the rope around your hand.

The halter and lead rope are the main tools of equine restraint and should always be used when leading or working on a horse. Check the halter and lead rope for splits or fraying because a horse can easily break a defective lead rope or halter with a sharp jerk of its head.

After you have caught the horse and it has settled down, place the neck strap and the buckle end of the halter in your left hand. Standing on the near side, hold the buckle in your right hand and the neck strap in your left hand, then move up to the horse's muzzle (Fig. 13-14). Gently slide the noseband around the horse's nose, flip the strap over the poll and on your side of the neck (Fig. 13-15), and secure the halter by buckling it to the neck strap (Fig. 13-16). Untie the lead rope from around the horse's neck and find the center ring on the bottom of the halter. Attach the clip to the center ring (Fig. 13-17).

Check to make sure the halter is settled correctly on the horse's face. There should be no pressure points from rings or rivets, and the straps should not be close to or over the horse's eyes.

If you must approach a horse from the rear, as in a box stall or if the animal is tied, always let the horse know you are approaching. Begin to talk quietly to the horse before you get close. Remember that a horse's kicking range is 6 to 8 feet straight back, and these kicks are usually very accurate. Talk to the horse before and as you approach it, so you do not surprise or startle it. It is safest to pass behind the horse about 10 to 12 feet or more or to stay in direct physical contact by keeping your hand on the horse's rump when passing around the rear (Fig. 13-18). This does not guarantee that you will not get kicked; however, if you are kicked, the blow will be reduced and further down on your body, where it is less life threatening.

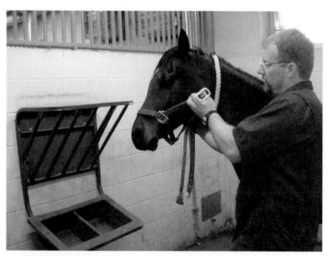

FIGURE 13-14 Standing on the near side, hold the buckle in your right hand and the neck strap in your left hand as you move up to the horse's muzzle (From Sheldon CC, Topel J, Sonsthagen BS: Animal restraint for veterinary professionals, St Louis, 2006, Mosby.)

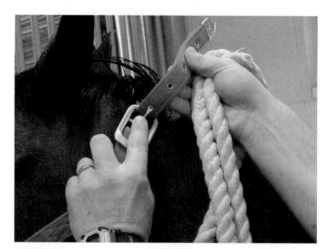

FIGURE 13-16 Secure the halter by buckling it to the neck strap (From Sheldon CC, Topel J, Sonsthagen BS: Animal restraint for veterinary professionals, St Louis, 2006, Mosby.)

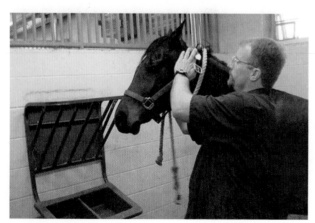

FIGURE 13-15 Gently slide the noseband around the horse's nose and flip the strap over the poll on your side of the neck. (From Sheldon CC, Topel J, Sonsthagen BS: Animal restraint for veterinary professionals, St Louis, 2006, Mosby.)

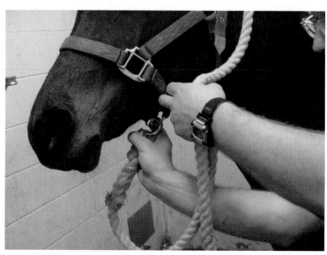

FIGURE 13-17 Attach the clip to the center ring. (From Sheldon CC, Topel J, Sonsthagen BS: Animal restraint for veterinary professionals, St Louis, 2006, Mosby.)

LEADING A HORSE

Once you have haltered the horse, grasp the lead rope where it connects to the halter with your right hand and use your left hand to hold the loose end of the rope in neat loops, with the entire rope held in front of you (Fig. 13-19). Never wrap the loose end of the lead rope around your hand or have the rope running behind you. If the horse bolts, you will be pulled along with it and could be seriously injured. Always walk on the near side of the horse, close to the shoulder, and hold the lead rope with your right hand about 1 foot away from the base of the halter.

After you stop leading a horse, stand as close to its shoulder as possible and face the same direction as the horse. Be careful not to stand too far in front of the horse, as it can rear up and strike with its front foot. Also, do not stand too near or the horse can accidentally step on the back of your heels as you are walking. Never move under a horse's neck to get

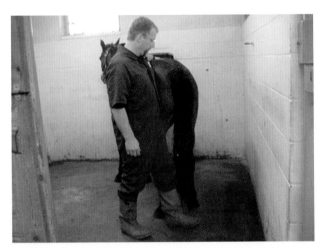

FIGURE 13-18 It is safest to pass behind the horse about 10 to 12 feet or more or to stay in direct physical contact by keeping your hand on the horse's rump when passing around the rear. (From Sheldon CC, Topel J, Sonsthagen BS: Animal restraint for veterinary professionals, St Louis, 2006, Mosby.)

to the other side. This is very dangerous and could result in injury if the horse is suddenly frightened.

Some horses may try to bite you while being led or handled. Deliver punishment at the time of the bite by rapping the horse firmly on its muzzle. You do not have to cause pain with such a rap; only convey the impression that you will not tolerate bad behavior. Punishment given too long after the fact is futile.

TYING A HORSE

If a horse is to be left unattended, it should always be tied to a sturdy object with a properly fitting halter and suitable lead rope. The knot used to tie the lead rope should be a quick-release knot, such as the halter tie. Pass the rope around a sturdy post, ideally a vertical post that is placed in the ground (Fig. 13-20). Allowing 2 to 3 feet of lead for the horse, make a loop that opens up in the end as close to the post as you can and lay it on top of the standing part (Fig. 13-21). Make a bight in the end; pass it under the standing part and through the loop (Fig. 13-22). Pull the bight to tighten the knot (Fig. 13-23). The quick-release knot allows the horse to be released quickly if it panics, catches its foot, or falls down. To release the knot, simply pull on the end.

The horse should be allowed about 2 to 3 feet of lead rope so it can adjust the angle of its neck and shift position as it desires. Allowing more slack than that may cause the horse to tangle its front feet in the rope. Any less slack may frustrate the horse enough for it to try to escape. Do not tie a horse's head too high or too low so it is at an unnatural angle. Rather, tie it so the horse's head is held in a natural position about level with its withers. Always check the area around a tied horse for possible hazards that could cause serious injuries if the horse were suddenly frightened.

CROSS TYING

Cross tying is another way to secure a horse's head and to keep it from rearing. To cross tie, clip one lead rope to the

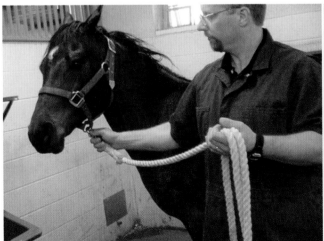
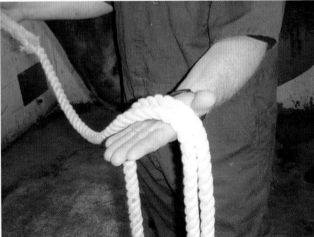

FIGURE 13-19 Once the horse is haltered, grasp the lead rope where it connects to the halter with your right hand; your left hand holds the loose end of the rope in neat loops, with the entire rope held in front of you. (From Sheldon CC, Topel J, Sonsthagen BS: Animal restraint for veterinary professionals, St Louis, 2006, Mosby.)

lateral cheek rings on the left side of the horse's halter. Tie the left lead, using the halter tie. Then walk safely around to the horse's right side and affix the second lead to the lateral cheek ring and tie the horse, again using the halter tie (Fig. 13-24). Do not stand directly in front of the horse. Even with its head secured, the horse can still toss its head or strike out with its front foot.

RESTRAINT OF THE HEAD

For almost every veterinary procedure done on a horse, the head must be restrained. The standard equipment for head restraint is the halter and lead rope. You can use these to hold the horse still, direct its attention elsewhere, and secure it to one spot. Therefore, it is important to examine this equipment for worn or broken parts before use. In addition, while using the halter, be sure to maintain a firm hold.

You must follow three important rules when restraining a horse. First, always stand on the same side of the horse as the person who is working on the animal. If the horse tries to escape, it usually will move away from you. If there are people on both sides of it, the animal will pick the smaller of the barriers and move over that, possibly resulting in injury to a person bending or kneeling down. You will also have to pay attention to the horse as well as what is going on with the procedure. Too often handlers become so wrapped up in what is going on with the procedure that they miss the signs of the horse getting restless or agitated. Then it is too late to try to calm the horse or warn the other person to be ready to get out of the way.

The second rule is to keep the horse's head down so that its eye is looking into your eye. If the horse raises its head up above your shoulders, you will not be able to keep it from moving either up or away. To keep the horse's head down, place one hand over the poll, applying a gentle pressure, and pull down on the lead rope. Watch the horse carefully; some horses resist this pressure and get agitated. If that is the case,

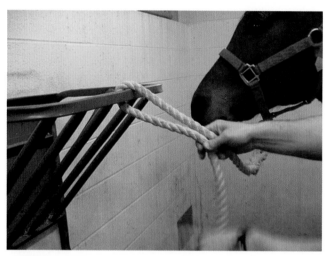

FIGURE 13-20 Pass the rope around a sturdy post, ideally a vertical post that is placed in the ground (From Sheldon CC, Topel J, Sonsthagen BS: Animal restraint for veterinary professionals, St Louis, 2006, Mosby.)

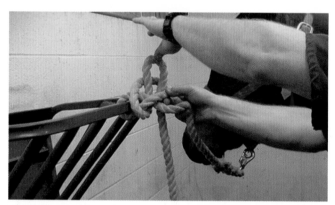

FIGURE 13-22 Make a bight in the end; pass it under the standing part and through the loop (From Sheldon CC, Topel J, Sonsthagen BS: Animal restraint for veterinary professionals, St Louis, 2006, Mosby.)

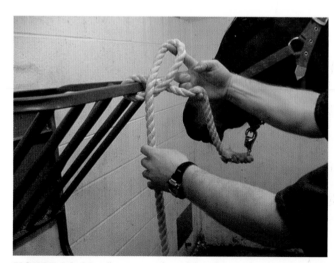

FIGURE 13-21 Allow 2 to 3 feet of lead for the horse and make a loop that opens up in the end as close to the post as you can. Lay it on top of the standing part. (From Sheldon CC, Topel J, Sonsthagen BS: Animal restraint for veterinary professionals, St Louis, 2006, Mosby.)

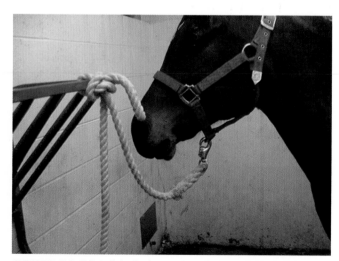

FIGURE 13-23 Pull the bight to tighten the knot. (From Sheldon CC, Topel J, Sonsthagen BS: Animal restraint for veterinary professionals, St Louis, 2006, Mosby.)

ease up on the pressure over the poll but maintain the pressure on the lead rope.

The third rule is to never stand directly in front of a horse. It can rear up and come down on top of you. It can strike out with its front feet or can run you down in an effort to escape. Always stand to the side of the horse, and be prepared for a sudden reaction.

DISTRACTION TECHNIQUES

Sometimes a halter alone is not adequate restraint, and you must rely on other devices to distract the horse's attention. Distraction techniques can help, but if distraction is not enough, a twitch or a chain shank may be necessary.

ROCKING AN EAR

Stand on the left side of the horse. Hold the halter with your left hand over the lateral ring. With your right hand grasp the horse's ear at the base and gently rock it or bend it back and forth. Do not do this too vigorously because you can damage the cartilage and cause the horse's ear to droop. Show horses often are trimmed up around the ears. You may also wish to ask the owner if it is okay to use this technique because it could make them resist having their ears handled.

SKIN ROLL

Grasp as much skin on the shoulder as you can get with one or both hands. Rocking it back and forth or jiggling it provides enough distraction to allow you or another person to accomplish intravenous (IV) and intramuscular (IM) injections.

HAND TWITCH

Stand on the left side of the horse, and hold its halter in your right hand so that you have good head control. Grasp the upper lip with your left hand, and rock the lip back and forth. Be careful not to close off the horse's nostrils.

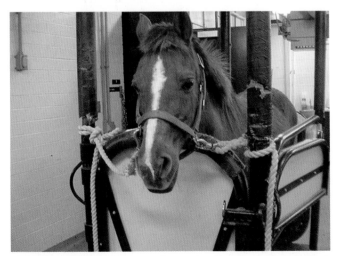

FIGURE 13-24 To cross tie, clip one lead rope to the lateral cheek rings on the left side of the horse's halter. Tie the left lead, using the halter tie. (From Sheldon CC, Topel J, Sonsthagen BS: Animal restraint for veterinary professionals, St Louis, 2006, Mosby.)

BLINDFOLDS

If a horse is afraid to enter a trailer, stock rack, or box stall, or is simply obstinate, using a towel as a blindfold may help. The blindfolded horse usually calms down and then depends on you to guide it. Work slowly and talk constantly to reassure the blindfolded horse.

LEG LIFT

The last technique is quite useful when trying to take a radiograph of a leg. If the horse moves or is unwilling to stand still, lift and hold the leg opposite of the one being radiographed. This will often make the horse stand still. With all techniques, remember the distraction must be intermittent.

TWITCHES

Common types of twitches used on horses are the chain, humane (or clamp), and rope twitches. All have advantages and disadvantages. Often a client's attitude about twitches dictates which one, if any, is used in a particular situation. Twitches should be used only if you know how to apply them and often as a last resort.

Twitches work only for a short time before the muzzle loses feeling, so the greatest effect is when it is first applied. To maximize the twitch's usefulness, tightening and loosening the loop around the muzzle keeps the circulation flowing and keeps the horse's attention on the twitch longer. Be aware that many horses try to get away or resist the twitch when it is first applied; stay with them by moving with their motions. If they shake you off the first time, it becomes more difficult to place the twitch on again. However, if a horse continues to struggle or escalates the struggle, try another distraction technique.

After the twitch is removed, massage the muzzle to restore circulation. This also lets the horse know that a person can touch its muzzle without hurting it.

The twitch can be applied to the lower lip of a horse as well, but this method should be used only if the horse raises strong objections to using the upper lip. Always curl the lip inward to protect the inner surface.

The **chain twitch** is a flat chain loop attached to the end of a stout wooden handle to form a loop. To apply the twitch, hold onto the halter and the twitch handle with your right hand and place the loop of chain over your left hand. Catch one side of the loop between your little finger and ring finger to prevent it from slipping down onto your wrist (Fig. 13-25). Grasp as much of the horse's upper lip with your left hand as possible, pressing the bottom edges together to protect the delicate inner surface (Fig. 13-26), and quickly slide the handle up so the chain loop rests high up around the lip. Tighten the chain around the upper lip by twisting the handle (clockwise if on the left side of the head and counterclockwise if on the right) before letting go of the muzzle (Fig. 13-27). Hold the twitch in your left hand and the halter with your right.

An advantage of a chain twitch is that it slips off easily when the chain is loosened. The length of the handle is usually long enough for the restrainer to stand back beside the horse and hang onto the halter as well. The chain can be loosened and tightened or gently wiggled for added distraction. If steady pressure is constantly applied, the muzzle loses circulation and becomes numb, rendering the twitch ineffective. A disadvantage is that sometimes the horse learns to wiggle its upper lip to dislodge the twitch. Another disadvantage occurs if the horse pulls the handle out of the handler's hands. The free handle can then become a dangerous weapon if the horse throws its head.

The **humane twitch** is a metal clamplike device that pinches the upper lip between two bars. The twitch usually has a length of cord with a clasp attached to it that can be wrapped around the end of the twitch and then attached to the halter. Regardless of its name, this twitch is not any more humane or inhumane than the chain or rope twitch.

The primary disadvantage of this twitch is that it applies steady pressure that can cause the lip to lose feeling and the twitch to lose its effectiveness. Also, the twitch can be dislodged

and become a hazardous flying object if it is attached to the halter. This can scare the horse, causing it to fight to get away from this strange object. Unfortunately, it cannot get away because the twitch is attached to its halter. For this reason, it is not recommended that the twitch be clipped to the halter.

To apply the humane twitch, start by reaching your left hand through the handles. Grasp the horse's upper lip to roll the lips in before placing the twitch around the muzzle. Close the twitch by bringing the handles together firmly (Fig. 13-28). Hold the twitch with your left hand and the halter with your right. Do not twist the muzzle while it is in the twitch because this causes more pain than is necessary.

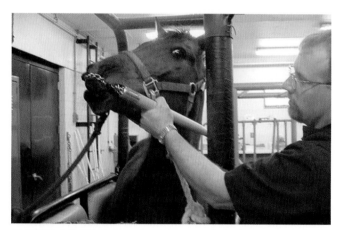

FIGURE 13-27 Tighten the chain around the horse's upper lip by twisting the handle (clockwise if on the left side of the horse's head and counterclockwise if on the right) before letting go of the muzzle. (From Sheldon CC, Topel J, Sonsthagen BS: Animal restraint for veterinary professionals, St Louis, 2006, Mosby.)

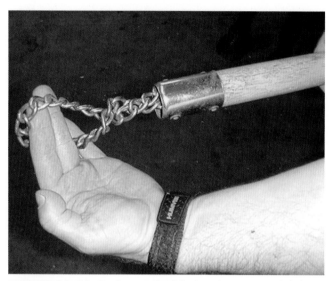

FIGURE 13-25 Catch one side of the loop between your little finger and ring finger to prevent it from slipping down onto your wrist. (From Sheldon CC, Topel J, Sonsthagen BS: Animal restraint for veterinary professionals, St Louis, 2006, Mosby.)

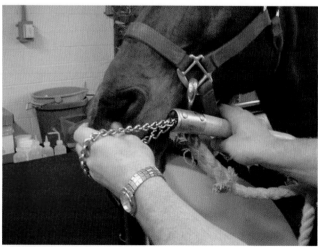

FIGURE 13-26 Grasp as much of the horse's upper lip with your left hand as possible, pressing the bottom edges together to protect the delicate inner surface. (From Sheldon CC, Topel J, Sonsthagen BS: Animal restraint for veterinary professionals, St Louis, 2006, Mosby.)

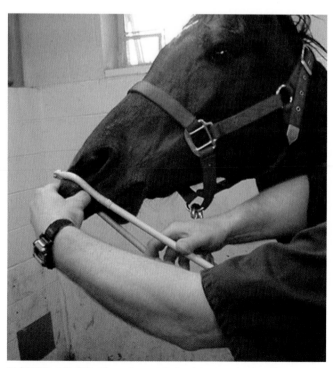

FIGURE 13-28 Close the twitch by bringing the handles together firmly (From Sheldon CC, Topel J, Sonsthagen BS: Animal restraint for veterinary professionals, St Louis, 2006, Mosby.)

Simply squeeze or jiggle the muzzle to achieve the desired effect. The humane twitch will lose its effectiveness in 10 minutes because the muzzle will lose circulation and go numb.

A rope twitch is made from small-diameter cord attached to a stout handle or ring. It is applied to the horse's muzzle in the same manner as the chain twitch. The advantage of a rope twitch is that it is relatively inexpensive and easily made. Also, the loop tends to stay on the horse's muzzle better than a chain. The disadvantage of the rope muzzle is that it tends to pinch the horse's muzzle more than the chain, often causing unnecessary pain.

CHAIN SHANK

The chain shank (also stud shank) is a long leather or nylon strap with about 2 feet of flat chain at its end, attached to a snap. It can be used as another distraction device or on horses that need more restraint than just a halter, such as many stallions. You can use a chain shank in a number of ways.

The first method is the most common. With the halter in place, pass the chain end through the ring on the cheek piece of the near side (Fig. 13-29) and pass it across the bridge of the horse's nose to the ring on the off side of the head (Fig. 13-30). The chain is held in the same hand that holds the lead rope. When the horse tosses its head or rears up, you can snap the chain to make the horse stop or pay attention (Fig. 13-31).

Another way to use the chain shank is to attach the chain as previously described, but instead of leaving it across the bridge of the horse's nose, pass it under the horse's top lip (Fig. 13-32). This really gets the horse's attention when you

snap the chain. Please use it sparingly and only when a horse is being extraordinarily naughty.

You can also put the chain shank under a horse's chin. This is not recommended, however, because it can cause the horse to throw its head up when the chain is snapped instead of keeping its head down, where you can maintain control.

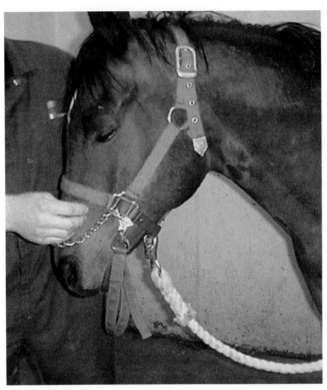

FIGURE 13-30 Next, pass it across the bridge of the horse's nose to the ring on the off side of the horse's head. (From Sheldon CC, Topel J, Sonsthagen BS: Animal restraint for veterinary professionals, St Louis, 2006, Mosby.)

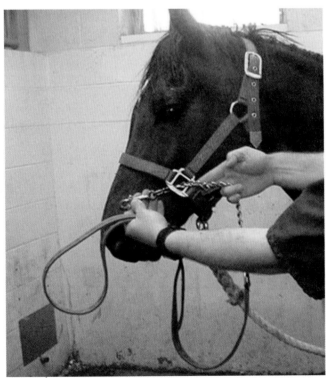

FIGURE 13-29 With the halter in place, pass the chain end through the ring on the cheek piece of the near side. (From Sheldon CC, Topel J, Sonsthagen BS: Animal restraint for veterinary professionals, St Louis, 2006, Mosby.)

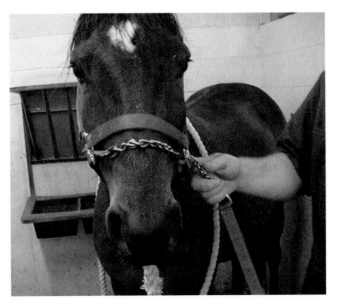

FIGURE 13-31 Hold the chain in the same hand that holds the lead rope. (From Sheldon CC, Topel J, Sonsthagen BS: Animal restraint for veterinary professionals, St Louis, 2006, Mosby.)

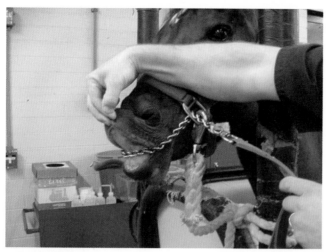

FIGURE 13-32 Another way to use the chain shank is to attach the chain as previously described, but instead of leaving it across the bridge of the horse's nose, pass it under the horse's top lip. (From Sheldon CC, Topel J, Sonsthagen BS: Animal restraint for veterinary professionals, St Louis, 2006, Mosby.)

STOCKS

Stocks are narrow enclosures with removable or semiopen sides and a gate at both ends. They can be made of steel pipes or wooden planks, with the top bar or plank no higher than the horse's shoulder. The front of the stocks should have the necessary hooks for cross tying so the horse cannot jump forward or to the side if it tries to escape. A gate is included at both ends because horses do not like narrow, confined areas. The opened front gate gives the appearance of an escape route as the horse is walked into the stocks.

After opening both gates, lead the horse up to the back gate and step to the outside of the stocks. Do not go into the stocks. Pass the rope around the bars as needed to keep the horse moving. Have someone gently close the front and back gates as soon as the horse is properly situated inside. A horse should not be left unattended when placed in the stocks.

TAIL TYING

Much of a horse's weight can be raised or moved by its tail, which is quite strong. This makes the tail a handy object to use when you need to move an anesthetized horse. However, the tail can also be a nuisance that must be tied out of the way for certain procedures. Remember to always tie the tail to the animal's own body because severe injury may result if the tail is tied to an immovable object and the horse suddenly bolts.

To secure a cord or rope to the tail, first find the last coccygeal vertebra of the tail. Gather the hair up and make a bight with the hair so that the vertebra is on one side and the gathered hair is on the other side of the bight. Support the tail in your hand while you bring the end of the rope through the bight. Pass the end of the rope around the bight so it ends up on top. Bring the end under the rope that is looped around the tail. Tighten by pulling the short end and the long end together. You can now tie the long portion of the rope to one of the horse's front legs or its neck using a bowline knot (Fig. 13-33).

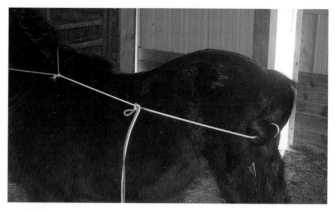

FIGURE 13-33 Tie the long portion of the rope to one of the horse's front legs or the neck using a bowline knot. (From Sheldon CC, Topel J, Sonsthagen BS: Animal restraint for veterinary professionals, St Louis, 2006, Mosby.)

HOBBLES

Breeding hobbles are used to prevent obstinate mares from kicking the stallion when mounting. These hobbles can also be used for rectal or vaginal palpation if stocks are unavailable. Start with a long rope with a bowline on a bight tied in the center. Place the loop around the horse's neck and tie the long ends to each leg above the hock with a halter tie or clove hitch. Place a couple of bales of straw or hay behind the horse for added security just in case the horse can still move its back legs.

RESTRAINT OF FOALS

The easiest way to catch a foal is to back the mare into the corner of a large box stall and secure her in place. The foal naturally tries to hide behind the mare's flank. When it begins to move, grasp the foal around the front of its chest with one arm and quickly around the rump, or grasp its tail with your other hand. Once you have stopped the foal's forward motion, it will typically try to escape by moving backward.

After you have caught the foal, press it up against the wall or a sturdy partition. If this is not feasible, have another person hold the foal in the same manner on the opposite side. Before capturing the foal, make sure the wall or partition does not have holes through which the foal might put its legs, which could cause injuries.

Do not hold onto the foal's tail too tightly or press it down between the legs because this sometimes makes the foal sit down. Also, never lift a foal off its feet. This makes foals very nervous, and they struggle fiercely to regain their feet.

Always talk to and comfort a foal when handling it. Rough handling leads to behavior problems later in life.

Finally, never remove a foal from the sight of the mare. Both mare and foal will fret until they are reunited, and both may injure themselves trying to get back together. Securely tying the dam and keeping the foal within the mare's sight can prevent such problems.

CATTLE RESTRAINT

Dairy cattle are usually used to human handling and can be vaccinated or medicated while haltered and in a stanchion or head gate. However, care should be taken at all times to protect the handler from harm. Beef cattle are not used to being handled and so should be placed in a chute and haltered for most procedures (Fig. 13-34). If available, vaccinations or medications can be given IM or SQ to cattle that are in an alley, as long as they are crowded in fairly tightly so they can't move forward or backward. Serious injuries can occur by being kicked. While working on the back end, place a bar or bale of hay behind their rear legs. Dairy cattle will tolerate antikicking chains being placed just above the hocks, or you can tie a foot up with a long rope (Fig. 13-35).

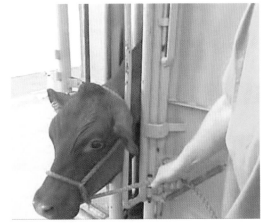

FIGURE 13-34 Cattle restrained in a squeeze chute. A rope halter has also been placed to allow further control of the head. (From Sheldon CC, Topel J, Sonsthagen BS: Animal restraint for veterinary professionals, St Louis, 2006, Mosby.)

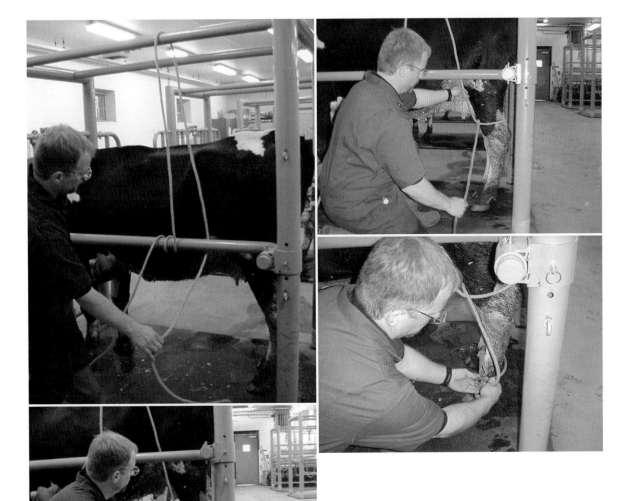

FIGURE 13-35 Lift the leg to the desired height so that the hock is above or level with the stifle, and secure the rope by using a quick release knot to prevent injury if the cow falls. (From Sheldon CC, Topel J, Sonsthagen BS: Animal restraint for veterinary professionals, St Louis, 2006, Mosby.)

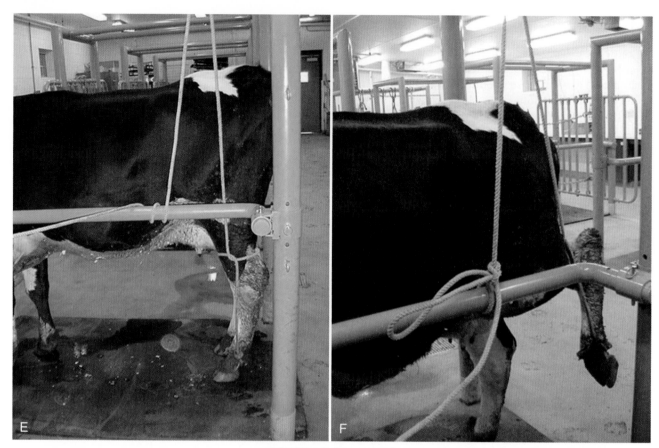

FIGURE 13-35, cont'd

MECHANICAL DEVICES

SQUEEZE CHUTE

The **squeeze chute** is a restraint device used almost exclusively on beef cattle (Fig. 13-36). Nearly all medical procedures can be facilitated by use of a properly constructed chute. A chute usually has three mechanical working parts: the head gate, tailgate, and squeeze. An animal is run into a chute by means of an alleyway.

Cows will usually settle if they feel they are confined in this way. The head gate is closed tight enough so that the animal cannot put a foot through, but not so tight as to clamp the cow's neck to occlude the airway. There are side panels that can be opened to allow access to the cow's side or feet. The tailgate acts as a barrier between you and the cow's rear legs. This allows access to the perineal area for pregnancy checking, tail bleeding, or assistance during calf delivery. The head gate allows you to approach the cow to place a halter or administer oral medications.

Be aware that a cow can still stretch its neck quite a way out and can move it from side to side. The danger is being butted with the head, which is usually not fatal, unless there is direct contact to your head. If the cow's head needs to be controlled, a halter should be applied.

HALTER

The halter used on cattle is usually a rope halter that can be adjusted to fit any sized cow or bull. Two things to remember

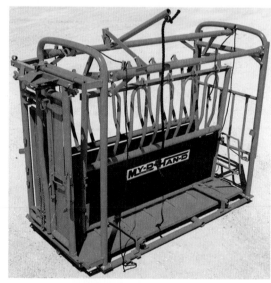

FIGURE 13-36 Cattle squeeze chute. (From Sirois M: Principles and practice of veterinary technology, ed 3, St Louis, 2011, Mosby.)

when applying a halter are that the part that tightens when the lead is pulled goes around the nose and the lead comes off the left side of the cow's head. Before applying the halter, be sure the head stall is large enough to go behind the ears but not so large that you have to make major adjustments while standing close to the cow's head. Most people slip the nose band on first, then the headstall behind the ears (Fig. 13-37).

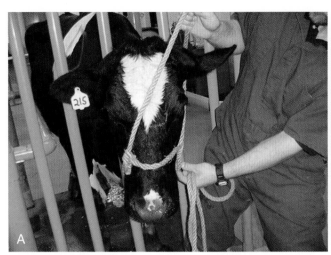
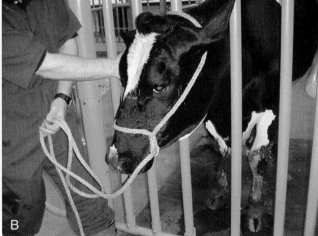

FIGURE 13-37 A, Placing a halter on a cow. **B,** Halter in position on a cow. (From Sirois M: Principles and practice of veterinary technology, ed 3, St Louis, 2011, Mosby.)

Pulling the lead will cause the halter to tighten up, and the cow's head can be tied to the side of the chute. Make sure that you adjust the side straps so they are not resting over the eyes. Halter and tying the head to the chute allows jugular venipuncture or injections, ear tag placement, and ophthalmic procedures to be performed.

STANCHIONS

A stanchion usually consists of a head gate without sidebars to restrict lateral movement. Dairy cattle are often placed in stanchions and are comfortable being worked on in them. They are usually not substantial enough to handle beef cattle. The handler must be aware that even though the head is secured, the cow can kick you.

HOBBLES

Hobbles are usually used on dairy cattle that have tendency to kick the milkers. Hobbles can be either a metal clip that is placed on each hock or a padded strap that is buckled around the lower leg. With both types, it is important to keep the cow's legs squared under her. If the back legs are brought in too close, she could lose her balance and fall.

TILT TABLE

Cattle, especially bulls, often need their feet trimmed. This can be done in a chute, but it is easier to do on a tilt table (Fig. 13-38).

Lead the animal or use an alleyway to put the animal near the table in its vertical upright position. Then sedate the animal and strap it to the table. Tilt the animal so it is in lateral recumbency. This allows access to all four feet at a comfortable height.

APPROACHING AND MOVING

Cattle have the same wide-angle vision as horses. This can be used to the handler's advantage when getting them to move in a desired direction. Cattle have a "pressure point" at the shoulders. If you move past the shoulder going toward

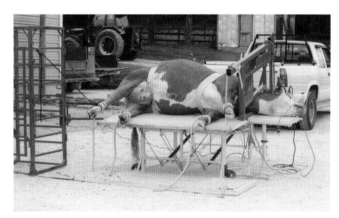

FIGURE 13-38 Tilt table for hoof trimming. (From Sirois M: Principles and practice of veterinary technology, ed 3, St Louis, 2011, Mosby.)

the rear of the cow, it prompts the cow to move forward. If you move toward the head it will make the cow stop. Use this information to move cattle into a pen or down an ally without a lot of prompting with a whip or paddle.

To move a herd or group of cattle into a pen or ally, do not push them too hard. Rather, allow them to look inside and inspect the area. Place one person toward the opening of the gate and one behind the group you need to move. The person in the back puts pressure on the group by stepping forward; the person toward the front puts pressure on the group by walking toward the rear of the group from directly behind their shoulders toward the rear. As the cattle start to move into the pen, the person at the front of the group continues the forward motion by stepping behind the group as he or she moves in that direction. Be aware that cattle will kick if frightened or pushed too hard. They seldom kick straight out, having an arch from front to back. This is important to remember because you can get kicked standing to the side of a cow as well as behind it. Either stand right next to the rear of the cow or back at least 6 to 8 feet. You can be kicked standing next to the animal, but it will not be as deadly as inside the 6-foot range.

Sometimes it is difficult and even dangerous to separate a cow and her calf away from the herd. Instinctively they try to remain with the herd for protection. The best scenario is to move a small group, containing the intended cow and calf, into a pen that has a gate into another pen. One person operates the gate, opening and closing it as the appropriate animal approaches. Two other people are placed in the same positions as described for pushing a group into a pen. Move the mother and her calf along the fence opposite to the person at the gate. This allows the gate to close behind the cow and calf.

Remember that mothers are very protective of their calves and may chase after you if they feel threatened. Have escape routes in mind and watch the cattle carefully. Do not turn your back on the group.

It is also important to lock up any dogs that may be around, even if they are trained cattle dogs. Cows with young at their side will get very upset when a dog is in the pen with them and often charge the dog. Unfortunately, the dog often looks to people for protection and will run behind the closest person. The cow will not differentiate between you and the dog.

SHEEP RESTRAINT

Remember that sheep have a strong flocking instinct and can be moved easily as a group. A singled-out sheep may panic and hurt itself or the handler while trying to get back to the flock. Using small pens that can either crowd the sheep together or moving a single sheep out of the pen in view of the rest of the flock is a good way to handle these sensitive animals. Sheep have a frail skeletal system and can be injured easily if they are chased into fences. Rough handling can break their back and legs. Never grab sheep by the wool; it is easily pulled out and the skin tears easily, causing bruising, which devalues the carcass and pelt.

Setting a sheep up on its rump is often used for venipuncture, ID injections, and foot trimming (Fig. 13-39). Backing the sheep into a corner and pinning its body up against a wall with a hand under the chin will usually suffice for most procedures.

Sheep become hyperthermic easily because of their wool and normally high body temperature (102° to 104° F). Use caution when working with sheep in ambient temperatures greater than 50° F and high humidity. Working in the early part of the morning with good ventilation is a must to keep sheep from overheating.

GOAT RESTRAINT

Goats can often be handled like sheep; however, many milking goats are halter broken and can be led to a small stanchion or tied to a post for procedures. They do not like to be set up like sheep; therefore, lateral recumbency, like a big dog, is often used if they need to be off their feet. Goats can be crowded into a pen, and then an individual goat can be caught and moved out to a work area. You can catch a goat by placing an arm around its neck and the other hand on its tail, much like a foal, and then direct its movements with forward

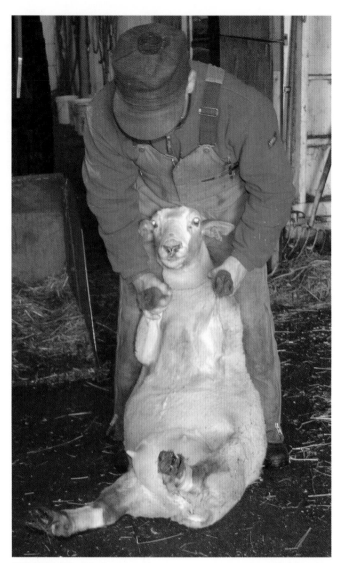

FIGURE 13-39 Setting a sheep up on its rump. (From Sheldon CC, Topel J, Sonsthagen BS: Animal restraint for veterinary professionals, St Louis, 2006, Mosby.)

or backward pressure. Goats that are handled frequently may have a collar that can be used to lead it to the work area. If the goats are in a panic and you cannot get an arm around the neck, grasp a front leg and hold it off the ground. Most goats will stop and allow you to encircle them with your arms or place a collar or halter on them. Some may throw themselves to the ground and cause a disturbance. Be careful not to wrench the leg if this happens.

Once caught, place the goat's rear end in a corner to prevent it from backing up, and press its body against a wall to prevent lateral movement. Hands can be wrapped around either side of the face to lift the head for medications, IM or SQ injections, or jugular venipuncture (Fig. 13-40). Never grab hold of a goat's horns; they resent this and will resist violently. They will either run at you and butt you or shake their heads vigorously. This is especially true of billy goats. Also it is advisable not to grasp the beard on intact male goats. They urinate on their beards as a means of attracting females and the musky scent is difficult to remove. Goats also remember people and rough handling, so be kind. Their payback can be an unpleasant knock with their heads.

SWINE HANDLING AND RESTRAINT

A significant animal welfare and production concern is the potential for stress from improper handling of pigs. Proper handling reduces stress during routine production practices, such as moving of swine, blood sampling, vaccinating, clipping tails and teeth, ear notching, detusking, castration, and administration of therapeutics. Pigs are not herd animals, but they tend to follow other pigs. When one pig becomes distressed and screams, the others may react as a group and panic, or they may come to the rescue of the "injured" pig. Pigs are extremely protective of their young and will come running if a piglet cries out. Pigs are also extremely stubborn, which can be used to advantage with various restraint procedures, particularly the hog snare.

Pigs can become hyperthermic if chased or roughly handled, even in cool weather. Overheated pigs must be cooled immediately or they are likely to die of heat stroke.

Pigs' main defensive weapons are their teeth. They can tear flesh easily and have very strong jaws; the tusks of boars can be very dangerous. Enter all adult swine enclosures with caution and be prepared to exit quickly. Sows are very dangerous when there are piglets at their side; a handler should never get into the same pen with a sow and piglets.

DRIVING AND CATCHING

Pigs can be difficult to drive in an open pen. Solid-paneled hurdles work well to move pigs, as well as pieces of PVC piping or a cane. Pigs stop when confronted with a solid barrier, such as hurdles, and pigs will move along when tapped on the rear quarters. Pigs should be driven into a small pen with solid walls at least as high as a pig's shoulder. They can be separated from the group again using the hurdles and pipe or cane.

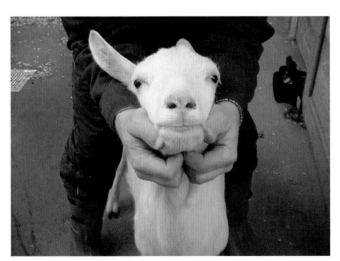

FIGURE 13-40 Holding the head for jugular venipuncture. (From Sirois M: Principles and practice of veterinary technology, ed 3, St Louis, 2011, Mosby.)

DIRECTING A SINGLE PIG

When moving a single pig, walk behind it with a hurdle in front of you (Fig. 13-41). Use a cane or paddle to direct the pig by tapping it on the flank to move it forward or on the shoulder to move it right or left. If it turns and moves toward you, set the edge of the hurdle on the ground and tilt it forward. This prevents the pig from getting its snout under it and lifting, allowing it access to or through your legs. The solid barrier will make the pig turn around.

HOG SNARE

A **hog snare** is used for restraining pigs for venipunctures or other injections. The snare is usually a metal pipe with a cable loop on one end. The free end of the cable runs through the hollow pipe, so the size of the loop can be controlled. Excessive tightening can injure the pig's snout. A snare should be in place for a maximum of 20 to 30 minutes. A rope can be used in place of the pipe and cable snare. If using a snare on a boar with tusks, it is important to get the snare behind the tusks. However, this creates a possible hazard if the snare gets hung up on the tusks as it is removed. The pig is strong enough to jerk the snare from your hands and then swing it around. If the snare hits you or becomes airborne, someone is going to get hurt. Be advised that once a pig has experienced a snare, it is difficult to capture it again.

It is advisable to wear ear protection when using a hog snare because they scream the entire time they are held. Even employing a hog snare for the short time it takes to complete one procedure can cause your ears to ring for the rest of the day.

RESTRAINING PIGLETS

Baby pigs weighing less than 50 pounds are captured by grasping a back leg and holding the pig upside down until it can be held on your forearm close to your body or placed in a holding pen. If removing piglets from a sow, do it quickly

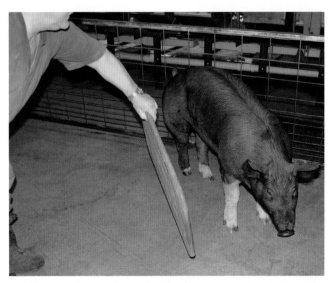

FIGURE 13-41 Moving a pig with a hurdle. (From Sirois M: Principles and practice of veterinary technology, ed 3, St Louis, 2011, Mosby.)

and move to a different room to perform the procedure so you do not agitate the sow. Many farms have a cart to place the piglets in so they can be together, which makes them quiet down faster. Another way to quiet a piglet while holding it is to cradle its body against yours. This gives it a sense of security, and it will not squeal.

Piglets can be restrained by holding both hind legs (Fig. 13-42) or placing them in a V-trough for such procedures as castration, ear notching, and cutting needle teeth. Piglets weighing more than 30 pounds can be held the same way, but it may take two people to hold them upside down by their hind legs.

RESTRAINING POTBELLIED PIGS

Potbellied pigs are usually kept as pets and have a docile temperament; however, some potbellied pigs may show aggression. Small pet pigs tend to squirm, jump, and climb on whomever is trying to restrain them. Ear protection is important for the handler because they can squeal as loud as a full-sized pig. Chemical restraint is sometimes the best choice.

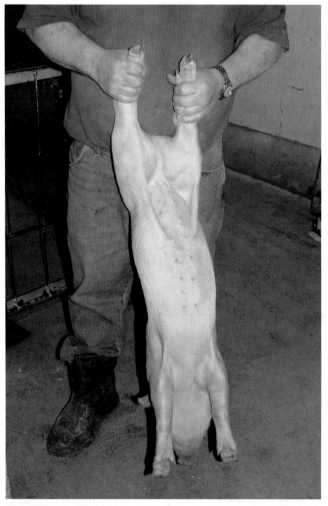

FIGURE 13-42 Holding a pig for transportation. (From Sirois M: Principles and practice of veterinary technology, ed 3, St Louis, 2011, Mosby.)

COMMON PROCEDURES IN LIVESTOCK

HOOF TRIMMING

Periodic trimming of the hooves of is required for the comfort and humane treatment of the animals. Damaged or overgrown hooves can be trimmed and shaped by using various types of knives, shears, and electric grinders.

Cattle must be properly restrained for hoof trimming by using, at least, a squeeze chute. Hydraulically operated tilt tables made specifically for trimming cattle feet make the task safe and efficient. The cattle are secured to the table then laid over on their side (tilted), so the operator has the legs safely restrained and the hooves at a comfortable working height.

Sheep and goats that are not allowed to graze or that are raised in confinement tend to develop overgrown feet. Typically the sidewalls and the toes overgrow. Sheep can be set up on their rumps, and goats can be done standing. The sidewalls should be trimmed to keep the sole flat and the toes pointing forward. Toes are normally squared off. Trimming is done with heavy scissors, hoof rot shears, or a sharp knife (Fig. 13-43). If bleeding occurs, apply hemostatic powder or copper naphthenate solution. Severe bleeding may require bandaging.

CRUTCHING (OR TAGGING)

Ewes close to parturition should be **crutched** or tagged. This procedure removes the wool from around the vulva and the udder. A clean vulva area facilitates passage of the lamb and allows the birthing process to proceed easily. Removing the wool from around the udder assists the lambs in finding and suckling the teats. Lambs suck on anything on the ewe's body, including wool and fecal tags. Trimming this debris from around the vulva and udder areas prevents the lambs from sucking inappropriately.

TAIL DOCKING AND CASTRATING

The tail of lambs is commonly docked to reduce the incidence of fecal material collecting on and around the anus. This in turn causes scalding. Flies will lay eggs in the skin that hatch into maggots. This can cause serious injury to the lamb and even death. The tail is docked or banded below the webbing on the tail using a clean tail-docking instrument, or an elastrator with an elastic band is placed around the tail, which impairs the circulation and causes the tail to fall off in a about 1 week. If the tail is docked too short, it can cause prolapse of the rectum. Castration can also be done with the elastrator at the same time as the tail docking. The restraint technique is the key, holding the lamb against your body and both legs on one side in each hand (Fig. 13-44).

The tail of piglets is commonly clipped to reduce the incidence of tail biting later in the grower-finisher stage. This behavioral vice may result in stress, lameness, and paralysis. The tail is docked approximately 2 cm from the base of the tail using clean, slightly dull side cutters to crush the tail.

Cauterizing clippers tend to reduce the amount of bleeding. Cutting the tail too short may result in anal prolapse.

After puberty male pigs may have an offensive odor or "boar taint" that is evident in pork during cooking. There are various techniques of castration, each determined by the age and size of the pig. The best time to castrate is before 3 weeks of age. However, one disadvantage to early castration is reduced detection of inguinal hernias. A knife blade can be used in boars of any size. A hooked blade (No. 12) works well with pigs weighing less than 15 kg.

Pigs castrated between 2 weeks and 16 weeks of age can be held by the back legs, with the abdomen toward the operator and the back of the pig cradled between the restrainer's legs.

Male calves are usually castrated at a fairly young age depending on the owner's preferences. They can be castrated using an emasculator, which will surgically remove the testicle from the body. Some producers will use the elastrator, an elastic band that goes around the testicle causing circulation loss, which will make the testicles fall off in about a week; however, this should not be used on calves over 1 month old. The band can fall off, and they are more prone to tetanus. Dehorning is also done on young stock; the use of chemicals or a heated iron that burns the horn nub is a common technique. The use of lidocaine for pain control during the burning has been found to greatly reduce the stress of this method of dehorning.

CLIPPING TEETH

The newborn piglet has eight very sharp canine teeth (Fig. 13-45). These are also referred to as wolf or **needle teeth**. In large litters, if the needle teeth are left intact, the piglets scratch each other, causing infection and significant irritation to the sow's teats. Cutting the teeth in smaller litters may be unnecessary, but many producers clip teeth as a precaution. Using clean, sharp side cutters, position the side cutters parallel to the gum line and clip off the distal half of each tooth. Take care not to cut the pig's gum or tongue. Cutting too short may shatter the teeth, leading to gum infection.

UMBILICAL CORD CLIPPING

The umbilical cord can act as a portal of entry for bacteria. If the piglet is bleeding from the umbilical cord, tie off the cord immediately using string. Using disinfected side cutters, cut the cord 4 to 5 cm from the abdominal wall. Spray with or dip the end of the cord in 2% povidone-iodine.

> ### CRITICAL CONCEPT
> Before attempting to deliver medication by any method, be sure the animal is adequately restrained for the method used.

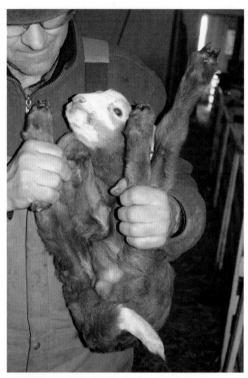

FIGURE 13-44 Holding a lamb for tail docking and castration. (From Sirois M: Principles and practice of veterinary technology, ed 3, St Louis, 2011, Mosby.)

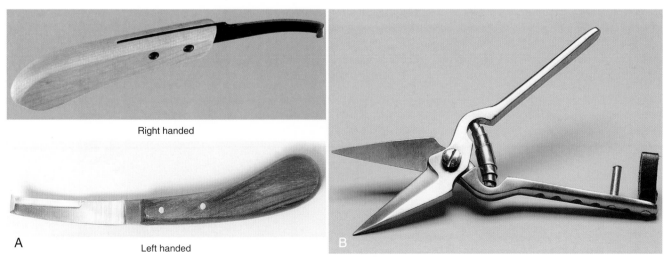

Right handed

Left handed

A   B

FIGURE 13-43 A, Hoof knife. B, Hoof trimmer. (From Sirois M: Principles and practice of veterinary technology, ed 3, St Louis, 2011, Mosby.)

MONITORING HOSPITALIZED PATIENTS

Hospitalized patients must be monitored regularly for changes in their condition. Horses only slightly ill can develop more severe and even life-threatening illness while receiving treatment. For instance, a horse receiving antibiotic therapy for a mild respiratory infection can develop life-threatening diarrhea from changes in bowel microflora. A horse receiving nonsteroidal anti-inflammatory drugs for an orthopedic problem can develop gastrointestinal ulceration

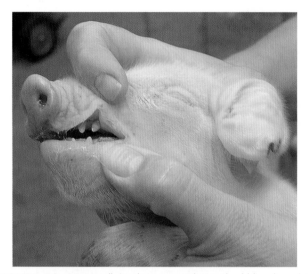

FIGURE 13-45 Needle teeth in neonatal pigs should be clipped to prevent bite injuries to the dam and littermates. (From Bassert J, Thomas J: McCurnin's clinical textbook for veterinary technicians, ed 8, St Louis, 2014, Saunders.)

or renal dysfunction secondary to the anti-inflammatory medication, particularly if the animal is not eating and drinking normally.

The heart rate, respiratory rate, rectal temperature, mucous membrane color (Fig. 13-46), capillary refill time, attitude, digital pulses, urine and fecal output, gastrointestinal motility, and appetite should all be monitored at least once or twice daily. Critically ill neonates require more frequent monitoring, sometimes as often as every 2 hours, because their condition can deteriorate rapidly. Adult horses should be weighed at admission with a walk-on scale, if available, or a weight tape can be used to estimate the horse's weight. Neonates should be weighed at admission and then daily. Most newborn animals can be weighed by picking them up and weighing the handler and animal together on a conventional scale and then subtracting the handler's weight. This may not be feasible with large foals.

CARE OF RECUMBENT HORSES

Nursing care for recumbent animals must be meticulous. Caring for a horse that is unable to rise is tedious and often unrewarding. Horses that remain recumbent for prolonged periods eventually develop various complications, regardless of the primary disease. Because of the weight of the animal, several people are needed to frequently turn the animal from one side to the other. This is usually done with long ropes looped, not tied, around the pasterns so that the handlers can stand farther from the limbs of the horse, or by using a winch and harness when available. If the size of the

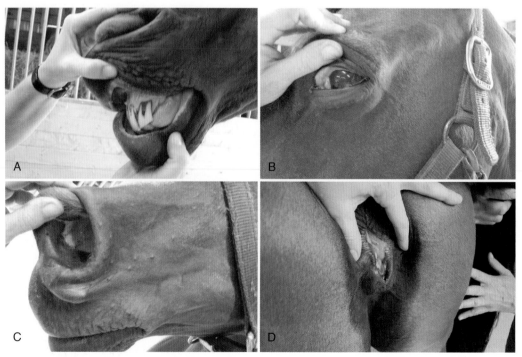

FIGURE 13-46 Examination of mucous membranes. **A,** Examination of the gums. **B,** Examination of the conjunctiva. **C,** Examination of the mucosa of the nares. **D,** Examination of the vulva in the female. (From Sirois M: Principles and practice of veterinary technology, ed 3, St Louis, 2011, Mosby.)

horse permits, it would be preferable to flex the legs up next to the body then roll the horse's torso over the flexed legs rather than roll the horse over on its back. Rolling the horse on its back may cause a twisted intestine and add another unneeded complication to an already sick or injured animal. When a horse is turned from one side to another, the animal often kicks, which can be very dangerous for anyone standing in the vicinity. The animal must be turned as frequently as possible to prevent development of decubital ulcers on the skin and edema and congestion in the dependent portion of the lung. Helmets can be applied to horses that tend to flail about and hit their head against the wall or ground. The technician and assistant should also pay particular attention to the eyes of a recumbent animal because the corneas can become ulcerated if the animal rubs its eyes on the ground.

> ### CRITICAL CONCEPT
> No one should stand within striking distance of the limbs of a recumbent horse.

The primary disease must be resolved as quickly as possible so that the animal may once again stand. If the horse can stand but only with assistance, the hind limbs can be supported by suspending a rope attached to the tail from a ceiling beam. The head may also need to be supported. Commercial slings are available that provide support for horses that have some ability to support themselves but require additional help. A sling cannot be used for horses with flaccid paralysis or other conditions that make them unable to support themselves at all because they can only slump down in the sling. Slings must be well padded to prevent development of pressure sores.

No matter how meticulous the nursing care, decubital ulcers may develop over bony prominences, such as the tuber coxae, carpus, hock, shoulder joint, or elbow. These must be cleaned with a mild antibacterial soap. Topical antibacterial powders or sprays can also be used. A spray that creates a "breathable" bandage may provide the best protection. Any bony protuberance that can be protected by wraps should be wrapped. It is important to keep the animal clean and dry. Frequent cleaning can help to prevent urine scalding and reduce the severity of decubital ulcers. Additional bedding may also help minimize the formation of decubital sores.

The recumbent animal may not eat or drink well. Soft, highly palatable feeds should be offered. If mashes are offered but not eaten, they must be replaced frequently to ensure palatability. Fresh, clean water should be offered to the recumbent animal every 2 hours, if possible. The food and water may have to be given by nasogastric tube because the animal may aspirate feed or water into the lungs when trying to eat or drink in lateral recumbency. If possible, it is preferable to feed the horse while it is in a more sternal position. Infusion of IV fluids may be required in more debilitated or dehydrated animals.

BANDAGING

Materials needed to bandage the distal limbs include cotton quilts or sheet cotton (three sheets) and track wraps, brown roll gauze, or some type of conforming bandage material. Leg wraps can be used to protect a wound, to give additional support, or to cover a medicated area. The wrap should be applied with even pressure so that the tendons running along the caudal aspect of the leg (superficial and deep digital flexor tendons) are protected and pressure is evenly applied over the entire length of the tendons.

To start, a quilt or some other thick padding is wrapped around the leg. Sheet cotton can be used; at least three sheets are needed for sufficient padding. Start the wrap at the front portion of the leg and then bring the quilt across the outside of the leg, around the back, and then inside of the leg, maintaining even tension at all times (Fig. 13-47). Once the quilt is in place, a track wrap brown gauze roll or other type of outer wrap is used. The same principle is followed, with the wrap being placed from lateral toward medial across the back of the leg. It is best to start this part of the wrap near the bottom of the leg (distally) and work up (proximally).

The outer wrap is secured with Velcro attachments, ties, or adhesive tape. If adhesive tape is used, the ends should not overlap because the tape is relatively inelastic and may produce uneven pressure across the tendons. If roll gauze is used, this can be secured with adhesive tape; alternatively, an additional layer can be applied using a conforming bandage wrap. When the wrap is finished, a small strip of padding should be visible in the innermost layer of the wrap both proximally and distally (Fig. 13-48). Care must be taken to make sure that the wrap is snug but not too tight. Two fingers should be able to fit snugly between the leg and the wrap, but the wrap should feel firm and should not slip down the leg. If the wrap is applied to protect a wound, antibacterial ointment and a nonstick dressing must first be applied to the area and held in place with a layer of stretch gauze.

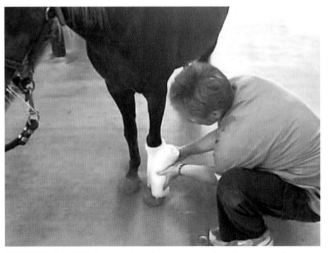

FIGURE 13-47 Application of sheet cotton for placement of a wrap to the distal limb of a standing horse. (From Sirois M: Principles and practice of veterinary technology, ed 3, St Louis, 2011, Mosby.)

If the full length of the leg must be wrapped, an additional wrap can be applied so that it overlaps the lower limb wrap to some extent. This additional wrap is applied in a similar manner. The proximal wrap should overlap the distal wrap and extend to the midradius area. Often a piece of the wrap is cut out over the accessory carpal bone to prevent development of pressure sores over this bone. This is more difficult to do on the hind leg because special consideration must be given to the highly movable hock joint. Often the conforming bandage material is applied in a figure-8 around the hock so that only the sheet cotton contacts the point of the hock.

FOOT WRAPS

There are many different ways to wrap feet. The foot is first picked clean and then washed and dried if needed. If the foot requires medication, this can be applied and then covered with a gauze sponge secured with a layer of rolled gauze. If padding is needed for protection, roll cotton or two to three sheets of cotton are used to wrap around the foot. Next, rolled brown gauze or stretch gauze can be used to secure the sheet cotton. This is applied in figure-8 fashion to make the sheet cotton lie flat across the bottom of the foot. Finally, elastic tape or duct tape is applied to provide additional support and protection, and secure the bandage in place. It is very important to have the ground surface of the foot wrap flat, rather than convex and bulging, so that even pressure is applied to the bottom of the foot. If no padding is needed and the foot wrap is being used to apply medication to an area of the foot, the duct tape or a conforming bandage material can be applied directly to the foot after a nonsticking dressing or gauze sponge is placed over the medication.

Be careful not to wrap up over the coronary band if no protective padding is in place. Excessive pressure directly on the coronary band can reduce circulation to hoof tissues and cause damage or sloughing of the hoof. If there is any question about the amount of pressure on the coronary band, one or more vertical slits can be cut in the bandage where it covers the coronary band to relieve pressure.

TAIL BANDAGES

Tail wraps can consist of stall bandages, rolled brown gauze, or even commercial tail bags. If the tail wrap is intended to be left on the horse for many days, it is important that the wrap not extend proximally to include the tail bones (coccygeal vertebrae) because the tail has little muscular padding and a tight wrap can occlude blood circulation to the tail and create a tissue slough or even loss of the entire tail. If it is necessary to wrap more proximally on the tail, a nonconstricting wrap should be loosely applied and changed daily.

At times it is necessary to wrap the tail of a horse with severe diarrhea to keep the tail clean. This can be done using a plastic rectal sleeve. Holes can be cut in the sleeve to help keep the tail from "sweating." The tail hair should first be braided and the sleeve slid over the tail and tied at the most proximal part of the braid. The sleeve can also be anchored to the most proximal part of the tail with a strip of adhesive tape or duct tape placed lengthwise from the sleeve cranially along the midline of the back.

The tail may also need to be wrapped when a mare is about to foal or for a reproductive examination. Rolled brown gauze is applied, starting at the tail head (proximal area) and working distally, being sure to incorporate all of the tail hairs within the wrap. When the wrap reaches just distal to the last tail bone, the remaining tail hairs can be folded and incorporated within this section of the wrap (Fig. 13-49). The brown gauze is then tied to itself to end and secure the wrap.

SAMPLE COLLECTION

URINE COLLECTION

A female generally urinates just after standing. However, urine samples for bacteriologic, chemical, and microscopic testing can be collected directly from the bladder by inserting a catheter using aseptic technique.

The animal should be suitably restrained and the vulva cleaned. For goats a double-bladed small animal vaginal speculum is inserted into the vagina. Under visual control

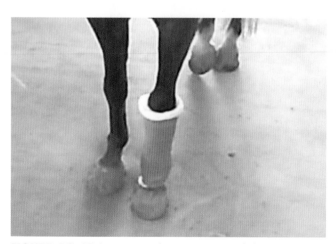

FIGURE 13-48 Leg wrap with outer covering of elastic wrap over sheet cotton. (From Sirois M: Principles and practice of veterinary technology, ed 3, St Louis, 2011, Mosby.)

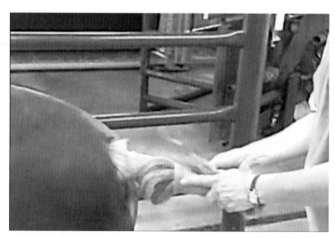

FIGURE 13-49 Tail hairs should all be incorporated into the wrap. (From Sirois M: Principles and practice of veterinary technology, ed 3, St Louis, 2011, Mosby.)

with illumination from a light, a sterile curved metal urinary catheter is inserted into the urethra. For cattle a catheter is guided in with one hand in the rectum, so the feces needs to be raked out and the vulva cleaned thoroughly before placing the catheter.

Urethral catheterization of males cannot be performed. The presence of a urethral diverticulum at the level of the ischial arch makes it impossible to introduce a catheter into the urinary bladder.

Collecting urine from sheep is easier than with many other animals. Have a specimen cup ready before starting. Hold the sheep in a standing position and pinch the nostrils closed until urination occurs. Generally the sheep will urinate within 30 seconds. The nostrils may be held closed for up to 1 minute. If the sheep does not urinate in that minute, allow the animal to rest for 1 or 2 minutes. Repeat the procedure as necessary to obtain a sample.

BLOOD COLLECTION

Sites for venous blood sampling in horses include the jugular vein (Fig. 13-50), cephalic vein, lateral thoracic vein, saphenous vein, and coccygeal vein. Any vein that can be identified, occluded, and accessed safely may be used.

For cattle, the jugular vein is one of the most common locations for venipuncture. It is the largest-diameter and most accessible vein. Proper restraint of the head is critical to ensure safety of personnel. The tail vein is another common location for blood collection because it is easily accessed if the animal has limited side-to-side mobility. Cattle are generally more tolerant of venipuncture in the tail than in the neck.

The jugular vein is commonly used for blood collection in sheep and goats. The cephalic vein on the forearm or the femoral vein on the hindleg can also be used.

In swine, blood collection from the tail vein is limited to adult pigs without docked tails. The tail vein is found on the ventral midline of the tail at the junction of the tail with the body. The volume of blood typically obtained is approximately 2 to 5 mL. The cranial vena cava is commonly used for blood collection (Fig. 13-51). Because the jugular vein is not as deep a structure as the cranial vena cava, it is a safer structure for access with a needle. However, the jugular veins are not as large in diameter and may be difficult to find, especially in large or heavy animals.

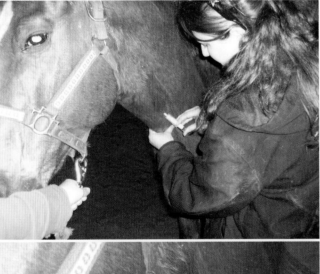

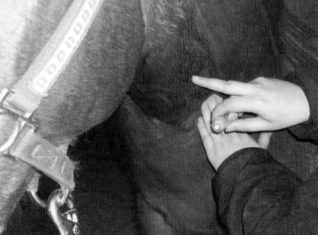

FIGURE 13-50 Location of the jugular vein. (From Holtgrew-Bohling K: Large animal clinical procedures for veterinary technicians, ed 2, St Louis, 2012, Mosby.)

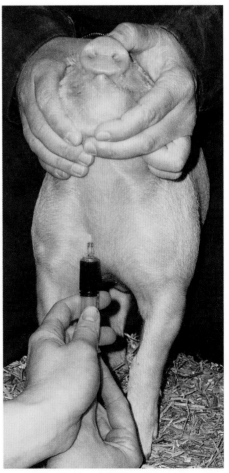

FIGURE 13-51 A blood sample from the right anterior vena cava is taken with the needle directed into the jugular fossa just lateral to the manubrium sterni. (From Bassert J, Thomas J: McCurnin's clinical textbook for veterinary technicians, ed 8, St Louis, 2014, Saunders.)

ADMINISTRATION OF MEDICATION

ORAL ADMINISTRATION

Medications that are in liquid form and required in only small doses may be administered with a dose syringe or a syringe with the locking tip removed. The syringe is placed through the side of the mouth in the area of the **diastema**, or interdental space (space between the incisors and premolars) (Fig. 13-52). The medication is deposited on the caudal portion of the tongue if possible. Medications in pill form can be crushed with a mortar and pestle and then mixed with something sweet, such as molasses, and given in a similar manner. It is best not to mix medication with the feed because horses often eat around the medication and do not consume the full dose. Medication that must be given in large volumes requires use of a nasogastric tube for delivery into the stomach.

BALLING GUN

Boluses (large tablets), capsules, or magnets may be given per os (PO) with a balling gun. This instrument is available in various sizes for use in different species. Cattle require a balling gun with a large metal or flexible plastic head and a long handle. The plastic head produces less trauma to the pharyngeal tissue than a metal head but is easily damaged by teeth. Small balling guns are manufactured for use in calves, sheep/lambs, and goats/kids.

The methods of introducing a balling gun, dose syringe, drench bottle, or Frick's speculum are similar in all species. For cattle, sheep, and goats: stand cranial to the animal's shoulder and, facing the same direction as the animal, reach across the bridge of the nose with the animal's head positioned on your hip. Insert the fingers of this hand into the mouth at the interdental space and apply pressure to the hard palate, which causes the animal to open its mouth. Lubricate the bolus and balling gun before inserting it into the animal's mouth. Insert the balling gun or similar instrument straight in over the incisors on the bottom jaw; the fingers inside the mouth can guide it as it moves to the center of the tongue. Once it reaches the tongue you'll feel it bump over the esophageal groove; advance the balling gun until the rings of the handle touch the lips (Fig.13-53). This ensures that the balling gun is back far enough in the mouth to deposit the bolus, forcing the animal to swallow and preventing expulsion of the medication. Depress the plunger a couple of times to eject the bolus, then remove the instrument. Observe the animal to be sure the medication was swallowed. It is not necessary to elevate the head until the bolus is swallowed if the bolus was deposited correctly. If working on sheep that are short enough, straddle them to insert the balling gun.

Commercially prepared paste syringes containing medication are inserted the same as for the balling gun. The paste is usually deposited on the tongue and not down the esophagus.

FRICK'S SPECULUM

A **Frick's speculum** may be used to give two or more boluses to cattle. Insert the speculum in the same manner as the balling gun. Once the speculum is placed over the base of the tongue, the boluses are inserted into the speculum. Allow the boluses to travel down the speculum and into the esophagus. Remove the speculum and observe for swallowing. This method is used to save time but has the added danger of aspiration of medication.

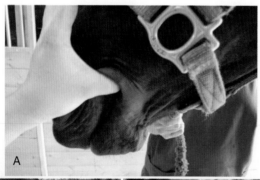

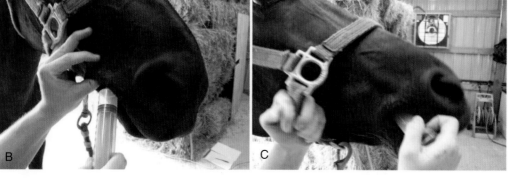

FIGURE 13-52 **A,** Opening the lips before placing the oral syringe in the mouth. **B,** Placement of the dose syringe near the commissure of the lips. **C,** Proper positioning of the oral syringe. (From Sirois M: Principles and practice of veterinary technology, ed 3, St Louis, 2011, Mosby.)

DRENCHING

Giving small volumes of liquids PO is often referred to as **drenching**. Drenching is done with a dose syringe with various-sized nozzles to fit the animal or a drench bottle (Fig. 13-54). A 60-mL catheter-tipped syringe or a bulb syringe may be used as a dose syringe in calves, lambs, and kids. The drench bottle should be made of strong glass and have a long, tapered neck and smooth mouth.

The technique for drenching is similar to that described for the balling gun except you insert the bottle at the **commissure** of the lips in the interdental space. The animal's head should be held slightly elevated so that the nose is level with the animal's eye. If the head is raised excessively, the animal could aspirate some of the medication. Give the medication slowly, allowing the animal to swallow at its own pace. The Drench-Matic dose syringe can be used to medicate a herd of animals. When the handles are squeezed, a set amount of medication is delivered to each animal. It is attached to a hose that is inserted into a gallon container that holds the medication. If administering medications in a crowd pen, make sure to mark each animal as it is done so you don't double-dose or miss one.

OROGASTRIC INTUBATION

Orogastric administration, also called "stomach tubing," is a quick and relatively painless method to deliver large quantities of liquid medication or fluids. A stomach tube may be passed through the nasal cavity (nasogastric administration)

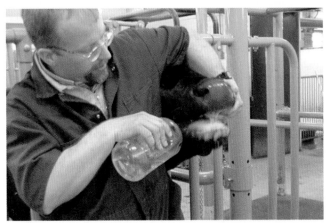

FIGURE 13-54 Drenching a cow with the animal restrained in a stanchion. (From Sheldon CC, Topel J, Sonsthagen BS: *Animal restraint for veterinary professionals,* St Louis, 2006, Mosby.)

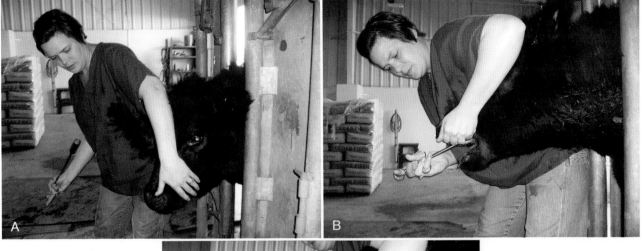

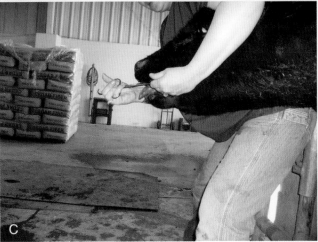

FIGURE 13-53 **A,** Preparation for insertion of the balling gun. The balling gun must be held tipped up to prevent the pill from falling out. **B,** Insertion of the balling gun into the oral cavity. **C,** Administration of medication by depressing the plunger. (From Holtgrew-Bohling K: *Large animal clinical procedures for veterinary technicians,* ed 2, St Louis, 2012, Mosby.)

in horses, but this method is not commonly used in food animals. In food animals, the stomach tube is usually passed through the oral cavity with the aid of a mouth speculum (Fig. 13-55).

An oral speculum is required to prevent damage to the soft stomach tube from the animal's teeth or be closed off by the animal biting down on the tube. The Frick's, Drinkwater, or Bayer speculum is inserted into the mouth and held in place by an assistant or the person inserting the tube.

Stomach tubes are available in different lengths and diameters. Choose an appropriately sized tube for the individual animal. A tube with an outside diameter of ⅝ to 1 inch is the average size used for adult cattle. A foal stomach tube is often used for "tubing" calves, sheep, and goats. A 14-French feeding tube will work on neonate lambs and kids. A stomach pump, syringe, or funnel can be used to facilitate administration.

Measure the distance externally from the mouth to the rumen, and insert the tube approximately this distance. The first 3 feet of the tube should be lubricated with water or water-soluble lubricating jelly before intubation. With the veterinary assistant holding an oral speculum in place, the veterinary technician inserts the tube into the speculum and advances it with gentle pressure.

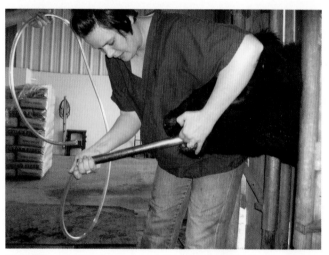

FIGURE 13-55 Placement of Frick's speculum. (From Holtgrew-Bohling K: Large animal clinical procedures for veterinary technicians, ed 2, St Louis, 2012, Mosby.)

PARENTERAL INJECTIONS

Drugs and other liquids can be injected into a muscle (IM) or vein (IV), under the skin (SQ), or into a layer of the skin (ID). Some medications can be given by multiple routes, either intravenously or intramuscularly. It is very important to know which routes of administration are acceptable for each drug administered because injection by an inappropriate route can have harmful or even lethal effects on the horse. For example, procaine penicillin should be given only in the muscle (IM). If this medication is given in the vein (IV), the procaine component may cause excitation, seizures, and death. Some medications should be administered intravenously only. These medications can be very caustic and cause tissue sloughing if administered outside the vein (**perivascular**) or in the muscle.

Whenever the efficacy of treatment is not compromised, drugs and vaccines should be given subcutaneously rather than intramuscularly to minimize damage to muscle tissue and decrease the incidence of abscesses.

SUBCUTANEOUS INJECTIONS

Occasionally medications are injected subcutaneously in horses. These medications are usually given in smaller doses, such as for allergy desensitization. A 20- or 21-gauge, 1-inch needle should be used. Any area where the skin can easily be lifted from the underlying muscle and fascia may be used; the lateral aspect of the neck where IM injections are also given is a suitable site in horses. The skin is first cleaned with alcohol if necessary and then pulled laterally to form a "tent." The needle is then inserted under the skin (Fig. 13-56). Always aspirate to make sure no blood enters the syringe and then inject.

Subcutaneous (SC) injections are given in the lateral aspect of the neck, over the ribs, or in front of the shoulder in cattle, sheep, and goats. Subcutaneous injections in pigs less than 25 kg are given primarily in the loose skin of the flank or caudal to the elbow. If injecting into the flank, inject into the folds of the skin and not into the peritoneal cavity. In larger pigs the preferred injection site is the loose skin caudal to the ear. It is not necessary to tent the skin as we do in small animals if you use a short enough needle. This technique is used if vaccinating numerous animals in an alley or crowd pen; otherwise, pinching the skin to make a tent works well.

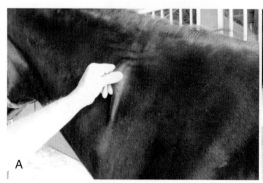 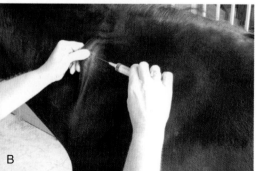

FIGURE 13-56 A, Elevating the skin for subcutaneous injection. **B,** Injection technique for subcutaneous injection. (From Sirois M: Principles and practice of veterinary technology, ed 3, St Louis, 2011, Mosby.)

For sheep, limit the volume of medication to 5 mL per site. If a large volume is to be injected, divide the dose into several portions injected at different sites. If done correctly, subcutaneous injection should leave a bleb under the skin.

INTRAMUSCULAR INJECTIONS

Various sites can be used for IM injections in horses. The safest muscle to use is in the lateral neck area. The neck muscles of the horse can be used for administering only small volumes of medication. The area to be used is a triangular portion on the side of the neck formed by the ligamentum nuchae dorsally, the spine ventrally, and the scapula caudally. Another common area for IM injection is in the semitendinosus and semimembranosus muscles of the hind leg. This is the preferred site for IM injections in neonatal foals because they are usually the largest muscle masses available in young and minimally developed foals. However, this is a very vulnerable position for the handler, and horses that are known to kick should not be injected at this site. Yet another available site would be the pectoral muscles found on the cranial chest wall between the front legs. There should always be an experienced handler available to properly restrain the horse when administering any IM injections in the horse.

A 16- or 18-gauge, 1.5-inch needle should be used for IM injections in adults. A 20-gauge, 1-inch needle should be used for small equines and neonates. The site is cleaned with alcohol if necessary, and the needle, without an attached syringe, is inserted with a quick jab. Intramuscular (IM) injections are not as commonly used in food animals. The movement to reduce injection abscesses and scarring in the muscles used for prime cuts of meat has prompted the medical community to limit IM injections to the lateral cervical muscles. These muscles are cranial to the scapula, dorsal to the cervical vertebrae, and ventral to the ligamentum nuchae. With pigs, the area of the neck muscle caudal to the ear is used.

Dairy cattle can be given IM injections in a stanchion or head gate; a halter is usually not necessary. Beef cattle should be placed in a chute and, if running a large group of cattle at one time, the injection can be given in the alleyway as they are waiting to go through the chute. Calves, sheep, and goats are backed into a corner and the head is restrained by placing an arm around their necks. Pigs will require a hog snare if they are adults; if under 40 to 50 pounds, they can be picked up by their back legs or crowded into a small pen with a marker crayon to mark each pig after an injection.

INTRAVENOUS INJECTIONS

When administering medication IV, the blood dilutes the medication, causing it to become less caustic. The jugular vein is the only appropriate vein for IV injections in horses. The jugular vein runs caudally along the jugular furrow from the head and then enters the thoracic inlet on its way to the heart. The carotid artery runs deep to the jugular vein in the same vicinity, but it courses deeper into the neck and is separated from the jugular vein in the more cranial portion of the neck.

The veins most often used for IV injections in cattle, sheep, and goats are the jugular veins; in cattle, the coccygeal (tail) vein and subcutaneous abdominal (milk) veins also can be used. The jugular veins are most often used for large-volume IV injections. In addition to their accessibility, there is less chance of being kicked when using these veins. The jugular vein is always used for IV injections in calves, sheep, and goats because it is the largest accessible vessel. The auricular vein is used in pigs.

The coccygeal (tail) vein is used for IV injection of small volumes (0.3 to 0.5 mL) of drugs that are noncaustic to the surrounding tissues in case it goes perivascular (Fig. 13-57). Most dairy cattle are tolerant of tail injections; however, there is a chance of being kicked. This can be minimized with proper restraint, including placing a bar or bale of hay behind the back legs.

The subcutaneous abdominal vein, also called the mammary or milk vein, is used mainly when the jugular veins are thrombosed (occluded) or cannot be located. There are several disadvantages to milk vein injections. The technician has an increased risk of being kicked. A second person may be required to provide additional restraint. The milk vein rolls easily under the skin, making it hard to puncture the vein and thread the needle. Finally, hematomas are easily formed and may result in thrombosis of the vein.

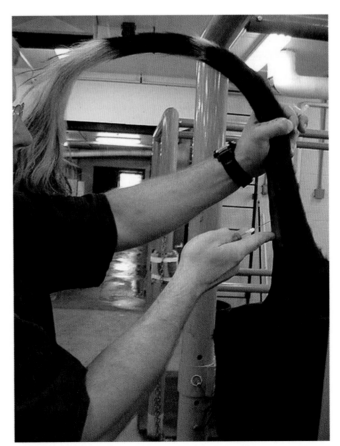

FIGURE 13-57 Coccygeal venipuncture. (From Sheldon CC, Topel J, Sonsthagen BS: Animal restraint for veterinary professionals, St Louis, 2006, Mosby.)

The auricular vein in pigs is often used to deliver IV medications. A winged (butterfly) infusion set can be used to access the vein and be secured with Tegaderm, a transparent dressing that adheres well to bare skin. The injection should be fairly slow because the vein will often balloon out if it is given too fast.

Preparation for IV injection is similar for all veins. Cotton soaked in 70% alcohol should be applied to the injection site to remove gross contamination and increase visibility of the vein. IV injections should not be made through dirt or fecal material because phlebitis, septicemia, and/or contamination of medication and samples may result. Clipping the hair over the injection site may be necessary if it cannot be readily visualized.

RESTRAINT. Beef cattle are placed into a chute and their heads are haltered for the jugular vein injection. For tail injections, a bar should be placed behind their back legs to prevent kicking. The subcutaneous abdominal vein is rarely used on beef cattle but can be accessed by lowering the side panels on the chute. Tying the back legs may be necessary because they can kick forward with their rear legs. Dairy cattle can be given IV injections in a stanchion. Using the other restraint devices and techniques as previously discussed is also a good idea to ensure your safety.

The veins can be easily accessed on sheep if the animal is set up on its rump. Goats, adult sheep, and small calves can be backed into a corner and pinned up against the wall with the restrainer's body. Reach both hands around the head and grasp the jaws with each hand. The cephalic and femoral veins may be used also, with the sheep and goats in a standing or lateral recumbency position.

The needle selected for IV injection of large volumes of fluids varies according to personal preference and the flow rate desired. It also depends on the viscosity of the drug to be administered. Use the smallest needle possible because this reduces discomfort to the patient and minimizes trauma. A 14-, 16-, or 18-gauge, 1.5- to 2-inch needle is best for giving large volumes to adult cattle. A correctly placed needle is not likely to slip from the vein if the cow thrashes around, decreasing the chances of perivascular infiltration of irritants and hypertonic solutions. For injections of small volumes into the jugular vein, use of a 16-, 18-, or 20-gauge, 1.5-inch needle is recommended for cows and calves. Depending on the size of the sheep or goat, an 18- or 20-gauge, 1- to 1.5-inch needle and syringe can be used.

A rubber IV line, referred to as a simplex, is used for IV infusions. A syringe may also be used to inject medication. Its size depends on the volume of medication to be injected.

Cotton and 70% alcohol are also needed to clean the injection site of manure and dirt.

Intravenous injections are commonly given in the auricular vein (Table 13-4) on pigs and some large cattle. Pigs

TABLE 13-4	Recommended Needle Sizes, Injection Volumes, and Blood Sample Volumes, Based on Pig Size								
	INJECTIONS			**BLOOD SAMPLING**					
IM	**SC**	**IV**	**CRANIAL VENA CAVA**	**JUGULAR VEIN**	**EAR VEIN**	**MEDIAL CANTHUS**	**TAIL VEIN**	**CEPHALIC VEIN**
Piglet									
Needle	18-20 gauge, 11 mm	21 gauge, 11 mm	20 gauge, 38 mm	20 gauge, 38 mm		20 gauge, 25 mm		
Quantity	1-2 mL/site		Unlimited			5-10 mL		
Weaner									
Needle	18-20 gauge, 18 mm	21 gauge, 25 mm	20 gauge, 38 mm	20 gauge, 38 mm		20 gauge, 25 mm		20 gauge, 38 mm
Quantity	1-2 mL/site		Unlimited			5-10 mL		5-10 mL
Grower-Finisher									
Needle	16 gauge, 18-25 mm	18 gauge, 25 mm	18 gauge, 65 mm	20 gauge, 38 mm	20 gauge, 25 mm	16 gauge, 38 mm		
Quantity	1-3 mL/site		Unlimited		1-2 mL	5-10 mL		
Breeding Stock									
Needle	14-16 gauge, 38 mm	18 gauge, 38 mm	16 gauge, 90 mm	20 gauge, 38 mm	20 gauge, 25 mm	14 gauge, 38 mm	20 gauge, 25 mm	
Quantity	1-3 mL/site		Unlimited		1-2 mL	5-10 mL	5-10 mL	

From Sirois M: Principles and practice of veterinary technology, ed 3, St Louis, 2011, Mosby.

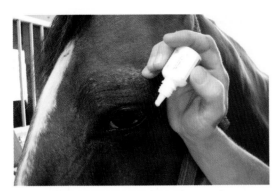

FIGURE 13-58 Proper technique for medicating the eye. Note that the hand is stabilized against the horse's head. (From Sirois M: Principles and practice of veterinary technology, ed 3, St Louis, 2011, Mosby.)

less than 15 kg can be held, whereas larger pigs should be restrained using a snare. The auricular vein, near the lateral border of the ear, is prominent when held off using thumb pressure or a rubber band as a tourniquet at the base of the ear. After a minute the ear veins become engorged. A 20- to 22- gauge, ¾- to 1-inch infusion set (butterfly catheter) works very well for administration of solutions. If you need to leave the catheter in, a Tegaderm bandage is a clear bandage that works well on the bare skin of the ear.

EYE MEDICATION

Topical ointments or solutions can be applied directly to the eye in horses and other livestock. Once the animal is adequately restrained, gently pry the eye open with clean fingers, being careful to touch only the outer lids (Fig. 13-58). Ointments can be applied by placing a small bead of ointment into the lower conjunctival sac. Care must be taken not to scratch the surface of the cornea. Ophthalmic drops can be placed in the lower conjunctival sac using the plastic dispenser vial provided or using a sterile tuberculin syringe without an attached needle if the solution is to be used on multiple horses.

Severe corneal ulcers may require topical treatments as often as every 1 to 2 hours. For horses that become head shy and resentful with this frequent treatment schedule, alternative medication delivery systems can be used. Lavage systems can be placed in the upper eyelid (subpalpebral) or inserted into the tear duct (nasolacrimal duct), and liquid medications can then be delivered easily through either of these systems. Severe corneal ulcers and some other abnormalities may require extra protection for the eye. A protective eye cup can be used to protect the eye and keep the horse from dislodging the lavage system. The black plastic cup also protects the eye from direct sunlight, which could cause pain. This may be very important because many corneal ulcers require treatment with atropine to inhibit ciliary spasm. This makes the horse unable to constrict the pupil when exposed to direct sunlight. Netted fly masks can also be used to provide some protection for the eyes. Horses that spend a lot of time lying down may accumulate shavings or bedding in the eyes. Eye cups or netted fly masks can also be used to help keep the shavings out.

RECOMMENDED READINGS

Church DC: *Livestock feeds and feeding*, ed 3, Englewood Cliffs, NJ, 1991, Prentice-Hall.

Cohen ND, et al.: Medical management of right dorsal colitis in 5 horses: a retrospective study (1987-1993), *J Vet Intern Med* 9:272–276, 1995.

Hanie EA: *Large animal clinical procedures for veterinary technicians*, St Louis, 2006, Mosby.

Howard JL: *Current veterinary therapy 3: food animal practice*, St Louis, 1993, Saunders.

Orsini JA, Divers TJ: *Manual of equine emergencies*, ed 3, St Louis, 2009, Saunders.

Pond WG, Mersmann HJ: *Biology of the domestic pig*, Ithaca, NY, 2001, Comstock Publishing Associates.

Pugh DG: *Sheep and goat medicine*, St Louis, 2002, Mosby.

Radostits OM: *Herd health: food animal production medicine*, ed 3, St Louis, 2001, Saunders.

Reed SR, Bailey WM, Sellon DC: *Equine internal medicine*, ed 3, St Louis, 2010, Saunders.

Sirois M: *Principles and practice of veterinary technology*, ed 3, St Louis, 2011, Mosby.

Smith BP: *Large animal internal medicine*, ed 4, St Louis, 2009, Mosby.

Spurlock SL, et al.: Long-term jugular vein catheterization in horses, *J Am Vet Med Assoc* 196:425–430, 1990.

Glossary

A

Abduction Movement of a limb or part away from the median line or middle of the body.

Abrasion An injury in which the epithelium is removed from the tissue surface.

Absolute leukocyte value The number of each type of leukocyte in peripheral blood; calculated by multiplying the relative percentage from the differential count by the total white blood cell count.

Absorption The movement of drug molecules from the site of administration into the systemic circulation.

Academy Organization that establishes its own bylaws, leaders, application committee, testing committee, and credentialing committee, testing only those candidates who meet specific requirements.

Acariasis Infestation with mites.

Accuracy The closeness with which test results agree with the true quantitative value of the constituent.

Acid-fast A staining procedure for demonstrating the presence of microorganisms that are not readily decolorized by acid after staining; a characteristic of certain bacteria, particularly *Mycobacterium* and *Nocardia*.

Acidosis A condition in which the blood pH is less than 7.35.

ACTH stimulation Test designed to evaluate the response of the hormone that stimulates adrenocortical growth and secretion (adrenocorticotropic hormone).

Activated clotting time A test of the intrinsic and common pathways of blood coagulation that uses a diatomaceous earth tube to initiate clotting.

Active immunity Refers to an animal's production of antibody as a result of infection with an antigen or immunization.

Acupressure Use of finger pressure instead of needles on acupoints along the body's meridians.

Acupuncture Placing of small, sharp, sterile needles into specific points on the body.

Ad libitum Free choice, as much as desired (also called ad lib).

Ad libitum feeding Offering food at all times so that the animal can eat at its leisure.

Adaptive immunity A component of the immune system that responds to specific antigens.

Adduction Movement of a limb or part toward the median line or middle of the body.

Aerobic In the presence of oxygen.

Aerosolized The form of ultramicroscopic solid or liquid particles dispersed or suspended in air or gas.

Agammaglobulinemic Without immunoglobulins.

Agar A seaweed extract used to solidify a culture medium.

Agglutination Clumping of particles.

Aggression Behavior that is intended to harm another individual.

Agonist A chemical substance that can combine with a cell receptor and cause a reaction or create an active site.

Agonistic Referring to a behavior shown in situations of social conflict to defuse aggressive behavior.

Agranulocyte White blood cell group that has no visible cytoplasmic granules.

Air sacs Found in avian species; nine thin, transparent membranes connected to the primary and secondary bronchi that act as reservoirs for air entering and leaving the lungs.

ALARA Acronym for *as low as reasonably achievable*; a program in place by the National Committee on Radiation Protection ensuring that radiation exposure is as low as possible by wearing safety protection and using nonmanual restraint for veterinary patients.

Albumin A group of plasma proteins that composes most of the protein in plasma.

Alcohol Disinfectant that must remain in contact with a site for 15 to 20 minutes to be effective.

Alkaline phosphatase A group of enzymes that functions at alkaline pH and catalyzes reactions of organic phosphates.

Alkalosis A condition in which the blood pH is higher than 7.45.

Allergen An antigen that evokes an allergic or hypersensitivity reaction.

Allopathic medicine Another term used to describe Western medicine.

Alopecia Loss of hair.

Alpha hemolysis Characterized by partial destruction of blood cells on a blood agar; evident as a greenish zone around the bacterial colony.

Alphanumeric system A dental charting system that identifies each tooth with letters that directly correlate with the type of tooth and numbers that correlate with the placement of the tooth in the dental arcade.

ALT Alanine aminotransferase; cytoplasmic enzyme of hepatocytes released when hepatocytes are damaged.

Alternative therapy A practice that deviates from the Western approach.

Alveolus A tiny, grapelike cluster of thin cells in the lungs, the site of gas exchange.

American Animal Hospital Association (AAHA) An organization that has set standards for veterinary practice facilities.

American Association for Laboratory Animal Science (AALAS) Organization founded in 1950; dedicated to the humane care and treatment of laboratory animals and the quality research that has led to scientific gains that have benefited humans and animals.

American Society for the Prevention of Cruelty to Animals (ASPCA) Organization founded by Henry Bergh in 1866 to enforce animal anticruelty laws.

American Veterinary Medical Association (AVMA) Accreditation Policies and Procedures Manual Guidelines created by the Committee on Veterinary Technician Education and Activities (CVTEA) for veterinary technician programs to follow, outlining standards for education of veterinary technicians (http://www.avma.org).

American Veterinary Medical Association–Professional Liability Insurance Trust Organization that provides services to protect the assets and reputations of the participants and enhances the image of the profession; in the near future, may offer professional insurance to technicians.

Amylase Enzyme derived primarily from the pancreas that functions in the breakdown of starch.

Anaerobic In the absence of oxygen.

Analgesia Pain relief, in the form of oral, transdermal, or injectable medication; the inability to feel pain while still conscious. The word is derived from the Greek *an-*, meaning without, and *algesis,* meaning sense of pain.

Analgesic Drug that reduces the perception of pain without loss of other sensations.

Anamnesis Information gained from the patient and others regarding the patient's medical history; derived from the Greek word meaning loss of forgetfulness.

Anaphylaxis A severe hypersensitivity reaction characterized by profound hypotension, pulmonary edema, and collapse caused by massive exposure to an antigen.

Anatomic timed scrub Surgical personnel preparation accomplished by repeating the scrub protocol for 5 minutes.

Anemia Reduction in the oxygen-carrying capacity of blood caused by a reduced number of circulating red blood cells (RBCs), reduced packed cell volume (PCV), or a reduced concentration of hemoglobin.

Anesthesia Loss of feeling or awareness. Literally means "no feeling"; may be local, regional, spinal-epidural, or general (supraspinal).

Angiotensin-converting enzyme (ACE) inhibitor Medication that blocks the angiotensin-converting enzyme and prevents formation of angiotensin II and aldosterone.

Angiotribe Large crushing instrument used to clamp blood vessels.

Animal model An animal whose anatomy and/or physiology make it suitable for research for studying a specific human disease.

Animal Welfare Act U.S. federal law that regulates the treatment of animals in research, exhibition, and transport and by dealers. Other laws, policies, and guidelines may include additional species coverage or specifications for animal care and use, but all refer to the Animal Welfare Act as the minimum acceptable standard.

Anion Negatively charged ion.

Anisocoria Uneven pupil size.

Anisodactyl The foot shape of passerines; three toes point forward and one toe points to the rear.

Anisokaryosis Variation in size of nuclei in cells of a sample.

Anisonucleoliosis Variation in size of nucleoli.

Anode A positively charged electrode in the x-ray tube consisting of a tungsten target that produces x-rays when hit with electrons from the cathode.

Antagonist A drug or other chemical substance capable of reducing the physiologic activity of another chemical substance; refers especially to a drug that opposes the action of a drug or other chemical substance on the nervous system by combining with and blocking the nerve receptor.

Anthelmintic General term used to describe compounds that kill various types of internal parasites.

Anthropomorphism Attributing human characteristics and emotions to animals.

Antibiotic See antimicrobial; the terms are interchangeable.

Antibloat medication Pharmacologic agent that acts by reducing the number of gas-producing rumen microorganisms or by breaking up the bubbles formed in the rumen with frothy bloat.

Anticholinergic Medication that inhibits the transmission of parasympathetic nerve impulses, thereby reducing smooth muscle spasms (e.g., in the bladder).

Anticonvulsant A drug used to control seizures.

Antiemetic A drug given to prevent vomiting; derived from the Greek *emesis,* meaning vomiting.

Antigen Any substance capable of eliciting an immune response.

Antigenic determinant (epitope) The particular part of the antigen that binds the antibody.

Anti-inflammatory A drug that relieves pain or discomfort by blocking or reducing the inflammatory process.

Antimicrobial A drug that kills or inhibits the growth of microorganisms such as bacteria, protozoa, or fungi.

Antisepsis The prevention of infectious agent growth on animate (living) objects; the destruction of most living pathogenic microorganisms on animate (living) objects.

Antiseptic Chemical agent that kills or prevents the growth of microorganisms on living tissue.

Anuria Absence of urine.

Anxiolysis A drug given to prevent anxiety; suffix derived from the Greek *lysis,* meaning breakdown, destruction, separation.

Aortic thromboembolism An aggregation of platelets and fibrin that acutely migrates and lodges at a distant site in the circulatory system.

Apnea Suspension of external breathing.

Apnea monitor Sensor placed between an endotracheal tube (ETT) connector and breathing circuit to determine whether the patient is breathing.

Apteria The featherless tracts of birds.

Arch Row of teeth, such as the mandibular/maxillary arch.

Aromatherapy Therapeutic use of pure essential oils derived from aromatic plants to help balance and heal the mind, body, and spirit.

Arrhythmia Any abnormal pattern of electrical activity in the heart; abnormal heart rhythm; irregular heartbeat.

Arthropod Ectoparasite belonging to the phylum Arthropoda (insects).

Artifact A structure or feature not normally present, but visible, that diminishes the quality of a radiograph.

Asepsis A condition of being free from infection.

Aseptic technique All precautions taken to prevent contamination and ultimately infection.

Aspartate aminotransferase (AST) An enzyme of hepatocytes found free in the cytoplasm and attached to the mitochondrial membrane that is released when hepatocytes are damaged.

Assertive communication Acting confidently, confident in stating a position or claim.

Ataxia A wobbly or uncoordinated gait.

Atelectasis The lack of gas exchange within alveoli, usually caused by alveolar collapse or fluid consolidation.

Atlas First cervical vertebra.

Audition Listening carefully.

Auditory sense A mechanical sense. Through a complex set of auditory passageways and ear structures, vibrations of air molecules are converted into impulses that the brain decodes as sounds.

Auscultation Listening to heart and lung sounds using a stethoscope; listening to sounds produced by the body directly (with the ear and no instrument) or indirectly (using a stethoscope to amplify sounds).

Autoclave A sterilization unit that creates high-temperature pressurized steam.

Autoimmune disease Humoral or cell-mediated response against antigens found in a body's own cells (e.g., systemic lupus erythematosus, rheumatoid arthritis).

Autoimmunity Any condition that results in production of antibody against a body's own tissues.

Autotomize Breaking away of part of the lizard tail at points of fracture planes of cartilage through the vertebral bodies.

Axon Projection of a nerve cell that conducts impulses away from the cell body, to other neurons, or to effector organs, such as muscle cells.

Ayurveda East Indian philosophy of diet, herbs, and exercise used to promote health and vitality.

Azotemia An increase in waste products in the blood, specifically blood urea nitrogen (BUN) and creatinine; increased retention of urea in the blood.

B

Bacilli Rod-shaped bacteria.

Bactericidal Kills bacteria.

Bacteriology Study of bacteria.

Bacteriostatic Inhibits bacterial replication.

Baermann technique Parasitology test used to recover larvae.

Bain coaxial circuit A type of nonrebreathing circuit, also referred to as the modified Mapleson D system, in which the tube supplying fresh gas is surrounded by the larger corrugated tubing that conducts gas away from the patient.

Balanced fluid solution Fluid that is similar in composition to plasma.

Balfour retractor Self-retaining retractor with a set screw to maintain tension on tissues, commonly used to retract abdominal wall.

Ballottement Rhythmically pressing the fist into an area of the abdomen in an attempt to detect any large underlying masses or organs.

Band cell Immature granulocyte with parallel sides and no nuclear lobes or indentations.

Bandage scissors Scissors with a blunt tip that can safely be introduced under a bandage for removal.

Barbering Refers to an action that occurs when a dominant mouse chews the fur of a subordinate mouse.

Barotrauma Respiratory system injury following excessive circuit pressure changes; may also refer to injury to the eustachian tube, ear drum, and stomach.

Basal metabolic rate (BMR) The minimum amount of energy necessary for daily maintenance.

Base narrow canines When the angle of canine growth is directed inward from a normal occlusion.

Base wide canines When the angle of canine growth is directed outward from a normal occlusion.

Basophilia Increase in the number of basophils in a cell; also refers to the bluish-gray appearance of cells or their components that have a high affinity for stains with an alkaline pH (e.g., methylene blue).

Beer's law Describes the relationship among light absorbance, transmission, and concentration of a substance in solution.

Behavior Any act done by an animal; exhibited for a reason and with purpose.

Benign A tumor or growth that is not malignant; can refer to any condition that is not life threatening.

Beta hemolysis Complete destruction of red blood cells on a blood agar that creates a clear zone around the bacterial colony.

Bile acids Group of compounds synthesized by hepatocytes from cholesterol that aid in fat absorption.

Bilirubin Insoluble pigment derived from the breakdown of hemoglobin, which is processed by hepatocytes.

Biologics Wide range of medicinal products such as vaccines, blood and blood components, allergenics, somatic cells, gene therapy, tissues, and recombinant therapeutic proteins created by biologic processes, as opposed to chemical processes. Biologics can be composed of sugars, proteins, or nucleic acids or complex combinations of these substances, or may be living entities such as cells and tissues. Biologics are isolated from a variety of natural sources—human, animal, or microorganism—and may be produced by biotechnology methods and other technologies.

Biopsy Removal of cells or tissues for microscopic or chemical examination.

Biosafety level I Refers to substances that ordinarily do not cause disease in humans (e.g., most soaps and cleaning agents, vaccines administered to animals, infectious diseases that are species-specific). It should be noted, however, that these otherwise harmless substances may affect individuals with an immune deficiency.

Biosafety level II Refers to substances that have the potential to cause human disease if handled incorrectly. At this level, specific precautions are taken to avoid problems. The hazards in this level include mucous membrane exposure, possible oral ingestion, and puncture of the skin.

Biosafety level III Refers to substances that can cause serious and potentially lethal disease. The potential for aerosol respiratory transmission is high.

Biosafety level IV Refers to substances that have a high risk of causing life-threatening diseases. Facilities that handle these substances exercise maximum containment. Personnel shower in and shower out and dress in full body suits equipped with a positive air supply.

Biotransformation The alteration of a drug by the body before being eliminated.

Bisecting angle technique   A radiographic technique in which the film is placed as close to the intended tooth as possible. (The shape of the oral cavity usually prevents parallel placement.) The cone is then directed midway between the angle of the tooth and the film.

Bladderworm   Fluid-filled larval stage of some cestodes.

Blend   Refers to combinations of herbs.

Blood agar   An enriched medium that supports the growth of most bacterial pathogens; usually composed of sheep blood.

Blood crossmatch   Complex testing that is performed prior to a blood transfusion to determine if the donor's blood is compatible with the blood of an intended recipient.

Blood group antigens   Antigens on the surface of red blood cells that characterize the blood as being of a certain type.

Blood type   A classification of blood based on the presence or absence of inherited antigens on the surface of red blood cells.

B lymphocyte (B cell)   A type of lymphocyte that can be transformed into plasma cells on antigenic stimulation to produce antibodies.

Boar   A pig or male guinea pig.

Board of Veterinary Medical Examiners   A state body that interprets the act governing the practice of veterinary medicine that reviews cases brought against a veterinarian or layperson performing surgery, prescribing medicine, or diagnosing disease. The board is charged with protecting consumers and their pets and livestock. They review cases to determine whether the standard of care has been met and if there has been negligence or malpractice causing injury or death to an animal.

Body condition scoring   Method of subjectively quantifying subcutaneous body fat reserves.

Body language   Body mannerisms, postures, and facial expressions that can be interpreted as unconsciously communicating someone's feelings or psychological state.

Bolus   A drug given intravenously as a single volume at one time; a large tablet or ball of food that is intended to be swallowed or a large amount of fluid or liquid medication given quickly, intravenously (as opposed to being given slowly, or titrated).

Brachycephalic   Condition of having a short face; more specifically, a short, wide muzzle (e.g., short-nosed dogs).

Brachygnathism   Maxillary underbite; the mandibular arcade is longer than the maxillary arcade.

Bradyarrhythmia   Any disturbance of the heart's rhythm resulting in fewer than normal heartbeats. The prefix is derived from the Greek *brady,* meaning slow.

Bradycardia   Abnormally low heart rate, decreased heart rate.

Brainstem   In the brain, forms the stem to which the cerebrum, cerebellum, and spinal cord are attached; maintains the vital functions of the body such as respiration, body temperature, heart rate, gastrointestinal tract function, blood pressure, appetite, thirst, and sleep-wake cycles.

Breathing circuit   That part of the anesthetic machine in which the flow of gases is directed through two unidirectional valves, one in an expiratory and one in an inspiratory tube. The rebreathing bag and the canister of soda lime for CO_2 absorption are located between the two tubes.

Bronchial sounds   Sounds produced by the movement of air through the trachea and large bronchi; usually heard over the area of the trachea and carina, most noticeably during expiration.

Bronchodilator   Drug that inhibits bronchoconstriction.

Brown-Adson tissue forceps   Tissue forceps with small serrations on the tips that cause minimal trauma but hold tissue securely.

Buccal   Referring to the cheek.

Buck   A male rabbit.

Buffy coat   A layer of material above the packed erythrocytes following centrifugation; consists primarily of leukocytes and thrombocytes.

Bulk laxative   Substance that acts to pull water into the bowel lumen via osmosis or helps retain water in the feces.

Bumblefoot (pododermatitis)   An inflammation of the ball of the foot of birds and guinea pigs; usually caused by infection with *Staphylococcus* spp.

Bursa of Fabricius   The lymphoid organ in birds in which B lymphocytes were first discovered.

Byproduct feeds   Residues of the feed-processing industry; are found in a wide array of feedstuffs.

C

Calculus   Hardened, or calcified, plaque.

Capillary refill time   The time required for blood to refill capillaries after displacement by finger pressure.

Capnometer   A device that determines respiratory rate and end-tidal CO_2 by estimating partial CO_2 in the bloodstream at the end of expiration, when CO_2 levels of the expired gas are approximately equal to alveolar and arterial CO_2 ($Paco_2$).

Capnophilic   Refers to an organism requiring high levels of carbon dioxide for growth or enhancement of growth.

Capsid   Protein coat that surrounds the genetic material of viruses.

Carapace   The upper or dorsal shell of chelonians.

Carcinoma   Describes tumors of epithelial cell origin.

Cardiopulmonary arrest (CPA)   The cessation of functional ventilation and effective circulation.

Caseous exudate   Exudate formed when a purulent material changes into a thick, pasty material.

Cast   Structure formed from the protein precipitate of degenerating kidney tubule cells; may contain embedded materials.

Castroviejo needle holders   Needle holders with a spring and latch mechanism for locking.

Catabolic   A destructive metabolic process whereby complex substances are converted by living cells into simpler compounds, with release of energy.

Catalase   An enzyme that catalyzes the breakdown of hydrogen peroxide to oxygen and water.

Catchpole   Rigid pole with a loop at one end used to move an aggressive or fearful dog to or from a run or cage.

Cathode   A negatively charged electrode that produces electrons in the x-ray tube.

Caudal   Pertaining to the tail end of the body or denoting a position more toward the tail or rear of the body than another reference point (body part).

Cavy   A common name for a guinea pig.

Celiotomy   An incision into the abdominal cavity, also called a laparotomy.

Cell-mediated immunity   An immune system mechanism involving actions of the cells of the immune system rather than antibodies.

Cementoenamel junction (CEJ) The division of the tooth between the crown and root of the tooth.

Cementum The substance that covers the root of the tooth. It is more similar to bone (45% to 50% inorganic) and is formed by cementoblasts. The cementum is able to regenerate.

Centers for Disease Control and Prevention (CDC) One of the major divisions of the U.S. Department of Health and Human Services. It serves as the national focus for developing and applying disease prevention and control, environmental health, and health promotion and education activities designed to improve the health of the U.S. population. The CDC's major departments include the office of the director, six coordinating centers and offices, and the National Institute for Occupational Safety and Health.

Centesis The act of puncturing a body cavity or organ with a hollow needle to draw out fluid.

Central catheter A long catheter left in place for extended periods; composed of materials designed to produce little if any tissue reaction.

Central nervous system The brain and spinal cord.

Central venous pressure (CVP) The pressure of blood in the thoracic vena cava, near the right atrium of the heart. CVP reflects the amount of blood returning to the heart and the ability of the heart to pump blood into the arterial system.

Cercaria Life cycle stage of trematodes that develops in the intermediate host.

Cere The flesh-colored skin located at the base of the upper beak in many bird species.

Cerebellum Located just caudal to the cerebrum. The cerebellum does not initiate movements but serves to coordinate, adjust, and generally fine-tune movements directed by the cerebrum.

Cerebrovascular accident (CVA) A stroke.

Cerebrum The largest, most rostral part of the brain. It is the center of higher learning and intelligence; it functions in perception, maintenance of consciousness, thinking and reasoning, and initiating responses to sensory stimuli.

Certification Credential generally conferred by a private or professional organization (e.g., a state veterinary technician association).

Cervical vertebrae Vertebrae located in the neck region.

Cervix The round, muscular structure that separates the uterus (cranially) from the vagina (caudally).

Cesarean section The surgical removal of a newborn via an abdominal incision.

Cestode Organism in the order Cestoda; tapeworm.

Chelonian Referring to turtles and tortoises.

Chemical name Describes the chemical composition of a drug.

Chemical sterilization indicators Generally, paper strips or tape that change color when a certain temperature, pressure, or chemical exposure has been reached, indicating that conditions for sterility have been met.

Chief complaint The reason why the client has sought veterinary care for the animal; the primary medical problem.

Chiropractic Spinal adjustments performed to reverse a variety of nerve, muscle, and motion problems.

Chisel Instrument used to shape bone and cartilage.

Choana The V-shaped notch in the roof of the mouth of birds that provides communication between the nasal cavity and oropharynx.

Choanal papillae Sharp, fingerlike projections that surround the choana in most healthy psittacines.

Cholestasis Any condition in which bile excretion from the liver is blocked.

Cholesterol Plasma lipoprotein produced primarily in the liver, as well as ingested in food; used in the synthesis of bile acids.

Chromic surgical gut Surgical gut suture that has been exposed to chrome or aldehyde to slow absorption.

Chylomicron A small fat globule composed of protein and lipid.

Cicatrix A scar; the contracted area of fibrous tissue that remains under the dermis after the healing of a wound.

Cloaca In birds, the terminal end of the urinary, reproductive, and gastrointestinal tracts.

Closed-suction drains Drains that use vacuum bottles and plastic conduits to draw fluid away from the wound by producing a negative pressure.

Cocci A bacteria with a round shape.

Coccygeal vertebrae Vertebrae found in the tail.

Coelom A body cavity; in birds and reptiles, the coelom makes up the thoracic and abdominal cavities.

Colic Severe abdominal pain of sudden onset caused by a variety of conditions, including obstruction, twisting, and spasm of the intestine.

Collimator A device on an x-ray machine used to restrict the x-ray beam to reduce scatter.

Colloidal gold assay A type of immunochromatographic test that uses a colloidal gold-antibody conjugate in the test system.

Colonic Drug or function related to the colon.

Colostrometer A tool that measures the specific gravity of colostrum.

Columella The middle ear bone in birds.

Coma An unconscious patient that does not respond to any stimuli.

Combining form A word or root word that might use the connecting vowel "o" when it is used as an element in a medical word formation. The combining form is the combination of the root word and combining vowel.

Combining vowel A vowel, usually an "o," used to connect a word or root word to the appropriate suffix or to another root word.

Committee on Veterinary Technician Education and Activities (CVTEA) A group of individuals with varying backgrounds in veterinary medicine and veterinary technology who oversee the curricula and guidelines outlined in the AVMA Accreditation Policies and Procedure Manual.

Common law Laws developed by judges through decisions of courts and similar tribunals (called case law), rather than through legislative statutes or executive action, and corresponding legal systems that rely on precedent case law.

Companion Animal Parasite Council Organization that fosters animal and human health, while preserving the human-animal bond, through recommendations for the diagnosis, treatment, prevention, and control of parasitic infections.

Complement A group of plasma proteins that function to enhance the activities of the immune system.

Complementary therapy Practice used in conjunction with or as complement to the Western approach.

Compound word Two or more words or root words combined to make a new word.

Comprehensive Drug Abuse Prevention and Control Act   A law created in 1970 by Congress to regulate the manufacture, distribution, dispensing, and delivery of certain drugs that have the potential for abuse.

Compress   Cold herbal tea on a cloth.

Computed radiography (CR)   A type of digital radiography that uses a cassette screen (imaging plate) system.

Computed tomography (CT)   An imaging modality that uses an x-ray tube that freely rotates around a patient, creating a data set of images that can be manipulated in sagittal, transverse, and axial planes.

Concentrates   Feeds that are low in fiber and high in energy and/or protein.

Conclusion   The result or outcome.

Concussion   A brain injury that is a violent shock or jarring of brain tissue.

Congenital disease   A disease present at birth.

Congestive heart failure   Increased pulmonary or systemic venous capillary pressure resulting in fluid leakage and subsequent pulmonary edema or effusion.

Consent form   An educational tool explaining treatment, procedures, anesthesia, risks, and the possibility of death. When signed by the educated client, the form acts as a tool that provides some evidence that the client understood the diagnosis, treatment, and outcome as well as payment methods acceptable at end of services rendered if litigation arises.

Contamination   The presence of microorganisms within or on an object or wound.

Continuous rate infusion   Drug(s) given over a long period of time, ranging from hours to days, as a slow injection or drip.

Contour feathers   The largest external feathers of adult birds. These are found on the wings, tail, and body surface and are the feathers of flight.

Control   A biologic solution of known value used for verification of accuracy and precision of test results.

Controlled substance   A drug that has been deemed by the Drug Enforcement Administration (DEA) as potentially abusive; a substance with potential for physical addition, psychological addiction, and/or abuse; also referred to as a schedule drug.

Controlled Substance Act (CSA) of 1970   A law most applicable to the veterinary community regarding the drugs used by veterinarians.

Contusion   A bruise or injury with no break in the surface of the tissue.

Coombs test   An immunologic test designed to detect antibodies on the surface of erythrocytes (direct Coombs test) or antibodies in plasma against erythrocytes (indirect Coombs test).

Co-pay   A specified dollar amount of a covered service that is the policy holder's responsibility.

Coprodeum   The terminal end of the rectum in the cranial compartment of the cloaca.

Corticosteroid   A glucocorticoid.

Cortisone   A glucocorticoid.

Cotton suture   An organic nonabsorbable suture material with less tissue reaction than silk; cotton supports bacterial growth.

Counted brush stroke method   A surgical personnel preparation accomplished by dividing the skin into surface areas and applying a set number of brush strokes to each surface.

Coupage   A technique used in conjunction with nebulization to promote removal of respiratory secretions.

Coverts   Smaller feathers that cover the remiges and rectrices of birds. They are for covering the body and play no role in flight.

Cranial   Pertaining to the cranium or head end of the body, or denoting a position more toward the cranium or head end of the body than another reference point (body part).

Cranial cruciate ligament repair   The surgical stabilization of the stifle joint following cranial cruciate ligament rupture.

Cranial sacral   Type of hands-on therapy that uses subtle manipulation of the skull and spine to relax and align the body for optimal energy flow.

Cream   A semisolid dosage form of a medicinal agent that is applied to the skin.

Creatinine   Waste product formed during normal muscle cell metabolism.

Credentialed veterinary technician   A person who has graduated from an AVMA-accredited program, has passed the Veterinary Technician National Examination, and maintains certification, registration, or licensure in the state in which he or she lives.

Crile forceps   Hemostatic forceps with transverse serrations that extend the entire jaw length.

Critical care   Intensive monitoring and treatment of an unstable patient with a life-threatening or potentially life-threatening illness or injury.

Crop   In birds, an outpocketing of the esophagus; the outcropping or dilation of the esophagus located at the base of the neck, just cranial to the thoracic inlet.

Crossbite, anterior   Maxillary incisors caudal to mandibular incisors.

Crossbite, posterior   Mandible wider than the maxilla.

Crown   The exposed, or visible, portion of the tooth above the gingival tissue.

Cryoprecipitate   A blood product that is prepared from plasma and contains von Willebrand factor, factor VIII, fibrinogen, and fibronectin.

Cryosupernatant plasma   Plasma from which cryoprecipitate has been removed.

Curette   An instrument used to scrape the surface of dense tissue.

Curved needle   Suture needle manipulated with needle holders.

Cusps   Flaps.

Cutaneous exudate   See serous exudate.

Cutting needles   Suture needles with two or three opposing cutting edges; used in tissues that are difficult to penetrate.

Cyanosis   A blue coloration of the skin and mucous membranes caused by the presence of deoxygenated hemoglobin.

Cyclozoonosis   A zoonosis in which several cycles of disease usually occur sequentially in several different vertebrate species, one of which is human.

Cysticercus   A larval form of tapeworm consisting of a single scolex enclosed in a bladderlike cyst.

Cytokine   Soluble molecule that serves as a mediator of cell responses.

Cytotoxic T cell   A type of lymphocyte that searches for and destroys pathogen in infected body cells on stimulation by cytokines.

D

Débridement phase   A process of entering of the neutrophil into a wound to scavenge debris and kill bacteria, therefore decontaminating the wound of foreign debris.

Deciduous teeth   The primary or first set of teeth; often referred to as baby teeth. They fall out and are replaced by permanent teeth.

Declawing   Onychectomy, the surgical removal of a claw.

Decongestant   A pharmacologic agent that reduces congestion of the mucous membranes.

Decubital ulcer   Pressure sores exacerbated by recumbency, increased skin moisture, and irritation; pressure sores (bed sores) that result from an animal lying on a bony prominence for too long.

Deductible   The dollar amount an individual must pay for services before the insurance company's payment. Clients may have a choice of per-incident deductible or annual deductible with a pet health insurance policy.

Definitive host   The host that harbors the adult, mature, or sexual stages of a parasite.

Delta foramina   The entry point for the nerves and blood vessels into the pulp cavity; also called the apical delta because it is located at the apex, root tip, of the tooth.

Dendrites   Parts of a neuron that conduct impulses received from other neurons toward the nerve cell body.

Dental pad   An area of dense tissue that replaces the upper incisors in most ruminant species.

Dentin   The layer beneath the enamel and cementum (70% inorganic, 30% organic collagen and water); formed by odontoblasts from pulpal tissue that continue to manufacture dentin in a tubular pattern throughout the life of the tooth.

Department of Labor   The federal agency that fosters and promotes the welfare of job seekers, wage earners, and retirees that administers a variety of labor laws, including those that guarantee workers' rights to safe and healthful working conditions, a minimum hourly wage and overtime pay, freedom from employment discrimination, unemployment insurance, and other income support.

Depressed   Condition when a patient is conscious but slow to respond to stimuli.

Dermatophyte   A group of cutaneous mycotic organisms commonly known as ringworm fungi.

Developer   A chemical solution that converts the exposed silver halide crystals of an exposed x-ray film to black metallic silver.

Diabetic ketoacidosis (DKA)   A potentially life-threatening complication in patients with diabetes mellitus, wherein the body switches to burning fatty acids and produces harmful ketone bodies.

Diapedesis   The process whereby cells, especially neutrophils, exit the blood vessels, usually at a site of inflammation, by squeezing through the microscopic spaces between the endothelial cells lining the blood vessels.

Diastema   A gap in the dental arcade, as seen between the incisors and cheek teeth of some species.

Diastole   Relaxation of heart chambers to receive the blood.

Diastolic blood pressure   The minimum force during the relaxation phase, or when the aortic and pulmonic valves are closed; the pressure of blood in the artery when the heart relaxes between beats.

Differential cell count   Procedure for classifying cells to determine the relative percentages of each cell type present in a peripheral blood or bone marrow sample.

Differential diagnoses   Diagnostic possibilities.

Differential medium   Bacterial culture method that allows bacteria to be identified based on their biochemical reactions on the medium.

Diffusion   Movement of molecules across a semipermeable membrane from an area of high concentration to an area of low concentration of solutes.

Digital imaging and communications in medicine (DICOM)   The universal standard whereby medical images are stored and transferred.

Dipteran   An insect of the taxonomic order Diptera (flies); most adults contain a single pair of wings.

Direct digital radiography (DDR)   A type of digital radiography that uses an imaging plate of detectors connected directly to a computer system.

Direct marketing   The most popular form of marketing. The Yellow Pages are a typical example of direct marketing.

Disinfectants   Chemical agents that kill or prevent the growth of microorganisms on inanimate objects.

Disinfection   The destruction of pathogenic microorganisms or their toxins; the destruction of vegetative forms of bacteria on inanimate or nonliving objects; may not necessarily include spores or spore-forming bacteria.

Dispensing fee   A fee added to medication that is dispensed through the hospital to recover the cost of the pill vial, label, and team members' time to fill the prescription.

Disseminated intravascular coagulation (DIC)   Also referred to as consumption coagulopathy and defibrination syndrome. It is an acquired, secondary coagulation disorder characterized by depletion of thrombocytes and coagulation factors.

Distal   Farther from the center of the body relative to another body part or a location on a body part relative to another closer location; away from the center of the dental arch.

Distraction technique   The use of mild pain to distract the attention of an animal so that a procedure can be performed.

Distribution   Movement of a drug from the systemic circulation into the tissues.

Diuretic   A drug that increases urine formation and promotes water loss.

Diurnal   Pertaining to those species that forage or hunt in the daytime.

Doe   A female rabbit.

Dolichocephalic   The condition of having a long face; more specifically, a long, narrow muzzle.

Dorsal   Pertaining to the back area of a quadruped (animal with four legs) or denoting a position more toward the spine than another reference point (body part).

Dorsal recumbency Restraint technique whereby the animal is held in position resting on its back; may require use of a V trough to keep the patient in position.

Dosage form The form in which the drug is supplied—solid, semisolid, liquid.

Dosage interval The time between administration of separate drug doses.

Dosage regimen The dose and dosage interval of a specific drug.

Dose The amount of drug administered at one time.

Dosha The metabolic body type, one of three bodily humors, used in Ayurvedic medicine to determine balances and imbalances.

Dosimetry badge Used for monitoring cumulative exposure to ionizing radiation.

Down feathers The layer of fine feathers under the exterior feathers.

Drug elimination Removal of a drug from the body.

Drug Enforcement Agency (DEA) The primary federal law enforcement agency responsible for combating the abuse of controlled drugs.

Drug metabolism The alteration of a drug by the body before elimination.

Dry cow A dairy cow that is not being milked during her dry period. The dry period usually consists of a 60-day window between the end of one lactation cycle and the expected birth of another calf, which will start a new lactation cycle.

Ductus deferens A convoluted structure in which sperm storage and maturation occur.

Dullness A thudlike sound produced by encapsulated tissue, such as the liver or spleen.

Dysphagia Difficulty eating.

Dyspnea Increased respiratory effort or difficulty breathing.

Dystocia An abnormal or difficult labor.

E

Ecchymosis A small hemorrhagic spot, larger than petechiae, in the skin or mucous membranes, that forms a nonelevated, rounded or irregular, blue or purplish patch.

Economic order quantity Method for determining the correct amount of inventory to order.

Ectoparasite A parasite that resides on the surface of its host.

Effective renal plasma flow (ERPF) A clearance study to evaluate kidney function; uses test substances eliminated by glomerular filtration and renal secretion.

Effector cells Collective term for lymphocytes that act in the immune system to enhance the functions of other cells.

Effleurage A massage technique using the palm and fingers in a light and slow motion.

Effusion Excess fluid in a tissue or body cavity.

Electrocautery A device containing a needle tip or scalpel that is heated before it is applied to tissue to provide hemostasis in vessels smaller than 2 mm.

Electrocoagulation A process that involves generating heat in tissue with a high-frequency current to provide hemostasis in vessels smaller than 2 mm.

Electrolyte Any substance that dissociates into ions when in solution.

Elimination The passing of urine or feces.

ELISA Enzyme-linked immunosorbent assay, an immunologic test.

Elixir A solution of drug dissolved in sweetened alcohol.

Emasculatome A castrating instrument to accomplish closed castration, keeping the skin intact.

Emasculator An instrument used to perform open castration by crushing and severing the spermatic cord.

Emergency care An action directed toward the assessment, treatment, and stabilization of a patient with an urgent medical problem.

Emetic Drug that induces vomiting.

Employee handbook A document created in well-managed veterinary hospitals to outline policies and procedures (e.g., labor expectations, sexual harassment, overtime, vacation, benefits); hospital philosophy and mission, vision, and value statements. At the time of hire and annually, the employee handbook is reviewed with the employee and updated.

Enamel Substance that covers the crown of the tooth. It is 96% inorganic and made of hydroxyapatite crystals.

Endemic Refers to a disease that is commonly found in a given geographic area.

Endoparasite A parasite that resides within a host's tissues.

Endospore The dormant form of a bacterium; intracellular refractile bodies resistant to heat, desiccation, chemicals, and radiation; formed by some bacteria when environmental conditions are poor.

Endotoxin A chemical substance that causes disease; produced in the cell walls of gram-negative bacteria and often stimulates the release of pyrogens by the host's cells.

End-tidal Pertaining to or occurring at the end of expiration, when CO_2 levels of the expired gas are approximately equal to the concentration of alveolar and arterial CO_2 ($Paco_2$).

Energy-producing nutrients Substances that have a hydrocarbon structure that produces energy through digestion, metabolism, or transformation.

Enrichment medium A type of culture medium formulated to meet the requirements of the most fastidious pathogens.

Ensiling A harvesting process whereby forage is chopped and placed into a storage unit (e.g., silo) that excludes oxygen.

Enteric Refers to a drug or function related to the duodenum, jejunum, or ileum (small intestines).

Enteric bacteria Bacteria inhabiting the intestinal tract.

Enteric-coated tablet A tablet that has a special covering that protects the drug from the harsh acidic environment of the stomach and prevents dissolution of the tablet until it enters the intestine.

Enterotomy An incision into the intestine.

Enzootic A normal level of animal disease over time in a given geographic area.

Eosinophil A cell of the inflammatory system that contains pink to reddish-orange staining granules when stained with Wright-Giemsa stain; usually prominent in inflammation associated with parasitic infestations and allergic reactions.

Eosinophilia An increase in circulating eosinophils; also used to describe the reddish appearance of cells or components of cells that have a high affinity for stains with an acidic pH.

Eosinophilic exudates Exudates composed primarily of eosinophils.

Epidemic An increase over the normal expected number of disease cases in a geographic area or certain period of time.

Epidemiology The study of the occurrences of disease and the risk factors that cause disease in a population.

Epidural anesthesia   A form of regional anesthesia involving injection of drugs through a catheter placed into the subarachnoid or epidural space of the spinal cord to block the transmission of signals through nerves in or near the spinal cord.

Epiglottis   A flap of cartilage that acts as a trap door to cover the opening of the larynx during swallowing.

Epitheliotropic   A term used to characterize pathogens, especially viruses, that infect epithelial cells, such as the respiratory, intestinal, or urinary epithelium.

Epizootic   An increase over the normal expected number of animal disease cases in a geographic area or certain period of time.

Epizootiology   The study of the occurrences of disease and the risk factors that cause disease in an animal population.

Equal employment opportunity   Refers to law that promotes equal opportunity in employment through the administrative and judicial enforcement of federal civil rights laws and through education and technical assistance.

Erythrocyte indices   Calculated values that provide the average volume and hemoglobin concentrations of erythrocytes in a peripheral blood sample.

Eschar   Necrotic layers of tissue that slough off.

Esophageal stethoscope   An instrument placed in the esophagus during anesthesia at the level of the heart to amplify the heartbeat, audible from a distance.

Essential amino acids   Amino acids that cannot be synthesized in the body and therefore must be supplied by the diet.

Estrogen   A steroid compound, named for its importance in the estrous cycle, that functions as the primary female sex hormone.

Ethics   The system of moral principles that determines appropriate behavior and actions in a specific group.

Ethmoturbinate   Delicate bony scroll located in the nasal cavity of some species.

Ethology   The study of animal behavior.

Ethylene oxide   The organic compound with the formula C_2H_4O; a carcinogenic. It is used to sterilize substances that would be damaged by high-temperature techniques. The gas kills bacteria (and their endospores), mold, and fungi.

Etiologic diagnosis   The causal description of a lesion, such as enteric salmonellosis.

Etiology   The study of causes of disease.

Eukaryote   An organism whose cells have a membrane-bound nucleus; includes most plant and animal cells.

Euthanasia   The act of ending a patient's life in a humane manner.

Evaluation   Sorting data to determine which is important and which is irrelevant.

Evisceration   The protrusion of an organ (viscera) through an incision.

Excretion   The removal of a drug from the body.

Exempt employees   Those who are exempt from certain wage and hour laws (e.g., overtime pay); usually applies to administrative, executive, or professional employees.

Exfoliative cytology   The study of cells shed from body surfaces.

Exotoxin   A chemical substance that causes disease; often produced by gram-positive bacteria and secreted into the surrounding medium.

Expectorant   Compound that increases the fluidity of mucus in the respiratory tract by generating liquid secretions by respiratory tract cells.

Extension   The act of straightening, such as a joint; also, the act of pulling two component parts apart to lengthen the whole part

External marketing   A marketing technique that targets potential clients.

Extracellular fluid (ECF)   Body fluid outside the cells, such as plasma and interstitial fluid.

Exudate   The visible product of the inflammatory process; usually composed of cellular debris, fluids, and cells that are deposited in tissues and on tissue surfaces.

Eyed needles   Suture needles in which suture material must be threaded.

F

Facial   Referring to labial and buccal surfaces of the face.

Facultative anaerobe   Bacteria that do not require oxygen for metabolism but can survive in the presence of oxygen.

Fair Debt Collection Practices Act   An act that was passed to protect the public from unethical collection procedures.

Fair Labor Standards Act   A federal law that sets minimum wage and overtime regulations.

Fastidious organism   A bacterial species with complex growth or nutritional requirements.

Fat-soluble vitamins   Metabolized in a manner similar to fats and stored in the liver.

Federal law   A law established by the U.S. government and legislators (congresspeople and senators), enforced by different departments and agencies.

Feed analysis   A chemical analysis that determines the proportion of specific components of a feedstuff.

Feedstuff   Any dietary component that provides some essential nutrient or serves some other function.

Femoral head ostectomy   The surgical amputation of the femoral head.

Fever (pyrexia)   An abnormal increase in body temperature caused by the release of agents that increase the body's biologic setting to a higher temperature.

Fibrin   An insoluble protein that is essential to the clotting of blood.

Fibrinous exudate   An exudate composed mostly of fibrin, which is derived from a plasma protein, fibrinogen.

Fibrosis   Scarring; the end result of tissue repair.

Finochietto retractor   A self-retaining retractor with a set screw to maintain tension on tissues; commonly used to retract the thoracic wall.

First-intention healing   Also called primary healing, the healing of injured tissue directly without the intervention of granulation tissue.

Fixer   A chemical solution that clears the unchanged silver halide crystals on the x-ray film after developing and hardens the gelatin layer.

Flank incision   An incision oriented perpendicular to the long axis of the body, caudal to the last rib.

Flanking   Placing a calf in lateral recumbency.

Flatness   An extremely dull sound produced by very dense tissue, such as muscle or bone.

Flexible endoscope   An instrument used for gastrointestinal endoscopy, duodenoscopy, colonoscopy, and bronchoscopy.

Flexion   The act of bending, such as a joint.

Flowmeter   Part of the anesthetic machine that receives medical gases from the pressure regulator. The purpose is to measure and deliver a constant gas flow to the vaporizer, common gas outlet, and breathing circuit.

Fluoroscopy   An imaging technique that uses an x-ray tube and image intensifier to produce a continual stream of images.

Focal-film distance (FFD)   The distance measured from the target of the x-ray tube to the radiographic film or plate; now commonly referred to by the term *source-image distance* (SID).

Fomentation   A hot compress.

Fomite   An inanimate object or surface (cage, food bowl, countertop) that may be contaminated with infectious agents and capable of transmitting such agents.

Forage   Feed made up of most or all of the plant.

Formaldehyde, formalin   A chemical compound with the formula CH_2O; it exists in water as the hydrate $H_2C(OH)_2$. Aqueous solutions of formaldehyde are referred to as formalin; exposure to formaldehyde is a significant consideration for human health because it is carcinogenic.

Fractional clearance of electrolytes   A mathematic manipulation that describes the excretion of specific electrolytes relative to the glomerular filtration rate.

Fresh-frozen plasma   The liquid portion of blood that has been harvested and frozen within 8 hours from the time of blood collection, preserving all coagulation and other proteins in the plasma.

Fresh whole blood   A unit of blood that is less than 8 hours postcollection and has been kept at room temperature, preserving all components in the blood.

Friction massage   A fast, invigorating circular massage.

Fructosamine   A molecule formed as a result of the irreversible reaction of glucose bound to protein.

Fungicidal   A substance that kills fungi.

Furcation   The junction at which multiple roots join the neck of the tooth.

G

Gait   The manner of walking, stepping, or running.

Gastric   Drugs or functions related to the stomach.

Gastroenteropathies   Any disease of the stomach and intestines.

Gastropexy   The surgical fixation of the stomach to the abdominal wall.

Gastrotomy   An incision into the stomach.

Gauntlets   Heavy leather gloves used to restrain animals.

Gavage   Feeding with a feeding tube passed through the oral cavity into the stomach.

Gelpi retractor   A self-retaining retractor with a box lock to maintain tension on tissues, commonly used in orthopedic surgeries.

GEM   Genetically engineered mice.

General anesthesia   A purposeful derangement of a patient's normal physiologic processes to produce a state of unconsciousness, relaxation, analgesia, and/or amnesia.

General appearance   The patient's facial expression, size and position of the eyeballs, general body condition (flesh and hair coat), response to commands, and temperament.

General senses   Tactile, temperature, kinesthetic, and pain senses. They are distributed generally throughout the body or over the entire skin surface.

Generic equivalent   A copycat drug that has properties equivalent to the original compound.

Generic name   See "nonproprietary name."

Gingival margin   An epithelial collar often not directly attached to the tooth; also called the free gingiva.

Gingival sulcus   The space between the free gingiva and the enamel of the tooth; often called a pocket. A pocket is the abnormal or additional depth to the sulcus.

Gingivitis   Inflammation of the gingiva.

Globulins   A complex group of plasma proteins designated as alpha, beta, or gamma; includes immunoglobulins, complement, and transferrin.

Glomerular filtration rate (GFR)   The rate at which substances are filtered through the glomerulus and excreted in the urine.

Glucose   A monosaccharide that represents the end product of carbohydrate metabolism.

Gonadotropins   Protein hormones secreted by gonadotropic cells of the pituitary gland, including follicle-stimulating hormone (FSH) and luteinizing hormone (LH).

Granulation tissue   Highly vascularized connective tissue produced after extensive tissue damage.

Granulocyte   Any cell with distinct cytoplasmic granules.

Granulomatous   An inflammatory condition characterized by high numbers (more than 70%) of macrophages.

Gray (Gy)   The measured unit of radiation dose that is absorbed because of ionized radiation.

Grid   A device that is made up of lead strips interspaced with a radiolucent material that allows most of the primary radiation to pass through; absorbs the scatter radiation.

Gustatory sense   A chemical sense that detects substances that are in the mouth and dissolved in saliva.

H

Hands-on therapy   Treatment by practitioners who use their own hands or body to move, adjust, or manipulate the patient to help facilitate the healing process.

Hay   Forage that is cut and allowed to dry before being collected into bales for storage.

Hazardous materials plan   An identified, detailed plan explaining how toxic materials are to be treated; may include safety training and contact numbers for local hazardous materials teams, authorities, and physicians.

Healing crisis   A temporary worsening of symptoms followed by overall improvement.

Heel effect   Refers to visible differences in the density produced on a radiograph; there is greater radiation intensity on the cathode side because of the angle of the target on the anode side.

Helper T cell   A type of lymphocyte that binds to the antigen on a macrophage surface and then secretes specific cytokines to activate other elements of cell-mediated immunity.

Hematuria   The presence of intact erythrocytes in the urine.

Hemoglobinuria   The presence of free hemoglobin in the urine.

Hemolysis   The rupture of a red blood cell; the destruction of erythrocytes.

Hemoprotozoans   Parasites located in peripheral blood.

Hemorrhagic exudate   Exudates that consist primarily of erythrocytes that have collected in a tissue after disruption of the vascular system.

Hemostasis The arrest of bleeding by the physiologic properties of vasoconstriction and coagulation.

Herbal therapy The use of specific plant leaves, roots, and/or flowers to assist healing.

Herniorrhaphy The surgical repair of a hernia by suturing the abnormal opening closed.

Heterophil A leukocyte of avian, reptile, and some fish species containing prominent eosinophilic granules; functionally equivalent to the mammalian neutrophil.

Hexacanth The infective stage of some cestodes.

Histopathology The evaluation of tissue samples; the microscopic study of diseased tissues.

Hob A male ferret.

Hobble A device used to fasten together the legs of an animal to prevent straying.

Hog snare A mechanical restraint device consisting of a metal pipe with a cable loop on one end.

Homeopathy Remedies based on the principle of like curing like; refers to a system of healing that uses dilute substances known to cause the same symptoms as the illness.

Homeostasis A constant internal environment in the body.

Horizontal nystagmus Recurrent, flickering, back-and-forth eye movements.

Host A living being that offers an environment for maintenance of the organism; not always necessary for the organism's survival.

Human-animal bond The interaction between humans and animals, the special interactive bond that actually enhances human quality of life.

Human carcinogen Any substance, radionuclide, or radiation agent directly involved in the promotion of cancer or the increase of its propagation.

Humoral immunity An immune response involving the production of specific antibody.

Husbandry The production, housing, and management of animals.

Hyaline cast A structure formed from the protein precipitate of degenerating kidney tubule cells with no embedded materials.

Hydatid cyst Larval cyst stage of the tapeworms *Echinococcus granulosus* and *E. multilocularis,* which contains daughter cysts, each of which contains many scolices.

Hydrocephalus An abnormal buildup of cerebrospinal fluid in the brain.

Hydrosol Water left behind after the steam distillation process of aromatherapy. Hydrosols are dilute, gentle, and only subtly aromatic.

Hydrotherapy Use of water as physical therapy; can be passive hydromassage or active walking or swimming therapy.

Hypercapnia Derived from the Greek, *hyper,* plus *kapnos,* meaning vapor. It is the excess of carbon dioxide in the blood, indicated by an elevated PCO_2 as determined by blood gas analysis and resulting in respiratory acidosis; also known as hypercarbia or hypercarbemia.

Hyperechoic A structure in an ultrasound image that appears bright or white compared with adjacent structures.

Hyperkalemia An increased concentration of potassium in the blood.

Hypermotility An increased frequency or intensity of intestinal sounds.

Hypernatremia An increased concentration of sodium in the blood.

Hyperplasia An increased number of cells of an organ or tissue.

Hyperresonance A booming sound heard over a gas-filled area, such as an emphysematous lung.

Hypersegmented Describes a neutrophil with more than five nuclear lobes.

Hypersensitivity Immune system reactions that damage a body's own tissues.

Hyperthermia An increase above the body's normal temperature caused by drugs, toxins, or external temperature, such as in heat stroke; increased body temperature.

Hypertonic A solution that has a greater solute concentration than cells located in it; causes cells to lose water because of osmotic pressure.

Hyphae The body of a fungus created as a result of the linear arrangements of cells that cause multicellular or multinucleate growth.

Hypoadrenocorticism A deficiency in the production of mineralocorticoid and/or glucocorticoid steroid hormones.

Hypochlorite A sanitizing agent found in products such as laundry bleach, which has a wide spectrum of antimicrobial activity.

Hypochromic Erythrocytes with decreased staining intensity because of decrease in hemoglobin concentration.

Hypokalemia A decreased concentration of potassium in the blood.

Hypomotility A decreased frequency or intensity of intestinal sounds.

Hyponatremia A decreased concentration of sodium in the blood.

Hypothermia Decreased body temperature.

Hypothermic Refers to abnormally low body temperature.

Hypotonic A solution that has a lower solute concentration than cells located in it, which causes cells to gain water (swell); caused by osmotic pressure.

Hypovolemia Abnormally low circulating blood volume.

Hypovolemic shock Physiologic compensatory mechanism caused by decreased intravascular volume.

Hypoxemia Deficiency in the amount of oxygen reaching body tissues.

I

IACUC Institutional Animal Care and Use Committee.

Icterus Abnormal yellowish discoloration of skin, mucous membranes, or plasma as a result of increased concentration of bile pigments.

IgA An antibody isotype important in mucosal immunity; secreted onto the mucosal surface of organs such as the lungs and gastrointestinal tract and found in secretions such as milk and tears.

IgE The primary immunoglobulin associated with allergic and parasitic reactions.

IgG The most common antibody, found in the highest concentration in the blood.

IgM The second most common antibody in the blood; major immunoglobulin isotype produced in a primary immune response.

Immunodeficiency The inability to build up a normal immune response; a state in which the immune system's ability to fight disease is compromised or entirely absent.

Immunodiffusion   An immunologic test performed by placing reactants onto an agar plate and allowing them to migrate through the gel toward each other.

Immunoglobulin (Ig)   An antibody; plasma proteins produced against specific antigens.

Immunologic tolerance   A state of nonresponsiveness to antigens, whether self or foreign.

Implant   A solid dosage form of drug that is injected or inserted under the skin and dissolves or releases that drug over an extended period of time.

Imprinting   A rapid learning process that enables a newborn animal to recognize and bond with its owner.

Inactivated vaccine   A vaccine that consists of a noninfectious agent, such as whole killed pathogens or selected antigenic subunits; enough to induce immunity.

Indemnity insurance   A type of pet health insurance in which the client is reimbursed for services after they have been provided.

Indirect marketing   A marketing technique that is used by practitioners on a daily basis; clean facilities, genuine service, and excellent customer care are a few examples.

Infection   Microorganisms in the body or a wound that multiply and cause harmful effects.

Inflammatory phase   Healing phase in which bacteria and debris are phagocytized and removed and factors are released that cause the migration and division of cells involved in the proliferative phase.

Informed consent   A person's agreement to allow something to happen, such as a medical treatment or surgery, which is based on full disclosure of the facts necessary to make an intelligent decision.

Injectable   A medication that is administered via a needle and syringe.

Innate immunity   The nonspecific components of the immune system that function the same way, regardless of which antigen is present.

Inquiry   Probing into significant areas that require more clarification.

Insensible water loss   Water loss that is difficult to measure and/or cannot be seen (e.g., losses from the respiratory tract).

Inspection   An active process in which the technician visually examines the patient's entire body in a systematic manner for structure and function, paying close attention to deviations or abnormalities.

Instincts   Inherited or genetically coded responses to environmental stimuli.

Integrative veterinary medicine (IVM)   A combination of natural and holistic therapies with conventional veterinary therapies.

Intensifying screens   Plates in the x-ray cassette composed of phosphorescent crystals (phosphors) that function to emit light.

Interdental space   A space, void of teeth, found in the upper and lower arcades that extends from the corner incisors to the first premolars.

Interferons   Small soluble proteins that enhance the function of the immune system.

Intermediate-acting glucocorticoid   Glucocorticoid that exerts an anti-inflammatory effect for 12 to 36 hours.

Intermediate host   The host that harbors the larval, immature, or asexual stages of a parasite.

Internal marketing   A marketing technique that targets current or existing clients for services offered in the practice.

Interproximal   The surface between two teeth.

Interstitium   Between cell layers.

Intervertebral disc fenestration   The surgical removal of prolapsed intervertebral disc material that is causing pressure on the spinal cord.

Intestinal resection and anastomosis   The surgical removal of a segment of intestine, and suturing the cut ends together.

Intra-arterial   Into an artery.

Intracellular fluid (ICF)   Fluid located within the cells.

Intradermal injection (ID)   Injecting a drug within (not beneath) the skin with a very small needle.

Intramedullary bone pinning   The surgical insertion of a metal rod or pin into the medullary cavity of a long bone to fix fracture fragments into place.

Intramuscular (IM) administration   Injecting a drug into a muscle mass.

Intraosseous   Referring to route of injection directly into the bone marrow.

Intraperitoneal (IP) injection   Injecting a drug into the abdominal cavity.

Intravenous (IV) injection   Injecting a drug into a vein.

Inventory turns per year   The number of times an item must be reordered within a stated period; 8 to 12 turns per year should be a goal of each practice.

Iris scissors   Delicate scissors designed for fine, precise cuts, often used in ophthalmic procedures.

Irritant laxative   Substance that acts to irritate the bowel to increase peristaltic motility.

Isoenzymes   A group of enzymes with similar catalytic activities but different physical properties.

Isoerythrolysis   An uncommon complex disorder of newborns that results from a blood group incompatibility between mother and offspring resulting in destruction of the RBCs of the offspring.

Isosthenuria   A condition in which the urine specific gravity approaches that of the glomerular filtrate.

Isotonic   A solution with the same solute concentration as cells, so that the cells neither gain nor lose water.

Isotype   A class of antibody based on molecular weight; examples include IgG, IgM, IgA, IgE, and IgD.

J

Jackson-Rees circuit   A type of nonrebreathing circuit, also referred to as the Mapleson F system. As with other Mapleson circuits, it contains a fresh gas flow that is used to remove exhaled carbon dioxide, a fresh gas inlet at the patient's end of the breathing tube, and a reservoir bag at the opposite end. As with an Ayre's T piece, the fresh gas inlet of a Jackson-Rees circuit enters the breathing tube at a 45- to 90-degree angle.

Jill   A female ferret.

K

Karyolysis   Degeneration or dissolution of a cell nucleus.

Karyorrhexis   Fragmentation of a cell nucleus.

Keel   The bony ridge on the sternum of birds to which the flight muscles attach.

Kelly forceps Hemostatic forceps with transverse serrations that extend over only the distal portion of the jaws.

Ketoacidosis Accumulation of ketone bodies in the body tissues and fluids.

Ketonuria The presence of detectable ketone bodies in urine.

Kinetic assay A chemical test that measures the rate of change of a substance in the test system.

kVp (kilovoltage peak) The maximum voltage applied across an x-ray tube that determines the energy of the electrons produced.

L

Labial The surface toward the lip.

Laceration A tear or jagged wound.

Lagomorphs Gnawing mammals that have two pairs or incisors in the upper jaw, one behind the other; rabbits.

Laminitis Inflammation of the hoof lamina, a cause of lameness; also called founder.

Laparotomy An incision into the abdominal cavity, also called celiotomy.

Laryngoscope A medical instrument used to obtain a view of the vocal folds and glottis, which is the space between the cords; often used to help place the endotracheal tube.

Laryngospasm An uncontrolled or involuntary muscular contraction (spasm) of the laryngeal cords. The spasm can happen often without any provocation but tends to occur after tracheal extubation.

Larynx Commonly called the voice box; a short, irregular tube of cartilage and muscle that connects the pharynx with the trachea and controls airflow to and from the lungs.

Latent image The invisible image in the emulsion of an x-ray film produced after the film has been exposed to light.

Lateral Denoting a position farther from the median plane of the body or a structure, on or toward the side away from the median plane, or pertaining to the side of the body or a structure.

Lateral ear resection The surgical removal of the lateral wall of the vertical portion of the external ear canal.

Lateral intercostal thoracotomy An incision into the lateral thorax, oriented between two ribs.

Lateral recumbency A restraint technique whereby the animal is held in position resting on the side of the body.

Lavage To irrigate or wash.

Laws These set the maximum limits from which we can deviate from the acceptable norm; enforced by authorized officers.

Left shift The presence of increased numbers of immature cells in a peripheral blood sample.

Lethargy Sluggish or drowsy.

Leucopenia A decreased number of leukocytes in the blood.

Leukemia The presence of neoplastic cells in the blood or bone marrow.

Leukocyte A white blood cell.

Leukocytosis Increased numbers of leukocytes in the blood.

Licensure This is maintained by the state government or veterinary state board and may be mandatory.

Lignin An inert compound that increases rigidity of the plant cell wall.

Lingual A surface toward the tongue.

Lipase A pancreatic enzyme that functions in the breakdown of fats.

Lipemia The presence of fatty material in plasma or serum.

Local or municipal law Legislation created by townships, counties, or cities that governs the rules and regulations in a municipality authorizing officers to enforce the laws.

Long-acting glucocorticoids Glucocorticoids that exert an anti-inflammatory effect for more than 48 hours.

Loop diuretics Medications that produce diuresis by inhibiting sodium resorption from the loop of Henle in nephrons.

Lumbar vertebrae Bones located in the abdominal region that serve as the site of attachment for the large sling muscles that support the abdomen.

Lymphadenitis Inflammation of one or more lymph nodes.

Lymphocyte A leukocyte involved in the inflammatory process; also has roles in humoral and cell-mediated immunity.

Lymphokine A type of cytokine produced by T lymphocytes.

Lysis The destruction or decomposition, as of a cell or other substance, under the influence of a specific agent or force.

M

M:E ratio Relative percentages of myeloid and erythroid cells in the bone marrow.

mA (milliamperage) The current produced by the x-ray tube during an exposure.

Macrophage An important cell in the inflammatory process; functions to phagocytize pathogens and then presents antigen on its surface for recognition by immune cells; a phagocytic cell derived from the monocyte.

Magill circuit A semiclosed breathing circuit, also known as the Mapleson A system, in which rebreathing is prevented by having the gas flow rate from the cylinders slightly in excess of the patient's minute respiratory volume.

Magnetic resonance imaging (MRI) An imaging modality using a magnetic field that recognizes the natural resonance of the atoms within the body to produce images.

Maintenance energy requirement (MER) The BMR plus the additional energy needed for normal physical activity.

Maintenance fluid solution Fluid with a composition different than plasma; low-sodium, high-potassium concentration.

Major blood crossmatch Process that detects antibodies in the recipient plasma against the donor red blood cells.

Malocclusion The improper positioning of teeth.

Malpractice A type of negligence in which a physician fails to follow generally accepted professional standards, causing injury to the patient.

Mandible The lower jaw or arcade of the teeth.

Margin The difference between the selling price and cost per unit.

Markup A term commonly used to price a product based on a percentage of cost, such as per tablet, per mL, or per bottle.

Mast cell Tissue cell characterized by abundant, small, metachromatic cytoplasmic granules that functions in the immune system.

Mastectomy The surgical removal of part or all of one or more mammary glands.

Material safety data sheet Informational material that must be kept in all businesses; contains detailed product safety information on hazardous materials found in that place of a business; an OSHA mandate.

Mathieu needle holders   Needle holders with a ratchet lock at the proximal end of the handles of the holder, permitting locking and unlocking with just a progressive squeezing of the instrument.

Maturation phase   Wound healing process during which collagen is remodeled and realigned along tension lines and cells that are no longer needed are removed by apoptosis.

Maxilla   The upper jaw or arcade of the teeth.

Mayo-Hegar needle holders   Needle holders with a ratchet lock just distal to the thumb, with a blade for cutting sutures.

Mayo scissors   Tissue scissors designed for cutting heavy tissue, such as fascia.

Mayo stand   An instrument stand that is movable and has a removable tray top.

Mean arterial pressure   Defined as the average arterial pressure during a single cardiac cycle; considered to be the perfusion pressure experienced by organs in the body.

Medial   Denoting a position closer to the median plane of the body or structure, toward the middle or median plane, or pertaining to the middle or a position closer to the median plane of the body or structure.

Median sternotomy   An incision along the midline of the ventral thorax.

Megakaryocyte   Bone marrow cell from which blood platelets arise.

Mentation   The mental state or status of a patient; the patient's attentiveness or reaction to its environment; mental function.

Meridians   Rivers or channels that travel throughout a body connecting and regulating different body parts and organs.

Merozoite   Life cycle stage of a protozoal parasite that results from asexual reproduction.

Mesaticephalic   A condition of having a medium face; more specifically, a medium length and width muzzle; mesocephalic.

Mesenchymal   Cells or tissues derived from the embryonic mesoderm.

Mesial   Toward the center of the dental arch (rostral).

Mesophile   Organisms with an optimal growth temperature between 25° and 40° C (77° and 104° C).

Mesothelial   Cells that line body cavities; derived from the embryonic mesoderm.

Metabolite   An altered drug molecule.

Metastasis   Neoplastic cells present in areas other than the location in which they originated.

Metazoonosis   A zoonosis that is maintained by invertebrate (e.g., tick, mosquito) and vertebrate species.

Metzenbaum scissors   Delicate scissors designed for cutting fine, thin tissue.

Microaerophilic   An organism requiring oxygen for growth at a level below that found in air.

Microbial fermentation   Process whereby herbivores break down cellulose.

Microfilaria   Larval offspring of the group of filarial worms in the phylum Nematoda.

Minimum prescription fee   The minimum amount charged to a client for a prescription fill; for example, if a client needed only two pills, a minimum prescription fee may be instituted.

Minor blood crossmatch   Process that detects antibodies in the donor plasma against the recipient red blood cells.

Miracidium   Ciliated larval stage of a digenic trematode.

Mixed nerves   A combination of sensory and motor nerves.

Modified live   A vaccine that consists of a weakened version of the pathogen, which will induce an immune response but is attenuated enough so that it will not cause disease.

Molting   The process of feather replacement that occurs one to several times a year, depending on the species.

Monocyte   A precursor cell in the stage of development of tissue macrophage; after a monocyte leaves the bloodstream and enters tissue at a site of inflammation, it becomes an activated macrophage.

Monofilament suture   A suture made of a single strand of material, creating less tissue drag than multifilament suture.

Monokine   A type of cytokine produced by macrophages.

Morphologic diagnosis   A physical description of a lesion, such as "acute necrotizing enteritis."

Mosquito hemostats   A small hemostatic forceps with transverse jaw serrations.

Mother tincture   A natural source combined with alcohol, term used in homeopathy and flower essences.

Motor nerves   Carry instructions from the central nervous system out to the body.

Mott cells   Plasma cells containing multiple globular cytoplasmic inclusions composed of immunoglobulin (Russell bodies).

Mouthing   A beaking phase of neonatal development.

Mucogingival line   The border between the attached gingiva and looser mucosa.

Mucopurulent exudate   This consists of a mixture of purulent and mucous exudates.

Mueller-Hinton media   Standard culture media used to evaluate the susceptibility of microorganisms to antimicrobial agents.

Multifilament suture   A suture made of several strands of material twisted or braided together; more pliable and flexible than monofilament.

Multimodal therapy   The use of several analgesic drugs, each with a different mechanism of action resulting in lower dosages and thus increasing safety for the animal.

Murine   Pertaining to mice or rats.

Muzzle   Nylon, leather, or gauze covering placed over an animal's mouth to prevent biting.

Mycology   The study of fungi.

Myelography   An examination that involves injecting a contrast medium into the subarachnoid space to visualize the spinal cord.

Myiasis   Infestation with larvae (maggots) of dipterans.

Myoclonus   A brief, involuntary twitching of a muscle or a group of muscles.

Myopathy   A muscular disease in which the muscle fibers do not function for one of many reasons, resulting in muscular weakness; derived from the Greek *myo-*, meaning muscle, and *-pathy*, meaning suffering.

N

Narcosis   Unconsciousness induced by a narcotic drug.

Nares   The nostrils; the external openings of the nasal cavity.

Nasogastric Pertaining to the nose and stomach, particularly placement of a feeding tube into the stomach via the nares.

National Fire Protection Association An authority on fire, electrical, and building safety.

Natural immunity An immunity conferred to the body by exposure to a pathogen by natural means rather than through vaccination.

Natural killer (NK) cell A subpopulation of lymphocytes capable of direct lysis of cells infected with antigen.

Nebulization Humidification of inspired gases to promote mobilization and removal of unwanted secretions in patients with respiratory disease.

Necropsy Postmortem examination of an animal body.

Negative contrast agent Gas such as oxygen or carbon dioxide that is radiolucent on radiographs used to outline organs during diagnostic imaging procedures.

Negligence Finding that a practitioner's actions were below the level of competence expected of the professional.

Negri body Eosinophilic-staining inclusion body found in cells that have been infected with rabies.

Neoplasia The process of abnormal and uncontrolled growth of cells; generic term to describe any growth; often used to describe a tumor, which may be malignant or benign.

Neuroleptanalgesia A state of CNS depression (sedation or tranquilization) and analgesia induced by a combination of a sedative, tranquilizer, and analgesic.

Neuron Nerve cell; the basic structural and functional unit of the nervous system.

Neuropathic pain A complex, chronic pain state that is usually accompanied by tissue injury in which the nerve fibers may be damaged, dysfunctional, or injured and send incorrect signals to other pain centers.

Neurotransmitter Molecules that diffuse across the synapse to contact the cell membrane of the adjacent nerve cell.

Neurotropic A term used to characterize pathogens, especially viruses, that infect cells of the central nervous system.

Neutropenia Abnormal decrease in the number of neutrophils in a peripheral blood sample.

Neutrophil Leukocyte that functions to phagocytize infectious agents and cellular debris; plays a major role in the inflammatory process.

Neutrophilia An abnormal increase in the number of neutrophils in a peripheral blood sample.

Nit The egg stage of lice bound to the hair or feather shaft of the host.

Nitrogen-free extract (NFE) The nonfiber carbohydrate portion of the feed.

Nociception The neural processes of encoding and processing noxious stimuli. It is the afferent activity produced in the peripheral and central nervous systems by stimuli that have the potential to damage tissue; initiated by nociceptors, or pain receptors.

Nocturnal species Animals that forage and hunt at night.

Non–energy-producing nutrients Nutrients that play an important role throughout the body; often called the gatekeepers of metabolism.

Nonessential amino acids Building blocks of proteins that are synthesized in the body.

Nonexempt employee Employee who receives hourly wages; subject to wage and hour laws (e.g., overtime pay; usually applies to nonprofessional employees not in administrative positions).

Non-nutritive feed additives Buffers, hormones, binders, and medications added to feeds.

Nonproductive cough A dry and hacking cough with no mucus produced.

Nonproprietary name Also known as generic name; a concise name given to a specific compound.

Nonrebreathing system Anesthetic breathing circuits in which exhaled gases are discharged to the environment and do not pass back to the patient.

Nonsuppurative exudate An exudate composed primarily of lymphocytes and monocytes; usually restricted to exudates in the central nervous and integumentary systems (skin).

Nonsystemic antacids Medications that neutralize acid molecules in the stomach or rumen directly.

Nonverbal communication Communication by means other than by using words (e.g., through facial expressions, hand gestures, tone of voice).

Norman mask elbow A nonrebreathing circuit that is almost identical to a Jackson-Rees, except that the endotracheal tube connector is at right angles to the breathing tube. This is considered a Mapleson F system. This circuit may slightly reduce mechanical dead space as compared with an Ayre's T piece or Jackson-Rees.

Normochromic Cells that stain with their characteristic color.

Normocytic Cells that appear with their characteristic morphology.

Normothermia Normal body temperature.

Nosocomial infection A hospital-acquired infection.

NSAID Nonsteroidal anti-inflammatory drug.

Nuclear medicine An imaging modality that uses a gamma camera and radioisotopes to visualize metabolic, physical, and functional processes.

Nuclear molding A deformation of nuclei by other nuclei within the same cell or adjacent cells.

Nutrient Any constituent of food that is ingested to support life.

Nystagmus Involuntary eye movement.

O

Object-film distance (OFD) That distance between the object being radiographed and the film or plate. Object-image distance (OID) is the term now used.

Oblique At an angle, or pertaining to an angle.

Observation Observing nonverbal communication, body language, and facial expressions.

Occlusion The surface of the tooth that touches the opposing tooth.

Occupational Safety and Health Act (OSHA) A federal law designed to provide a safe workplace for all persons working in any business engaged in commerce.

Ointment A semisolid dosage form that is applied to the skin.

Olfactory sense A chemical sense that detects chemical substances in inhaled air.

Oliguria Decreased urine production.

Olsen-Hegar needle holders Needle holders with a ratchet lock just distal to the thumb.

Onychectomy   Declawing; surgical removal of a claw.

Oocyst   The resistant spore phase of some parasitic protozoans.

Operant conditioning   A behavioral theory based on the principle that the consequences of a behavior will influence its frequency.

Operculum   A lid or flap covering an opening; common structure on the eggs of some trematodes; a keratinized flap of tissue inside the nares of some birds.

Opisthotonus   A state of a severe hyperextension and spasticity in which a patient's head, neck, and spinal column enter into a complete arching position.

Opsonization   The coating of the outer surface of pathogens by antibodies to allow easier phagocytosis by macrophages.

Orally administered   Drugs given by mouth.

Orchiectomy   The surgical removal of the testes.

Organophosphates   Compounds that are commonly used as insecticide dips; may result in toxicity if used inappropriately.

Orogastric tube   A flexible tube that is passed through the mouth (*oro-*), down the esophagus and into the stomach (*-gastric*), for the purpose of delivering fluids and liquid medication directly into the stomach.

Oropharynx   The oral cavity in birds.

Oscillometer   An instrument used for measuring the changes in pulsations in the arteries, especially of the extremities.

Osmolality   Concentration of particles in a solution; unit expressed as mOsm/kg.

Osmosis   The movement of water across a semipermeable membrane from the side with a higher water concentration to the side with a lower water concentration.

Osmotic diuretic   A medication that helps retain water in the renal tubular lumen via osmosis by altering the solute concentration.

Osmotic pressure   The pressure required to stop the movement of water into a solution containing solutes when the solutions are separated by a semipermeable membrane.

Osteotome   An instrument designed to cut or shape bone and cartilage.

Outstanding accounts   Client accounts that owe money to the veterinary practice; money owed to a creditor.

Ovariohysterectomy   The surgical removal of the uterus and ovaries.

Overtime   Any time accumulated while on the time clock; over 40 hours in any 1 week (7 consecutive days).

Oxidase   An enzyme present in some groups of bacteria involved with the reduction of oxygen during normal bacterial metabolism.

Oxygen saturation   Also known as dissolved oxygen (DO); a relative measure of the amount of oxygen that is dissolved or carried in a given medium.

P

Packed cell volume   Ratio of red blood cells to total plasma volume.

Packed red blood cells   A unit of packed red blood cells; begins as a volume of whole blood, from which platelets and plasma have been removed, leaving a preparation of mostly red blood cells.

Pain   An unpleasant sensory or emotional experience associated with actual or potential tissue damage; classified as peripheral (visceral or somatic), neuropathic (originating from damaged nerves), clinical (ongoing pain), and idiopathic (unknown cause).

Palatal   A surface toward the mouth.

Palisade   A parallel arrangement of some species of bacteria; often described as looking like a picket fence.

Palmar   The caudal surface of the front foot distal to the antebrachiocarpal joint; also pertains to the undersurface of the front foot.

Palpation   Using the hands and sense of touch to detect tenderness, altered temperature, texture, vibration, pulsation, masses or swellings, and other changes in body integrity; can be classified as light or deep.

Pancytopenia   Decreased numbers of all blood cells and platelets in a peripheral blood or bone marrow sample.

Paracostal incision   An incision oriented parallel to the last rib.

Parakeet   A small, slender parrot, usually having a long, tapering tail and often kept as a pet; also referred to as a budgerigar.

Parallel technique   A radiographic technique in which the film is placed in the mouth parallel to the teeth and the cone is aimed perpendicular to the film and tooth.

Paramedian incision   An incision located lateral and parallel to the ventral midline of the animal.

Parasite   An organism that has adapted to live on or within a host organism, deriving all its nutrients from that host, ideally without killing the host.

Parasympathetic system   This is the so-called rest and restore system; predominates during relaxed, routine, business as usual states.

Parenterally administered   Drugs given by injection.

Parthenogenic   A condition in which female organisms produce eggs that develop without fertilization.

Partial intravenous anesthesia (PIVA)   Combining intravenous and inhalation anesthesia to achieve balanced anesthesia.

Passerines   A bird of the order Passeriformes, which includes perching birds and songbirds such as canaries, finches, and sparrows.

Passive exercise   Type of physical therapy in which no voluntary muscle activity is used.

Passive immunity   Receiving antibodies from colostrum or synthesized antibodies.

Paste   A semisolid dosage form that is given orally.

Pathogen   An infectious organism that can cause disease in a host.

Pathologist   One who studies disease.

Pathology   The study of disease.

Pecten   A dark, ribbonlike structure attached to the retina and extending into the vitreous humor; thought to provide nourishment to the eye.

Pediculosis   Infestation with lice.

Peer assistance   Service provided by veterinary professional organizations offering wellness programs to veterinary professionals experiencing substance abuse.

Penrose drain   A surgical device placed in a wound to drain fluid; consists of a soft rubber tube placed in a wound area.

Penumbra   The partial or imperfect shadow of an object outside the complete shadow, where the light from the source is partially cut off.

Per os   By mouth.

Percussion Tapping the body's surface to produce vibration and sound; commonly used on the thorax for examining the heart and lungs; the creation of waves of air to loosen secretions in the lungs, typically accomplished by clapping hands across the thorax to elicit a cough.

Perfused Having a blood supply.

Perfusion Blood flow across all tissues in an individual's body; derived from the Latin *perfundere*, meaning to pour over; refers to the passage of oxygenated blood through body tissues.

Peridontium The supporting structures around the tooth.

Perineal urethrostomy An incision into the urethra and suturing of the splayed edges to the skin to create a larger urethral orifice.

Periodic parasite A parasite that lives part of its life cycle on its host and part off its host.

Periodontal ligament A ligament that holds the tooth into the alveolar bone; attached to cementum and to the alveolar socket; absorbs the shock of pressures applied to the occlusal surface of the tooth.

Periodontitis Inflammation of the peridontium.

Periosteal elevator An instrument designed to remove the periosteum.

Peripheral Pertaining to or situated near the periphery, the outermost part, or surface of an organ or body part.

Peripheral nervous system Carries impulses between the central nervous system and the rest of the body.

Peritonitis An infection in the abdominal cavity.

Perivascular Pertaining to around a blood vessel.

Permanent teeth A secondary, or second, set of teeth; often referred to as adult teeth.

Personal protective equipment (PPE) Any item used to protect against undue harm; includes ear plugs, lead gloves, lead apron, safety glasses, examination gloves, and hot mitts.

Petechia Small red or purple spots on the body, caused by minor hemorrhage or broken capillary blood vessels.

Petrissage A deep massage used on the back, flank, and chest in which the skin is lifted, pulled, and kneaded.

Phagocytosis The ingestion of substances, including pathogens, by cells.

Pharmacokinetics Refers to how a drug moves into, through, and out of the body.

Pharynx The throat, a common passageway for the digestive and respiratory systems.

Phenol Disinfecting product that kills vegetative forms of many gram-negative and gram-positive bacteria.

Pheromone A natural or synthetic chemical that may influence the behavior of an animal.

Phlebitis Local venous inflammation.

Phosphors A substance that phosphoresces, or emits light, when exposed to electromagnetic radiation.

Photostimulable Able to store a latent image that may be released as light when stimulated by a scanning laser such as a computed radiography (CR) or directed digital radiography (DDR) plate.

Picture archival computing system (PACS) Dedicated computer systems (servers) used for storage, retrieval, transferring, and manipulating images.

Pili A component of some bacterial cells that allows bacteria to attach more easily to and colonize host tissues and minimize the host's immune response.

Plain surgical gut A suture material made from the submucosa of sheep intestines or serosa of bovine intestines.

Plantar The caudal surface of the back foot distal to the tarsocrural joint; also pertains to the undersurface of the rear foot.

Plaque A soft mixture of bacteria and mucopolysaccharides (carbohydrates) that adheres to the tooth.

Plasmacyte (plasma cell) A cell derived from a B lymphocyte that has been transformed to produce and secrete antibodies.

Plastron The lower or ventral shell of chelonians.

Platelet Irregular, disc-shaped fragment of megakaryocytes in the blood that assists in blood clotting.

Pleuritis An infection in the thoracic cavity.

Pneumatized Filled with air.

Pneumonia Inflammation of the lungs with tissue consolidation.

Poikilocytosis Any abnormal cell shape.

Pollakiuria Increase in the frequency of urination.

Polychromasia A variable staining pattern; basophilia.

Polycythemia An increase in the number of circulating erythrocytes.

Polymerase chain reaction The method used to replicate and amplify DNA molecules in a sample.

Polyuria An increase in the total volume of urine produced.

Porous adhesive tape A tape that allows evaporation of fluid from the bandage and also allows movement of fluid into the wound.

Positive contrast medium Compound such as barium or iodine that is radiopaque on radiographs; used to visualize organs in the body.

Positive inotropic drug Drug that increases the strength of contraction of a weakened heart.

Posture The position or carriage of the body.

Potassium-sparing diuretic Drug that promotes secretion of sodium and conservation of potassium in the body.

Potentiometer A type of electrochemical analyzer used to evaluate ionic activity in a solution.

Poultice A wet herbal pack.

Precision The magnitude of random errors and reproducibility of measurements.

Preemptive analgesia Refers to taking steps to predict and prevent pain before it occurs.

Prefix A syllable, group of syllables, or word joined to the beginning of another word to alter its meaning or create a new word.

Preliminary data Information gathered from the client, such as patient characteristics (e.g., age, breed, sex, reproductive status).

Premium The amount paid annually or monthly for a policyholder to maintain an insurance policy for a pet.

Prepatent period The time interval between infection with a parasite and demonstration of the infection.

Preprandial samples Samples from an animal that has not eaten for some time.

Prescription An order from a licensed veterinarian directing a pharmacist to prepare a drug for use in a client's animal.

Presenting complaint What the client perceives the patient's problem to be; the primary medical problem.

Pressure manometer A device that measures the pressure of gases in the breathing circuit and the patient's lungs.

Presumptive diagnosis   To make a diagnosis without having all the facts or proof.

Primary flight feathers   Also known as the remiges; the contour feathers on a bird's wing that emerge from the periosteum of the metacarpus; numbered from the carpus distally and proximally.

Primary healing   Also called first-intention healing; the healing of injured tissue directly without intervention of granulation tissue.

Primary hemostasis   The formation of the primary platelet plug following injury to the vessel involving the blood vessel, platelets, and certain adhesive proteins (e.g., von Willebrand factor, collagen).

Primary hyperalgesia   Describes pain sensitivity that occurs directly in the damaged tissues.

Problem-oriented medical record (POMR)   A common type of record system in which each entry follows a distinct format—the defined database, problem list (also referred to as master list), plan, and progress section. In the progress section, a standard SOAP format is followed.

Proctodeum   The caudal part of the cloaca, which empties its contents into the vent.

Productive cough   A cough that produces mucus and other inflammatory products that are coughed up into the oral cavity.

Progestin   A reproductive hormone similar to progesterone.

Proglottid   Segments that comprise the body of a cestode.

Prognathism, maxillary   Overbite; the maxillary arcade is longer than the mandibular arcade.

Prokaryote   A single-celled organism, usually a bacterium; contains a cell wall, lacks a nucleus and organelles; DNA consists of one double-stranded chromosome.

Prophylaxis   The process whereby the teeth are cleaned to prevent disease.

Proprietary name   Also known as trade name; a unique name given by a manufacturer to its particular brand of drug.

Proprioception   The sense of body part position.

Proteinuria   An abnormal presence of protein in the urine.

Protozoistatic   Inhibits protozoal replication.

Proud flesh   Excess granulation tissue formation on the leg of a horse; the formation of excessive granulation tissue.

Proventriculus   The glandular portion of the stomach responsible for production of the gastric juices and propulsion of food into the ventriculus (gizzard).

Proximal   Nearer to the center of the body, relative to another body part, or a location on a body part relative to another, more distant, location.

Proximate analysis   Determination of dry matter (DM), crude protein (CP), ether extract (EE, crude fat), crude fiber (CF), and ash.

Pruritus   Itching.

Psittacine   Bird belonging to the family Psittacidae, which includes the parrots, macaws, and parakeets.

Psychrophiles   Organisms with optimal growth at cold temperatures (15° to 20° C [59° to 68° F]).

Pterylae   The feather tracks on the skin of birds; specific tracts located on the surface of the body where feather follicles are located.

Pulp cavity   Consists of the pulp chamber, in the crown and the root canal, in the tooth root; the cavity surrounded by the dentin; contains blood vessels, nerves, and connective tissue.

Pulse deficit   Presence of a difference between the heart rate and pulse rate, as in atrial fibrillation.

Pulse oximeter   A device that detects changes in the oxygen saturation of hemoglobin by calculating the difference between levels of oxygenated and deoxygenated blood; also determines heart rate.

Pulse oximetry   A noninvasive technique that continuously measures arterial oxygen saturation in the blood.

Pulse pressure   The difference between systolic and diastolic arterial pressures.

Pulse quality   A series of pressure waves within an artery caused by contractions of the left ventricle and corresponding with the heart rate; easily detected over certain superficial arteries.

Punishment   An action that decreases the likelihood of a behavior occurring.

Purulent   Containing, discharging, or causing the production of pus; refers to a cytology sample characterized by the presence of neutrophils representing more than 85% of total nucleated cells in the sample.

Pyknosis   Condensed nuclear chromatin in a degenerating cell.

Pyogenic   A characterization of bacteria that causes the host to produce a purulent or suppurative exudate.

Pyogranulomatous   A cytology sample characterized by the presence of macrophages representing more than 15% of total nucleated cells in the sample.

Pyometra   An infection in the uterus.

Pyrogen   An agent in the body that increases the body's biologic setting to a higher temperature.

Q

Qi   The Chinese term for central life force.

Quaternary ammonium compound   A sanitizing agent most effective against gram-positive bacteria but less effective against gram-negative bacteria.

Queen   A female cat, intact; mother cat.

R

Rare earth element   Photosensitive element such as lanthanum oxybromide and gadolinium oxysulfide in an x-ray intensifying screen.

Rebreathing system   Anesthetic breathing circuits in which the exhaled gas is recirculated to the patient with CO_2 removed.

Receptor   A specific protein molecule on or in the cell with which a drug will combine.

Recipe   The full chemical compound of the drug being prescribed.

Recombinant vaccine   A vaccine that consists of a live nonpathogenic virus into which the gene for a pathogen-related antigen has been inserted.

Recumbent   Lying down; a modifying term is needed to describe the surface on which the animal is lying.

Redia   A secondary larval form of some digenic trematodes that develops within a mollusk's intermediate host.

Reflexology   The use of hand and finger pressure to massage and stimulate pressure points located in the paws.

Refractive index   Measure of the degree of light bending as it passes from one media to another, relative to air; function of the dissolved material in the sample.

Refractometer   Instrument used to measure the refractive index of a solution.

Regional or segmental anesthesia Achieved by blocking the nerve or nerves that supply a region or segment of the body by injecting an anesthetic around the nerves that supply the area to block conduction from the area.

Registration Maintained by the state government, veterinary state board, or state veterinary technician association; may be mandatory.

Reiki A Japanese hands-on energy healing practice that promotes the flow of energy to aid in the healing process.

Reinforcement Something that increases the likelihood of a behavior occurring.

Releasability The ability for a wild animal to be released on recovery based on the injuries sustained.

Remiges Contour feathers found on the wing of a bird.

Reorder point The inventory level at which additional product is ordered.

Repair phase Wound-healing phase characterized by angiogenesis (blood vessel formation), collagen deposition, granulation tissue formation, epithelialization, and wound contraction.

Replacement fluid solution Fluids with a composition similar to plasma; high-sodium, low-potassium concentration.

Rescue remedy A combination of five flower essences used to calm an individual experiencing shock, trauma, panic, or mental paralysis.

Reservoir A location in which a pathogenic agent is maintained prior to transmission; a reservoir is often a living organism.

Reservoir bag A rebreathing bag that provides a gas volume sufficient for the patient to inhale maximally without creating negative pressure in the circuit.

Residue An accumulation of a drug or chemical or its metabolites in animal tissues or food products, resulting from drug administration to the animal or contamination of food products.

Resonance A hollow sound, such as that produced by air-filled lungs.

Respiration The transport of oxygen from the outside air to the cells within tissues, and the transport of carbon dioxide in the opposite direction.

Respondeat superior Describes an employer who is responsible for the actions of the employees performed during the course of their employment.

Rete pegs Interdigitations of connective tissue that provide a firm attachment to the periosteum of the alveolar bone.

Reticulocyte An anuclear, immature erythrocyte.

Reticulopericarditis A disease that can occur when a cow ingests a metallic foreign body that penetrates the forestomach, diaphragm, and pericardium; also known as hardware disease.

Retrices Contour feathers found on the tail of a bird.

Rhinotheca The upper beak of a bird or chelonian.

Right to Know Law A federal law mandating that all workplaces educate employees regarding the hazards that they will encounter while on the job.

Rigid endoscope Instrument comprised of a metal tube, glass rods, lenses, and light source; used for rhinoscopy, cystoscopy, laparoscopy, arthroscopy, vaginoscopy, colonoscopy, and thoroscopy.

Rochester-Carmalt forceps A large crushing instrument often used to control large tissue bundles.

Rodents Relatively small gnawing mammals that have a single pair of incisors with a chisel-shaped edge in the upper jaw (e.g., mice, rats).

Roentgen equivalent mean (rem) Unit that expresses the dose equivalent that results from exposure to ionizing radiation.

Rongeurs An instrument designed to cut and remove bone pieces.

Root The unexposed, or submerged, portion of the tooth below the gingival tissue.

Root word The subject part of a word consisting of a syllable or group of syllables, or word that is the basis (or word base) for the meaning of the medical word.

Rostral Pertaining to the nose end of the head or body, or toward the nose.

Rouleaux The arrangement of erythrocytes in a column or stack.

Rumenotomy An incision into the rumen.

Ruminatoric Drug used to stimulate an atonic rumen.

S

Sacral vertebrae Fused vertebrae in the pelvic region; sacrum.

Saddle thrombus An embolus that breaks loose and occludes one or more branches of the aorta at the aortic trifurcation.

Safelight Light produced that will not affect radiographic film; consists of a low-wattage light bulb and special filter.

Sanitizer Another term for an antiseptic or disinfectant.

Saprozoonosis A zoonotic disease that depends on an inanimate reservoir to maintain the cycle of infection.

Sarcoma A generic term to describe any cancer arising from connective tissue cells.

Scatter radiation Radiation created as a result of the interaction of primary beam x-ray photons and body parts or matter that travel in a different direction and have lower energy.

Scavenging system Component of an anesthetic machine that functions to discard excess gas properly; some located on machines as a filter canister, others set up as a central unit with a fan to direct gases out of the building.

Schedule drug See "controlled substance."

Schistocyte Fragmented erythrocytes usually formed as a result of shearing of the red cell by intravascular trauma.

Schizont Life cycle stage of some protozoal organisms; arises from multiple asexual fission.

Scolex The head of a cestode by which it attaches to its host.

Scutes Pertaining to chelonians, the bony shell covered by a superficial layer of keratin shield; pertaining to snakes, the large scales found on the ventral aspect of the body.

Secondary container labeling Mandated by OSHA, all materials dispensed out of the primary storage unit must be properly identified with Material Safety Data Sheet (MSDS) information to include health hazard, flammability, reactivity, and personal protection.

Secondary flight feathers Also known as the remiges; the contour feathers that emerge from the ulna, are numbered from the carpus proximally.

Secondary hemostasis Formation of fibrin involving certain coagulation factors in the extrinsic, intrinsic, and common coagulation pathways.

Second-intention healing Closure of a wound using granulation tissue.

Sedation   A mild to profound degree of CNS depression in which the patient is drowsy but may be aroused by painful stimuli.

Seizures   Periods of altered brain function characterized by loss of consciousness, altered muscle tone or movement, altered sensations, or other neurologic changes.

Selective media   A type of culture media that contains antibacterial substances that inhibit or kill all but a few types of bacteria.

Semiclosed breathing system   A circle system in which some rebreathing occurs in which there is adequate fresh gas flow and the pop-off settings are at intermediate values.

Senn (rake) retractor   Double-ended retractor, one end with fingerlike curved prongs (sharp or blunt) and the other end with a flat, curved blade.

Sensible water loss   Water loss that is easy to measure and can be seen (e.g., urine).

Sensitivity testing   A method used to determine the resistance or susceptibility of a microorganism to specific antimicrobials.

Sensory nerves   Nerves that carry information only toward the central nervous system.

Sentinel   A surveillance animal housed for the purpose of identifying abnormal occurrences.

Serology   The study and application of antibody detection in the serum.

Serous exudate   An exudate that consists primarily of fluid with a low protein content.

Short-acting glucocorticoid   A glucocorticoid that exerts an anti-inflammatory effect for less than 12 hours.

Shrinkage   The unexplained loss of inventory.

Sievert (Sv)   The dose of radiation equivalent to the dose absorbed by tissue; 1 Sv equals 100 rem.

Sig   On a written prescription, this indicates directions for the client when treating the animal.

Silage   A partially fermented forage state.

Silk suture   Braided, multifilament, organic, nonabsorbable suture material.

Sinus rhythm   The normal conduction sequence of the heart.

Snake hook   A piece of equipment used to restrain the head of an aggressive or venomous snake temporarily for the purpose of capturing it.

Snubbing   A restraint technique in which the animal is held in position using a leash through a wall anchor or the hinges or bars on a low cage.

SOAP medical record   An acronym (*s*ubjective, *o*bjective, *a*ssessment, *p*lan) that identifies the most common data entry formats used by veterinary practices.

Socialization   The exposure of a young animal to new experiences, people, other animals, and places with the goal of preventing fearful or anxious behavior as adults.

Society   Group of individuals with a common interest in a veterinary technician discipline.

Solid   Powdered drugs compressed into pills, discs, or capsules.

Soluble factor   An enzyme or protein produced by bacteria that inhibits host functions and provides the bacteria with a foothold in the host.

Solution   A drug dissolved in a liquid vehicle that does not settle out if left standing.

Somatic pain   Generally well-localized pain that results from the activation of peripheral nociceptors without injury to the peripheral nerve or central nervous system.

Sow   A female guinea pig or pig.

Special senses   Gustatory, olfactory, auditory, vestibular, and visual senses; concentrated in certain areas, rather than being generally distributed.

Specific   Any herb known for its effectiveness in the treatment of a particular condition.

Specific gravity   Ratio of the density of a substance to the density of a reference substance; in veterinary practice, density of a quantity of liquid compared with that of an equal amount of distilled water.

Specificity   The ability of a test to evaluate a given parameter correctly.

Spectrophotometer   Instrument designed to measure the amount of light transmitted through a solution.

Sphygmomanometer   Also called a blood pressure meter; a device used to measure blood pressure comprised of an inflatable cuff to restrict blood flow and a mercury or mechanical manometer to measure the pressure. The word comes from the Greek *sphygmós* (pulse), plus manometer (pressure meter).

Splenectomy   The surgical removal of the spleen.

Spoilage   The forage harvested at a given stage of development and fed directly to an animal.

Sporocyst   The larval stage of a digenic trematode that develops in a mollusk intermediate host.

Sporozoite   The infective stage of some protozoal parasites.

Squeeze chute   A capture device made of metal or wood that restrains cattle.

Standard   A nonbiologic solution of an analyte, usually in distilled water, with a known concentration.

Standard operating procedure (SOP)   A written set of directions and policies; a practice may abbreviate medical record annotations, but an SOP must be kept on the premises detailing the procedure.

Stasis   The congestion of blood vessels caused by sludging of blood flow in the vessels caused by fluid loss through exudation.

State veterinary medical association   A nonprofit professional organization of veterinarians establishing bylaws, nominating officers, and enhancing the professional experience through volunteerism.

State veterinary technician association   A nonprofit professional organization of veterinary technicians establishing bylaws, nominating officers, and enhancing the professional experience through volunteerism.

Sterilization   The destruction of all organisms, including bacteria and spores.

Sterilization indicator   Indicators that undergo a chemical or biologic change with some combination of time, temperature, or chemical exposure, allowing for monitoring the effectiveness of sterilization.

Sterilizer   Another term for an antiseptic or disinfectant.

Sternal recumbency   A restraint technique in which the animal is held in position resting on its breastbone.

Stimulus   An internal or external change that exceeds a threshold causing stimulation of the nervous or endocrine system.

Stock   A small, square restraining pen with a front and back gate.

Stored whole blood A unit of blood that is older than 8 hours postcollection that has been refrigerated, adversely affecting certain components in blood.

Strabismus A condition in which the eyes are not properly aligned with each other.

Straight (Keith) needles A suture needle used in accessible places in which the needle can be manipulated directly with the fingers.

Struvite A common crystal seen in alkaline to slightly acidic urine; sometimes referred to as triple phosphate crystals or magnesium ammonium phosphate crystals.

Stupor Condition in which a semiconscious patient can respond to noxious (painful) stimuli.

Subcutaneous injection (SQ or SC) Injecting a drug deep to (beneath) the skin, into the subcutis.

Subgingival Below the gingiva.

Subluxation Misalignment of vertebrae causing compensation in posture or movement.

Substrate Material selected or preferred by an animal for urination and defecation.

Subtherapeutic level Refers to a dose of a drug below the ideal range of concentration; therefore, the beneficial effect is not achieved.

Suffix A syllable, group of syllables, or word added at the end of a root word to change its meaning, give it grammatical function, or form a new word.

Superficial Situated near the surface of the body or a structure; the opposite of deep.

Supine Lying face up, in dorsal recumbency.

Suppository A drug that is inserted in the rectum, dissolved and released to be absorbed across the membranes of the intestinal wall.

Suppurative Purulent.

Supragingival Above the gingiva.

Surgical biopsy The evaluation of tissue that has been surgically removed from the body.

Suspension A drug in which the particles are suspended but not dissolved in the liquid vehicle.

Suture Any strand of material used to approximate tissues or ligate blood vessels.

Sutures Immovable joints in the skull.

Suture scissors Scissors with a concavity at the top of one blade, designed for removing skin sutures after wound healing.

Swaged needle Suture needle that is joined with suture into a continuous unit.

Symmetry To observe closely for complementary (balanced) or noncomplementary conformation of the thorax and abdomen. Note any difference in the size or shape of the extremities.

Sympathetic system This produces the fight-or-flight reaction in response to real or perceived threats.

Sympatholysis Inhibition of the postganglionic functioning of the sympathetic nervous system (SNS).

Synapse The junction of an axon with another nerve cell.

Syrinx The voice box of birds; analogous to the mammalian larynx.

Syrup A solution of a drug with water and sugar.

Systemic antacid Medication that decreases acid production in the stomach.

Systole The contraction of heart chambers to pump the blood into body tissues and lungs.

Systolic blood pressure The maximum force caused by contraction of the left ventricle of the heart.

T

Tachyarrhythmia An abnormally rapid heartbeat accompanied by an irregular rhythm; derived from the Greek *tachy*, fast, and *a + rhythmos*, rhythm.

Tachycardia Abnormally rapid beating of the heart.

Tachypnea Rapid breathing.

Tail jacking Restraint technique used to relax the hindquarters for rectal palpation and tail bleeding of cows whereby the base of the tail is lifted straight up.

Tapered needle A suture needle with a sharp tip that pierces and spreads tissues without cutting them.

Target cells Leptocyte with a peripheral ring of cytoplasm surrounded by a clear area and dense, central, rounded area of pigment.

Tellington TTouch A gentle manipulation therapy used as a realignment technique.

Telodendron The branched end of an axon.

Tenesmus Straining to defecate.

Tenotomy scissors Delicate scissors designed for ophthalmic procedures.

Therapeutic index The lethal dose of a drug for 50% of the population (LD_{50}) divided by the minimum effective dose for 50% of the population (ED_{50}); also known as the therapeutic ratio.

Therapeutic range The ideal range of a drug concentration in the body.

Thermal therapy The use of heat or cold to facilitate circulation and pain relief.

Thermophile Organism with optimal growth at elevated temperatures.

Third-intention healing The treatment of a grossly contaminated wound by delaying surgical closure until after contamination has been markedly reduced and inflammation has subsided.

Thoracic vertebrae Bones in the chest region that form joints with the dorsal ends of the ribs.

Thoracotomy An incision into the thorax.

Thorax The area located between the neck and diaphragm.

Thrombocyte Platelet; cytoplasmic fragment of bone marrow megakaryocyte.

Thrombocytopenia Decrease in circulating platelets.

Thrombophlebitis The inflammation of a vein associated with clotting.

Thrush A degenerative condition of the hoof that may occur secondary to a bacterial infection; appears as black, malodorous material in the region of the frog.

Thymus A lymphoid organ of birds and mammals.

Tick paralysis A condition resulting from introduction of a neurotoxin into the body during attachment of and feeding by the female of several tick species.

Tidal volume The lung volume representing the normal volume of air displaced between normal inspiration and expiration, when extra effort is not applied.

Tincture An alcohol solution meant for topical application; liquid herbal extract usually preserved with alcohol or vegetable glycerin.

Tisane An herbal infusion.

Titer The greatest dilution at which a patient sample no longer yields a positive result for the presence of a specific antibody.

T lymphocyte (T cell) A type of lymphocyte involved in cell-mediated immunity.

Tonicity The osmotic pressure between two solutions determined by solute concentration.

Topical anesthesia Numbing of the area by reversible block nerve conduction near the site of administration, thereby producing temporary loss of sensation in a limited area.

Topical application or administration Applied onto the skin.

Total body water (TBW) The total water content of the body; accounts for 60% of lean body weight.

Total daily dose The amount of drug delivered to the animal in 24 hours.

Total intravenous anesthesia (TIVA) Balanced anesthesia achieved by using two or more injectable drugs in combination.

Toxic Containing or being poisonous material, especially when capable of causing death or serious debilitation; refers to waste, radiation, or chemicals.

Toxic neutrophil A neutrophil characterized by the presence of cytoplasmic basophilia, Döhle bodies, vacuoles, heavy granulation, and/or giantism.

Toxoid Inactivated antigenic toxin molecules that stimulate development of the animal's own antibodies.

Trachea Also known as the windpipe; carries air from the larynx to the lungs.

Trade name See "proprietary name."

Traditional Chinese medicine (TCM) The ancient practice of acupuncture and herbal therapy originating in China.

Tranquilization A state of relaxation and calmness characterized by a lack of anxiety or concern, without significant drowsiness.

Transducer A device on an ultrasound machine that emits and receives a sound wave signal that converts the waves into electrical impulses.

Transduction Part of the nociception and pain pathway; signal begins with tissue trauma, where the nociceptors are stimulated, and is converted into electrical impulses once the threshold is exceeded.

Transgenic Refers to animals containing foreign DNA that was injected directly into the pronucleus of the zygote.

Transmission Part of the nociception and pain pathway in which a noxious stimulus exceeds the nociceptor's threshold and travels along peripheral nerves to the spinal cord (dorsal horn) and brain (thalamus).

Transudate An effusion characterized by a low protein concentration and low total nucleated cell counts.

Trematode Organism in the phylum Trematoda; commonly referred to as a fluke.

Trephine An instrument designed to bore holes in bone.

Triadan charting system A method of dental charting that identifies each tooth with a three-digit number.

Triage From the French for "to sort"; used to classify patients according to the severity of illness or injury to determine their relative priority for treatment.

Trophozoite The motile form of a protozoal parasite.

Twitch A rope, strap, or chain that is tightened over a horse's lip as a restraining device.

Tympany A musical or drumlike sound produced by an air-filled organ, such as with gastric dilation, volvulus.

U

Ultrasonic Doppler A device that monitors heart rate and rhythm by detecting blood flow through small arteries.

Ultrasound An imaging modality that uses sound waves that interact with tissues and are reflected back to create an image.

Unbalanced fluid solution Fluid that differs in composition from plasma.

Urates The end product of nitrogenous waste production from the liver; excreted by the kidney as a pasty white to yellow material found in bird droppings.

Urea The principal end product of amino acid breakdown in mammals.

Urethrotomy An incision into the urethra.

Uric acid A metabolic byproduct of nitrogen catabolism.

Urochrome Pigment that imparts color to a urine sample.

Urodeum The middle compartment of the cloaca that is the terminal end of the ureters and genital ducts.

Urolithiasis The presence of calculi (stones) in the urinary tract.

Uropygeal gland In the bird, an oil-producing gland used to waterproof feathers—a bilobed gland with one duct opening that empties into a lone papilla, found dorsally at the base of the tail; secretes a lipoid sebaceous material that is spread over feathers during preening to help with waterproofing.

Urticaria A relatively mild cutaneous hypersensitivity reaction such as hives.

V

Vaccine A biologic product representing a pathogenic organism that stimulates immunity toward the pathogen.

Vaporizer A component of the anesthetic machine; produces a controlled and predictable concentration of anesthetic vapor in the carrier gas by delivering a diluted anesthetic to the patient.

Vasoconstriction Narrowing of the blood vessels resulting from contraction of the muscular wall of vessels, particularly the large arteries, small arterioles, and veins.

Vasodilation The dilation of blood vessels.

Vasodilator Any substance that opens (dilates) constricted vessels.

Vector Any organism that transmits a disease-causing organism to new hosts.

Vehicle A mode of transmission of an infectious agent from the reservoir to the host.

Venipuncture Puncture of a vein for the purpose of withdrawing blood.

Vent The external opening of the cloaca.

Ventilation Maintains normal concentrations of oxygen and carbon dioxide in the alveolar gas and, through the process of diffusion, also maintains normal partial pressures of oxygen and carbon dioxide in the blood flowing from the capillaries; measured as the frequency of breathing multiplied by the volume of each breath.

Ventral   Pertaining to the underside of a quadruped or denoting a position more toward the abdomen than another reference point (body part).

Ventral midline incision   An incision located on the ventral midline of the animal.

Ventriculus   The second stomach of birds; the site of protein digestion and mechanical breakdown of food.

Vermicide   An anthelmintic that kills a parasitic worm.

Vermifuge   A drug that paralyzes a worm but does not kill it.

Vertebrae   A series of individual bones in the spinal column.

Vertebral canal   A long, flexible tube formed by the vertebrae.

Vesicular sounds   Heard over normal lung parenchyma; produced by movement of air through small bronchi, bronchioles, and alveoli; best heard on inspiration.

Vestibular disease   Disorders of the body's balance system in the inner ear.

Vestibular sense   A mechanical sense that monitors balance and head position.

Veterinarian   A person who has graduated from a 4-year AVMA-accredited program and who has received a Doctor of Veterinary Medicine (DVM) degree.

Veterinary assistant   A person with the training of a clinical aide, less than that required of a veterinary technician.

Veterinary behaviorist   A veterinarian who is board-certified in animal behavior by the American College of Veterinary Behaviorists.

Veterinary Practice Act   A statute enacted as an exercise of the powers of the state to promote the public's health, safety, and welfare by safeguarding the people of the state against incompetent, dishonest, or unprincipled practitioners of veterinary medicine.

Veterinary team   Usually consists of a veterinarian, technician, assistant, receptionist, and hospital manager.

Veterinary technician   A person who has graduated from a 2-year AVMA-accredited program.

Veterinary technician specialist   A technician who is credentialed and has met all the requirements established by the testing agency and passed the examination according to the organization's guidelines; must be a member in good standing of the specialty group.

Veterinary technologist   A person who has graduated from a 4-year AVMA-accredited program.

Veterinary technology   The science and art of providing professional support service to veterinarians.

Virology   The study of viruses.

Virucidal   Refers to a substance that kills viruses.

Virus   An extremely small, nonliving infectious agent, ranging from 30 to 450 nm in diameter; can cause disease in a wide variety of animals.

Visceral larva migrans   The migration of certain nematode through an organism's tissues and organs.

Visual sense   An electromagnetic sense (sight). Its receptor organ, the eye, has a complex organization of component parts that function together to gather and focus light rays on photoreceptor cells.

Vomiting center   The group of neurons in the medulla of the brainstem that control the complex process of emesis.

W

Warble   Common name for the larvae of some species of flies; often in swollen, cystlike subcutaneous sites, with a fistula or pore communicating to the outside environment.

Water-soluble vitamin   Vitamin that is passively absorbed from the small intestine; excess amounts excreted in the urine.

Weitlaner retractor   A self-retaining retractor with a box lock to maintain tension on tissues, commonly used in neurologic surgery.

Wheal   A fluid-filled, raised area on the surface of the skin caused by an allergic or hypersensitivity reaction to an irritant; a small, but palpable, amount of fluid that was injected into the top layers of the skin by using a syringe and small-gauge needle.

Withdrawal time   The minimum length of time that must pass from the last administration of the medicine until the time that the animal is slaughtered for food or the milk is collected for human consumption.

Wound   An injury caused by physical means, with disruption of normal structures.

Wry bite   Right and left, mandible and maxilla, are different lengths and widths.

X

X-ray   A form of electromagnetic radiation.

Y

Yang energy   Traditional Chinese medicine term describing male energy—insistent, unyielding activity, brightness, fire, and sun.

Yin energy   Traditional Chinese medicine term describing female energy—calm, yielding, stillness, darkness, water, and moon.

Z

Zone of inhibition   An area of no bacterial growth around an antimicrobial disc; indicates some sensitivity of the organism to the particular antimicrobial.

Zoonosis   Any disease or infection that is naturally transmissible between vertebrate animals and humans.

Zoonotic   Capable of being transmitted between animals and humans.

Zoonotic diseases   Infectious agents shared by humans and animals; approximately 150 zoonotic diseases exist.

Zygodactyl   The foot shape of psittacines; the second and third toes face forward, and the first and fourth toes are directed backward.

Appendices

| APPENDIX A | Normal Physiologic Data in Adult Dogs and Cats |

SPECIES	HEART RATE (BEATS/MIN)	RESPIRATORY RATE (BREATHS/MIN)	RECTAL TEMPERATURE
Dogs	60-140	10-30	37.5°-39° C (99.5° -102° F)
Cats	140-250	20-30	38°-39° C (100° -102° F)

| APPENDIX B | Summary of Lengths of Estrous Cycle and Gestation Periods in Dogs and Cats |

PUBERTY	ESTROUS CYCLE LENGTH	ESTROUS DURATION (DAYS)	OVULATION	OPTIMAL BREEDING (FRESH OR FROZEN)	GESTATION
Canine (Dog or Bitch)					
6 mo	No true cycle (estrus is 2 times/yr)	9	2-4 days after onset of cytologic estrus	Days 3 and 5 or 4 and 6 after LH peak; day 5 or 6 after LH peak	57 days from day 1 of cytologic diestrus, 63 days from ovulation, or 65 days from LH peak
Feline (Cat or Queen)					
6-12 mo	Seasonally polyestrous; depends on whether ovulation occurs	8	Induced ovulators after coitus	After day 3 of estrus and >2 hr apart for at least three breedings	65 days

LH, Luteinizing hormone.

| APPENDIX C | Normal Daily Urine Production for Dogs and Cats |

SPECIES	DAILY URINE OUTPUT (ML/KG)
Dogs	20-40
Cats	20-40

| APPENDIX D | Normal Blood Gas Values* |

BLOOD SAMPLE	PH	P_{CO_2} (MM HG)	HCO_3 (MM HG)	P_{O_2} (MM HG)
Dog, venous	7.32-7.40	33-50	18-26	
Dog, arterial	7.36-7.44	36-44	18-26	85-100
Cat, venous	7.28-7.41	33-45	18-23	
Cat, arterial	7.36-7.44	28-32	17-22	85-100

*In-house normal values should be established if the machine does not come with a published reference range.

| APPENDIX E | Normal Heart Rate and Blood Pressure in Dogs and Cats |

SPECIES	NORMAL HEART RATE (BEATS/MIN)	NORMAL BLOOD PRESSURE (MM HG)		
		SYSTOLIC	DIASTOLIC	MEAN
Dogs (large)	60-100	100-160	60-90	80-120
Dogs (medium)	80-120			
Dogs (small)	90-140			
Cats	140-250	100-160	60-90	80-120

| APPENDIX F | Hematology Reference Range Values | | |

PARAMETER	ADULT DOG	ADULT CAT	UNITS
Red blood cell, total	5.3-7.8	6.68-11.8	$\times 10^6$ cells/mm^3
Hemoglobin, Hb	13.5-19-5	11.0-15.8	Grams
Hematocrit, Hct	39.4-56.2	33.6-50.2	%
Mean corpuscular volume, MCV	65.7-75.7	42.6-55.5	fL
Mean corpuscular hemoglobin, MCH	22.6-27.0	13.4-18.6	Pg
Mean corpuscular hemoglobin concentration, MCHC	34.3-36.0	31.3-33.5	g/dL
Mean platelet volume, MPV	8.8-14.3	11.3-21.3	fL
White blood cell	4.36-14.8	4.79-12.52	$\times 10^3$ cells/mm^3
Platelet count	194-419	198-405	$\times 10^3$ cells/mm^3
Segmented neutrophils	3.4-9.8	1.6-15.6	$\times 10^3$ cells/mm^3
Nonsegmented neutrophils (bands or non-segs)	0-0.01	0-0.01	$\times 10^3$ cells/mm^3
Lymphocytes (lymphs)	0.8-3.5	1.0-7.4	$\times 10^3$ cells/mm^3
Monocytes (monos)	0.2-1.1	0-0.7	$\times 10^3$ cells/mm^3
Eosinophils (eos)	0-1.9	0.1-2.3	$\times 10^3$ cells/mm^3
Basophils (basos)	0	0	$\times 10^3$ cells/mm^3

| APPENDIX G | Normal Chemistry Values | | |

PARAMETER	ADULT DOG	ADULT CAT	UNITS
A : G ratio	0.6-2.0	0.4-1.5	mEq/L
Alanine aminotransferase, ALT	16-73	5-134	IU/L
Albumin, Alb	2.8-4.0	3.0-4.2	g/dL
Alkaline phosphatase, SAP or Alk Phos	15-146	0-96	IU/L
Amylase	347-1104	489-2100	mOsm/kg
Anion gap	16.3-28.6	15-32	mEq/L
Bicarbonate, venous	20-29	22-24	mEq/L
Bilirubin, total	0-0.2	0.1-0.5	mg/dL
Blood urea nitrogen, BUN	8-27	15-35	mg/dL
Calcium, Ca	9.2-11.6	7.5-11.5	mg/dL
Chloride, Cl	104-117	113-122	—
Cholesterol, Ch	138-317	42-265	mg/dL
Creatine kinase, CK; formerly CPK	48-380	72-481	IU/L
Creatinine, Cr	0.5-1.6	0.5-2.3	mg/dL
Gamma glutamyltransferase, GGT	3-8	0-10	IU/L
Globulin, glob	2.0-4.1	2.8-5.3	g/dL
Glucose	73-116	63-150	mg/dL
Ionized calcium, iCa	1.15-1.39	—	mg/dL
Lipase	22-216	0-222	IU/L
Na : K ratio	27.4-38.4	30-43	—
Osmolality, calculated	292-310	290-320	—
Phosphorus, P	2.0-6.7	2.7-7.6	mg/dL
Potassium, K	3.9-5.2	3.3-5.7	mEq/L
Sodium, Na	147-154	147-165	IU/L
Total protein, TP	5.5-7.2	5.4-8.9	g/dL
Triglyceride, TG	19-133	24-206	mg/dL

APPENDIX H | Normal Urinalysis Findings

TEST	DOG	CAT
Specific gravity (SpGr)	Variable	Variable
Color	Pale to dark yellow	Pale to dark yellow
pH	5.0 to 8.5	5.0 to 8.5
Protein	Negative to +1	Negative to +1
Glucose	Negative	Negative
Ketones	Negative	Negative
Bilirubin	Negative to trace	Negative
Blood	Negative	Negative

Microscopic

Red blood cell (RBC) count	<5 RBCs/HPF	<5 RBCs/HPF
White blood cell (WBC) count	<3 WBCs/HPF	<3 WBCs/HPF
Epithelial cells	Negative	Negative
Casts	Negative	Negative
Bacteria	Negative	Negative
Special: Urine protein-to-creatinine ratio	<0.3	<0.6

APPENDIX I | Hemostasis Reference Range Values

TEST	CANINE	FELINE
Platelet count	$166\text{-}600 \times 10^3/\mu L$	$230\text{-}680 \times 10^3/\mu L$
Prothrombin time (PT)	5.1-7.9 sec	8.4-10.8 sec
Activated partial thromboplastin time (APTT)	8.6-12.9 sec	13.7-30.2 sec
Fibrin degradation products (FDPs)	$<10\,\mu g/mL$	$<10\,\mu g/mL$
Fibrinogen	100-245 mg/dL	110-370 mg/dL
Activated clotting time (ACT)	60-110 sec	50-75 sec

VETERINARY ASSISTANT MODEL CURRICULUM ASSOCIATION OF VETERINARY TECHNICIAN EDUCATORS

I. Office & Hospital Procedures
1. Prepare appropriate certificates for signature
2. Perform basic filing & retrieving of medical records
3. Perform basic veterinary medical record keeping procedures
4. Demonstrate elementary computer skills
5. Utilize medical terminology
6. Recognize & respond appropriately to veterinary medical emergencies by notifying the appropriate personnel
7. Inventory supplies
8. Restock shelves
9. Maintain x-ray, surgery logs
10. Prepare appropriate hospital information packets.
11. Perform basic filing & retrieving of radiographs, lab reports, etc.

II. Communication & Client Relations
1. Develop effective client communication skills
2. Demonstrate professional ethics
3. Greet clients
4. Demonstrate proper appointment scheduling & make appointments
5. Admit & discharge patients
6. Answer & direct phone calls
7. Demonstrate an understanding of the human/animal bond
8. Describe the roles & responsibilities of each member of the veterinary health team & the important part that each plays in the delivery of excellent care
9. Demonstrate commitment to high-quality animal care & the team approach to veterinary medicine

III. Pharmacy & Pharmacology
1. Recognize legal issues involving drugs in the workplace
2. Recognize general types & groups of drugs & demonstrate proper terminology
3. Differentiate prescription drugs from over-the-counter drugs
4. Describe proper prescription label requirements
5. Label & package dispensed drugs correctly
6. Store, safely handle & dispose of biologic & therapeutic agents, pesticides, & hazardous waste
7. Perform inventory control procedures including restocking supplies
8. Reconstitute vaccines & know proper vaccination protocols
9. Describe appropriate routes & methods of drug & vaccine administration that the veterinarian or veterinary technician may choose

IV. Examination Room Procedures
1. Place & restrain small animals on tables
2. Apply dog & cat safety muzzle
3. Determine & record temperature, pulse, respiration, & weight of pets
4. Trim nails (dogs, cats, & birds)
5. Express anal sacs
6. Recognize common external parasites such as mites, lice, fleas, and ticks
7. Recognize common dog & cat breeds
8. Bathe & groom animals
9. Discuss canine & feline nutrition requirements for well animals
10. Maintain sanitation of the veterinary facility
11. Demonstrate knowledge of basic normal & abnormal canine & feline behavior
12. Discuss routine preventive care protocols for dogs & cats

V. Surgical Preparation & Assisting
1. Prepare surgical equipment/supplies
2. Sterilize instruments & supplies using appropriate methods
3. Identify common instruments
4. Identify common suture materials, types, & sizes
5. Assist with preparation of patients using aseptic techniques
6. Operate & maintain autoclaves
7. Describe operating room sanitation & care
8. Assist with positioning of surgical patients
9. Maintain proper operating room conduct & asepsis
10. Perform postsurgical cleanup of animals & equipment
11. Fold surgical gowns & drapes
12. Identify & care for common surgical equipment & supplies
13. Properly dispose of hazardous medical wastes

VI. Small Animal Nursing
1. Implement patient & personnel safety pleasures
   a. Name potential zoonotic diseases
   b. Describe isolation procedures
   c. Describe hazardous waste disposal
2. Describe basic sanitation in a small animal veterinary clinic
3. Provide routine record-keeping & observation of hospitalized patients, taking particular care to make notations when cleaning & feeding
4. Demonstrate familiarity with common preventable diseases & medical conditions of dogs & cats
5. Monitor and restrain patients for fluid therapy & record observations
6. Hand pilling (dog, cat)
7. Restrain patients for injections
8. Apply & remove support bandages on healthy animals
9. Perform therapeutic bathing, basic grooming, & dipping of small animals

10. Clean ears
11. Prepare feed & prescription diets & be aware of any special dietary requirements
12. Clean & disinfect cages, kennels, & stalls
13. Provide care & maintenance of nursing equipment
14. Place small animals in cages & remove them from cages
15. Place & restrain small animals on tables
16. Apply dog & cat safety muzzle
17. Apply Elizabethan collar
18. Apply restraint pole

VII. Laboratory Procedures
1. Collect voided urine samples
2. Determine physical properties of urine
    a. Color
    b. Clarity
    c. Specific gravity
3. Restrain animals for collection of blood samples
4. Collect fecal samples for parasitologic exam
5. Prepare fecal flotation solutions
6. Assist in necropsy procedures

7. Laboratory Record Keeping
    a. Ensure all lab results are accurately recorded
    b. Stock lab supplies
    c. File lab reports
    d. Maintain laboratory log books

VIII. Radiology & Ultrasound Imaging
1. Implement & follow recommended safety procedures
2. Describe the purpose of a radiographic technique chart
3. Assist in completion of diagnostic radiographs
    a. Measure patient using x-ray caliper
    b. Assist in the positioning of large & small animal patients
4. Process diagnostic radiographs
    a. Use hand processing
    b. Maintain quality control
    c. Label, file, & store film
    d. Use automatic processing
5. Properly care for equipment
    a. Clean screens

APPENDIX K Policy on Assistant Training Curriculum Approval

INTRODUCTION*

Credentialed veterinary technicians work more efficiently when they have an individual who can assist them in the completion of their responsibilities. Therefore, NAVTA recognizes the vital role of assistants on the veterinary health care team and further understands that assistants may be more effective/efficient if they are provided formal training in certain tasks. Veterinary Assistant Training programs must emphasize the role of all members of the team and are responsible for educating both students and their potential employers on proper delegation to the assistant. Any tasks delegated to the assistant must be under the direct supervision of the veterinarian or veterinary technician.

ROLE OF THE MEMBERS OF THE VETERINARY HEALTH CARE TEAM

NAVTA supports the following terminology pertaining to the titles of the members of the veterinary health care team.

"Veterinary Technician Specialists" (VTS). These individuals possess advanced certification from a specialty Organization recognized by NAVTA.

"Veterinary Technology" is the science and art of providing professional support service to veterinarians in the practice of their profession.

"Veterinary Technician" is a person who has graduated from a two- or three-year, AVMA-accredited program in

veterinary technology and passed the Veterinary Technician National Examination. They are credentialed as a Licensed Veterinary Technician (LVT), Registered Veterinary Technician (RVT), or Certified Veterinary Technician (CVT), depending on the jurisdiction.

"Veterinary Technologist" is a graduate of a four-year, AVMA-accredited program who holds a baccalaureate degree from such study and holds credentials per the state or jurisdiction.

"Laboratory Animal Technician" is a person whose academic training, knowledge, and skills have been limited to laboratory animals.

The adjectives, "animal," "veterinary," "ward," or "hospital" combined with the nouns "attendant," "caretaker," or "assistant" are titles sometimes used for individuals where training, knowledge, and skills are less than that required for identification as a veterinary technician, veterinary technologist, or laboratory animal technician.

NAVTA firmly believes the term "Veterinary Technician" is limited to those individuals who have obtained:

- Education from an AVMA accredited Veterinary Technology program, AND
- Passing score on the Veterinary Technician National Examination (VTNE), AND
- Holds current credentials as a Licensed, Registered, or Certified Veterinary Technician.
- **OR** holds credentials by passing the VTNE **PRIOR** to the change instituted by the American Association of Veterinary State Boards (AAVSB) January 1, 2010 (utilized the grandfathering allowance to sit for the VTNE for experienced individuals--No longer an option).

*From NAVTA Policy on Veterinary Assistant Training Programs Curriculum and Assessment of Skills. NAVTA. 2014. http://c.ymcdn.com/sites/www.navta.net/resource/resmgr/Policy_on_VA_programs_rev_7-.pdf?hhSearchTerms=%22policy+and+veterinary+and+assistant%22. Accessed December 8, 2015.

ESSENTIAL REQUIREMENTS FOR ASSISTANT PROGRAMS

1. Courses to accomplish the training of assistants may be offered through high schools, informal short courses, and certificate programs at community colleges, and distance-learning programs.

2. Minimum requirements include an affiliation with an AVMA-accredited program in veterinary technology. This affiliation should be one which facilitates the acquiring of additional education from the assistant level to veterinary technician for those individuals that choose to continue on with a career in veterinary technology. The letter should outline the VT program's recognition of the Assistant Program curriculum and training; visits from the VT program students or faculty are encouraged.

3. A working relationship should be developed with the national, state, and local veterinary technician association and individuals from these associations should be appointed to the program's Advisory Committee.

4. The assistant program courses must be taught by credentialed veterinary technicians and/or licensed veterinarians.

5. The program should encompass a minimum of 150 contact hours, including a significant number of hours devoted to hands-on training with live animals in the workplace or classroom laboratory.

6. The curriculum should be task oriented. and additional basic tasks may be added to the skills list but must not encroach on essential areas of study for veterinary technicians.

7. A mechanism must be in place to evaluate the student's progress both on the didactic material and with hands-on skills **prior** to the student moving to clinical experience.
   - Hands on experience during the program must involve exposure to the equipment and supplies needed to adequately train the assistant with the Vet Assistant Essential Skills listed below.
   - Hands-on experience and skill demonstration must also include the handling of live small animals during the program coursework with proper supervision to ensure safety for the animal handler and to the animal.

   In order for the novice Veterinary Assistant to learn proper restraint and handling skills and to ensure the graduate is competent at a beginner level, NAVTA firmly believes the Veterinary Assistant student should be exposed to the handling of live small animals as part of the curriculum and training.

8. It is vital the program have a policy in place to ensure all students/graduates are competent in the skill set and that individuals who cannot meet the minimum requirements are not allowed to graduate until the minimum academic and clinical experience is met.

9. NAVTA encourages the program to expose veterinary assistant students to certain large and exotic animals; however, the committee recognizes the limitation of availability for all programs, thus the notation optional on the Essential Skills regarding these species.

10. It is vital the Veterinary Assistant Program Director have the ability to initiate change in Curriculum, Hands-on training protocols, and have the authority to correct any deficiencies noted.

TASKS APPROPRIATE TO DELEGATE TO THE ASSISTANT

When identifying those tasks which are appropriate for an assistant to complete, the determining factor in assigning tasks to the assistant is the impact of the task on a positive patient outcome.

In developing the following list of tasks which the assistant may be trained to perform, each task was evaluated for appropriateness based on, but not limited to, the following criteria:

1. What is the impact of the task on a positive patient outcome?
2. Could/would the average client perform the task?
3. Does it change the physiologic state of the patient?
4. Does the information obtained, impact the veterinarian's diagnosis?

It is essential to remember that the completion of all assistant tasks requires some degree of supervision either by the veterinarian or the credentialed veterinary technician.

The following delineation of tasks, appropriate for delegation to the assistant on the veterinary health care team, was developed through a cooperative effort between NAVTA, the Association of Veterinary Technician Educators (AVTE), and the AVMA's Committee on Veterinary Technician Education and Activities.

Educating assistants on tasks beyond the scope of this list is discouraged and may impact the ability of the program to receive the status of NAVTA Approved Veterinary Assistant Program. Graduates of non-approved programs will not be able to sit for the Approved Veterinary Assistant Examination and will not be able to receive Certification from NAVTA.

ESSENTIAL SKILLS FOR ASSISTANT TRAINING*

I. Office and Hospital Procedures
   A. Front Desk
      1) Greet clients
      2) Demonstrate proper appointment scheduling and make appointments
      3) Prepare appropriate forms and certificates for signature
      4) Admit patients
      5) Discharge patients
      6) Perform basic filing and retrieving of medical records

*From Essential Skills for Assistant Training. NAVTA. 2014. http://c.ymcdn.com/sites/www.navta.net/resource/resmgr/ Essential_Skills_for_VA_Rev_.pdf?hhSearchTerms=%22 Essential+and+Skills+and+Assistant+and+Training%22. Accessed December 8, 2015.

7) Perform basic veterinary medical record keeping procedures

8) Demonstrate elementary computer skills

9) Utilize basic medical terminology and abbreviations

10) Perform basic invoicing, billing, and payment on account procedures

B. Telephone

   1) Answer and direct phone calls

   2) Recognize and respond appropriately to veterinary medical emergencies by notifying the appropriate hospital personnel

   3) Request records and information from other veterinary facilities

C. Maintain basic cleanliness and orderliness of a veterinary facility

   1) Inventory supplies

   2) Restock shelves

   3) Perform basic filing and retrieving of medical records, radiographs, lab reports, etc.

   4) Demonstrate knowledge of basic cleaning techniques of animal kennels and bedding, examination rooms, hospital facilities, and surgical suites.

II. Communication and Client Relations

A. Develop effective client communication skills

B. Write business letters and professional electronic communication with clients

C. Understand ethical conduct in relationship to the day to day operations of a veterinary hospital

D. Describe the roles and responsibilities of each member of the veterinary health team and the important part that each plays in the delivery of excellent care

E. Professional Conduct

   1) Understand the human-animal bond

   2) Demonstrate professional and appropriate appearance and language in the workplace

   3) Demonstrate appropriate use of electronic communication in the workplace (cell phone usage, text messaging, social networking, digital photography, etc.)

III. Pharmacy and Pharmacology

A. Legal issues

   1) Recognize legal issues involving drugs in the workplace

   2) Recognize general types and groups of drugs and demonstrate proper terminology

   3) Differentiate prescription drugs from over-the-counter drugs and describe proper prescription label requirements

B. Filling medications and inventory control

   1) Label and package dispensed drugs correctly

   2) Store, safely handle, and dispose of biologic and therapeutic agents, pesticides, and hazardous waste

   3) Perform inventory control procedures, including restocking supplies and checking expiration dates

C. Vaccinations

   1) Reconstitute vaccines and be familiar with proper protocols.

   2) Describe possible routes and methods of drug and vaccine administration that the veterinarian or veterinary technician may choose

IV. Examination Room Procedures

A. Restrain patients

   1) Small animals

     a. Place and remove small animals from cages

     b. Place and restrain small animals on tables

     c. Apply dog and cat safety muzzle

     d. Apply Elizabethan collar

     e. Apply restraint pole

     f. Demonstrate standing, sitting, lateral, sternal, and dorsal restraint positions

     g. Recognize when to alter normal restraint for compromised patients in the exam room (i.e. Ringworm, Contagious diseases, Ectoparasite infestation) and describe appropriate action or personnel to notify

   2) Restrain birds, Rabbits, Pocket Pets, Reptiles, and other exotics—optional

   3) Large animals—optional

     a. Halter, tie, and lead horses and cattle

     b. Restrain cattle & horses

     c. Apply twitch

     d. Apply nose tongs/leads

     e. Restraint sheep & swine

     f. Load large animals

B. Basic Procedures

   1) Determine and record temperature, pulse, respiration, body condition score, and weight of pets

   2) Trim nails (Required: Cats and Dogs. Optional: Birds and Exotics)

   3) Express anal sacs using the external method

   4) Recognize AKC dog breeds and CFA cat breeds.

   5) Be able to properly identify the gender of small animal species, particularly felines.

   6) Perform exam room grooming (i.e., trimming nails, external ear canal cleaning, etc.)

   7) Be familiar with small animal nutritional requirements, pet food labeling standards, dry matter basis calculations, and the differences between pet food products

   8) Apply ear medication

   9) Apply eye medication

   10) Take an accurate history and report chief complaint

V. Small Animal Nursing (Large Animal Nursing--Optional)

A. Safety Concerns

   1) Demonstrate knowledge of basic normal and abnormal animal behavior

   2) Utilize patient & personnel safety measures

3) Identify potential Zoonotic diseases

4) Describe isolation procedures

5) Describe hazardous waste disposal

6) Describe basic sanitation

7) Be familiar with OSHA standards

B. Animal Care

  1) Provide routine record-keeping, and observation of hospitalized patients (i.e., stress importance of notations made when cleaning and feeding)

  2) Demonstrate a basic understanding of:

    a. small animal anatomy

    b. common diseases

    c. medical conditions

  3) Monitor/restrain patients for fluid therapy and record observations

  4) Perform hand pilling (dog, cat)

  5) Administer oral liquid medication (dog and cat)

  6) Demonstrate understanding of a treatment plan

  7) Apply and remove bandages to healthy animals (equine leg and tail wraps optional)

  8) Perform therapeutic bathing, basic grooming, and dipping of small animals

  9) Clean external ear canals

  10) Prepare food & prescription diets - be aware of any special dietary needs

  11) Clean & disinfect cages and kennels (stalls - optional)

  12) Provide care & maintenance of nursing equipment

  13) Demonstrate an understanding of euthanasia and post mortem care

  14) Capillary refill time and normal mucous membrane evaluation

VI. Surgical Preparation and Assisting

A. Assist in performing surgical preparations

  1) Prepare surgical equipment/supplies

  2) Sterilize instruments & sanitize supplies using appropriate methods

  3) Operate and maintain autoclaves

  4) Identify common instruments

  5) Identify common suture materials, types, and sizes

  6) Assist the veterinarian and/or veterinary technician with preparation of patients using aseptic technique

  7) Assist with positioning of surgical patients

  8) Aid the veterinarian/and or veterinary technician with physical monitoring of recovering surgical patients

  9) Maintain the Surgical Log

B. Facility and Equipment Cleanliness

  1) Maintain proper operating room conduct and asepsis

  2) Perform post-surgical clean up

  3) Fold surgical gowns and drapes

  4) Maintain operating room sanitation and care

C. Have knowledge of:

  1) Surgical equipment

  2) Surgical room and prep area

  3) Instrument cleaning and care

  4) Proper disposal of hazardous medical wastes

VII. Laboratory Procedures

A. Assistance in the laboratory

  1) Collect voided urine samples

  2) Determine physical properties of urine, including color and clarity

  3) Assist in the collection of blood samples with restraint and supply preparation

  4) Identify common blood tubes used in veterinary medicine

  5) Collect voided fecal samples for examination

  6) Prepare fecal flotation solutions and set up fecal flotations and direct smears

  7) Assist the DVM or veterinary technician in necropsy procedures

  8) Explain how to handle rabies suspects & samples safely

  9) Handle disposal of deceased animals

  10) Identify external parasites: mites, lice, fleas, and ticks

  11) Assist in the preparation of various specimen staining techniques

B. Laboratory Record Keeping

  1) Ensure all laboratory results are accurately recorded

  2) Stock laboratory supplies

  3) File laboratory reports

  4) Maintain laboratory log

VIII. Radiology & Ultrasound Imaging

A. Follow recommended safety measures.

B. Assist the veterinarian and/or the veterinary technician in the completion of diagnostic radiographs and ultrasound including the restraint, preparation, and positioning of patients

C. Maintain quality control

D. Label, file, and store film and radiographs

E. Properly care for radiography equipment

F. Care and maintenance of film cassettes and screens

G. Know safety techniques for handling processing chemicals

H. Process diagnostic radiographs using:

  1) Manual dipping tank processing OR

  2) An automatic processor OR

  3) Digital processing

I. Maintain x-ray log

Index

A

AAHA. *see* American Animal Hospital Association

AAHA canine vaccination guidelines, for general veterinary practice, 197t–201t

Abbreviations, commonly used in prescriptions, 110b

Abdominal incisions, 260, 280f

Abduction, 63

Absorbable sutures, 251, 251f

Absorption, of drugs, 114

Abyssinian cat, 132f

Academy, 6

Acanthocephela, 323

Acariasis, 327

Accordion pleat-folding technique, 259f

Accounts receivable, 35

Acid phosphatases, 306

Acid-fast stains, 314

Acoustic shadowing, 356

Activated clotting time, 304, 473t

Activated partial thromboplastin time, 304–305, 305f, 473t

Active dogs, 178

Active immunity, 308

Ad libitum, 176

Adduction, 63

Adjacent, 63

Adrenal glands, 96

Adrenal medullary hormones, 96

Adrenocortical hormones, 96

Adrenocorticotropic hormone, 95, 96t

Adsorbents, 115b, 116–117

Adult cats, 178

Adult dogs, 178

African Greys, 386t

A:G ratio, 472t

Agammaglobulinemic, defined, 412–413

Agglutination test, 310, 310f

Aggression
  castration and, 147
  defensive, 147–148, 148f
  prevention of, 147
  puppy tests for, 147
  signs of, 156
  types of, 147t

Aggressive dogs, 156
  body language associated with, 151
  description of, 156
  handling of, 156
  removing of, from cages or runs, 156–157, 156f–157f, 157b

Agonistic behaviors, 147

Agranulocytes, 82

Alanine aminotransferase, 306, 472t

Albumin, 305, 472t

Alcohols, 129, 129t

Alkaline phosphatases, 306, 472t

Allergic skin diseases, 310

Allergies, food, 187t–190t

All-in-one bag, 186

Alpha globulins, 305

Alveolus, 85

Amazon parrots, 386t

American Animal Hospital Association, 243

American Association of Feline Practitioners, feline vaccination guidelines, 203t–204t

American College of Veterinary Radiology, 352

American Kennel Club, 132, 133t–136t

American Society for the Prevention of Cruelty to Animals (ASPCA), 14

American Veterinary Medical Association (AVMA)
  history of, 10b–11b
  veterinary technician program, 5

Americans with Disabilities Act, 12

Amino acids
  crystalline, 186
  essential, 175, 175b

Aminoglycosides, 124b, 125

Amitraz, 127

Ammonium urate, 187t–190t

Amphibians. *see also* Reptiles
  capture and restraint of, 403
  determining gender of, 403
  diseases in, 406, 406b
  euthanasia of, 407
  parasitology in, 405
  radiology in, 405, 405f
  venipuncture in, 404

Amphotericin B, 126

Amylase, 306–307, 472t

Anal sacs
  anatomy of, 221–222, 222f
  care of, 221–222
  expression of
    external, 222
    internal, 222
    technique for, 222

Analgesia, 235, 282

Analgesics, 123, 123b

Anatomic planes, 63f, 352f

Anatomy, 69–103

Anechoic, 355

Anemia, 187t–190t

Anesthesia, 235, 242–283, 276f
  adverse events during, 278
  cardiovascular monitoring during, 278
  checklist for, 263b
  endotracheal intubation for, 275
  equipment and supplies used in, 267–274
    breathing circuits, 269, 272–274

Anesthesia *(Continued)*
    daily inspection checklist, 269b
    endotracheal tubes, 267–268, 269f
    intravenous fluid administration, 267
    laryngoscope, 268
    medical gas, 268–269
    monitoring of, 277t–278t, 277b
  gases, waste, personnel exposure to, 275b
  general, 275
  induction of, 275
  maintenance of, 275–276
  monitoring of, 276–278
  physiologic conditions monitored during, 277
  preanesthetic medication, 274
  recovery from, 280–283
  respiratory function monitoring during, 277–278

Anesthesia machines, 269–272, 271f
  diagram of, 272f
  flow meters, 269–271, 271f
  vaporizers, 271–272, 272f

Anesthetics, 122, 123b
  hazards associated with, 21–22

Anestrus, 100

Anger stage, of grief, 52

Angry clients, 49

Animal behavior, 131–170

Animal Behavior Society, 150

Animal bites, 193

Animal body regions, 65t–67t

Animal care and nursing, 208–241

Animal handling hazards, 19–20

Animal husbandry, 171–207

Animal identification, 173, 173f

Animal rights activists, 14

Animalia, 320–323

Anion gap, 472t

Anisodactyl, 372

Annual deductible, 41

Annular array, 355

Anode, 337

Anode heel effect, 338f

Anorexia, 187t–190t

Anorexic patients, 185

Antacids, 115b, 117

Anterior pituitary gland, 95

Anthropomorphism, 142

Antiarrhythmic drugs, 117–118, 118b

Antibiotics, small mammal administration of, 372

Antibodies, 82–83

Antibody titers, 310

Anticoagulants, 299

Anticonvulsants, 123, 123b

Antidiarrheals, 115b, 116

Page numbers followed by "b", "f" and "t" indicate boxes, figures and tables respectively.

Antidiuretic hormone, 95, 96t
Antiemetics, 115b, 116
Antifungals, 124b, 126
Antigen, 308
Anti-inflammatories, 128–129
Antimicrobials, 124–126
　disinfectant use of, 245, 245t
Antiparasitics, 126–127, 126b
Antiseptics, 129–130, 129t
Antitussives, 119–120, 119b
Antiulcer drugs, 115b, 117
Antivenin, 195–196
Apnea monitor, 277t–278t
Appendicular skeleton, 74–76, 75t
Appetite, 281
Appetite stimulants, 115b, 117
Appointments
　length of, 28
　reminders and recall systems for, 28–30, 29f
　scheduling of, 27–28, 27f
Arrector pili muscle, 77f, 78–79
Arrhythmias, 215, 215f
Arthropoda, 323–325
Articular surface, 73
Artifacts
　radiographic, 350, 350b–352b
　ultrasound, 356
As low as reasonably attainable
　(ALARA), 346
Ascites, 187t–190t
Asepsis, principles of, 244–247
Aseptic technique, 244
　microbiology use of, 314
　rules of, 244–245
　sterilization. see Sterilization
Aspartate aminotransferase, 306
ASPCA. see American Society for the
　Prevention of Cruelty to Animals (ASPCA)
Assistant programs, essentials requirements
　for, 475–476
Assistant training
　curriculum approval, policy on, 475–478
　essential skills for, 476–478
Assisted gloving, 266, 267f–268f
Association of American Feed Control
　Officials, 182
Association of Pet Dog Trainers, 150
Association of Veterinary Technician
　Educators, veterinary assistant model
　curriculum, 474–475
Atelectasis, 240
Attending, 54
Attitude, 280–281
Auditory sense, 92–93, 92f
Auscultation, 213–214, 214f
Australian shepherd, 140f
Autoantibodies, 310
Autoclave
　sterilization uses of, 247, 247f
　surgical instruments cleaned with, 254–255
AVMA. see American Veterinary Medical
　Association (AVMA)
Axial skeleton, 73–74, 75f
Azotemia, 306

B
B lymphocytes, 82
Bacitracins, 125

Bacteria, 192
　characteristics of, 311
　description of, 310–311, 314f
Bacterial cell shapes, 311f
Bacterial infections, 20
Baermann technique, 333–334
Bags, for feline restraint, 161–163, 161b, 162f–163f
Ball bandage, 396
Balling gun, medication administration with, 440, 441f
Bandage application, principles of, 237–238, 238b
Bandage components, 238–240, 238f–239f
Bandaging, 437–438, 437f–438f
　figure-of-eight, 392, 396
Barbering, 366
Bargaining stage, of grief, 52
Barium sulfate, 354
Barking
　noise caused by, 20
　reduction of, 141, 142f
Basophils, 303, 472t
Bathing, 219
Beagle, 137f
Beak, 373
　injuries to, 395
　overgrowth of, 381
　trimming of, 381, 381f
Bed sores. see Decubital ulcers
Bedding, for horses, 416
Behavior
　definition of, 141
　imprinting of, 141, 141f
　negative reinforcement, 141
　positive reinforcement, 141
　stimulus for, 141
　submissive, 141f, 151, 152f
Behavior modification plan, 149, 149t
Behavior problems
　aggression, 142, 147
　destructive behavior. see Destructive
　　behavior
　in exotic animals, 151
　house training, 142–144, 143b
　medication for, 149–150, 149f
　prevention of, 142–148, 142f
　providing services for, 148–151
　resolution of, 148–150, 150f
　socialization to prevent, 147–148, 148f
　specialist referral for, 150–151, 150b
Bereavement, 51
Beta globulins, 305
Bicarbonate, 472t
Biguanides, 130
Bile acids, 306
Bilirubin, 305, 472t
Binocular microscope, 287–288, 287f
Biochemical test materials, 315
Biologic value, of protein, 175
Biologics, 21
Biotransformation, 115
Birds
　amputation in, 395–396
　anatomy of, 373–378
　bandaging of, 392
　beak of, 373
　behavior of, 378–380, 378f

Birds (Continued)
　biting by, 379
　bleeding emergencies in, 394, 394b
　blood collection in, 386–387, 387f
　capture and restraint, 383–385, 385f
　　procedure before, 383
　chewing by, 378, 379f
　circulatory system of, 377
　client education about, 380
　crop, 374–375
　diagnostic sampling techniques in, 386–387
　digestive system of, 374–376, 376f
　dominance behavior of, 379
　ears of, 377–378
　Elizabethan collar placement in, 392–393, 392f
　emergencies in, 393b
　　aerosol toxicity, 394
　　animal bites, 395, 395f
　　beak injuries and repair, 395
　　bleeding, 394, 394b
　　burns, 396
　　egg stasis or binding, 394–395
　　foreign bodies, 395
　　fractures, 395–396, 395f–396f
　　head trauma, 396
　　heavy metal toxicosis, 397, 397b
　　ingested poisons, 397
　　leg fractures, 396
　　lower airway, 394, 394b
　　respiratory, 394
　　space-occupying masses, 394, 394f
　　upper airway, 394b
　　wing fractures, 396
　endoscopy for, 389, 389f
　ethical euthanasia techniques, 398
　euthanasia, 398
　eyes of, 377, 377f
　fear behavior of, 378, 378f
　feathers of, 373
　fecal examination of, 387
　figure-of-eight bandaging of, 392, 396
　fluffing by, 393, 393f
　gastrointestinal contrast study in, 388–389
　gavage feeding in, 391, 391f
　gender determination in, 382, 382f
　housing and husbandry of, 380–381
　imaging in, 387–389
　inappropriate bonding with, 380
　infectious disease in, 390–391, 390b
　integument of, 373
　intramuscular injections in, 392, 392f
　medication administration in, 391
　microchipping in, 382–383
　musculoskeletal system of, 373
　nail trimming of, 382, 382f
　nursing care of, 389–393
　　hospitalization, 389–393, 390f
　nutrition for, 381
　overview of, 372–398
　oxygen cage for, 389–390, 390f
　passerines, 372, 373b
　physical examination of, 383–386, 384f, 386f
　pododermatitis in, 395–396, 396f
　psittacines, 372, 373b
　radiography in, 387–388, 388f
　reproductive system of, 377
　respiratory distress in, 393–394, 393b, 394f

Birds *(Continued)*
  respiratory system of, 374, 375f
  self-mutilation by, 379–380, 379f–380f
  skin of, 373
  smell sense of, 378
  special senses of, 377–378
  standing radiograph of, 388
  stress in, 383
  subcutaneous injections in, 392, 392f
  supportive care for, 391
  tape splints for, 395f
  urinary system of, 376–377, 376f
  venipuncture in, 387f
  vision of, 377, 377f
  vital signs for, 386t
  vocalization by, 379
  weighing of, 386, 386f
  zoonotic diseases in, 390, 390b
Bismuth-glucose-glycine yeast, 313
Bitches. *see also* Dog(s)
  estrous cycle and gestation period in, 471t
  handling of, 155
  parturition in, 102
Biting, by birds, 379
Biting midges, 326
Bladder, 98
Bleeding emergencies, in birds, 394, 394b
Blindfolds, 425
Bloat, 187t–190t
Blood, 81
  collection of, 439, 439f
  composition of, 81, 81f
Blood agar, 313
Blood film. *see* Differential blood film
Blood gases, normal values, 471t
Blood glucose, 307
Blood pressure, normal, in dogs and cats, 471t
Blood smear, 302, 302b
Blood tests
  coagulation testing, 303–305
  complete blood count, 299–303
    automated analyzers used in, 299
    components of, 299
    differential blood film. *see* Differential blood film
    packed cell volume, 299–300
    total plasma protein, 301
  plasma, 298–299, 301b
  sample for
    collection of, 297–298
    type of, 298–299
  whole blood, 298
Blood typing card, 310f
Blood urea nitrogen (BUN), 306, 472t
Blood vascular system, 79–80, 79f
Bloodhound, 137f
Blue-sensitive film, 342–343
Board of Veterinary Medical Examiners, 15
Boarding
  admitting patients for, 38
  form for, 39f
Body condition scoring system
  for cats, 177f
  for dogs, 176, 177f
  for livestock, 412, 412t
Body language
  of client, 49–50
  of dogs, 151

Body parts, anatomy and, combining forms for, 59–61, 60t–61t
Body regions, 64, 65t–67t
Body temperature
  maintenance of, 214–215
  monitoring of, 214–215, 214f
  postoperative evaluation, 280
  rectal measurement of, 215
Body weight, 280
  assessment of, 214, 214f
Boluses, 440
Bone. *see also* Skeleton
  composition of, 73
  features of, 73
  flat, 73
  irregular, 73
  of limbs, 75t
  long, 73
  neck of, 73
  pneumatic, 73
  pneumatized, 373
  radiopaqueness of, 338
  sesamoid, 73
  shapes of, 74f
  small, 73
  types of, 73
Bone loss, 187t–190t
Bordetella bronchiseptica, 193
Borrelia burgdorferi, 20
Borreliosis, 20
Boston terrier, 139f
Botflies, 326
Bouvier des Flandres, 140f
Bowman's capsule, 97–98, 98f
Box turtles, 402
Boxer, 132, 138f
Brachycephalic dogs, description of, 210
Bradyarrhythmias, 215
Bradycardia, 215
Breathing circuits, 269, 272–274
Breathing control, 85–86
Bronchodilators, 119b, 120
Buccal, 64
Buccal mucosal bleeding time, 304, 304f
Bucks, 363
Bucky, 341
Buffy coat smear, 334
Bulb syringe, 226, 226f
Bull's eye culture medium, 313f
BUN. *see* Blood urea nitrogen (BUN)
Burmese, 132f
Burns
  in birds, 396
  in reptiles, 399, 400f
Burrito technique, for restraint, 161b
Burrowing mites, 328
Butterfly catheters, 229
Byproduct feeds, 411

C
Cages
  bedding in, 362, 399
  description of, 172–173
  lighting of, 399
  removing cats from, 164–165, 165f
  removing dogs from, 156–157, 156f–157f, 157b

Cages *(Continued)*
  reptile housing, 399
  rodent housing, 361
Calcitonin, 95, 96t
Calcium, 472t
Caloric requirements, 184–186
Cancer, 187t–190t
Canine (teeth), 86
Canine body language, 151
Canine distemper, in ferrets, 364
Canine infectious respiratory disease, 193
Capillaries
  blood, 79–80
  lymph, 83
Capillary refill time, 216, 218f
Capnometer, 277t–278t
Capsid, 192
Capture
  of amphibians, 403
  of birds, 383–385
    procedure before, 383
  of chelonians, 401–402
  of lizards, 402–403
  of snakes, 401
Carbohydrates, 175
Carbon dioxide-absorbent canister, 273, 273t
Cardiac cycle, 80–81, 80f
Cardiac murmur, 215
Cardiac muscle, 90, 91f
Cardiocentesis, 404
Cardiovascular system. *see also* Heart
  drugs affecting, 117–119
CareCredit, 36
Carrier, removal of cat from, 164
Castration, 147
Cat(s), 143–144, 144f. *see also* Queens; specific feline entries
  aggression by, 147, 147t
  behavior of, 160
  blood gas values in, 471t
  breeds of, 132
  in cages, 172f
  cestode in, 322t
  chemistry values in, 472t
  daily energy requirements, 181f
  danger potential of, 160
  dental formula for, 87
  destructive behavior by, 144–146
  distraction techniques for, 164
    caveman pats, 164
    puffs of air, 164
  endocrine glands in, 95f
  endotracheal intubation in, 275
  estrous cycle and gestation period in, 471t
  gestation in, feeding during, 181
  handling of, 160–169
  hematology reference range values in, 472t
  house training of, 143–144
  intramuscular injections in, 169f
  lactation in, feeding during, 181
  litter box training of, 143
  nail trimming of, 221f
  nematodes in, 323t
  normal heart rate and blood pressure in, 471t
  normal physiologic data in, 471t

Cat(s) (*Continued*)
normal ranges of heart rate, respiratory rate, and rectal temperature in, 213t
nutrient considerations for different life stages in, 179t–180t
psychological needs of, 174
recommended feeding practices for, 178b
removal of
from cage, 164–165, 165f
from carrier, 164
restraint of, 160–169
cat lasso, 169, 169f
for cephalic venipuncture, 165–166, 166f–167f
chemical, 169
dorsal recumbency, 169, 169b
gauntlets, 164
for jugular venipuncture, 166–168, 167f–168f
lateral recumbency, 168–169, 168b
muzzles, 163–164, 163f–164f
removal from cage, 164–165, 165f
removal from carrier, 164
scruffing technique, 168
sitting recumbency, 165–168, 165f
sternal recumbency, 165–168, 165f
towel and blanket, 160–161
scratching by, 145, 145f
tourniquet for cephalic venipuncture for, 166, 167f
urinalysis in, 473t
urine production in, 471t
Cat lasso, 169, 169f
Catchpole, 153, 155f
Catheter(s)
bandage for, 231
central, 229
intravenous, 229–231, 229f
care of, 230–231
over-the-needle peripheral, 229–230, 230f
parenteral nutrition administration using, 186
securing of, 230f
urinary, 231–232
winged infusion (butterfly), 229
Catheter tip, 107, 107f
Cathode, 337
Cattle
beef, 412
care of, 418–419, 418f–419f
dairy, 411–412
restraint of, 429–432, 429f–430f
approaching and moving in, 431–432
halter for, 430–431, 431f
hobbles for, 431
squeeze chute for, 430, 430f
stanchions for, 431
tilt table in, 431, 431f
Caudal, 63, 352
Caveman pats, 164
Celiotomy, 261
Cell-mediated immunity, 308
Cellophane tape preparation, 333, 334b
Cells, 70, 71f. *see also* specific cell
Central, 63
Central catheter, 229
Central nervous system, 88–89, 88f

Central nervous system stimulants, 123–124, 123b
Central venous pressure, 277t–278t
Centrifugal flotation, of fecal specimens, 331, 333b
Centrifuge, 289–290, 289f
Centrifuged hematocrit tube, 301f
Cephalosporins, 124–125, 124b
Cere, 373, 376f
Cervix, 99f, 100
Cesarean section, 260
Cestodes, 321–322, 321f, 322t
Chain shank, 427, 427f–428f
Chain twitch, 425, 426f
Chelonians. *see also* Reptiles
capture of, 401–402
description of, 400
emergency and critical care of, 406
feeding of, 400
handling of, 401–402
intravenous catheter sites in, 406t
radiology in, 405
restraint of, 401–402, 402f
venipuncture in, 404, 404f, 404t
Chemical(s)
developing, 21
hazards associated with, 22–23
mixing of, 23
storage of, 20
Chemical indicators, 246, 246f
Chemical restraints, 169
Chemical spills, 23
Chemistry analyzers, 291–293, 292f
Chemoheterotrophic, 311
Chewing, by birds, 378, 379f
Chihuahua, 138f
Chinchillas, 369–370, 370f
Chinese hamsters, 366–367
Chlamydiosis, 390
Chlamydophila psittaci, 390
Chloramphenicol, 126
Chlorhexidine, 129t, 130
Chlorhexidine diacetate solution, 234
Chloride, 472t
Chlorine compounds, 129–130, 129t
Choana, 374
Cholesterol, 472t
Chromogen, 309
Circuit manometer, 273
Circulation
fetal, 83, 84f
pulmonary, 80
systemic, 80
Circulatory system, 79–84
of birds, 377
blood vascular system, 79–80, 79f
functions of, 79
pathways of, 80–81
Citronella collars, 141, 142f
Classical conditioning, 141
Claws, scratching use of, 144, 145f
Clean surgical wounds, 233
Cleaning
of ears, 222, 223b
kennel assistant's role in, 4
Clicker training, 143

Clients
angry, 49
attending to, 54
body language of, 49–50
body posture of, 50
communication with, 49, 209, 209f
education of, during visit, 38, 38f, 38b
eye contact with, 50
first impression for, 26
greeting of, 30
grief counseling for, 51–54
information forms for, 31f
introduction to, 210b
invoicing of, 35–37
listening to, 54
loss. *see* Loss
mental health professional referral for, 55–56
monthly statements for, 36–37
relations with, 48–50
Clinical chemistry, 305–308
Cloaca, 375–376
prolapsed, 395, 395f
Closed-suction drains, 236
Clostridium tetani, 195–196
Closure, 54
Coagulation disorders, 303–304
Coagulation testing, 303–305
Cockatiels, 386t
Cockatoos, 386t
Cocker spaniel, 137f
Coelom, 374, 399
Cold chemical sterilization, 256–257, 256f, 256t
Colitis, 187t–190t
Collar, Elizabethan, 392–393, 392f
Collimators, 340
Colorimeter, 291
Colostrometer, 412–413
Colostrum, for debilitated calf, 412–413
Columella, 377–378
Combining form, 58
Combining vowel, 58
Commissure, 441
Common law
malpractice, 16
negligence, 17
Communication, 49, 209, 209f
Companion animals. *see also* Cat(s); Dog(s); Small mammals
as family members, 51
veterinary practice specializing in, 9
Complete blood count, 299–303
automated analyzers used in, 299
components of, 299
differential blood film. *see* Differential blood film
packed cell volume, 299–300
total plasma protein, 301
Compound light microscope, 287
Compound word, 58
word formation using, 59, 59t
Compounded loss, 55–56
Comprehensive Drug Abuse Prevention and Control Act, 18
Compressed gases, 22
Compressed medical gas cylinders, 269, 270f–271f

Compression smear, for sample preparation, 316
Computed radiography, 345
Computed tomography, 358
Computers
    appointment scheduling using, 27f, 28
    backing up, 48
    client education handouts from, 40
    inventory management using, 46–48, 46f
    management of, 48
    medical records on, 41–44, 42f
    reminder and recall systems, 28–30, 29f
Concentrates, 410–411
Concussion, 192
Conditions
    prefixes for, 62, 62t
    suffixes for, 61–62, 61t–62t
Congenital condition, 41
Connective tissue, 70–73, 72f
Consent forms
    anesthesia, 30
    blanket, 34f
    informed, 30, 33f–34f
Constipation, 187t–190t
Consultation rooms, 12
Contact, 64
Container caps, 23
Container labels, 23
Contamination, of wound, 244
Contour feathers, 373, 374f
Contrast studies, 354–355
    barium sulfate, 354
    double-contrast procedure, 355
    negative contrast media used in, 355
    positive contrast media used in, 354–355
    purpose of, 354
    water-soluble organic iodides, 354
Controlled Substance Act (CSA), 18, 18f
Controlled substances
    classifications of, 113, 113t
    definition of, 112
    labeling of, 112, 113f
    laws governing, 18
    prescribing of, 112–113
    prescriptions for, 113
    recordkeeping about, 112
    storing of, 112–113
Contusion, 192
Conures, 386t
Coombs test, 310
Co-pay, 41
Copper storage disease, 187t–190t
Coprodeum, 375–376
Coprophagic, 362–363
Corn, for livestock, 410–411
Cornea, description of, 93–94, 93f
Coverslip smears, 302, 303f
Cow's milk, 177
Cranial, 63, 352
Cranial nerves, 89, 89t
Crate training, 142
Creatine kinase, 307, 472t
Creatinine, 306, 472t
Credit cards, 35
Crile forceps, 249
Crop, 374–375
    burn, 396–397
    trauma, 396–397

Cross tying, of horse, 423–424, 425f
Crowding, 159
Crystalline amino acids, 186
CSA. see Controlled Substance Act (CSA)
Culture media, 313–314
    inoculating, 314
Culturette, 313f
Curry combs, horse grooming with, 417, 417f
Cutaneous larval migrans, 20
Cuterebra spp., larval, in subcutaneous fistula, 326f
Cyanoacrylates, 253
Cystocentesis, 318
Cystotomy, 261
Cytology, 315–317
    collection and preparation of samples
        fine-needle biopsy, 316
        for fluid samples, 317
        impression smears, 316
        swabbings, 316
    goal of, 315–316
    masses, 316–317
    scrapings, 316
    specimen, examination of, 317
    tissues, 316–317
    vaginal, 317

D
Dachshund, 137f
Darkroom
    cleanliness of, 348
    film identification, 348
    film processing in. see Radiographic film; processing of
    processing area, 347f
    safelights in, 348–349
    setup, 347–348, 347f
    techniques of, 347–350
    ventilation, 348
DEA. see Drug Enforcement Agency (DEA)
Dead space, 107
Debilitation, 187t–190t
Débridement, 235–236, 235f, 235b
Debt collection, 37, 37b
Decongestants, 119b, 120
Decubital ulcers, 416
    description of, 240
    in recumbent patients, 240, 240f
Deductible, 41
Deep, 63
Defecation, 281
Defensive aggression, 147–148, 152f
Definitive host, 319–320
Delta Society, 55–56
Demodectic mange, 328
Denial stage, of grief, 52
Dental formula, 87
Dental terminology, 64, 68f
Department of Labor, 18
Dermis, 78f
Destructive behavior
    aggression by, 147, 147t
    by cats, 144–146
    chewing, 146
    digging, 146
    by dogs, 146–147
    prevention of, 144–147
    scratching, 144

Developing chemicals, 21
Diabetes mellitus, 187t–190t, 307
Diagnostic imaging, 336–359
    computed tomography, 358
    contrast studies. see Contrast studies
    endoscopy. see Endoscopy
    magnetic resonance imaging, 358–359
    nuclear medicine, 359
    radiographs. see Radiographic images
    ultrasound. see Ultrasound
Diaphragm (stethoscope), 213–214
Diarrhea, 218–219
    acute, 187t–190t
Diastema, 440
Diestrus, 100–101
Differential blood film, 301–303
    blood smear preparation, 302, 302b
    eosinophils, 303
    erythrocyte morphology and variations, 303
    evaluation of, 302, 303f
    leukocytes on, 303
    lymphocytes on, 303
    monocytes on, 303
    parasites on, 303
    performing of, 302–303
    platelets, 303
    white blood cell count, 303
Digestive system, 86–88
    accessory organs of, 87–88
    of birds, 374–376, 376f
    esophagus, 87
    function of, 86
    intestine, 87
    mouth, 86–87, 86f
    stomach, 87
Digital imaging and communications in medicine (DICOM) files, 345
Digital radiography, 345. see also Radiographic images
Dilutions, 287
Dimethyl sulfoxide (DMSO), 314
Dipstick testing, of urine, 318–319, 318f
Dipylidium caninum, 321, 321f–322f
Direct drop test, 334
Direct exposure film, 342–343
Directional terms, 63–64, 63f, 352f–353f
Dirofilaria immitis, 323f–324f
Discharge instructions, 40, 40f, 49
Discharging patients, 38–40, 40f
Diseases. see also specific disease
    of cats, 205t–206t
    dietary factors, 202
    of dog, 205t–206t
    environmental factors, 202
    factors predisposing to, 202–207
    genetic factors, 202
    infectious. see Infectious disease
    metabolic factors, 207
    nonpathogens that cause, 192
    prefixes for, 62, 62t
    suffixes for, 61–62, 61t–62t
    terminology associated with, 191–192
    transmission of, 4, 193–195
    zoonotic. see Zoonotic diseases
Disinfectants, 129–130, 174
Disinfection, 129, 174, 245–247
Dispensing fee, 47
Disseminated intravascular coagulation, 304

Distal, 63, 353
Distance enhancement, 356
Distraction techniques, for cats, 164
Distribution, of drugs, 115
Diuretics, 118b, 119
Doberman Pinscher, 138f
Does, 363
Dog(s). see also Bitches; Puppies; specific
   canine entries
  aggressive, 157
   body language associated with, 151
   description of, 147
   handling of, 156
  blood gas values in, 471t
  body language of, 151
  brachycephalic, description of, 210
  breeds of, 132, 133t–136t
  cestode in, 322t
  chemistry values in, 472t
  chewing by, 146
  confinement of, 172–173
  daily energy requirements for, 179f
  danger potential of, 151
  dental formula for, 87
  destructive behavior by, 146–147
   appealing toys, 146–147, 146f
  digestive apparatus of, 86f
  endotracheal intubation in, 275
  estrous cycle and gestation period in, 471t
  fearful, 151, 157
  gestating or lactating, feeding, 176
  handling of, 151–160
  hematology reference range values in, 472t
  house training of, 142–143
  lifting of, 157, 157f
  nail trimming of, 220–221
  nematodes in, 323t
  nonaggressive, 156
  nonfearful, 156
  normal heart rate and blood pressure in,
   471t
  normal physiologic data in, 471t
  normal ranges of heart rate, respiratory rate,
   and rectal temperature in, 213t
  nutrient considerations for different life
   stages in, 179t–180t
  oral administration of medications in, 224
  psychological needs of, 174
  rectal examination in, 158–159, 158f
  removing of, from cages or runs, 156–157,
   156f–157f, 157b
  restraint of, 151–160
   catchpole, 153, 155f
   crowding, 159
   dorsal recumbency, 160
   gauntlet, 153, 153f
   lateral recumbency, 160, 160b
   leash, 151–153, 153f
   mobility-limiting devices, 153–155, 155f
   muzzles, 153, 154b
   standing, 157–159, 158f
   sternal recumbency, 159, 159b
  urinalysis in, 473t
  urine production in, 471t
Dorsal, 64, 352
Dorsal recumbency
  in cats, 169, 169b
  in dogs, 160

Dosage forms, 106–108, 106t
Dosimetry badge, 21
Double-contrast procedure, 355
Down feathers, 373, 374f
Drainage, of wound, 236
Drapes, 258
Draping, 279–280
Dremel tool, 221, 221f, 381f, 382
Drench, medication administration and, 441,
  441f
Drug(s). see also Medication(s)
  absorption of, 114
  administration of, 114–115, 114f
  anesthetic induction, 275
  antifungals, 124b, 126
  antiparasitics, 126–127, 126b
  biotransformation of, 115
  chemical name of, 105
  components of, 106f
  continuous rate infusion of, 114
  distribution of, 115
  dose of, 113–114
  elimination of, 115
  endocrine system, 120–121
  generic name of, 105
  handling of, 112
  hyperthyroidism treated with, 120b, 121
  hypothyroidism treated with, 120–121, 120b
  injectable, 107–108, 107f
  metabolism of, 115
  names of, 105
  patent rights for, 105
  pharmacokinetics of, 114
  proprietary name of, 105
  reconstitution of, 108, 109b
  reproduction affected by, 121–122
  storage temperature, 112t
  storing of, 112
  therapeutic range of, 113
  toxic, 113
  trade name of, 105
Drug dosage
  calculations of, 111–112, 111b
  forms of, 106–108, 106t
  interval, 114
  regimen for, 113–114
Drug Enforcement Agency (DEA)
  certification number from, 113
  description of, 18
Dysecdysis, 399, 399f
Dyspnea, 216

E
Ear(s)
  of birds, 377–378
  cleaning of, 222, 223b
  disease of, 222
  external, 93
  hair growth in, 222
  inner, 93
  medication administration in, 226, 226f
  rocking, 425
Eccentric tip, 107, 107f
Echinococcus spp., 321
Echogenic, 355
Echoic, 355
Eclampsia, 187t–190t
Eclectus parrots, 382, 382f, 386t

Ectoparasites, 319–320
EDTA. see Ethylenediaminetetraacetic acid
  (EDTA)
EEO. see Equal Employment Opportunity
  (EEO)
Egg retention, 394–395
Egg stasis or binding, 394–395
Electrical hazards, 23–24
Electrocardiograph, 277t–278t
Electrocautery, 249
Electrochemical methods, 291, 292f
Electrolytes, 186, 307–308, 308f
  for debilitated calf, 413–414
Electromagnetic radiation, 342
Electronic cell counters, 293f, 294–295
Electronic funds transfer (EFT), 36
Electroscalpel, 248
Elixirs, 106
Elizabethan collar, 155, 155f, 392–393,
  392f–393f
Emetics, 115–116, 115b
Employee handbook, 17
Enclosures, 172–173
Endocrine glands, 70
Endocrine system, 94–97
  adrenal glands, 96
  description of, 94
  drugs that affect, 120–121, 120b
  gonads, 97
  hormones, 94, 96t
  hypothalamus, 95
  pancreas, 96–97
  parathyroid glands, 95–96
  pituitary gland, 95
  thyroid gland, 95
Endoparasites, 319–320
Endoscopy
  accessory instruments used in, 357, 357f
  for birds, 389, 389f
  description of, 356–358
  endoscopes, 356–357, 356f
  gastrointestinal, 358
Endoscopy room, 357
Endotracheal intubation, 275
Endotracheal tubes, 267–268, 269f
Enema, description of, 224
Energy requirements, daily, canine, 179f
Ensiling, 410
Enteral nutritional support, 183–186, 184f,
  184b–185b
Enteric-coated tablets, 106, 106t
Enterotomy, 261
Enzyme analyses, 306
Enzyme-linked immunosorbent assay
  (ELISA), 309, 309f
Eosin-methylene blue, 313
Eosinophils, 303, 472t
Epidermis, 78f
Epinephrine, 96t
Epithelial cells, in urine, 319f
Epithelial tissue, 70, 71f
Equal Employment Opportunity (EEO), 17
Erythrocyte indices, 301, 302t
Erythrocytes
  description of, 81
  morphology and variations of, 303
Eschar, 237
Esophageal stethoscope, 277–278, 279f

Esophagus, 87
Essential amino acids, 175, 175b
Essential fatty acids, 175b
Estrous cycle, in dogs and cats, 471t
Estrus, 100
Ethics, 14–15
    definition of, 14
    professional, 15
    public service, 15
    veterinary profession, 15
    of working with animals, 14–15
Ethology, 141
Ethylene oxide, 23, 256
Ethylenediaminetetraacetic acid (EDTA), 299, 299f
Etiology, 190–191
Euthanasia. see also Loss
    in amphibians, 407
    of birds, 398
    methods, 241
    release form for, 30–35, 35f
    of reptiles, 407
Evacuation, 24
Examination rooms, 12, 12f
Exercise, for horses, 416–417
Exocrine glands, 70, 96–97
Exotic animals
    amphibians. see Amphibians
    behavior problems in, 151
    birds. see Birds
    reptiles. see Reptiles
Expectorants, 119b, 120
Expiration, 85
Expiration dates, 47
Expiratory dyspnea, 216
Extension, 64
Extension cords, 24
External records, of laboratory, 297
Eye(s)
    anatomy of, 93, 93f–94f
    of birds, 377, 377f
    medication administration in, 225, 225f
    safety of, 19
Eye contact, 50
Eyelids, 94

F
Facet, 73
Fair Debt Collections Practices Act, 37
Fair Labor Standard Act (FLSA), 18
Falls, 18
Farrowing, 420
Fats, 175, 175b
Fear
    aggression induced by, 152f
    of birds, 378, 378f
Fearful dogs, description of, 151
Feathers
    anatomy of, 373, 374f
    destructive behaviors, 379–380, 379f–380f
    molting, 373
    trimming of, 381
    types of, 373, 374f
Fecal flotation, 330, 330f, 332b
    for birds, 387
Fecal occult blood testing, 334

Fecal specimens, for parasite diagnosis
    Baermann technique, 333–334
    cellophane tape preparation, 333, 334b
    centrifugal flotation of, 331, 333b
    collection of, 330
    direct smear of, 330, 331b
    evaluation of, 330–334
    flotation method, 330
    sedimentation, 333, 333b
Feces removal, 174
Feeding. see also Nutrition
    body condition scoring system, 176, 177f
    of cats
        adult cats, 178–180
        considerations for, 178–181
        geriatric cats, 179t–180t, 180–181
        life-stage recommendations, 179t–180t
        with lower urinary tract disease, 180
        recommended practices for, 178b
    of chelonians, 400
    colostrum, 412–413
    of dogs, 176–178
        active dogs, 178
        adult dogs, 178
        free choice method, 176
        geriatric dogs, 178
        in gestation, 176
        life-stage recommendations, 179t–180t
        overweight dogs, 178
        recommended practices for, 178b
    electrolytes, 413–414
    force
        in reptiles, 406f
        in small mammals, 371
    gavage, 391, 391f
    of kittens, 178, 179t–180t
    of lizards, 400
    management, 411–415
        beef cattle, 412
        dairy cattle, 411–412
        goats, 415
        horses, 414
        nutrition in debilitated calf, 412–414
        pigs, 414–415
        sheep, 415
    milk, 413
    portion control method, 176
    of puppies, 177–178, 179t–180t
    of reptiles and amphibians, 400
    of snakes, 400
    time control method, 176
Feeding tubes, eating by patients with, 185–186
Feedstuffs, 409–411
Feline behavior, 160
Feline restraint bags, 161–163, 161b, 162f–163f
Feline urinary tract disease, 180
Female reproductive system
    anatomy of, 99, 99f
    physiology of, 100–101
Femoral pores, 403, 403f
Ferrets
    canine distemper susceptibility in, 364
    color of, 363–364
    description of, 363–364
    housing of, 361–362
    restraint of, 364, 365f
    teeth of, 364
    vaccination of, 372

Ferrets (Continued)
    venipuncture in, 371, 371f
    vital signs of, 364
Fertilization, 101–102, 101f
Fetal circulation, 83, 84f
Fever, 191
Fiberoptic endoscopes, 357
Fibrin degradation products, 473t
Fibrinogen, 473t
Fibrosis, 191
Figure-of-eight bandaging, 392, 396
Film-focal distance (FFD), 339
Filter test, 334
Fine-needle biopsy, 316
Fire safety, 24
First cervical vertebra (C1), 73–74
First-intention healing, 191–192
Fistula, crop, 396–397, 397f
Fixatives, 317
Flank glands, 367
Flank incision, 260
Flat bones, 73
Flatulence, 187t–190t
Flea dirt, 326f
Fleas, 325–326, 325f–326f
Flexible endoscopes, 357
Flexion, 64
Flies, 326
Flight feathers, 373
    trimming of, 381
Flow meters, 269–271, 271f
FLSA. see Fair Labor Standard Act (FLSA)
Fluconazole, 126
Flucytosine, 126
Fluid therapy, 232
Fluid volume, for maintenance total parenteral nutrition, 186
Flukes, 322
Fluoroquinolones, 124b, 125
Fluoroscopy, 345
Foals, restraint of, 428
Focused grids, 340–341, 341f
Folded arms, as body language, 49–50
Folding, of gowns, 257–258, 257f–258f
Food, pet, 182, 182f
Food label, 182f
Foodborne disease, 193
Foot wraps, 438
Forages, 409–410
Force feeding
    in reptiles, 405–406, 406f
    in small mammals, 371
Forceps, 248–249
Foreign bodies, 395
Forelimb, 74
Foreseeable harm, 17
Foreshortening, of radiographic images, 339
Formalin, 23
Forms, 30–35, 31f
    blanket consent, 34f
    boarding, 39f
    consent, 30, 33f–34f
    euthanasia release, 30–35, 35f
    health certificates, 35
    informed consent, 30, 33f–34f
    medical record, 32f–33f
    patient history, 31f–32f
    rabies certificates, 35, 36f

Fractures
  in birds, 395–396, 395f–396f
  wing, 396
Free-choice feeding, 176
French bulldog, 140f
Frick's speculum, 440
Front office procedures, 26–38
  appointment scheduling, 27–28, 27f
  cleanliness, 30
  forms commonly used, 30–35, 31f–35f
  greeting clients, 30, 48, 48f
  invoicing of clients, 35–37
  mail processing, 37–38
  monthly statements, 36–37
  outstanding debt collection, 37, 37b
  telephone etiquette, 26–27, 26f
Fructosamine, 307
Fungal infections, 20
Fungi, 311, 312t

G
Gallbladder, 306
Gallop rhythm, 213–214
Gamma globulins, 305
Gamma glutamyltransferase, 472t
Gas(es)
  anesthetic, 21
  compressed, 22
Gas exchange, 85
Gas sterilization, 256
Gastric dilation, 187t–190t
Gastric intubation, 232
Gastrointestinal contrast study, in birds,
  388–389
Gastrointestinal drugs
  adsorbents, 115b, 116–117
  antacids, 115b, 117
  antidiarrheals, 115b, 116
  antiemetics, 115b, 116
  antiulcer drugs, 115b, 117
  appetite stimulants, 115b, 117
  drugs that affect, 115–117
  emetics, 115–116, 115b
  laxatives, 115b, 117
  lubricants, 115b, 117
  protectants, 115b, 116–117
  stool softeners, 115b, 117
Gastrointestinal endoscopy, 358
Gastropexy, 261
Gastrostomy tube, 184
Gastrotomy, 261
Gauntlets
  for cats, 164
  for dogs, 153, 153f
Gauze muzzle, 153, 154b
Gavage feeding, 391, 391f
Gecko, 399f
General anesthesia, 275
General senses, 91–92, 92t
Generic name, 105
Genesis hematology analyzer, 293f
Gerbils, 365f, 367
Geriatric cats, 179t–180t, 180–181
Geriatric dogs, 178, 179t–180t
German shepherd dog, 140f
Gestation. see also Bitches; Queens
  in cats, feeding during, 179t–180t, 181
  in dogs, feeding during, 176

Gestation (Continued)
  period of, 102, 102t
    for cattle, 418
    weight gain during, 177f
Giardia spp., 320, 321f
Gib, 364
Gilts, 420
Gingivitis, 187t–190t
Gizzard, 375, 376f
Glenoid cavity, 75
Globulins, 305, 472t
Glomerular filtration, 306
Gloving, assisted, 266, 267f–268f
Glucagon, 87–88, 307
Glucocorticoids, 128, 128b
Glucose, 307
  instrument for measuring, 293f
  insulin effects on, 307
  normal values for, 472t
Goats
  care of, 419
  feeding management for, 415
  restraint of, 432–433, 433f
Golden hamster, 366–367
Golden retriever, 137f
Goldendoodle, 132f
Gonadotropin-releasing hormone (GnRH),
  100, 121–122
Gonads, 97
Gown(s), folding of, 257–258, 257f–258f
Gowning table, 244f
Gram stain, 314, 314f
Gram-negative bacilli, 315t
Gram-positive bacilli, 315t
Granulation tissue, 191, 192f
Granulocytes, 81–82
Gravity displacement autoclaves, 247
Green chop, forage and, 410
Green iguana, 399–400
Green-sensitive film, 342–343
Greeting of clients, 26f, 30, 48, 48f
Greyhound, 138f
Grid cutoff, 340–341, 341f
Grids, for scatter radiation, 340–341, 341f
Grief, 52–53
Grief counseling, 51–54
Griseofulvin, 126
Groomers, 3, 3f
  responsibilities of, 3b
Grooming
  anal sacs, 221–222
  bathing, 219
  ear cleaning, 222
  for horses, 417, 417f
  nail trimming, 220–221, 220f
Gross lesions, 191
Ground fault circuit interrupter (GFCI), 23
Gruel, 178
Guilt stage, of grief, 52
Guinea pigs, 367–369, 369f, 372f
  normal ranges of heart rate, respiratory rate,
    and rectal temperature in, 213t
Gustatory sense, 92

H
Hair
  in ear canal, 222
  shedding of, 173

Halter, for cattle restraint, 430–431, 431f
Hamsters, 366–367, 367f
  normal ranges of heart rate, respiratory rate,
    and rectal temperature in, 213t
Hand twitch, 425
Hand washing, 390–391
Handling
  of aggressive dogs, 156
  of injured dogs, 156
  of nervous dogs, 156
  of old dogs, 156
  of pregnant bitches, 155
  of puppies, 155
Haustra, 362–363
Hay, 410
Hazardous materials plan, 22–23
Hazards
  anesthetic, 21–22
  animal handling, 19–20
  bathing, 20
  chemical, 22–23
  compressed gases, 22
  dipping, 20
  electrical, 23–24
  radiation, 21
  sharp objects, 22
  zoonotic. see Zoonotic hazards
Head trauma, 396
Healing, and repair of damaged tissues,
  191–192
Health certificates, 35
Health insurance, 40–41
Hearing, 92
Heart, 80
  anatomy of, 79f, 80
  blood flow in, 80f
Heart rate
  abnormalities in, 215
  in cats, 213t, 471t
  in dogs, 213t, 471t
Heat (estrus)
  in bitches, 101
  description of, 100
  in queens, 101
Heating devices, 19
Heavy metal toxicosis, 397, 397b
Heel effect, 337, 338f
Hematocrit, 294, 472t
Hematology analyzers, 293–295
  care and maintenance of, 294–295
  impedance analyzers, 293–294, 294f
  laser-based analyzers, 294, 295f
  maintenance of, 294–295
  quantitative buffy coat system, 294
  types of, 293–294
Hematology examination
  coagulation testing, 303–305
  collection equipment, 298
  complete blood count. see Complete blood
    count
  plasma, 298–299, 301b
  procedures, 297–305
  reference range values for, 472t
  sample for
    anticoagulants added to, 299
    collection of, 297–298
    type of, 298–299
  whole blood, 298

Hematoma, 282
Hemoglobin, 472t
Hemolysis, 298
Hemorrhage, 282
Hemostasis, 249
    assessment of, 304
    defects of, 303–304
    definition of, 303
    reference range values for, 473t
Hemostatic forceps, 249, 250f
Heparin, 299
Hepatobiliary function testing, 305–306
Hereditary condition, 41
Herniorrhaphy, 261
Hip glands, 367
Histology, 317
Histopathology, 190–191
History of presenting complaint, 211, 211b
Hobbles
    for cattle restraint, 431
    for horses, 428
Hobs, 364
Hog snare, 433
Hoof
    picking of, for horses, 417–418, 417f–418f
    trimming, 434, 435f
Hookworms, 20
Hooves, 79
Horizontal nystagmus, 211
Horizontal scratching, 145, 145f
Hormones, 94, 96t
Horses
    approaching and capturing of, 421–422,
        421f–423f
    care of, 416–418, 436–437
        bedding, 416
        exercise, 416–417
        fly control, 416
        grooming, 417, 417f
        hoof picking, 417–418, 417f–418f
    chain shank for, 427
    distraction technique for, 425
    feeding management for, 414
    handling of, 420–428
    hobbles for, 428
    leading of, 423, 423f
    restraint of, 420–428
        head, 424–425
    stocks for, 428
    tail tying in, 428, 428f
    twitches for, 425–428
    tying of, 423–424, 424f
Hospice, 51
Hospital
    admitting patients to, 38
    cleanliness of, 173
    discharging patients from, 38–40, 40f
    exterior appearance of, 174, 174f
Hospital administrators, 7–8, 7b
Hospitalization sheets, 44, 45f
House training
    of cats, 143–144
    clicker method for, 143b
    crate training used in, 142, 143f
    description of, 142
    of dogs, 142–143
    of puppies, 142, 143b
Housekeeping, 173–174

Housing
    birds, 380–381
    description of, 172–173
    small mammals, 361–362, 361f
Human-animal bond, 50–56
    decision making affected by, 50
    description of, 14
    grief counseling, 51–54
    hospitalization effects on, 51
    nurturing, 51
Humane twitch, 426, 426f
Humoral immunity, 308
Husbandry, 172–174
    animal identification, 173, 173f
    in birds, 380–381
    disinfection, 174
    housekeeping, 173–174
    housing, 172–173
    large animal nursing and, 408–446
    lighting, 172
    room temperature, 172
    ventilation of, 172
Hyperadrenocorticism, 121
Hypercarbia, 272–273
Hyperechoic, 355
Hyperlipidemia, 187t–190t
Hyperthermia, 215
Hyperthyroidism, 121, 187t–190t
Hypertrophic cardiomyopathy, 118
Hyphae, 311
Hypoadrenocorticism (Addison's disease), 121
Hypodermis, 77f, 78
Hypoechoic, 355
Hypokalemia, 186
Hypothalamus, 95
Hypothermia, 214–215
Hypothyroidism, 120–121

I
Icterus, 300–301, 301f
Iguana, 399–400
Imaging, in birds, 387–389
Immune response, 192–193
Immune system, 308
Immunity, 81–83, 308
Immunoassays, 308
Immunoglobulins, 82, 83f, 305
Immunology
    principles of, 308–310
    tests of, 308–310
Impedance analyzers, 293–294, 294f
Implantation, 101f
Impression smears, 316, 316b
Imprinting, 141
Incisions, 260, 260f
Incubators, 295, 295f
Indemnity insurance, 41
Infection, 282–283
    of wound, 244
Infectious disease
    in birds, 390–391, 390b–391b
    preventing the spread of, in clinic, 390–391
Inflammation, 191, 191b
Influenza, 364
Informed consent form, 30, 33f–34f
Infrared motion analyzer, 292f
Ingested poisons, 397
Inhalant anesthetics, 115

Injectable drugs
    administration of, 107
    needles, 108, 108f
    syringes, 107–108, 107f
Injured dogs, 156
Innocent murmurs, 215
Inoculating dermatophyte test media,
        314–315
Insect growth regulators, 127
Insect repellents, 127
Inspiration, 85
Instrument(s), suffixes for, 63
Instrument table, 279–280
Insulin, 121, 307
Insulin syringe, 107–108, 108f
Insurance, 40–41
Integument, 76–79, 77f. see also Skin.
    of birds, 373
    claws, 79
    definition of, 76–77
    function of, 76–77
    hair, 78–79
    hooves, 79
    skin, 77–78
Intensifying screens, 343, 343f
Intermediate host, 319–320
Internal records, of laboratory, 297
Internet, laboratory access to, 286,
        286b
Intervertebral spaces, 339, 340f
Interview, 209, 209f, 209b
Intestinal anastomosis, 261
Intestine, 87
Intra-arterial injection, of drugs, 114
Intradermal injections of drugs, 114, 227
    angle of injection and location of medication
        deposit for, 226f
Intradermal skin testing, 310
Intramuscular administration of drugs, 114,
        228, 443
    angle of injection and location of medication
        deposit for, 226f
    in birds, 392, 392f
    in cats, 169f
    in dogs, 157–158, 158f
    muscle groups used in, 228, 228f
    restraint for, 228
    snubbing for, 160
Intraosseous administration of drugs, 229
Intraperitoneal administration of drugs, 114,
        229
Intravenous administration of drugs,
        228–229, 443–445, 443f, 444t
    catheterization, 229–231, 229f
    injection, 114, 228b
Inventory
    management of, 46–48, 46f
    ordering of, 46
    reorder point for, 46–47
Invoicing of clients, 35–37
Iodophors, 129t, 130
Ionized calcium, 472t
Ionizing radiation, 345. see also Radiation
Iris, 93f, 94
Irregular bones, 73
Islets of Langerhans, 306
Isoechoic, 355
Itraconazole, 126

J

Jejunostomy tube, 184
Jills, 364
Joints, 76, 76f–77f
Jugular venipuncture, 166–168, 167f–168f, 370–371, 387f

K

Keel, 373
Kennel assistants, 4, 4f, 4b
Kennel cough, 193
Ketoconazole, 126
Kidney function testing, 306
Kidneys, description of, 97, 98f
Kilovoltage peak (kVp), 337, 342
Kittening, 102
Kittens, 143. *see also* Cat(s)
Kübler-Ross, Elizabeth, 52

L

Labeling prescription items, 47–48
Labor laws, 18
Laboratory
    design of, 285–286, 285f
    electrical supply in, 286
    internet access in, 286, 286b
    measurements and mathematics used in, 286–287
    safety concerns, 286
    sink in, 285–286
    storage space in, 286
    supplies, 286
Laboratory animal technician, 475
Laboratory equipment and instrumentation, 287–297
    accuracy of, 296
    centrifuge, 289–290, 289f
    chemistry analyzers, 291–293
    control materials, 296–297, 296f
    description of, 12
    incubators, 295, 295f
    microscope, 287–289, 287f, 288b
    pipettes, 295
    precision of, 296
    quality assurance of, 296–297
    quality control of, 297
    refractometer, 290, 290f, 291b
    reliability of, 296
    slide dryers, 296
Laboratory procedures, 284–335
    electrolytes, 307–308, 308f
    enzyme analyses, 306
    enzymes, 307
    hepatobiliary function testing, 305–306
    histology, 317
    kidney function testing, 306
    lactate, 307, 308f
    pancreatic function testing, 306–307
Laboratory records, 297
Labrador retriever, 132, 137f
Laceration, 192
Lactate dehydrogenase (LD), 307, 308f
Lactation
    in dogs, feeding during, 176
    feeding during, in cats, 181
Lactophenol cotton blue stain, 314
Lactulose, 117
Lagomorphs, 362

Laminitis, in horse, bedding and, 416
Laparotomy, 261
Laryngoscope, 268, 270f
Laser scalpel, 247–248
Laser-based analyzers, 294, 295f
Lasso, 169, 169f
Lateral, 64, 352
Lateral ear resection, 261
Lateral intercostal thoracotomy, 260
Lateral recumbency
    in cats, 168–169, 168b
    in dogs, 160, 160b
Latex agglutination, 310
Lavage, 234–235, 234f
Laws, 15–18
    controlled substances, 18
    Equal Employment Opportunity, 17
    labor, 18
    malpractice, 16
    medical waste management, 17
    negligence, 17
    Occupational Safety and Health Act, 16–17
    practice acts, 16
    veterinary service quality, 16
Laxatives, 115b, 117
Lead, 397
Lead aprons, 346
Lead shielding, 346, 346f
Leash, 151–153, 153f
Leg lift, 425
Lens, 93f, 94
Leukocytes
    agranulocytes, 82
    antibodies, 82
    description of, 81
    granulocytes, 81–82
Leydig cells, 97
Lhasa apso, 140f
Lice, 326, 326f
Lifting
    description of, 18–19
    of dog, 157, 157f
Ligating clips, 250f
Lighting
    for reptiles, 399
    room, 172
Lincosamides, 124b, 125
Lingual, 64
Linognathus setosus, 326
Lipase, 307, 472t
Lipemia, 297–298, 300–301
Lipids, 186
Liquid medications
    dosage forms
        description of, 106–108, 106t
        dispensing of, 110
    oral administration of, 224, 224f
Listening, 54
Litter boxes
    changing and cleaning of, 144
    checklist for, 144b
    substrate of, 143
    training to use, 143
Liver
    anatomy of, 88
    in birds, 375, 376f
    drug biotransformation by, 115
Liver disease, 187t–190t

Liver function tests, 305
Livestock
    body condition scoring classification for, 412t
    clinical nutrition of, 415, 416t
    common procedures in, 434–436
        clipping teeth, 435, 436f
        crutching (tagging), 434
        hoof trimming, 434, 435f
        tail docking and castrating, 434–435, 435f
        umbilical cord clipping, 435–436
    feeding management for, 411–415
        beef cattle, 412
        dairy cattle, 411–412
        goats, 415
        horses, 414
        nutrition in debilitated calf, 412–414
        pigs, 414–415
        sheep, 415
    feedstuffs for, 411t
    nutrition for, 409–411, 410f
Lizards. *see also* Reptiles
    capture of, 402–403
    description of, 400
    emergency and critical care of, 406
    feeding of, 400
    handling of, 402–403
    intravenous catheter sites in, 406t
    radiology in, 405
    restraint of, 402–403, 402f
    vagal response in, 405, 406f
    venipuncture in, 404
Loneliness stage, of grief, 52–53
Long bones, 73
Loop diuretics, 119
Loop of Henle, 97–98
Lories, 386t
Loss. *see also* Euthanasia
    acknowledging of, 53
    compounded, 55–56
    emotions associated with, 52
    grief counseling for, 51–54
    staff effects of, 54–55
    validating of, 54
Love birds, 386t
Lower airway emergencies, in birds, 394, 394b
Lower respiratory tract, 85, 85f
Lower urinary tract disease
    feeding cats with, 180
    urinary catheterization in, 217
Lubricants, 115b, 117
Luer-Lok tip, 107, 107f
Lufenuron (Program, Sentinel), 127
Lumbar vertebrae (L), 73–74
Lungs, gas exchange in, 84
Luteinizing hormone, 95
Lyme disease, 20, 196
Lymph, 83
Lymphangiectasia, 187t–190t
Lymphatic system, 83–84
Lymphocytes, reference range values for, 472t

M

Macaws, 386t
Machines, 63
Macrolides, 124b, 125
Magnetic resonance imaging (MRI), 358–359
Mail, 37–38

Male reproductive system, 98–99, 99f
Malleus, 93
Malocclusion, 363
Malpractice
    common law, 16
    description of, 15
    elements of, 16
Mange, 327
Markup, 47
Mastectomy, 261
Master lists, 42, 43f
Mastiff, 138f
Material safety data sheet (MSDS), 16–17, 22–23, 23f
Maximum permissible dose (MPD), 346
Mayo scissors, 248, 248f
Mayo stand, 278–279
Mean corpuscular hemoglobin, 301, 302t, 472t
Mean corpuscular hemoglobin concentration, 301, 302t, 472t
Mean corpuscular volume, 294, 301, 302t, 472t
Medial, 64, 352
Median sternotomy, 260
Medical gas, 268–269
Medical history, 210
Medical records, 41–44
    computer, 42, 42f
    copying of, 42
    definition of, 41
    format of, 42–44
    hospitalization sheets included in, 44, 45f
    master lists, 42, 43f
    medications listed in, 44
    mistakes in, 42, 42f
    ownership of, 41–42
    paperless, 42, 42f
    problem-oriented, 43–44
    SOAP format, 33f, 43–44, 44f
Medical terms, 59
Medical waste management, 17, 17f
Medication(s). see also Drug(s)
    administration of, 223–232, 440–445
        in birds, 391
        eye, 445, 445f
        gastric intubation, 232
        intradermal, 227
        intramuscular. see Intramuscular administration of drugs
        intraosseous and intraperitoneal, 229
        intravenous. see Intravenous administration of drugs
        nasal, 225, 225f
        ophthalmic, 225–226, 225f
        oral, 223–224, 223f, 440–442, 440f
        otic, 226, 226f
        parenteral, 226–227, 226f, 442–445
        rectal, 224–225, 224b
        subcutaneous, 78, 227–228, 227f
        topical, 223
        urinary tract catheterization, 231–232, 231f
    behavior problems managed with, 149–150, 149f
    dispensing of, 108–110
    medical record listing of, 44
    prescription of, 110b
    reconstitution of, 108, 109b
Megestrol acetate (Ovaban), 122, 122b

Melanocytes, 77
Mental health professionals, 55–56
Mentation, 216
Mesial, 64
Metabolism, of drugs, 115
Metallic sutures, 252
Metestrus, 100
Metric system, 110, 110t–111t, 111b
Metronidazole, 125
Metzenbaum scissors, 248, 248f
Mibolerone (Cheque Drops), 122, 122b
Mice, 364–366, 366f
Microbiology, 310–315
    bacteria, 311, 314f
    biochemical test materials, 315
    biochemical tests, 315
    definition of, 310–311
    fungi, 311, 312t
    mycology, 311
    procedures, 314–315
    quality control concerns, 315
    sample
        collection of, 311
        culture media for, 313–314
        processing materials for, 313
    stains, 314, 314f
Microchip, 173
Microchipping, in birds, 382–383
Microfilariae, 323
Microhematocrit, 299–300, 300b
Microscope, 287–289, 287f, 288b
    use, care, and maintenance, 288–289
Middle area, 12, 13f
Milbemycin oxime (Interceptor, Sentinel), 127
Milk, for debilitated calf, 413
Milk production, 102–103
Milliamperage (mA), 337–338, 341–342
Millirem (mrem), 346
Minerals, 176, 176b
Minimum prescription fee, 47
Mirror image artifact, 356
Mites, 327–328, 328f–329f
Mobile pet practice, 9
Mobility-limiting devices, for dogs, 153–155, 155f
Modified Knott's test, 334, 335b
Modified live vaccine, 196
Molting, 373
Monitor lizard, 402, 402f
Monocular microscope, 287–288
Monocytes, reference range values for, 472t
Monofilament sutures, 250
Monthly statements, 36–37
Morphologic diagnosis, 191
Motor unit, 90
Mouth, 86–87, 86f
Mouthing, 378
Movement terms, 63–64
Mucolytics, 119b, 120
Mucous membrane color, 216, 217f
Multifilament sutures, 250
Murmurs, 215
Muscle
    cardiac, 90, 91f
    function of, 90
    skeletal, 90, 91f
    smooth, 90, 91f
    types of, 91f

Musculoskeletal system, of birds, 373
Muzzles
    for cat restraint, 163–164, 163f–164f
    for dog restraints, 153, 154b
Mycology, 311
Myiasis, 326

N
Nail trimmers, 220–221, 220f
Nail trimming
    in birds, 382, 382f
    description of, 220, 221f
Na:K ratio, 472t
Nanophyetus salmincola, 322
Narcotics, 116
Nasal administration of medications, 225, 225f
Nasoesophageal tube, 184, 184f
Nasogastric tube, 183
National Association of Dog Obedience Instructors, 150
National Association of Veterinary Technicians of America (NAVTA), 6, 6b, 10b–11b
National Commission on Veterinary Economic Issues (NCVEI), 40
National Dog Groomers Association, 3
National Fire Protection Association, 24
NAVTA. see National Association of Veterinary Technicians of America (NAVTA)
NCVEI. see National Commission on Veterinary Economic Issues (NCVEI)
Necropsy, 190–191
Needle(s)
    disposal of, 17f
    gauge of, 108
    hazards of, 22
    length of, 108
    parts of, 107f–108f, 108
    recapping of, 22
    sizes of, 108
Needle holders, 248
Needle teeth, 435
Negative contrast media, 355
Negative reinforcement, 141
Negligence, 15, 17
Nematodes, 322, 323t
Nephrons, 97, 98f
Nervous dogs, 156
Nervous system, 88–90
    autonomic, 81
    central, 88–89, 88f
    definition of, 88
    drugs that affect, 122–124
        analgesics, 123, 123b
        anesthetics, 122, 123b
        anticonvulsants, 123, 123b
        central nervous system stimulants, 123–124, 123b
        sedatives, 122, 123b
        tranquilizers, 122, 123b
    neurons, 88
    peripheral, 89
Neurons, 88
Neurotransmitters, 88
Neutrophils, 303
Nitrofurans, 126
No-bite collar, 155, 155f
Nociception, 281
Nonabsorbable suture, 251–252, 251f

Nonburrowing mites, 328
Nonclosure, of wound, 236–237
Nonessential amino acids, 175
Nonexempt employees, 18
Nonnutritive feed additives, 411
Nonpathogens, 192
Nonrebreathing circuits, 273–274, 274f
Nonsegmented neutrophils, reference range
    values for, 472t
Nonsteroidal anti-inflammatory drugs,
    128–129, 128b
Norepinephrine, 96, 96t
Normothermia, 214–215
Nosocomial infections, 173
Nuclear medicine, 359
Nutrients
    carbohydrates, 175
    definition of, 175
    energy-producing, 175, 175b
    fats, 175, 175b
    minerals, 176, 176b
    non-energy-producing, 175–176, 176b
    proteins, 175, 175b
    vitamins, 176, 176b
    water, 175
Nutrition, 171–207. see also Feeding
    of cats, 179t–180t
    in debilitated calf, 412–414
        colostrum for, 412–413
        electrolytes for, 413–414
        milk for, 413
    of dogs, 179t–180t
    for livestock, 409–411
        clinical, 415, 416t
        feed analysis in, 411, 411t
        feedstuffs for, 409–411
    pet food, 182, 182f
Nutritional status, 183
Nutritional support
    enteral, 183–186, 184f, 184b–185b
    goal of, 219
    in hospitalized patients, 183
    for ill or debilitated patients, 183
    jejunostomy tube for, 184
    nasoesophageal tube for, 184, 184f
    nasogastric tube for, 183
    parenteral, 186–190
    percutaneous endoscopic gastrostomy tube
        for, 184
    pharyngostomy tube for, 184
    wound healing benefits of, 191–192
Nystagmus, 211
Nystatin, 126

O

Obesity, 178, 187t–190t
Object-film distance (OFD), 342
Object-image distance (OID), 339, 340f,
    342
Oblique, 64
Oblique projections, 353
Occupational Safety and Health Act,
    16–17
    Right to Know Law, 22
Occupational Safety and Health
    Administration, 286
Odors, 173
Office managers, 6–7, 7f, 7b

Office procedures
    client relations, 25–56. see also Clients
    front office. see Front office procedures
    grief counseling, 51–54
    inventory management, 46–48, 46f
    medical records. see Medical records
    pet health insurance, 40–41
    standard operating procedures, 46
Office visit, 38–40, 38f, 38b
Ointments, ophthalmic administration of,
    225–226
Old dogs, 156
Olfactory nerve (CN I), 89, 89t
Olfactory sense, 92
Oncicola canis, 323
Onychectomy, 261
Oocyst, 320
Open-ended questions, examples of, 212t
Operant conditioning, 141
Operculum, 374
Ophthalmic administration of drugs, 212f,
    225–226
Optic nerve (CN II), 89
Oral administration
    in birds, 391
    description of, 223–224
Orchiectomy, 260
Ordering of products, 46
Organic nonabsorbable sutures, 251
Orogastric intubation, 183, 441–442, 442f
Orogastric tubes, 232
Orthopedic disease, developmental, 187t–190t
Orthopnea, 216
Oscillometric blood pressure monitor,
    277t–278t
Osmolality, 472t
Osmotic diuretic, 119
Otic administration of medications, 225, 225f
Outstanding debt collection, 37, 37b
Ovaries, 97
Ovariohysterectomy, 260
Overfeeding, 178
Over-the-counter (OTC) products, 47
Over-the-needle peripheral catheters, 229–230,
    230f
Overweight, 178
Oviducts, 99f, 100
Oxygen cage, 389–390, 390f
Oxytocin, 95, 96t

P

Packed cell volume (PCV), 299–300
Pain
    analgesia for, 282
    definition of, 281
    effects of, 282b
    nociception versus, 281f
    relief modalities, 282
    signs of, 282b
Palatability, of pet food, 183, 183b
Palmar, 64, 352
Pancreas
    of birds, 375, 376f
    endocrine, 306
    exocrine, 306
    function testing of, 306–307
    hormone produced by, 306
Pancreatic drugs, 120b, 121

Pancreatic exocrine insufficiency, 187t–190t
Pancreatitis, acute, 187t–190t
Papillon, 138f
Paracostal incision, 260
Parakeets, 386t
Parallel grids, 340–341
Paramedian incision, 260
Parasites. see also specific parasite
    cestodes, 321–322, 321f, 322t
    classifications of, 320–328, 320b
    definition of, 192
    diagnostic techniques for, 328–330
        immunologic tests, 334–335
        microscopic examination, 329
        sample collection and handling, 330
    ectoparasites, 319–320
    endoparasites, 319–320
    fleas, 325–326, 325f–326f
    flies, 326
    intestinal bleeding caused by, 334
    lice, 326, 326f
    life cycle of, 319–320
    mites, 327–328, 328f–329f
    nematodes, 322, 323t
    protozoa, 320
    ticks, 327, 327f–328f
    trematodes, 322
    vector of, 319–320
    zoonotic, 329t
Parasitism, 20–21
Parasitology, 319–335
Parasitology, in reptiles and amphibians, 405
Parathyroid glands, 95–96
Parenteral administration
    drugs, 114, 226–227, 226f
    nutritional support, 186–190
Parturition, 95, 102–103
Passerines, 372, 373b
Passive immunity, 195–196, 308
Past medical history, 210–211
Pasteurella, 193
Pathogens, 192
Pathology, 190
Patient(s)
    admitting of, 38
    discharging of, 38–40, 40f
    hospitalized, monitoring of, 436, 436f
    loss of. see Loss
    preparation for ultrasound examination,
        355–356
    psychological needs of, 174
    recumbent
        nursing care for, 240–241
        padding, 240–241
        turning, 240
    transfer of, 220
Patient characteristics, 210
Patient evaluation, 261
Patient history, 209–211
    communication with clients in, 209, 209f
    conclusion of, 211
    current environment, 210, 210b
    interview, 209, 209f, 209b
    introductory statement, 210
    obtaining of, 210–211
    origin, 210
    past medical history, 210–211
    patient characteristics, 210

Patient history *(Continued)*
    presenting complaint, 211, 211b
    prior ownership, 210
Patient history forms, 30, 31f–32f
Payment methods, 35
Pecking order, 141
Pectoral muscle, in birds, injections in, 392, 392f
Pediculosis, 326
Penicillins, 124b
Penrose drains, 236, 236f
Penumbra effect, 338–339
Percutaneous endoscopic gastrostomy tube, 184, 185f
Per-incident deductibles, 41
Perineal urethrostomy, 261
Periodontitis, 187t–190t
Peripheral, 64
Peripheral nervous system, 89
Peritonitis, 282–283
Persian cat, 133f
Personal protective equipment, 19, 19f, 19t, 390–391
Personal safety, 24
Pet food, 182, 182f
Pet health insurance, 40–41
Phagocytosis, 82f
Pharmacokinetics, 114
Pharyngostomy tube, 184
Phenols, 129, 129t
Pheromone, 146
Phlebitis, 230–231, 230f
Phosphatases, 306
Phosphorus, 472t
Photo albums, 11
Photo labeler, 348
Photometry, 291, 292f
Physical examination
    form used in, 212f
    gastrointestinal monitoring, 217–219
    preanesthetic, 262t
    purpose of, 211–219
    systematic method of, 213b
Physiologic murmurs, 215
Physiology, 69–103
Picture archiving and communication system (PACS), 345
Pigs, feeding management for, 414–415
Pill gun, 223f
Pipettes, 295
Pituitary gland, 95
Plantar, 64, 352
Plants, poisonous, 397, 398b
Plasma, 298–299, 301b
Platelet count, 304, 472t–473t
Platelets, 303
Platyhelminthes, 321
Plural endings, 62–63, 62t
Pneumatic bones, 73
Pneumatized bones, 373
Pododermatitis, 395–396, 396f
Point of maximal intensity (PMI), 215
Poisons, ingested, 397
Polymorphonuclear cells, 303
Porous adhesive tape, 239
Portal vein, 88
Portion control, feeding methods, 176
Positional terms, 63–64

Positive contrast media, 354–355, 354f
Positive inotropic agents, 118, 118b
Positive reinforcement, 141
Posterior pituitary gland, 95
Postoperative evaluation, 280–281
Potassium, 472t
Potter-Bucky diaphragm, 341
Practice acts, 16, 47
Practice managers, 7, 7b
Precipitation tests, 310
Precision vaporizers, 271–272
Prednisolone sodium succinate (Solu-Delta-Cortef), 128
Preexisting health condition, 41
Prefix, 58
    for diseases or conditions, 62, 62t
    word formation using, 58
Pregnancy, 101–102. *see also* Gestation
Premium, 41
Preoperative evaluation, 261
Preparation area, in surgery suite, 243
Preprandial samples, 297–298
Prescriptions
    components of, 109–110, 110f
    controlled substances, 113
    definition of, 108
    labeling of, 47–48
    pricing of, 47, 47b
    writing of, 108–109
Presenting complaint, 211, 211b
Prevacuum autoclave, 247
Preventive medicine program, 172
Pricing of products, 47, 47b
Problem-oriented medical record (POMR), 43–44
Procedures, suffixes for, 63
Proctodeum, 375–376
Product pricing, 47, 47b
Productive cough, 119
Proestrus, 100
Professional ethics, 15
Professional negligence, 15
Professional organizations, 9, 10b–11b
Prokaryotes, 192
Pronation, 64
Prone, 64
Proprietary name, 105
Protectants, 115b, 116–117
Protein
    description of, 175, 175b
    parenteral nutritional support delivery of, 186
    plasma, 301
    serum, 305
Prothrombin time, 304–305, 305f, 473t
Protozoa, description of, 320
Proventriculus, 375–376, 376f
Proximal, 64, 353
Proximate analysis, 411
Psittacines, 372, 373b
Psychological needs, 174
Pterylae, 373
Public health, 193
Public service, ethics of, 15
Puffs of air, 164
Pug, 139f
Pulmonary circulation, 80
Pulse, 215, 215f

Pulse oximeter, 277–278, 277t–278t, 278f
Punishment, 141
    house training use of, 143
Puppies. *see also* Dog(s)
    aggression testing of, 147
    chewing by, 146f
    crate training of, 142, 143f
    feeding of, 177–178, 179t–180t
    handling of, 155
    neonatal, 178
    weaning of, 178
Pyrexia, 191
Pyrogens, 191

Q
Quantitative buffy coat system, 294
Quaternary ammonium compounds, 129, 129t
Queening, 102
Queens
    estrous cycle and gestation period in, 471t
    feeding of, 181
    parturition in, 102
    reproductive patterns in, 101

R
Rabbits
    antibiotics administration to, 372
    description of, 362–363
    handling of, 363, 363f
    housing of, 361–362
    intestinal tract of, 362–363
    malocclusion in, 363
    normal ranges of heart rate, respiratory rate, and rectal temperature in, 213t
    nutrition for, 362
    restraining of, 363, 364f
    sexing of, 363
    teeth of, 362
    venipuncture in, 370–371, 371f
Rabies
    safety issues, 20
    vaccinations, certificate, 35, 36f
Rad, 346
Radiation
    carcinogenic effects of, 346
    fetal sensitivity to, 346
    hazards associated with, 21
    occupational exposure to, 346, 347f
    safety considerations, 345–347, 347b
    scatter, 340–341
    terminology associated with, 346–347
Radiation protection supervisor, 347
Radioactive iodine, 121, 359
Radiodermatitis, 346
Radiographic contrast, 338
Radiographic density, 337–338
Radiographic film, 342–343
    contrast of, 338
    direct exposure, 342–343
    electromagnetic radiation effects on, 342
    emulsion layer of, 342
    fogging of, 338
    identification of, 348
    intensifying screens, 343, 343f
    latitude of, 343
    layers of, 342
    processing of, 349–350
        artifacts caused by, 351b–352b

Radiographic film *(Continued)*
automatic, 350, 351b–352b
developer, 349
equipment for, 349–350
fixer, 349
manual, 349, 351b–352b
silver recovery, 350
screen-type, 342–343
silver halide emulsion of, 342
speeds of, 343
storage of, 343
Radiographic images
artifacts, 350, 350b–352b
black crescents or lines on, 350b–351b
contrast studies, 354–355
barium sulfate, 354
double-contrast procedure, 355
negative contrast media used in, 355
positive contrast media used in, 354–355
purpose of, 354
water-soluble organic iodides, 354
detail of, 338–341
directional terms, 352f–353f
distortion of, 339–340
exposure variables that affect, 341–342
exposure time, 341–342
kilovoltage peak, 337, 342
milliamperage, 337–338, 341–342
object-image distance, 339, 340f, 342
source-image distance, 339, 339f, 342
foreshortening, 339
landmarks for, 353t
oblique projections, 353, 353f–354f, 353t
positioning for, 352–353
quality of, 337–342
radiation safety issues, 345–347, 347b
terminology associated with, 352–353
x-ray tube, 337, 337f
Radiography
in amphibians, 405, 405f
in birds, 387–388, 388f
in chelonians, 405
in lizards, 405
in snakes, 405
Radiolucent, 338
Radionuclides, 359
Radiopaque, 338, 338f
Radius, 75
Rapid immunomigration assay, 309
Ratio, 287
Rats, 366, 366f
Reasonable care, 17
Rebreathing circuits, 272–273
Reception area. *see also* Front office procedures
cleanliness of, 30
description of, 11, 11f
Receptionists, 6, 6f, 6b, 49
β₁ receptors, 118
Recombinant vaccine, 196
Reconstitution of medication, 109b
Records, laboratory, 297
Recovery, from surgery, 280–283
Rectal administration of medications, 224–225, 224b
Rectal examination, 158–159, 158f

Rectal temperature, 215
in adults of some domestic species, 213t
in cats, 471t
in dogs, 471t
Recumbency, 64, 64f
description of, 64
dorsal
in cats, 169, 169b
in dogs, 160
lateral
in cats, 168–169, 168b
in dogs, 160, 160b
Red blood cells
reference range values for, 472t
in urine, 319f
Red-tailed hawk, 388f
Referral practice, 9
Referrals, for behavior problems, 150–151, 150b
Reflection, 53–54
Refractometer, 290, 290f
use, care, and maintenance, 290, 291b
Release forms
euthanasia, 30–35, 35f
medical record, 32f–33f, 41–44
Reminders and recall systems, 28–30, 29f
Renal failure, 187t–190t
Reorder point, for inventory, 46–47
Replacement stage, of grief, 53
Reproductive system, 98–103
of birds, 377
drugs that affect, 121–122
female, 99–103, 99f
functions of, 98
male, 98–99, 99f
physiologic patterns of, 101
Reptiles. *see also* Chelonians; Lizards; Snakes
biology of, 398–399
burns in, 399, 400f
determining gender of, 403, 403f
diseases in, 406, 406b
feeding of, 400
force, 405–406, 406f
fluids administration, 406, 406t
heating for, 399
history taking for, 400
housing for, 399–400
humidity requirements for, 399–400
husbandry of, 399
medications administration in, 406, 406t
normal physiologic values for, 403
overview of, 398–407
parasitology in, 405
shedding of skin by, 399, 399f
terrarium for, 399
venipuncture of, 404, 404t
water quality for, 400
Reservoir bag, 273
Reservoirs, 193
Residue, 124
Resistance, 124
Resolution stage, of grief, 52
Respiration
control of, 85–86
description of, 84
measurement of, 215–216
mechanisms of, 85–86

Respiratory distress, in birds, 393–394, 393b, 394f
Respiratory drugs, 119b
Respiratory rate
in adults of some domestic species, 213t
in cats, 471t
in dogs, 471t
Respiratory sinus arrhythmia, 215
Respiratory sounds, 216, 216b
Respiratory system, 84–86. *see also* Lungs.
of birds, 374, 375f
description of, 84
Respiratory tract
lower, 85, 85f
upper, 84–85, 84f
Restraint
of birds, 383–385
procedure before, 383
of chelonians, 401–402, 402f
of ferrets, 364, 365f
of gerbil, 367, 368f
for intramuscular injections, 228
of lizards, 402–403, 402f
of mouse, 366f
of rabbits, 363, 364f
of rats, 366, 366f
of snakes, 401, 401f
Restraint board, 383–385, 385f, 389f
Retail area, 12, 12f
Retractors, 249–250
Reverberation, 356
Reward, 143
Rhinotheca, 401–402
Rhipicephalus sanguineus, 327, 328f
Rickettsial parasites, 323–328
Arthropoda, 323–324
definition of, 323
fleas, 325–326, 325f–326f
flies, 326
lice, 326, 326f
mites, 327–328, 328f–329f
ticks, 327, 327f–328f
Rifampin, 126
Right to Know Law, 22
Rigid endoscopes, 356–357, 357f
Ringworm, 20
Robert Jones bandage, 396
Rochester-Carmalt forceps, 249
Rocky Mountain spotted fever, 324t
Rodents
antibiotics administration to, 372
chinchillas, 369–370
description of, 364–370
gerbils, 367
guinea pigs, 367–369, 369f
hamsters, 366–367
housing of, 361–362, 361f
mice, 364–366
nutrition for, 362
rats, 366
sex of, 364, 365f
venipuncture in, 370, 371f
Roentgen equivalent in man (Rem), 346
Romanowsky-type stain, 302b
Room temperature, 172
Root word, 58
Rope leash, 151–153, 153f
Rostral, 64, 352

Roundworms, 322, 323t
Rule-ins, 44
Runs, 156–157

S

Sabouraud dextrose, 313
Safelights, 348–349, 348f
Safety
　eye, 19
　fire, 24
　magnetic resonance imaging, 359
　Occupational Safety and Health Act, 16–17
　personal, 24
　radiation, 21, 345–347, 347b
　workplace, 18
Salmonella spp., 400
Sample collection
　hematology examination, 297–298
　microbiology examination, 311
　parasites, 330
　urinalysis, 318
Sand flies, 326
Sanitation, 172
Sanitizers, 174
Sarcoptes scabiei, 328, 328f
Sarcoptic mange, 20–21
Scalpels, 247–248, 248f
Scatter radiation, 340–341, 341f
Scavenging system, 21, 273–274
Scheduling of appointments, 27–28, 27f
Schroeder-Thomas splint, 396
Scintigraphy, 359
Scissors, 248
Sclera, 93–94, 93f
Scottish terrier, 138f
Scrapings, 316
Scratching post, 145, 145f
Screen-type film, 342–343
Scrub area, 243
Scrubbing, 234
　of skin, 262–264, 265b
Scruffing technique, 168
Sedation, 282
Sedatives, 122, 123b
Segmented neutrophils, 303
　reference range values for, 472t
Seizures, 123
Selective breeding, 132
Self-mutilation, of birds, 379–380, 379f–380f
Semisolid dosage forms, 106, 106t
Senn retractors, 249–250, 250f
Senses, 90–94. *see also* Ear(s); Eye(s)
　auditory, 92–93, 92f
　function of, 90–91
　general, 91–92, 92t
　gustatory, 92
　olfactory, 92
　special, 92–94, 92t
　vestibular, 93
　visual, 93–94, 93f
Sepsis, 186
Serial dilutions, 287
Seroma, 282
Serum assays, 307–308
Serum creatinine, 306
Serum protein, 305
Sesamoid bones, 73
Sexual harassment, 17

Shampoo, 219
Sharp objects, 22
Shar-pei, 139f
Shedding, of hair, 173
Sheep (ovine)
　care of, 419
　feeding management for, 415
　restraint of, 432, 432f
Shetland sheepdog, 140f
Shock collars, 141
Shrinkage, 46
Siamese cat, 133f
Sievert (SV), 346
Silage, 410
Silk, 251
Silver nitrate applicators, 221, 222f
Sink, in laboratory, 285–286
Sinus rhythm, 215
Sitting recumbency, 165–168, 165f
Skeletal muscle, 90, 91f
Skeleton, 73–76. *see also* Bone
　appendicular, 74–76, 75t
　axial, 73–74, 75f
　definition of, 73
　visceral, 76
Skin
　anatomy of, 77, 78f
　care of, 219–220, 220f
　scrubbing of, 262–264, 265b
Skin roll, 425
Skin staples, 253, 253f, 283f
Slice thickness artifact, 356
Slide dryers, 296
Slip tip, 107, 107f
Slips, 18
Small animal practice, 9
Small bones, 73
Small mammals
　chinchillas, 369–370
　definition of, 361
　diagnostic and treatment techniques in, 370–372
　fecal analysis in, 372
　force feeding of, 371
　gerbils, 367
　guinea pigs, 367–369, 369f
　hamsters, 366–367
　housing, 361–362, 361f
　intravenous injection for, 372
　mice, 364–366
　nursing care of, 370
　nutrition for, 362–370
　rats, 366
　urinalysis in, 372
Smears
　blood, 302, 302b
　fecal, 330, 331b
　impression, 316, 316b
Smooth muscle, 90, 91f
Snakes
　capture of, 401
　determining gender of, 403, 403f
　emergency and critical care of, 406, 407f
　feeding of, 400
　handling of, 401, 401f
　intravenous catheter sites in, 406t
　radiology in, 405
　restraint of, 401, 401f

Snakes *(Continued)*
　shedding of skin by, 398f
　transport of, 401f
　venipuncture of, 404, 404t
SNAP test, 309, 309f
Snapping turtles, 401–402
Snubbing, 160
Socialization, behavior problem prevention
　　through, 147–148, 148f
Society, 6
Sodium, 472t
Sodium citrate, 299
Sodium fluoride, 307
Software, 48
Soiling, 220
Solid dosage forms, 106, 106t
Sonolucent, 355
Sorrow stage, of grief, 52
Source-image distance (SID), 339, 339f, 342
Sows, 369
Soybean meal, for livestock, 411
Space-occupying masses, in birds, 394, 394f
Special senses, 92–94, 92t
　of birds, 377–378
Specialist referrals, for behavior problems,
　　150–151, 150b
Specific gravity
　definition of, 287
　of fecal flotation, 330, 330f, 332b
　of urine, 318
Spectrophotometers, 291
　principles of, 292f
Spills, chemical, 23
Spinal nerves, 89
Spirochetes, 315t
Splenectomy, 261
Spoilage, forage and, 410
Sporozoal parasites, 320
Sprite, 364
Squeeze chute, 430, 430f
Staff, loss effects on, 54–55
Stainless steel sutures, 252
Stains
　acid-fast, 314
　Gram, 314, 314f
　Romanowsky-type, 302b
Stanchions, for cattle restraint, 431
Standard operating procedure, 46, 297
Standing radiograph, 388
Standing restraint, of dogs, 157–159, 158f
Staples, skin, 253, 253f, 283f
Steam sterilization, 247
Sterile items, unwrapping of, 280
Sterilization
　definition of, 245
　gas, 256
　mode of action of, 245–246
　quality control for, 246
　steam, 247
Sterilization indicators, 246, 246f–247f
Sterilizers, 174
Sternal recumbency
　of cats, 165–168, 165f
　of dogs, 159, 159b
Stertors, 216
Stethoscope, 213, 214f
　esophageal, 277–278, 277t–278t, 279f
Stimulus, 141

Stocks, 428
Stomach, 87
Stomach tubing, 441–442
Stool softeners, 115b, 117
Storage
  endoscope, 358
  in laboratory, 286
  of supplies, 18
Stress, in birds, 383
Stretch receptors, 85–86
Stridor, 216
Struvite, 187t–190t
Stud shank, 427. see also Chain shank
Students, on veterinary health care team, 3
Subcutaneous administration of medications,
    114, 227–228, 227f, 442–443, 442f
  angle of injection and location of medication
      deposit for, 226f
Subjective, objective, assessment, and plan
    (SOAP) format medical record, 33f,
    43–44, 44f
Submissive behavior, 141f, 151, 152f
Suckle reflex, development of, 413
Suffix
  combining vowel added to, 58
  definition of, 58–59
  for diseases or conditions, 61–62, 61t–62t
  for instruments, 63, 63t
  for machines, 63, 63t
  for procedures, 63, 63t
  for surgical procedures, 61, 61t, 260b
  word formation using, 58–59, 59t
Sulfonamides, 124b, 125
Superficial, 64
Supination, 64
Supine, 64
Supplies
  laboratory, 286
  storing of, 18
Surgery
  discharge instruction after, 49
  glove removal during, 266–267
  hematoma after, 282
  hemorrhage after, 282
  instruments used in. see Surgical
      instruments
  operative site
    hair removal, 262–264, 263f
    positioning, 264–265, 264f, 275b
    preparation of, 262–265
    scrubbing of skin, 262–264, 265b
    sterile preparation of, 265
  pain management after, 281–282
  patient preparation for, 261–262
  postoperative complications of, 282–283
  postoperative evaluation, 280–281
  preoperative evaluation, 261
  recovery from, 280–283
  seroma after, 282
  wound
    appearance of, 281
    dehiscence of, 283
Surgery room, 243–244, 244f
Surgery suite, 243–244
Surgical assisting, 242–283
  draping, 279–280
  instrument table organization by, 279–280
  unwrapping or opening of sterile items, 280

Surgical gut, 251
Surgical instruments, 247–250
  autoclaving of, 254–255
  blades, 247–248
  care of, 253–258
  cleaning of, 253–254
  forceps, 248–249
  instrument packs, 255–256, 255b
  lubricating of, 254–255
  maintenance of, 253–258
  miscellaneous, 250
  needle holders, 248
  packed, 254, 254f
  retractors, 249–250
  scalpels, 247–248, 248f
  scissors, 248
  sterilization of, 256–257
  storing sterilized items, 258, 259t
  ultrasonic cleaning of, 253–254, 254f
Surgical mesh, 253
Surgical procedures
  incisions, 260, 260f
  orthopedic, 261, 264f
  soft tissue, 260–261
  suffixes for, 61, 61t, 260b
  terminology associated with, 260–261
Surgical team
  attire of, 265–266, 266f
  gloving of, 266–267
  gowning of, 266–267
  preparation of, 265–267
  surgical scrubbing, 266
Suture(s), 250–253
  absorbable, 251, 251f
  characteristics of, 250–251
  metallic, 252
  monofilament, 250
  multifilament, 250
  nonabsorbable, 251–252, 251f
  removal of, 283, 283f
  sizes of, 250–251, 251t
Suture needles, 252–253, 252f
Swabbings, 316
Swine
  care of, 420
  handling and restraint, 433–434
    directing, 433, 433f
    driving and catching, 433
    hog snare, 433
    of piglets, 433–434, 434f
    potbellied, 434
Synthetic absorbable sutures, 251
Synthetic nonabsorbable sutures, 251
Syrian hamster, 366–367
Syringes
  disposal of, 17f
  insulin, 107–108, 108f
  parts of, 107f
  reading of, 108f
  tuberculin, 107, 107f
Syrinx, 374
Syrup of ipecac, 116
Systemic circulation, 80

T
T lymphocytes, 82
Tablets
  calculation of, 112b

Tablets (Continued)
  description of, 106, 106t
  oral administration of, 224f
Tachycardia, 215
Taco technique, for restraint, 161b
Tail bandages, 438, 438f
Tail tying, in horses, 428, 428f
Tail vein, for venipuncture, 404
Tape splints, 395f
Tapered needles, 253
Tapeworms, 321
TD pipettes, 295
Technetium-99m (^{99m}Tc), 359
Teeth
  anatomy of, 86, 86f
  dental formula for, 87
  terminology for, 64, 68f
Telephone etiquette, 26–27, 26f
Tenesmus, 219
Tesla (T), 359
Tetracyclines, 124b, 125
Therapeutic range, 113
Thiacetarsamide sodium (Caparsolate), 127
Thioglycollate broth, 314
Thirst, 281
Thoracic incisions, 260, 280f
Thoracotomy, 261
Thorax, 85
Thrombocytopenia, 304
Thrush, 417–418
Thyroid gland, 95
Thyroid-stimulating hormone, 95, 96t
Ticks, 327, 327f–328f
Tilt table, for cattle restraint, 431, 431f
Time-controlled feeding, 176
Tinctures, 106
Tissue
  connective, 70–73, 72f
  epithelial, 70, 72f
Tissue adhesives, 253
Tissue forceps, 248–249, 249f
Toenails
  obtaining blood sample from, 404
  trimming of. see Nail trimming
Tone of voice, 26
Topical administration, 223
Total nucleated cell count (TNCC), 317
Total parenteral nutrition, 186
Total plasma protein, 301
Total protein, 472t
Tourniquet, 166, 167f
Towel and blanket, for restraint of cats, 160–161
Toxascaris spp., 323
Toxic drugs, 113
Toxic substances, 19
Toxoid, 195–196
Toxoplasma gondii, 21
Toxoplasmosis, 21
Trace elements, 186
Tracheobronchitis, 119–120
Tranquilizers, 122, 123b
Transducers, ultrasound, 355
Transferases, 306
Trauma, head, 396
Treatment area, 12–14, 13f
Trematodes, 322
Triglyceride, 472t
Trimming, nail, 220–221

Trophozoite, 320
Tube feeding, 406f
Tuberculin syringes, 107, 107f
Twitches, for horses, 425–428
Typhus, 324t

U

Ulcers, decubital
    description of, 240
    in recumbent patients, 240, 240f
Ultrasonic cleaning, of surgical instruments,
    253–254, 254f
Ultrasonic Doppler, 277t–278t
Ultrasound
    definition of, 355–356
    echotexture terminology, 355–356
    instrument controls, 356
Ultraviolet (UV) lighting, 399
Umbilical cord, clipping of, 435–436
Upper respiratory tract, 84–85, 84f
Urates, 376
Ureters, 98
Urethra, 98
Urethral catheters, 231
Urethrotomy, 261
Uric acid, 306
Urinalysis, 317–319
    biochemical testing, 318–319
    complete, 318–319
    normal findings, 473t
    sample collection for, 318
    in small mammals, 372
    specific gravity, 318
Urinary bladder, 98
Urinary catheterization, 231–232
    catheters for, 231f
    description of, 217
Urinary system, 97–98
    of birds, 376–377, 376f
    description of, 97
    kidneys, 97–98, 98f
    parts of, 97f
    ureters, 98
    urethra, 98
Urination, 281
    frequency assessments, 216–217
Urine
    collection of, 438–439
    dipstick testing of, 318–319, 318f
    production of, 216–217, 218f, 471t
    specific gravity, 318
Urine sediment
    cells in, 319f
    microscopic examination of, 319
Urodeum, 375–376
Urolithiasis, 306
Uroliths, 180
Uropygial gland, 373, 373f
U.S. Department of Agriculture (USDA) health
    certificates, 35

V

Vaccinations, 196–202. see also specific
    vaccination
    of ferrets, 372
    status assessments, 211
Vaccine, 196
Vacutainer blood collection system, 298, 298f

Vagal response, 405, 406f
Vagina, 99f, 100
Vaginal cytology, 317
Vagus nerve (CN X), 89, 89t
Vaporizers, 271–272, 272f
Vasoconstriction, 267
Vasodilators, 118–119, 118b
Vector, 193, 319–320
Vehicle, of transmission, 193
Veins, 79. see also specific vein
Venipuncture
    in amphibians, 404
    basilic vein for, 387, 387f
    blood sample collection, 298
    cephalic
        cat restraint for, 165–166, 166f–167f
        sternal restraint for, 159b
        tourniquet for, 166, 167f
    in chelonians, 404, 404f, 404t
    in ferrets, 371, 371f
    in frogs, 404
    jugular, 370–371, 387f
        restraint for, 166–168, 167f–168f
    in lizards, 404, 404t
    in rabbits, 370–371, 371f
    in reptiles, 404, 404t
    in rodents, 370, 371f
    in snakes, 404, 404t
    tail vein for, 404
    in toads, 404
Vent, 376
Ventilation, 20, 172
Ventral, 64, 352
Ventral midline incisions, 260
Ventriculus, 375, 376f
Vertebrae, 73–74
Vertebral formula, 75t
Vestibular sense, 93
Veterinarians, 8, 8f
    history of, 2
    licensed, 16
    responsibilities of, 8b
Veterinary assistants, 4–5, 4b–5b
    model curriculum, 474–475
    tasks appropriate to delegate to, 476
Veterinary behaviorists, 144
Veterinary health care team, 2–9
    body language of, 49–50
    groomers, 3
    groups that support, 10b–11b
    hospital administrators, 7–8, 7b
    kennel assistants, 4, 4f, 4b
    members of, 3–8, 3b
    mixed practice, 11
    office managers, 6–7, 7f, 7b
    organizations that support, 10b–11b
    personal qualifications of, 9
    practice managers, 7, 7b
    receptionists, 6, 6f, 6b, 49
    role of, 475
    students, 3
    successful environment for, 9b
    teamwork among, 8, 8f
    veterinary assistants, 4–5, 4b
    veterinary technicians. see Veterinary
        technicians
    veterinary technologists, 5, 5b
    web sites that support, 10b–11b

Veterinary medicine, history of, 2
Veterinary practice
    cleanliness of, 172
    companion animals, 9
    consultation rooms, 12
    design of, 11–14
    examination rooms, 12, 12f
    exterior appearance of, 174, 174f
    housekeeping of, 173–174
    middle area of, 12, 13f
    mobile pet practice, 9
    odors in, 173
    reception area of, 11, 11f
    referral practice, 9
    retail area of, 12, 12f
    treatment area of, 12–14, 13f–14f
    types of, 9–11
Veterinary profession, overview of, 1–24
Veterinary State Practice Act, 15
Veterinary Support Personnel Network,
    10b–11b
Veterinary Technician National Examination, 5
Veterinary technician specialists, 475
Veterinary technicians, 475
    description of, 5, 5f
    history of, 2
    responsibilities of, 5b
    specialists, 6, 6b
    supervision of, 16
Veterinary technologists, 5, 5b, 475
Veterinary technology, 475
Video endoscopes, 357
Viruses, 192
Visceral larva migrans, 20
Visceral skeleton, 76
Visceral smooth muscle, 90
Visual sense, 93–94, 93f
Vital signs
    auscultation, 213–214, 214f
    in birds, 386t
    body temperature. see Body temperature
    capillary refill time, 216, 218f
    description of, 213
    in ferrets, 364
    heart rate, 213
    mucous membrane color, 216, 217f
    pulse, 215, 215f
    respiration, 215–216
    urine production, 216–217
    weight, 214, 214f
Vitamins, 176, 176b
Vitreous humor, 94
Voice, 26, 153
Vomiting, 217–218
Vomiting center, 115–116
von Willebrand disease, 303–304
Vulva, 99f, 100

W

Warbles, 326
Warfarin, 304
Water, 175
Weaning, of puppies, 178
Wedge smear, 302, 302b
Weight, assessment of, 214, 214f
Weimaraner, 137f
West Nile virus, 390
Wether, 419

Whelping, 102
Whipworm, 323
White blood cell count, 303
White blood cells
    agranulocytes, 82
    antibodies, 82–83
    description of, 81
    granulocytes, 81–82
    reference range values for, 472t
Whole blood, 298
Wing vein, 387
Winged infusion catheter, 229
Wings
    fractures of, 396
    trimming of, 381–382
Withdrawal time, 419
Wolf teeth, 435
Word analysis, 59
Word parts
    combining form, 58
    combining vowel, 58
    compound word, 58
    introduction to, 58
    prefix, 58
    root word, 58
    word formation using, 58–59
        compound word, 59, 59t
        prefix, 58, 58t
        prefix, root word, and suffix, 59, 59t

Word parts (Continued)
    prefix and suffix, 59, 59t
    suffix, 58–59, 59t
Workplace safety, 18
Wound
    acute, 232
    assessment of, 233–234
    categories of, 232, 233b
    chronic, 233
    clean, 233
    clipping, 233–234
    contamination and infection, 232
    covering of, 237–240
    definition of, 191
    dehiscence of, 283
Wound closure, 236–240, 237t
    sutures used in. see Suture(s)
    tissue adhesives for, 253
Wound healing, nutritional support benefits
    for, 183

X

X-ray(s). see also Radiographic images
    description of, 337
    digital, 344–345
    equipment used to produce, 343–344, 344f
    intensifying screens, 343
    lead shielding for, 346, 346f
    mobile unit, 344, 344f

X-ray(s) (Continued)
    portable unit, 343–344, 344f
    radiation safety during, 345–347
    scatter radiation caused by, 340–341,
        341f
    stationary unit, 344, 344f
X-ray tube, 337, 337f

Y

Yorkshire terrier, 139f

Z

Zinc, 397
Zoonoses, 193
    causative organisms, animal hosts, and
        modes of transmission for,
        194t–195t
Zoonotic diseases, 193–195
    of birds, 390b
    control of, 195
    transmission of, 193–195
Zoonotic hazards
    bacterial infections, 20
    biologics, 21
    fungal infections, 20
    parasitism, 20–21
    rabies, 20
Zygodactyl, 372
Zygote, 101